Arthroscopic Laser Surgery

Allen T. Brillhart
Editor

Arthroscopic Laser Surgery

Clinical Applications

With a Foreword by Lanny L. Johnson

With 208 Figures, 121 in Full Color

Springer-Verlag
New York Berlin Heidelberg London Paris
Tokyo Hong Kong Barcelona Budapest

Allen T. Brillhart, M.D.
Northeast Florida Orthopaedics, Sports Medicine, and Rehabilitation, Inc.
2021 Kingsley Ave.
Orange Park, FL 32073
USA

Cover illustration: A 2.1 μm holmium:YAG laser beam profile as it is emitted from a 30-degree angled delivery system. From Fig. 24.12, p. 156 of the text.

Library of Congress Cataloging-in-Publication Data
Brillhart, Allen T.
Arthroscopic laser surgery : clinical applications / Allen T. Brillhart.
p. cm.
Includes bibliographical references and index.

ISBN-13: 978-1-4612-7550-3 e-ISBN-13: 978-1-4612-2468-6
DOI: 10.1007/978-1-4612-2468-6

1. Joints—Endoscopic surgery. 2. Joints—Laser surgery. I. Title.
[DNLM: 1. Laser Surgery—methods. 2. Joints—surgery. 3. Joint Diseases—surgery. 4. Arthroscopy—methods. WE 312 B857a 1994]
RD686.B75 1994
617.4′72059—dc20
DNLM/DLC
For Library of Congress 93-38570
CIP

Printed on acid-free paper.

Softcover reprint of the hardcover 1st edition 1995

Production managed by Theresa Kornak; manufacturing supervised by Rhea Talbert.
Typeset by Asco Trade Typesetting Ltd., Hong Kong.
Color separations and printing by Walsworth Publishing Co., Marceline, MO, USA

9 8 7 6 5 4 3 2 1

Especially to my family
and
Also to the scientists and engineers who are responsible for the development of arthroscopic laser systems.

Trademarks

Coherent, Inc.: VersaPulse™ holmium laser; VersaPulse™ Select holmium laser; InfraTome™ handpiece; VersaLink™ delivery device; VersaTip™ probe tip

Eclipse Surgical Technologies, Inc.: Eclipse 3200™ holmium laser; Eclipse PowerSculptor™ probes

Laser Photonics, Inc. (distributed by *Surgilase, Inc.*): LPI ML210™ holmium surgical laser system; LPI ML210™ holmium surgical laser fiberoptic delivery system

Luxar, Inc.: Luxar Extend Systems™; Microguides™; Endoguides™; LX-20™ laser

Premier Laser Systems, Inc. (formerly *Pfizer Laser Systems, Inc.*): S.A.F.E. System™; Model 20CH™ carbon dioxide surgical laser system; Orthopac™; Laserguide™ Orthopaedic System

Sharplan Lasers, Inc.: SharpLase™ Contact Fibers; Sharplan Model 3000™ neodymium:YAG laser; Sharplan Model Surgicenter 40™, Models 1041S™, 1055S™ carbon dioxide lasers

Sunrise Technologies, Inc.: sLASE 210™ holmium lasers; sLASE 210 holmium laser delivery systems

Surgical Laser Technologies, Inc.: Contact Laser™ technology; Contact Laser™ probes; Wavelength Conversion™; Contact ArthroProbe™; Contact Laser™ Systems Models CLMD 110-25W, CLMD 110-40W, and CLMD/Dual

Trimedyne, Inc.: OmniPulse™ holmium laser systems; OmniPulse-MAX™ holmium laser systems; OmniPulse™ laser delivery systems; Tapertip™ orthopaedic handpieces

Carl Zeiss, Inc.: OPMILAS 144™ surgical lasers; OPMILAS 144 Plus™ surgical lasers; OPMILAS 144™ delivery systems

Foreword

When Dr. Brillhart asked me to write this foreword, I questioned his wisdom, but not his courage. I am often critical, but rarely by invitation. My qualifications to write this foreword include being well acquainted with controversy, arthroscopy, and lasers in that order. I have never used a laser in a patient, but have investigated its healing potential on articular cartilage. So, at Dr. Brillhart's invitation, here goes.

Light has always been a fascination to mankind. The ultimate accolade for light is when it is identified as one of the attributes of God.

If that were not enough, now comes the LASER with fascination and power based upon imagery from science fiction. Now this powerful concept is combined with a medical technology, arthroscopy. KAZAM!

I have followed the controversy of laser use in arthroscopy, but have not chosen sides. It has produced more heat than light. Like arthroscopy itself, it has attracted a few pioneers, the contributors to this text. The similarity to arthroscopy has been with patients' acceptance coming before the medical establishment's recognition. The criticisms included the fact that marketing preceded the scientific evidence. The medical establishment's response was best displayed in the initial AAOS policy statement on lasers; ill advised and quickly revised.

I would encourage every orthopaedic surgeon to recognize this is the start and not the finish of laser use in arthroscopy. You would not want to be remembered with those who criticized Henry Ford for his initial product, the horseless carriage. Laser use in arthroscopy is going to happen in some way, shape and form. Dr. Brillhart and his contributors should be congratulated for starting this journey. Because of their work, the reader has the luxury of starting closer to the light.

Dr. Brillhart's preface sets the tone. This textbook collects in one place everything you wanted to know, but never asked, about lasers, the physics, definitions, various types, and early studies of the pioneers. The authors' open discussion about the state of the art should reduce the heat of criticism. The book is well organized and easy to read.

Learn from these pioneers. Receive their cautions. Build on their observations. Finally, let us encourage and not impede.

I thank Dr. Brillhart and his contributors for initiating the move of the laser from fascination to facts. We all look forward to the day when the light at the end of the tunnel turns out to be the benefit of lasers in tissue healing.

Lanny L. Johnson, M.D.
Clinical Professor of Surgery
Michigan State University
College of Human Medicine
East Lansing, MI
USA

Preface

There has often been a sense of hope and implied, if not actual, "larger than life" results in the minds of the laser enthusiasts and their surgical patients. This feeling is natural and universal. Nevertheless, each surgeon and patient must eventually come to grips with the truths of laser applications. If the myths of arthroscopic laser surgery are addressed, it is easier to be realistic and professional about what the procedures can accomplish. It is a matter of ethics and is essential to the credibility of arthroscopic laser surgery. The idea that arthroscopic laser surgery is better than conventional methods is often not well presented. The problem is that the word "better" is not specific, leaving both the supporters and non-supporters reasons to be correct.

When speaking of patient outcomes, usually evaluated after 2 years, one must take care about drawing conclusions. Specific procedures must be analyzed before arthroscopic laser surgery can be deemed "better" than conventional arthroscopy, although short-term results are encouraging. The 2.1 μm holmium:YAG laser and the 1.06 μm contact neodymium:YAG laser, when used for lateral release in the knee, have decreased postoperative hemarthroses and shortened recovery times. Arthroscopic laser meniscectomy has been compared favorably to conventional arthroscopic meniscectomy, and chapters in this book support these claims.

The area of arthroscopic laser chondroplasty is controversial, as is conventional arthroscopic chondroplasty. The benefits of chondroplasty in the face of severe degenerative arthritis are unpredictable whether a mechanical tool or a laser is used to treat it. That we can stimulate fibrocartilage repair in laboratory settings has created much enthusiasm. However, cautious observers have pointed out that there is no published evidence that long-term effects of laser chondroplasty are more beneficial than those achieved with conventional methods. Nevertheless, many anecdotal reports exist that the 10.6 μm CO_2 laser, the 2.1 μm holmium:YAG laser, and the 0.308 μm Excimer laser produce good clinical results. The benefits of laser use seem to lie in the facilitation of the procedure and the relative ability to spare uninvolved cartilage, claims that are supported in this book. Some surgeons believe that the short-term results are improved, especially with the lower grades of chondromalacia. Despite these reports, the use of lasers as an improvement over conventional tools for chondroplasty is a topic that will be debated for years to come.

As single instruments, lasers can cut, coagulate, and ablate depending on the method by which the laser energy is applied. Lasers provide the most versatile instruments arthroscopists have had up to now. Mechanical methods require multiple instruments that are often larger than laser probes to accomplish these functions. It is the instruments themselves, not the procedures, that represent the most significant improvements. When used properly, lasers offer the arthroscopist the potential ability to decrease hemarthroses, minimize iatrogenic articular cartilage damage, and avoid postoperative morbidity. As a result, quicker postoperative recovery times using certain wavelengths have been reported by some of the authors in this text.

Despite the complexities of laser use, the most significant factor in accomplishing successful arthroscopic laser surgery is knowing how to perform arthroscopy. James Larson often uses the following quote, "Lasers will not make a poor surgeon a good surgeon. They will not make a good surgeon a poor surgeon. However, they will make a good surgeon a better surgeon."

The arthroscopist must realize that all wavelengths are not equal. When considering the benefits of arthroscopic laser surgery, the specific laser system must be mentioned. It is not possible to include every laser in one category or to list a general set of advantages and disadvantages. The surgeon is encouraged to note the wavelength in micrometers or nanometers when discussing arthroscopic laser surgery.

Finally, this text presents only limited knowledge at a fixed time. Though it is fairly comprehensive, it should not be misconstrued as a substitute for formal laser training and credentialing. As everyone should know, information and technology change at a rapid rate. Constant research and study are a must.

Allen T. Brillhart, M.D.
Orange Park, FL

Contents

Contributors

SANDRA ABBOTT
Coherent Medical Group, 3270 West Bayshore Road, Palo Alto, CA 94303, USA

STEPHEN P. ABELOW, M.D., F.A.C.S.
Medical Director, US Professional Ski Tour, and Medical Director, Lake Tahoe Sports Medicine Center, 937 San Francisco Avenue, South Lake Tahoe, CA 96150, USA

GREGORY T. ABSTEN, B.SC. ALLIED HEALTH, M.B.A.
Clinical Instructor, Department of Ophthalmology, The Ohio State University College of Medicine, University Health Center, 456 West 10th Street, Columbus, OH 43210, USA

O. SAHAP ATIK, M.D.
Professor and Chairman, Department of Orthopaedics and Traumatology, Gazi University, Besevler, Ankara, 06520, Turkey

JONATHAN D. BLACK, M.D.
Orthopaedic Surgical Resident, Medical College of Pennsylvania, 3300 Henry Ave., Philadelphia, PA 19129, USA

ALLEN T. BRILLHART, M.D.
Northeast Florida Orthopaedics, Sports Medicine, and Rehabilitation, Inc., 2021 Kingsley Avenue, Orange Park, FL 32073, USA

MICHELE COOK, R.N., CNOR
Orange Park Surgical Center, 2050 Professional Center Drive, Orange Park, FL 32073, USA

COLETTE COZEAN, PH.D.
President, Premier Laser Systems, Irvine, CA 92718, USA

ROBERT S. CUMMINGS JR., M.D.
Orthopaedic Surgical Resident, Medical College of Pennsylvania, 3300 Henry Avenue, Philadelphia, PA 19129, USA

SANFORD D. DAMASCO
Trimedyne, Inc., 2801 Barranca Parkway, Irvine, CA 92714, USA

CLEMENT R. DARROW, II, D.V.M., M.P.H.
Laser Photonics, 12351 Research Parkway, Orlando, FL 32826, USA

Douglas K. Dew, m.d.
Attending Orthopaedic Surgeon, Department of Orthopaedic Surgery, HCA Putnam Community Hospital, P.O. Box 8039, Palatka, FL 32178, USA

Michael F. Dillingham, m.d.
Clinical Professor, Department of Orthopaedic Surgery, Stanford University Medical Center, 2884 Sand Hill Road, Menlo Park, CA 94025, USA

Dietmar Eisel, ph.d.
Director, Manufacturing, Engineering and Development, Humprey Instruments, Inc., San Leandro, CA 84577, USA

Gary S. Fanton, m.d.
Clinical Assistant Professor, Department of Functional Restoration, Stanford University Medical Center, 2884 Sand Hill Road, Menlo Park, CA 94025, USA

Terry A. Fuller, ph.d.
Adjunct Clinical Assistant Professor, Department of Urology, Jefferson Medical College, and Chief Operating Officer, Surgical Laser Technologies, Inc., Oaks, PA 19456, USA

Shari Gabriel, m.d.
Orthopaedic Surgical Resident, Arthroscopy and Sports Medicine Center of Southern Wisconsin, 2025 West Oklahoma Avenue, Milwaukee, WI 53215, USA

James G. Garrick, m.d.
Director, The Center for Sports Medicine, Saint Francis Memorial Hospital, 900 Hyde Street, San Francisco, CA 94109, USA

Neil D. Glossop, b.a.sc., m.eng., ph.d.
Director of Orthopaedic Research, Department of Orthopaedics, Baylor University Medical Center, 3500 Gaston Avenue, Dallas, TX 75206, USA

James F. Guhl, m.d.
Assistant Professor, Department of Orthopaedic Surgery, Medical College of Wisconsin, 8900 West Wisconsin Avenue, Milwaukee, WI 53226, USA

Pedro Guillén, m.d.
Professor, Department of Traumatology and Orthopaedic Surgery, University Fremap, Cart. Majadahonda a Pozuelo, Km. 3,500, Majadahonda, Madrid 28220, Spain

Stuart D. Harman
Sunrise Technologies, Inc., 47257 Fremont Boulevard, Fremont, CA 94538, USA

Joan L. Hawver, lvn
Trimedyne, Inc., 2801 Barranca Parkway, Irvine, CA 92714, USA

Robert W. Jackson, m.d., m.s.(tor), frcs(c)
Chief, Department of Orthopaedic Surgery, Baylor University Medical Center, 3500 Gaston Avenue, Dallas, TX 75246, USA

Charles E. Kollmer, m.d.
504 Palmetto Street, New Smyrna Beach, FL 32168, USA

Kathy Laakmann, ph.d.
Luxar Corporation, 19204 Northcreek Parkway, Bothell, WA 98011, USA

GREGORY J. LANE, M.D.
Orthopaedic Surgical Resident, Medical College of Pennsylvania, 3300 Henry Avenue, Philadelphia, PA 19129, USA

JAMES R. LARSON, M.D.
Clinical Assistant Professor of Orthopaedic Surgery, University of Minnesota, Medical Director, Minimal Invasive Care Center, Abbott Northwestern Hospital, 920 East 28th Street, Suite 600, Minneapolis, MN 55407, USA

HAR CHI LAU, M.D.
General Surgical Resident, Medical College of Pennsylvania, 3300 Henry Avenue, Philadelphia, PA 19129, USA

RAUL A. MARQUEZ, M.D., B.S., F.A.A.N.O.S.
Chief, Department of Surgery, Edinburg Hospital, Director, Orthopaedic Surgery Center & Sports Medicine, 1522 South Ninth, Edinburg, TX 75839, USA

DOUGLASS MEAD, M.S., B.M.E.
Product Manager, Sharplan Lasers, Inc., Allendale, NJ 07401, USA

L. MONTGOMERY, M.D.
Orthopaedic Research Laboratory, Division of Orthopaedics, Department of Functional Restoration, Stanford University School of Medicine, Stanford, CA 94305-5326, USA

PEKKA MOOAR, M.D.
Assistant Professor, Chief of Sports Medicine, Department of Orthopaedic Surgery, Medical College of Pennsylvania, 3300 Henry Avenue, Philadelphia, PA 19129, USA

DOUGLAS R. MURPHY-CHUTORIAN, M.D.
President, Eclipse Surgical Technologies, Inc., Sunnyvale, CA 94089, USA

W. L. NIGHAN, PH.D.
Carl Zeiss, Inc., 1 Zeiss Drive, Thornwood, NY 10594, USA

C. L. PETERSEN, PH.D.
Carl Zeiss, Inc., 1 Zeiss Drive, Thornwood, NY 10594, USA

JAMES H. QUINN, D.D.S.
Professor of Oral and Maxillofacial Surgery, Louisiana State University Medical Center School of Dentistry, 1100 Florida Avenue, New Orleans, LA 70119, USA

ED REED, PH.D.
Engineer, Coherent Medical Group, Palo Alto, CA 94303, USA

VAHID SAADATMANESH, M.S.
Senior Vice President, Research and Development, Trimedyne, Inc., Irvine, CA 92714, USA

D. J. SCHURMAN, M.D.
Orthopaedic Research Laboratory, Division of Orthopaedics, Department of Functional Restoration, Stanford University School of Medicine, Stanford, CA 94305-5326, USA

T. SHEA
Laser Photonics, 12351 Research Parkway, Orlando, FL 32826, USA

HENRY H. SHERK, M.D.
Chairman, Orthopaedic Surgery, Medical College of Pennsylvania, 3300 Henry Ave., Philadelphia, PA 19129, USA

Naomi N. Shields, MAJ MC, USAF
Orthopaedic Surgical Resident, Arthroscopy and Sports Medicine Center of Southeastern Wisconsin, 2025 West Oklahoma Avenue, Milwaukee, WI 53215, USA

Werner E. Siebert, M.D.
Assistant Professor and Clinical Director, Orthopaedic Clinic Kassel, Wilhelmshöher Allee 345, Kassel 34131, Germany

Michael Slatkine, Ph.D.
Director of Market Development, Sharplan Lasers, Inc., Allendale, NJ 07401, USA

David H. Sliney, Ph.D.
Chief, Laser Branch, Laser Microwave Division, US Army Environmental Hygience Agency, Aberdeen Proving Ground, MD 21010, USA

Chadwick F. Smith, M.D.
Clinical Professor of Orthopaedic Surgery, Department of Orthopaedics, University of Southern California, 1127 Wilshire Boulevard, Los Angeles, CA 90017, USA

B. Smith, B.S.E.T.
Laser Photonics, 12351 Research Parkway, Orlando, FL 32826, USA

R. Lane Smith, Ph.D.
Associate Professor (Research), Department of Functional Restoration/Orthopaedics, Stanford University, R144, 300 Pasteur Drive, Stanford, CA 94305-5341, USA

James W. Stone, M.D.
Clinical Instructor in Orthopaedic Surgery, Medical College of Wisconsin, 2025 West Oklahoma, Milwaukee, WI 53215, USA

Larry Supik, M.D.
Attending Orthopaedic Surgeon, Hutchinson Medical Center, 100 Grove Crescent, Fort Oglethorpe, GA 30736, USA

William P. Thorpe, M.D.
Associate Clinical Professor, Department of Orthopaedic Surgery, Southern Illinois School of Medicine, 48 Doctor's Park, Cape Girardeau, MO 63701, USA

C. Thomas Vangsness Jr., M.D.
Associate Professor, Department of Orthopaedics, University of Southern California School of Medicine, LAC/USC Medical Center, 2025 Zonal Avenue, GNH-3900, Los Angeles, CA 90033, USA

Art Vassiliadis, Ph.D.
Chairman and CEO, Sunrise Technologies Inc., Fremont, CA 94538, USA

Thomas M. Walker, M.D., Ph.D.
1850 Town Center Pkwy, #400, Reston, VA 22090, USA

W. Williams, Ph.D.
Laser Photonics, 12351 Research Parkway, Orlando, FL 32826, USA

Glenn D. Yeik
Trimedyne, Inc., 2801 Barranca Parkway, Irvine, CA 92714, USA

1

History of Arthroscopic Laser Surgery

Allen T. Brillhart

The advantages of using lasers in arthroscopy are now obvious to an increasing number of surgeons, although skepticism remains. In 1984 Robert Metcalf stated that, "Lasers have no advantage in arthroscopic surgery." This statement represented a culmination of 5 years of frustration with the use of the 10.6 μm CO_2 laser for arthroscopic meniscectomies (Smith and Nance, 1983, 1988).

James Smith and T.A. Nance (Seattle, Washington), between 1982 and 1984, performed a series of arthroscopic laser meniscectomies with the 10.6 μm CO_2 laser (Smith and Nance, 1983, 1988). A continuous wave laser was used. They began their work with the encouragement of Terry Whipple (Richmond, Virginia) who had experimented with the 10.6 μm CO_2 laser for meniscectomy in the laboratory since 1978 (Whipple et al., 1980). Because the initial clinical results were disappointing, a moratorium was declared on the use of the 10.6 μm CO_2 laser for arthroscopic meniscectomy (Smith and Nance, 1983; Metcalf, 1984).

In 1985, Whipple et al. wrote, "Laser meniscectomy should be considered only by surgeons well versed in the principles of laser surgery and only in controlled settings according to strict protocols." This cautious attitude persists even today. As late as March 1991, at the Arthroscopy Association of North America's meeting, in Anaheim, California, which was adjoining the annual meeting of the American Academy of Orthopaedic Surgeons, Whipple seriously questioned the benefits of laser arthroscopy. At the same symposium, James Smith called the future of laser arthroscopy "hoopla," and many in the audience applauded (Brillhart, 1991).

Much credit is given to those surgeons who persisted through this period of rejection. Chadwick Smith of the University of Southern California continued studying, improving, practicing, and teaching laser arthroscopy. In 1985 he introduced a pulsed 10.6 μm CO_2 laser device with a hand-held resonator for arthroscopic use and performed many 10.6 μm CO_2 laser arthroscopies with good and excellent results (Smith, 1986). He did not experience the same problems using this system as did James Smith (Smith and Nance, 1989). For his work, Chadwick Smith (Fig. 1-1) should be recognized as the "father of arthroscopic laser surgery."

Among those who should receive credit is Henry Sherk of the Medical College of Pennsylvania. Sherk had the foresight to recognize the potential for laser use in orthopaedic surgery, not only for arthroscopy but for a wide variety of applications. His text *Lasers in Orthopaedics* (1990) is the first of its kind.

In Europe, much credit is given to Werner Siebert of the University of Hannover, who pioneered work with lasers for arthroscopy. He has also been an enthusiast of laser use for other aspects of orthopaedic surgery (Siebert and Wirth, 1991).

In 1987, Metcalf outlined the criteria he considered important if lasers were to be accepted for arthroscopic meniscectomy:

1. Torn menisci must be efficiently resected without damage to adjacent normal structures, such as articular cartilage, the capsule, and popliteal neurovascular structures.
2. Accurate, precise application of the laser beam must be possible through narrow joint spaces to the posterior horns and the middle and anterior areas of the menisci.
3. Laser excision must be an improvement on present resection instruments such as hand-operated forceps, knives, and motorized cutting devices in speed, accuracy, and ease of use.
4. Ideally, laser beam transmission should be built into the arthroscope to avoid separate punctures.

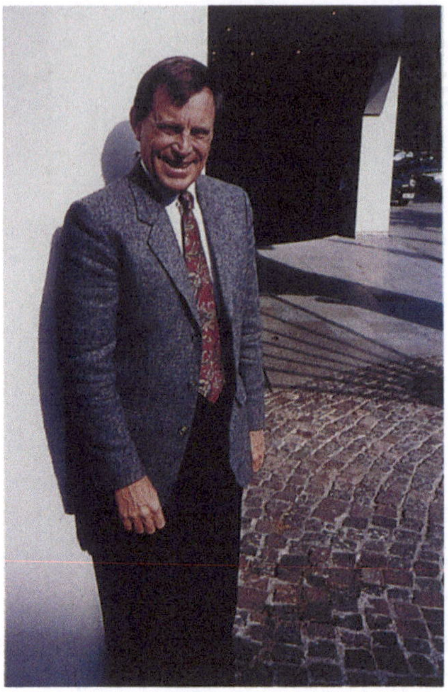

Figure 1-1. Chadwick Smith, father of arthroscopic laser surgery.

5. Low cost of present arthroscopic methods must not be exceeded.
6. Postoperative morbidity or complications must not be increased.

In my opinion, the most important of these criteria have been met with the exception of cost. Nevertheless, increased use and competition are driving laser prices down, a trend that should continue in the future (Abelow, 1993a).

The acceptance of laser arthroscopy parallels the acceptance of arthroscopy itself. In 1976 it was estimated that only 50 surgeons throughout the world performed arthroscopic procedures routinely. By 1986 that number was estimated to be 6000 (Metcalf, 1987). It is currently estimated that 80% of all orthopaedic surgeons practice arthroscopy.

In 1918 Kenji Takagi of Tokyo University invented the arthroscope (Jackson, 1991). Some 40 years later, in 1962, Watanabe and Ikeuchi performed the first arthroscopic meniscectomy (Jackson, 1991). Much criticism had to be overcome and new questions answered before arthroscopic meniscectomy became the procedure it is today. The first orthopaedic practice guidelines published by the American Academy of Orthopaedic Surgeons in 1989 (McCollough et al., 1989) clearly noted that arthroscopic partial meniscectomy is the surgical treatment of choice over arthrotomy and partial meniscectomy.

The most significant factors responsible for the acceptance of operative arthroscopy, according to Jackson (1983), were the improvements in instrumentation and the establishment of the video camera technique. One must stop and think that these two factors are, in the most part, attributed to the efforts of engineers.

As a parallel, in 1917 Albert Einstein was credited for the theory of stimulated emission. Some 41 years later, in 1958, Schawlow and Townes developed the laser principle. Townes received a Nobel Prize in physics for his work with masers and lasers in 1964. Schawlow, along with two others, subsequently received the Nobel Prize for his work in laser spectroscopy in 1981. In 1960, Maiman, working at Bell Laboratories, assembled the first laser device, a ruby red laser (Fuller, 1987; Ball, 1990). In 1961 the first clinical applications of this laser device were attributed to an ophthalmologist and to Goldman (1981) for his use of it as a dermatologic device.

Remarkably, the first orthopaedic surgeon interested in the laser principle was Robert Jackson (O'Brien et al., 1991), known to many as the "father of arthroscopy." His interest was engaged some 5 years prior to his visiting Watanabe in Japan and bringing the arthroscope to North America in 1964. Jackson, while a Fellow in Boston, visited a friend at the Massachusetts Institute of Technology who gave him one-half of a ruby bulb that was originally intended to be part of an early laser device.

The first 10.6 μm CO_2 laser was built by Patel in 1964 (Ball, 1990). Polyani in 1965 was the first to use the 10.6 μm CO_2 laser clinically for treatment of cancer (Ball, 1990). Appropriately, the first laser used for arthroscopic meniscectomy was the 10.6 μm CO_2 laser. Credit should be given to O'Connor (1977) for being the first to publish the fact that lasers could be used in arthroscopy.

In 1978 Whipple began research on the use of the 10.6 μm CO_2 laser for arthroscopy. His findings were presented at the 1981 Tri-annual Meeting of the International Arthroscopy Association in Rio de Janeiro. Smith and Nance (1983, 1988) began a series of 10.6 μm CO_2 laser meniscectomies on July 8, 1982. Independently, in December 1982 Philandrianos (1983, 1984a, b, 1992), in Paris, performed the first 10.6 μm CO_2 laser arthroscopy in Europe, during which he removed a portion of a torn meniscus.

The first 1.06 μm neodymium:YAG laser was built in 1964 (Geusic et al., 1964), but the first clinical application of the free beam 1.06 μm neodymium:YAG laser was not until 1977. Ackerman used it for a dental procedure (Ball, 1990) and subsequently Kiefhaber et al., (1977) for coagulation of gastrointestinal bleeding.

In 1978, Glick in San Francisco began to study the 1.06 μm neodymium:YAG laser in a free beam mode for meniscectomy. His findings were disappointing (Glick, 1981, 1984). Inoue et al. (1984) also performed some early work with the 1.06 μm neodymium:YAG and the 0.488 μm argon laser and found them to be ineffective. They recommended that the CO_2 laser be used.

In 1985, Siebert and other surgeons in Europe began to use the 1.06 μm neodymium:YAG laser in a free beam mode for arthroscopy. Early work with this method was not encouraging (Siebert et al., 1993). When applied to chondral surfaces of laboratory animals, Siebert (1991) noted that the laser had produced severe degenerative changes. This finding was later confirmed by Raunest (1991) in Dusseldorf. Cutting of meniscal tissue was found to be possible, however. Bradrick and Indresano (1991) later reported that fibrosis of subchondral bone can be caused when this laser is used in a noncontact mode.

The pulsed 10.6 μm CO_2 laser device developed by Chadwick Smith and others, gained U.S. Food and Drug Administration (FDA) "approval for marketing" for use in arthroscopic surgery in the mid-1980s. Since then, it has been estimated that more than 25,000 10.6 μm CO_2 laser arthroscopies have been performed, far more cases than with any other form of laser arthroscopy (O'Brien et al., 1991). This number is small when one considers that at least four thousand 10.6 μm CO_2 laser devices exist in U.S. hospitals today and that 10.6 μm CO_2 laser arthroscopic methods have been available during the first decade of laser arthroscopy.

In 1986 Fanton and Dillingham (Palo Alto, California) began work as chief clinical investigators for the development of the 2.1 μm holmium:YAG laser for arthroscopy (Fanton and Dillingham, 1992; Dillingham et al., 1993). This instrument is the first laser device specifically developed for use in arthroscopy. The first 2.1 μm holmium:YAG laser meniscectomies were performed in 1988. In February 1990, the FDA authorized marketing of the 2.1 μm holmium:YAG laser for arthroscopic procedures. Its small probe and versatility in terms of it being used in a liquid environment have made it increasingly popular.

Joffe and Daikuzono introduced contact laser technology for the 1.06 μm neodymium:YAG laser for use in general surgery. This technique allows the laser beam to deliver concentrated thermal energy at the point of contact. The free beam 1.06 μm neodymium:YAG energy is converted to thermal energy in the tip. It should not be confused with a free beam fiber that is used in tissue contact. This concept originally came from Japan but was first applied clinically in the United States.

During the late 1980s, O'Brien (Hospital of Special Surgery) and Miller (Massachusetts General Hospital) began using contact sapphire tips for arthroscopy (Miller et al., 1989). The sapphire tip probe was found to have unfavorable characteristics in an arthroscopic setting. A ceramic tip probe was subsequently developed predominantly for cutting and coagulating purposes. In 1991 the FDA released the ceramic tip probe with "approval for marketing" for use in arthroscopic surgery. This tip differed significantly from the 10.6 μm CO_2 laser delivery system in that it could be used in a liquid environment; moreover, it was much smaller and so could be more easily placed in tight joint spaces. Nevertheless, the search for the ideal tip for the contact 1.06 μm neodymium:YAG laser is still under way. Tip fragility remains a concern (Brillhart, 1992).

Also, during the late 1980s Löhnert (Dusseldorf, Germany) and his research assistant Raunest performed 0.308 μm Excimer laser arthroscopy (Raunest and Löhnert, 1990). The first systems were reported to be large and cumbersome, and the initial procedures were long. While in Canada, Robert Jackson performed experimental work with this laser device and reported that the first devices were slow in their application (Glossop et al., 1992). The 0.308 μm Excimer laser has not yet been approved for use in the United States but has been developed into a more practical system in Europe.

In 1992 I performed the first arthroscopic laser procedures with the free beam 1.44 μm neodymium:YAG (Brillhart, 1993). Its water absorption and tissue effects are similar to those of the 2.1 μm holmium:YAG laser. It should not be confused with the 1.06 μm neodymium:YAG laser.

Other wavelengths are currently being evaluated: the 0.532 μm KTP and the 2.0 μm thulium:YAG lasers. As with the 0.308 μm Excimer device, their approval for marketing in the United States may be forthcoming. The 2.94 μm erbium:YAG laser has received attention. No clinical studies were available at the time of this writing.

The contributions by James Garrick (1992) of the ambient air technique for 10.6 μm CO_2 arthroscopy and Stephen Abelow, who performed the first endoscopic laser-assisted carpal tunnel release, should be included in the history of laser arthroscopy. Laser-assisted spinal arthroscopy and temporomandibular joint arthroscopy using the laser for debridement are emerging procedures (Abelow, 1993b). Douglas Dew has made significant contributions in understanding laser tissue welding (Dew et al., 1993); Thomas Vangsness (1992) made early contributions in tissue spectroscopy; and T. Onomura and T. Yonezawa (Tokyo University) must be credited for their work in Japan (Yonezawa et al., 1991).

During early 1992 the American Academy of Orthopaedic Surgeons estimated that more than 3,000 orthopaedic surgeons had attended laser arthroscopy courses (McGinty, 1992), and more than 200 laser arthroscopy courses were scheduled in the United States that year. If this trend continues, there will be at least 6,000 surgeons trained in laser arthroscopy by 1996, representing an increase from 50 to 6,000 in 10 years, similar to the increase seen with the acceptance of arthroscopy itself.

In May 1993 Sherk stated:

"It is difficult to determine who are the experts in the application of lasers—the physicians or the manufacturers—and this raises questions as to how new procedures and unfamiliar technologies should be presented. Use of lasers in arthroscopy and discectomy appears to be reasonably well established, and the experienced investigators have been fairly well identified. As new applications become available, it is important that a mechanism be in place so that they may be introduced in a way that will offer maximum benefit, with least risk, to patients."

The following advisory statement was adopted by the Arthroscopy Association of North American in 1993:

AANA recognizes that the use of lasers in arthroscopic surgery is an alternative to mechanical techniques. There is no proven advantage of laser technique over other techniques. There is, however, the issue of cost effectiveness to be considered.

At the time of this writing, the current debates focused on these two issues, advantage and cost. Nevertheless, acceptance had reached a new level.

References

Abelow S (1993a) Arthroscopic laser surgery. Presented at the Annual meeting of the Arthroscopy Association of North America, Palm Desert, CA

Abelow S (1993b) Use of lasers in orthopedic surgery: current concepts. Orthopedics 16:551–556

Arthroscopy Association of North America (1993) Advisory statement. AANA Newsletter vol. 9, no. 2, p. 4

Ball KA (1990) Lasers: The Perioperative Challenge. Mosby, St. Louis

Bradrick JP, Indresano TA (1991) Laser-assisted arthroscopy of the temporomandibular joint. In Thomas M, Bronstein SL (eds), Arthroscopy of the Temporomandibular Joint. Saunders, Philadelphia, pp 327–335

Brillhart AT (1991) Lasers in arthroscopic surgery [letter to the editor]. Arthroscopy 7:411–412

Brillhart AT (1993) Ablation efficiency determination using the 1.44 micron neodymium:YAG laser. SPIE Proc 1880:29–30

Brillhart AT (1992) Technical problems of laser arthroscopy. [Abstracts]: Arthroscopy 8:403–404

Dew DK, Supik L, Darrow CR, Price GF (1993) Tissue repair using lasers: a review. Orthopedics 16:581–587

Dillingham MF, Price JM, Fanton GS (1993) Holmium laser surgery. Orthopedics 16:563–566

Einstein, A (1917) Zur Quantentheorie der Strahlung. Physiol Z 18:121–128

Fanton GS, Dillingham MF (1992) The use of the holmium laser in arthroscopic surgery. Semin Orthop 7:102–116

Fuller TA (1987) Fundamentals of lasers in medicine and surgery. In Surgical Application of Lasers (2nd Ed.) Year Book, Chicago, pp 16–33

Garrick J (1992) CO_2 laser arthroscopy using ambient gas pressure. Semin Orthop 7:90–94

Geusic JE, Marcos HW, van Uitert LG (1964) Laser oscillations in Nd-doped yttrium aluminum, yttrium gallium, and gadolinium garnets. Appl Phys Lett 4:182

Glick J (1984) Use of the laser beam in arthroscopic surgery. In Casscells SE (ed), Arthroscopy: Diagnostic and Surgical Practice, Lea & Febiger, Philadelphia 181–183

Glick J (1981) YAG laser meniscectomy. Presented at the Triannual Meeting of the International Arthroscopy Association, Rio de Janeiro

Glossop N, Jackson R, Randle J, Reed S (1992) The Excimer laser in arthroscopic surgery. Semin Orthop 7:125–130

Goldman L (1981) The Biomedical Laser: Technology and Clinical Applications. Springer-Verlag, Berlin

Inoue K et al (1984) Arthroscopic Laser Surgery. IAA, London, pp 29–30.9

Jackson RW (1991) History of arthroscopy. In Operative Arthroscopy. Raven Press, New York, pp 1–4

Jackson RW (1983) Arthroscopic surgery. J Bone Joint Surg 65A:416–520

Joffe S, Daikuzono N (1985) Artificial sapphire probe for contact photocoagulation and tissue vaporization with the nd:YAG laser. Med Instrum 19:173–178

Kiefhaber P, Nath G, Moritz K (1977) Endoscopic control of massive gastrointestinal hemorrhage by irradiation with high power neodymium:YAG laser. Prog Surg 15:140–145

McCollough III NC et al (1989) Academy publishes first clinical policies. Am Acad Orthop Surg Bull Oct:3–20

McGinty JB, Johnson LL, Jackson RW, et al (1992) Current concepts review: uses and abuses of arthroscopy: a symposium. J Bone Joint Surg 74A:1563–1577

Metcalf RW (1987) Lasers in orthopaedic surgery. In Dixon J (ed), Surgical Applications of Lasers (2nd Ed.) Year Book, Chicago pp 275–286

Miller DV, O'Brien SJ, Arnoczky SS, et al (1989) The use of the contact nd:YAG laser in arthroscopic surgery: effects on articular cartilage and meniscal tissue. Arthroscopy 5:245–253

O'Brien SJ, Garrick JG, Jackson RW, et al (1991) Symposium: lasers in orthopaedic surgery. Contemp Orthop 22:61–91

O'Connor RL (1977) Arthroscopy. Lippincott, Philadelphia, p 166

Philandrianos G (1992) A new arthroscopic surgery technique using CO_2 laser to treat intra-articular lesions. Am J Arthrosc 2:7–12

Philandrianos G (1984a) Le laser CO_2 en chirurgie orthopeédique premiers reésultants. Presse Med 18:1151

Philandrianos G, Deglise C (1984b) Laser CO_2 en arthroscopie du genou-technique-resultante preliminaires. J Med Lyon 1394:13–18

Philandrianos G (1983) Early comparative results of CO_2 laser surgery in knee pathology. In Proceedings, 5th International Congress of Laser Medicine and Surgery, Detroit

Raunest J (1991) Presented at the Third International Symposium on Lasers in Orthopaedics, Hannover

Raunest J, Löhnert J (1990) Arthroscopic cartilage debridement by excimer laser in chondromalacia of the knee joint: a prospective randomized clinical study. Arch Orthop Trauma Surg 109:155–159

Sherk HH (1990) Lasers in Orthopaedics. Lippincott, Philadelphia

Sherk HH (1993) Current concepts review: the use of lasers in orthopaedic procedures. J Bone Joint Surg 75A:768–776

Siebert W et al (1993) Lasers in arthroscopic surgery: experimental and clinical results. [Abstracts]. Lasers Surg Med Suppl 79A:37

Siebert W (1991) Lasers in orthopaedics in Europe. Presented at the Third International Symposium on Lasers in Orthopaedics, Hannover

Siebert WE, Wirth CJ (1991) Laser in der Orthopadie. Georg Thieme Verlag, Stuttgart

Smith CF (1986) Partial meniscectomy utilizing a pulsed handheld CO_2 laser system. Presented at the Annual Meeting of the American Academy of Orthopaedic Surgeons, New Orleans

Smith JB, Nance TA (1988) Laser energy in arthroscopic surgery. J. Serge Parisien (ed), Arthroscopic Surgery, McGraw-Hill, New York, pp 325–330

Smith JB, Nance TA (1983) Arthroscopic laser surgery. Presented in part at the annual meeting of the Arthroscopy Association of North America, Coronado, CA

Smith JB, Nance TA (1984) CO_2 laser energy for arthroscopic meniscus surgery. Presented to the American Academy of Sports Medicine, Anaheim, CA, July 25

Vangsness CT, Huang J, Boll J, Smith CF (1992) The optical

properties of the human meniscus. Semin Orthop 7:72–76

Whipple TL, Caspari RB, Meyers JF (1985) Arthroscopic laser meniscectomy in a gas medium. Arthroscopy 1:2–7

Whipple TL (1981) Applications of the CO_2 laser to arthroscopic meniscectomy in a gas medium. Presented at the Tri-annual Meeting of the International Arthroscopy Association, Rio de Janeiro

Whipple TL, Meyers JF, Caspari RB (1980) Arthroscopic meniscectomy: an effective, efficient technique. Orthop Transact 4:410

Yonezawa T, Onomura T, Atsumi K, Fujimasa I (1991) Third International Symposium in Lasers in Orthopaedics, Hannover

2

Introduction to the Basic Science of Arthroscopic Laser Surgery

Allen T. Brillhart

Laser light is electromagnetic radiation. Physics applies two models to describe the characteristics and propagation of electromagnetic radiation. That there are two ways to describe it explains why it is called "the dualism of light." One model describes light as a wave with a sinusoidal shape. Light waves from different parts of the electromagnetic spectrum have different wavelengths. The other model is a quantum model. A photon is the smallest quantum of electromagnetic radiation. A photon is also an elementary particle. It moves at the speed of light but has no rest mass. Light from different parts of the electromagnetic spectrum consists of photons that have different energies.

Electromagnetic radiation ranges from gamma radiation, x-rays, visible radiation, infrared radiation, microwaves, to the longest wavelength that can be detected. Radiation visible to the human eye, from 0.4 to 0.76 μm, covers a small part of the electromagnetic spectrum (Fig. 2-1). Today, most medical lasers operate in the range 0.25 to 10.60 μm.

There are two mechanisms by which light is created. Ordinary light emitted from a light bulb originates from a hot, thin wire. The distribution of wavelengths or photons is such that it has no discrete emission lines but contains all wavelengths within a certain range from the ultraviolet to the infrared. Another thermal light source is the sun. The type of radiation emitted from thermal sources is called "blackbody radiation."

In contrast to these thermal light sources there are "cold" light sources. For example, neon tubes do not radiate blackbody radiation but emit discrete wavelengths. The right admixture of wavelengths appears to be white. "Cold" light sources are used to build lasers.

Most clinical and research lasers used for arthroscopy operate in the infrared portion of the electromagnetic spectrum. Excimer lasers emit in the ultraviolet region. The 0.532 μm KTP and 0.632 μm helium-neon lasers emit visible radiation. The visible 0.632 μm helium-neon laser is a red aiming beam. The ultraviolet 0.308 μm Excimer laser is still considered experimental in the United States.

All electromagnetic waves have similar properties. They travel at the speed of light ($c = 3 \times 10^8$ m/s). In the wave model the following relation holds: $c = \lambda\nu$. Wavelength is abbreviated by the symbol lambda (λ) and is typically measured in meters, micrometers, nanometers, or angstroms. Nu (ν) is the frequency of the radiation and is measured in hertz, oscillations per second.

Atomic Transitions

To describe atomic and molecular transitions, it is preferable to use the quantum model. The basics of transitions for atoms and molecules are the same. Each atom has a specific energy level schema that relates to the ways electrons can orbit the nucleus. Usually only the outer electron can make a transition to another energy level, or orbit. *Ground state* is the lowest energy level from which transitions can take place; other, higher levels are called *excited states.*

If an electron transitions to a higher orbit, the electron will remain in an upper energy level for approximately 10^{-8} seconds, until it spontaneously returns to the ground state. As the electron spontaneously returns, one photon is emitted. This process is called spontaneous emission.

Alternately, if the same atom is struck by another photon while one of its electrons is in an excited state, the excited electron will be stimulated to return to the lower energy level. This process is called stimulated emission. Here two parallel or coherent photons will be emitted. Stimulated emission is the basic process for lasers.

ELECTROMAGNETIC SPECTRUM (laser portion)	ULTRAVIOLET	VISIBLE	INFRARED
WAVELENGTH μm	0.10	0.40 0.76	10^3

Figure 2-1. Electromagnetic spectrum.

The light, that originates from stimulated emission differs from light created by thermal light sources or via spontaneous emission. Laser light is monochromatic, highly directional or collimated, and coherent. *Coherence* means that the waves are in phase both temporally and spatially. *Spectral intensity* (intensity per wavelength interval) is high. The intensity and direction are essential for laser light to be useful for surgery.

Laser Device

Laser is the acronym for *l*ight *a*mplification by *s*timulated *e*mission of *r*adiation. In a laser device, a given energy source "pumps," stimulates, or excites electrons to go from a ground state to an excited state. When more electrons in an "active medium" are in the excited state than in the ground state, a population inversion has occurred.

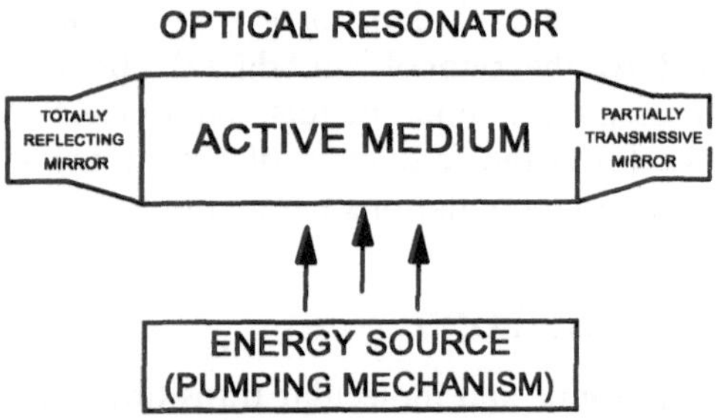

Figure 2-2. Laser device.

A single photon can stimulate the entire active medium to release its energy, resulting in laser light.

The three most important elements of a laser device are (l) the active or laser medium; (2) the energy source or pumping mechanism; and (3) an optical feedback system that is called the laser resonator (Fig. 2-2). The energy source varies depending on the type of active medium used. For solid-state media, such as the 1.06 or 1.44 μm neodymium:YAG laser, the energy source is usually a flashlamp. For gas lasers such as the 10.6 μm CO_2 laser, the energy source is a direct current discharge or a radiofrequency discharge. The resonator cavity usually has on one side a totally reflecting mirror and on the other side a partially transmissive mirror. When activated, the laser light is emitted from the partially transmissive mirror.

Delivery Systems

Laser beams are transmitted through delivery systems from the laser device to the target tissue. Usually a long articulating arm with a series of mirrors transmits the 10.6 μm CO_2 laser beam and allows it to propagate freely. Small, hollow waveguides are also available. Another version, a hand-held resonator, allows direct transmission to the waveguide. Flexible fiberoptic cables with rigid handpieces transmit the 1.06 μm and 1.44 μm neodymium:YAG wavelengths, and the 2.1 μm holmium:YAG wavelength. Wavelengths, from ultraviolet to 2 μm, are transmitted through quartz fibers with low water content. Special composite materials deliver the 2.94 μm erbium:YAG laser energy.

Spectroscopy

Spectroscopy is the study of the selective absorption or emission of electromagnetic energy. Laser beams selectively pass through some tissue and are highly absorbed

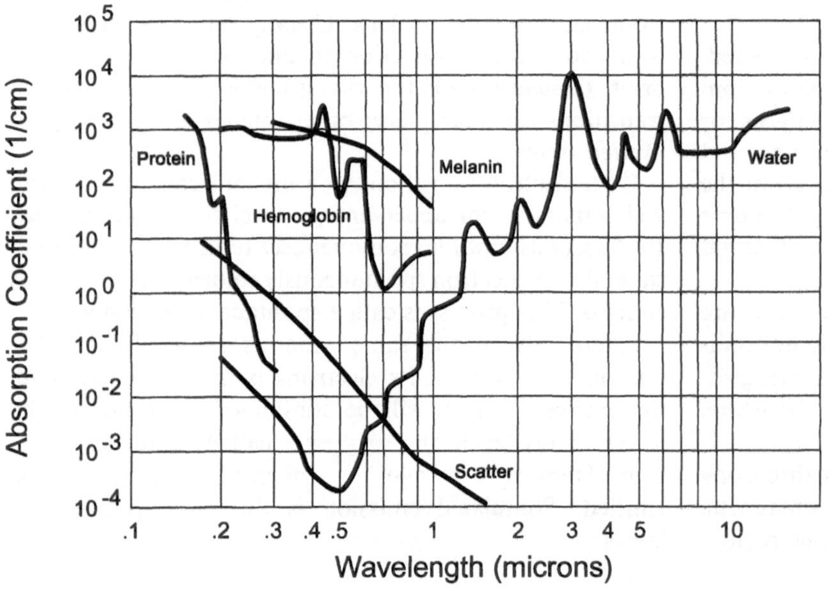

Figure 2-3. Laser absorption, absorption coefficient versus wavelength.

by others. Tissues differing in content of water, melanin or pigment, and hemoglobin absorb laser beams depending on their wavelength or frequency (Fig. 2-3).

These principles allow the surgeon to understand the unique applications of laser energy in arthroscopic surgery. Grasping the fact that the type of laser and the type of tissue are perhaps more important than the energy level used is essential for understanding laser arthroscopy.

Hyaline cartilage, meniscal tissue, synovial tissue, and ligaments contain different concentrations of intracellular water. The absorption of the water molecule of the 10.6 μm wavelength of the CO_2 laser, the 2.1 μm wavelength of the holmium:YAG laser, and the 1.44 μm wavelength of the neodymium:YAG laser make these instruments efficacious in the free beam mode.

The 1.06 μm free beam neodymium:YAG laser beam is absorbed readily by hemoglobin, making it attractive for coagulation but not for arthroscopy because of its poor water absorption. This free laser beam can partially pass through a meniscus or articular cartilage and be partially absorbed by the pigmented marrow elements of subchondral bone. A fiber tip is therefore needed that converts photons of energy directly into heat prior to effective application in the arthroscopic environment. On the opposite extreme, the 10.6 μm CO_2 laser beam is so well absorbed by water that it cannot be used in a liquid environment but must be used in a CO_2, ambient area, or a bubbled gas medium. The 2.1 μm holmium:YAG, 1.44 μm neodymium:YAG, and contact 1.06 μm neodymium:YAG lasers work well in the standard arthroscopic fluid mediums of saline and Ringer's lactate. With the 0.308 μm Excimer laser, tissue absorption is not dependent on the water molecule but on the biochemical composition of the tissue. This laser also works well in a fluid medium.

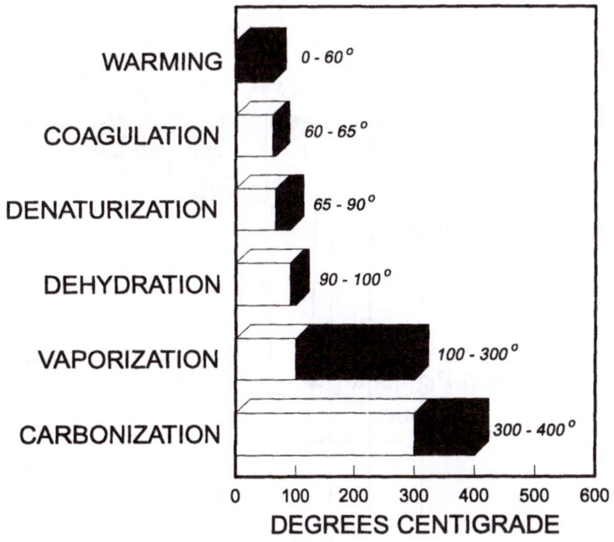

Figure 2-4. Photothermal tissue effects.

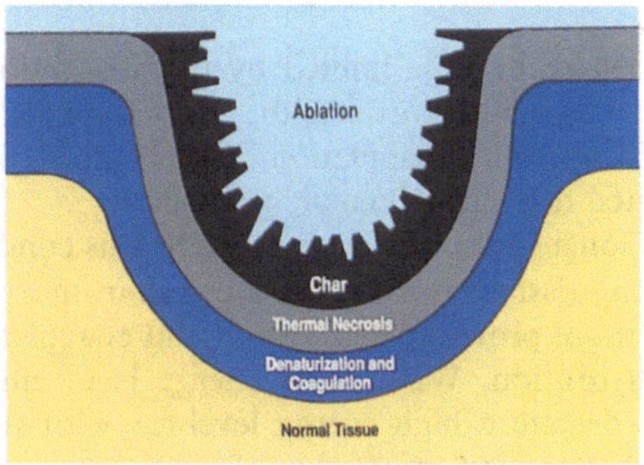

Figure 2-5. Variations of thermal effects, by zone. (From Brillhart AT, Arthroscopic laser surgery: first of four articles. *Am J Arthrosc* 1(1):9, 1991. With permission.)

Photothermal Tissue Effects

Laser energy is either totally or partially absorbed, scattered, reflected, or transmitted through tissue. Intracellular water is the target of most arthroscopic lasers. Light energy is converted to heat when absorbed by water. Depending on the heat generated, variations in tissue effects occur. Warming occurs before 60°C, coagulation at 60°C to 65°C, protein denaturization at 65°C to 90°C, dehydration at 90°C to 100°C, vaporization at 100°C to 300°C and carbonization at 300°C to 400°C (Fig. 2-4).

Variations of thermal effects are seen in zones. Ablation occurs in the first zone, char formation in the second zone, thermal necrosis in the third zone, denaturation and coagulation in the fourth zone, and normal tissue in the fifth zone (Fig. 2-5).

Absorption length refers to the depth that laser heat travels beyond the defect created (Fig. 2-6). It is important for the surgeon to remember that absorption length does not refer to the size of the "defect" created by the laser. Penetration depth refers to the depth of the defect created plus the absorption length. The defect depth relates to the desired primary ablation or cutting effect. The absorption length relates to secondary tissue effects. The penetration depth encompasses both effects.

Comparison of free beam tissue penetrations is important for evaluating the resultant tissue effects. The surgeon must keep in mind that these numbers are laboratory values and not in vivo values assimilated with variations of total contact areas, exposure times, total energy used, and mode and medium of application.

Thermodynamics

The laws of thermodynamics apply to laser tissue effects, primarily achieved through irradiation and heat conduction. The transfer of energy through photons of light occurs through irradiation. Once the light energy is converted to heat through warming of intracellular water, conduction of that heat is important. Even though the ab-

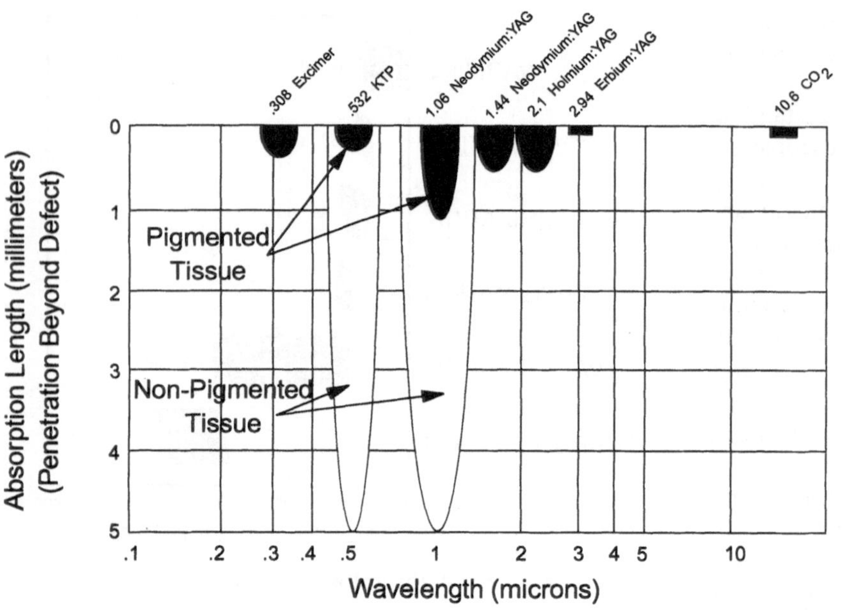

Figure 2-6. Laser absorption, aborption length versus wavelength.

sorption length may be limited by the absorption coefficients and specific wavelength, the secondary tissue effects of charring, coagulation, and necrosis are most often related to thermodynamic principles.

With a longer exposure time, more heat is conducted to surrounding tissues. It results in more char, more thermal necrosis, more protein denaturation and coagulation, and more dehydration. When laser energy is of short pulse duration, despite a high energy level (as with superpulsing) less conduction may occur if subsequent pulses are spaced apart in time so the tissue can cool down (*thermal relaxation*). If pulses follow each other faster than the thermal relaxation time, heat accumulates and the effect is close to that seen with a continuous wave laser. When coagulation is needed, increased pulses per second or longer pulse widths approaching a continuous wave are preferred. Alternately, true pulsing and superpulsing allow more precise cutting with fewer secondary tissue effects.

Photomechanical Tissue Effects

Rapid vaporization of both intracellular and extracellular water causes mechanical trauma to tissues. Increasing the energy setting results in more mechanical trauma, especially when pulsed lasers are used in a liquid medium. Increased photomechanical energy may be used to advantage to loosen debris that has been desiccated. However, it results in generation of a large quantity of particulate matter that clouds the arthroscopic medium. By reducing the photomechanical energy, the debris and "clouding" is minimized. In some instances, higher pulse rates with lower joules per pulse may ablate volumes of tissue more satisfactorily.

Biostimulation

Infrared lasers cause not only thermal changes but biophysiologic changes in tissue as well. With their usual application, high energy levels cause ablation of tissue and overshadow the biostimulating effects seen at much lower energy levels. Biostimulatory effects from light occur in nature every day, as is seen in photosynthesis, and vitamin D metabolism. The fact that specific photons of laser light can induce the production of fibrocartilaginous reparative tissue, though debated, should not be dismissed as inconceivable. The obvious questions of possible adverse effects of biostimulation should also not be dismissed even though they have not been seen over the first decade of arthroscopic laser use.

Mutagenicity

Interaction of photons with biomolecules can cause different effects, including electronic transitions, changes of vibration, and rotation. Photons absorbed by a molecule usually lead first to fluorescence with the molecule remaining in a higher energy state characterized by stronger vibration and faster rotation. As the molecule returns to its original state the excess energy is converted into motion of the entire molecule, which means increased kinetic energy, or heat. For photons of high energy, such as those in the short ultraviolet and x-ray region, interactions can lead to dissociation or ionization of the molecules. In the visible region, interactions predominantly involve electronic transitions with changes in vibration and rotation. If the number of photons at a time or the peak intensity of a pulse exceeds 1 to 10 megawatts, other interactions, such as optical breakdown, can take place and can lead to dissociation and ionization of molecules.

Infrared wavelength lasers have been used in surgery since the mid-1970s, and no case of resultant mutagenicity has been reported. The higher the frequency, the higher is the energy per photon ($E = h\nu$). Therefore in the ultraviolet, x-ray, or gamma ray ranges, the quantum energy ($h\nu$) that is absorbed by the tissue can result in ionization or irreparable modifications of biomolecular structures. With the lower frequencies, as in the infrared and visible ranges, absorption occurs without ionization. Excimer lasers raise the obvious question of ionization. Again, infrared lasers, the 10.6 μm CO_2, 2.1 μm holmium:YAG, 1.44 μm and 1.06 μm neodymium:YAG lasers, and so on, are nonionizing and nonmutagenic.

Acknowledgment. The author would like to thank Dr. Dietmar Eisel for his review of this chapter and his editorial comments.

Suggested Reading

Absten GT and Joffe SN (1989) Lasers in medicine: an introductory guide, second edition. Chapman and Hall, London

Brillhart AT (1991) Arthroscopic laser surgery: first of four articles. Am J Arth 1:5–12

Fisher J (1992) Photons, physiatrics, and physicians: a practical guide to understanding laser light interaction with living tissue, part i. Journal of Clinical Laser Medicine and Surgery 10:419–426

Koechner W (1988) Solid state laser engineering. 2nd ed. Springer-Verlag, New York, NY

Nave CR and Nave BC (1985) Physics for the health sciences, third edition. WB Saunders Company Philadelphia, PA

Serway RA (1990) Physics for scientists and engineers with modern physics, third edition. Saunders College Publishing Philadelphia, PA

3

Quantification of Energy Delivery for Arthroscopic Laser Surgery

Gregory T. Absten

Routine daily use of an arthroscopic laser does not usually require calculation and quantification of power density, total energy, or fluence. Control of the arthroscopic laser is generally based on visual cues, noting the geometries of the defects created and deciding whether to proceed faster or slower. In this sense, control of arthroscopic laser parameters is relative, and the surgeon learns to use it like any surgical instrument—by practice, not calculation. A knowledge of energy concepts is important to understand why a laser works as it does.

Light Energy: Joules

The total amount of light energy delivered to tissue is described in joules, which is simply the rate of delivery times the duration of the delivery:

$$\text{Joules} = \text{watts} \times \text{time} = \text{watts} \times \text{seconds}$$

Lasers that are truly pulsed, such as the 2.1 μm holmium:YAG and 1.44 μm neodymium:YAG have readouts of the joules of energy delivered, which is the parameter set by the operator. The average power then becomes a secondary readout determined by the joules per pulse and the pulse repetition rate. The 10.6 μm CO_2 lasers do not provide such a readout.

Although the concept is important, complete surgical procedures are not based on a light dose limit in terms of joules; that is, the procedure is terminated whenever the incision is finished or the correct amount of tissue is vaporized, regardless of the number of joules required. When trying to cut tough tissues, more joules per pulse may be beneficial, even if the average power delivered is not changed. Conversely, thin, or easier to cut tissues may allow use of lower energies per pulse. (Higher energies here may produce too much of a concussive or photomechanical explosive effect in the cut.)

Power

Power is simply the rate at which the energy is delivered in joules/second and is expressed in watts. The faster a given amount of energy may be delivered, the more confined is the resulting heat damage. As a general rule, the highest power with which one is comfortable controlling should be used if precision is desired. For arthroscopic use, lasers are designed that emit high peak power pulses.

Power Density

Power density is the single most important factor in the application of any laser. It is sometimes referred to as irradiance or spot brightness. Power density is the relation between the power and the spot size in which it is concentrated. It is a balance between these two parameters and is expressed in watts per square centimeter or power per surface area.

When the laser is operated as a continuously emitted beam, it is the power density that requires exquisite eye-hand coordination, not the power itself, as is commonly believed. Power density represents the speed at which the laser beam can penetrate the tissue. The higher the power density, the faster is tissue removal at that spot.

Considering the analogy of a magnifying glass and sunlight, it makes sense that the smaller the area in which the light is concentrated, the more intense and hotter it becomes. This relation is described by the formula

$$\text{Power density} = \frac{\text{watts} \times 100}{\pi r^2} = \text{watts/square centimeter}$$

It is useful to note that power density increases with either an increase in power or a decrease in spot size. Because the size contains a square function the tissue effect is changed more rapidly than the power.

Energy Fluence and Energy Density

Practically speaking, to vaporize target tissue effectively while minimizing unintentional thermal damage to the surrounding nontarget tissue, the clinician must first evaluate the absorption characteristics of the laser wavelength and then apply the concepts of energy fluence and energy density.

The magnitude of energy concentration is described most commonly as energy fluence (EA), or energy per unit area of the beam. Energy and spot diameter are considered together to produce the appropriate energy fluence to effectively vaporize all of the tissue in a determined area while minimizing thermal damage to surrounding tissue.

$$\text{EA} = \text{energy per pulse} \div \text{area (spot size)}$$
$$= \text{joules per square millimeter}$$

Energy fluence varies directly with energy and inversely with the diameter of the spot. Hence doubling the beam diameter (e.g., from 400 μm to 800 μm) increases the surface area by four times. Conversely, halving the spot size (e.g., from 400 μm to 200 μm) yields only one-fourth the area. Thus the energy fluence varies inversely with the square of the beam diameter.

The absorbed energy density (ED) measured in joules per cubic millimeter, determines the volume of tissue treated, or the size of the defect created by each pulse. Energy density can be calculated by dividing the energy fluence by the absorption length (L) of the laser.

$$\text{ED} = \text{EA/L} = \text{joules per cubic millimeter}$$

Pulsing Concepts

The way the laser energy is delivered to tissue is sometimes more important to the tissue effect than the wavelength selected. The rate at which the light is delivered determines the lateral extent of a burn, or its precision.

In particular it is useful to understand the basic differences between continuous wave, gated pulses, and true laser pulses.

Continuous Wave Operation

Most of the 10.6 μm CO_2 and most 1.06 μm neodymium:YAG lasers (nonophthalmic) operate in a continuous wave mode: The power output (rate of energy delivery) is steady and constant over the time during which it is delivered (Fig. 3-1).

The identifying characteristic of the continuous wave mode is that the maximum peak power delivered by the laser is never greater than the average power, which is what one reads on the power meter of the laser. In other words, a 40 watt maximum power 1.06 μm neodymium:YAG laser never produces higher power than the rated 40 watts, unlike true laser pulsing, the peak powers of which may go much higher.

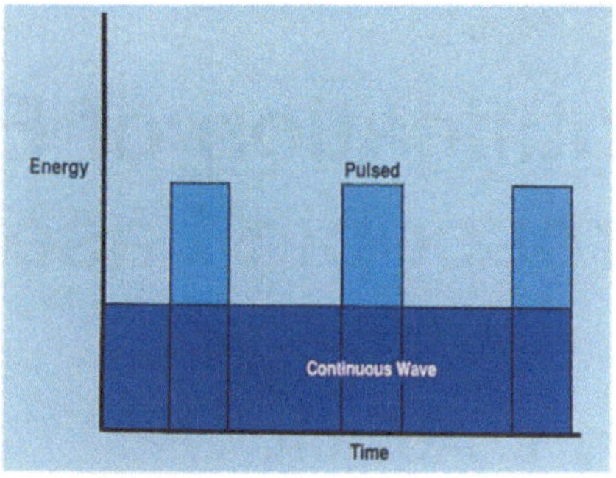

Figure 3-1. Comparison of continuous wave and pulsed mode. (From Brillhart AT Arthroscopic laser surgery, first of four articles. *Am J Arthrosc* 1(1):5–12, 1991. With permission.)

Continuous wave operation is also the most thermal way to use a laser in that the relatively long periods allow for more heat conduction to surrounding tissues. One gains hemostasis but at the expense of tissue precision.

A point of confusion on many lasers is that manufacturers sometimes label an operating button on the machine as continuous, although it does not necessarily mean a continuous wave mode. Rather, it may mean that the beam is emitted continuously so long as the foot pedal is depressed.

Gated (Timed) Pulse

When a laser such as continuous wave 10.6 μm CO_2 or continuous wave 1.06 μm neodymium:YAG are set on a pulse of fractions of a second to several seconds, it is generally a gated pulse and not a true pulse. Manufacturers of these lasers frequently label the button a pulse mode, either single or repeat. A gated pulse is simply a timer or shutter on a continuous wave beam.

The characteristic of a gated pulse is that the maximum peak power of the pulse is not any higher that the continuous wave setting. In other words, if a continuous wave 10.6 μm CO_2 laser is set at 40 watts for a 0.1 second pulse, the maximum power of that pulse does not exceed the 40 watts.

This type of pulsing may be achieved by either pumping the foot pedal while the laser is operating in a continuous wave mode or selecting a timer on the control panel. The foot pedal control is a faster way to work but does not provide the consistency the control panel pulse timer does. Pulsing a laser in this manner seems to be most useful in orthopaedics with a 10.6 μm CO_2 laser.

True Pulse

True laser pulses are found on many of the pulsed 0.308 μm Excimers, the superpulsed 10.6 μm CO_2, 0.532 μm

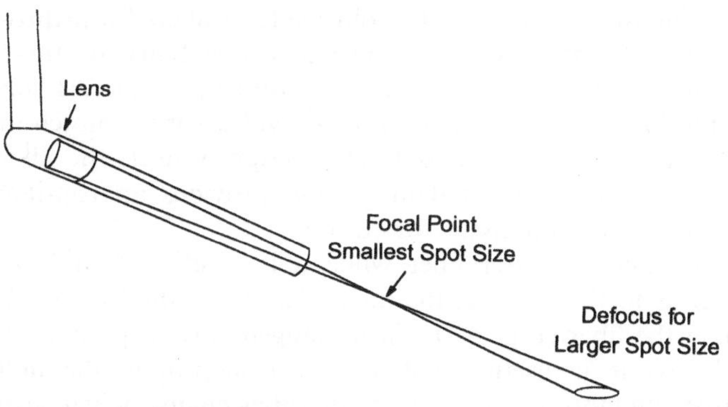

Figure 3-2. Focus/defocus of a 10.6 μm CO_2 laser beam.

KTP, 2.1 μm holmium:YAG, and 1.44 μm neodymium:YAG lasers. They are frequently used to limit the zone of thermal damage. Much of the cold cutting effects of 0.308 μm Excimer lasers have as much to do with their pulsing characteristics as with the wavelength of light (from 0.308 μm and up).

The identifying characteristic of a true laser pulse is that the maximum power output of the pulse far exceeds the maximum obtainable in a continuous wave mode. The power delivery is compressed to a short time frame. The 2.1 μm holmium:YAG laser, for instance, produces pulses of several thousand watts for only a few microseconds, which may be repeated 15 to 20 times per second to provide average powers of around 20 watts.

A pulsed 1.06 μm neodymium:YAG laser used in ophthalmology may produce power spikes of tens of millions of watts, but for only billionths of a second. This extreme pulsing leads to photoacoustic sparking effects.

True pulses may be emitted singularly, such as the pulsed dye laser for kidney stones or as a rapid series of pulses, such as the 0.308 μm Excimer laser in orthopaedics. The 0.532 μm KTP laser in orthopaedics also produces a series of pulses but of less individual energy than a 2.1 μm holmium:YAG laser. These rapid series pulses are referred to as high frequency pulsed lasers.

It is possible to squeeze so much energy into such a short pulse that the damage threshold for a fiber is exceeded. Shorter pulse widths usually lead to decreased fiber life when the same energy is used. It is for this reason that the ophthalmic 1.06 μm neodymium:YAG lasers, which produce a spark and snap, cannot be delivered down a fiber, as can an ordinary continuous wave 1.06 μm neodymium:YAG laser used in orthopaedics. The input energy would blow up the input end of the fiber. Some of the medical 0.308 μm Excimer lasers had so much energy compression in short pulses that the pulse widths had to be redesigned in the lasers to allow their use down fibers for cardiovascular use and potential orthopaedic use.

Contact Tip and Free Beam Methods of Energy Delivery

Given present technology, there are two modes of laser-tissue interaction: contact tip and the free beam mode. In the contact tip mode, the laser (usually a 1.06 μm neodymium:YAG laser) is used to heat a tip on the end of a fiber. The heated tip is then used to heat the tissue it touches. This mode works, or interacts with tissue, by conduction. The hot tip, rather than the laser light itself, cuts or cauterizes the tissue. The tissue interaction process in this case is somewhat similar to an electrocautery, except that a laser provides the source of heat.

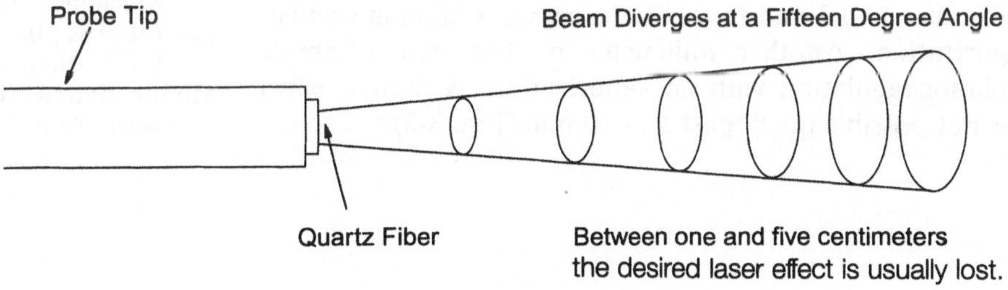

Figure 3-3. Divergence of a laser beam from a quartz fiber.

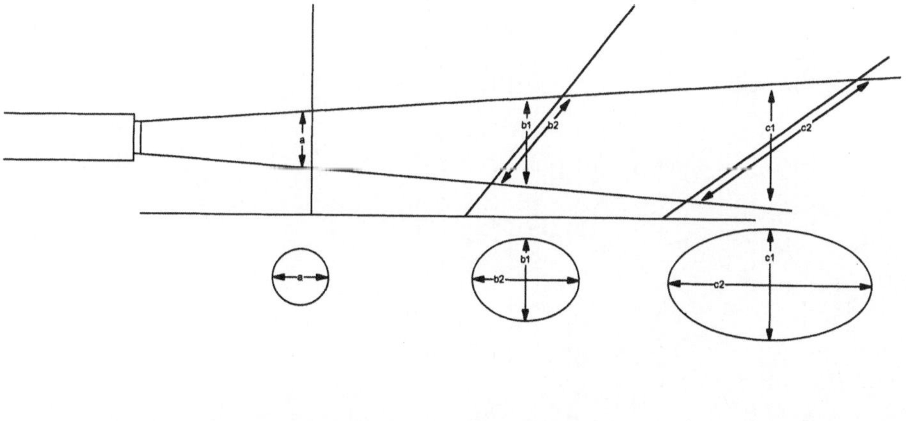

Figure 3-4. Profiles of a spot size relative to the angle of application and distance. (Courtesy A.T. Brillhart, 1993.)

Most surgical lasers use the free beam mode. With free beam mode lasers, it is the laser light itself that interacts with tissue. The 2.1 μm holmium:YAG laser, like the 10.6 μm CO_2 laser, is an example of a free beam laser. The laser light enters the tissue, is absorbed, and heats the tissue instantly to the vaporization temperature. If a laser interacts with tissue in this way, the laser is classified as free beam, even though the laser light may be delivered via an optical fiber.

Laser beams are unlike a physical instrument, such as a scalpel blade, in that they do not have definite sides. The beam is a concentration of energy in a spot that tends to fade at the edges. This characteristic affects the size of the spots created at different settings and the precision of incisions.

Furthermore, beams are emitted differently from fibers (0.532 μm KTP and 2.1 μm holmium:YAG lasers), than they are from an articulated arm (10.6 μm CO_2 lasers), which preserves the true shape of the beam. Figure 3-2 illustrates the focus/defocus effect of the 10.6 μm CO_2 laser beam. The biggest difference in using this apparatus, compared to a fiber system, is that this 10.6 μm CO_2 beam stays tightly focused for a greater distance than that of a fiber system. Though it is easy to control the 10.6 μm CO_2 laser beam, if one wanted to intentionally drill a hole through the side of the knee, aiming from the other side of the joint, it would be possible. This maneuver is not physically possible from such a distance with a fiber system.

Fibers tend to scramble the input beam resulting in a blended, homogeneous output, diverging immediately in a 10 to 15 degree cone (Fig. 3-3). There is no focal point to a fiber, which means that power density, and hence tissue effect, is highest at the tip of the fiber and falls off rapidly with short distances from the fiber tip. Cutting is achieved with the fiber just off the tissue (<1 mm). Another 1 to 2 mm further back creates sculpting and vaporization. Another millimeter or two causes simple photocoagulation with no vaporization. A desired effect is not possible much past 5 to 10 mm (Fig. 3-3).

Handpieces designed to hold the laser fibers for arthroscopic use provide some mechanical stability to these slender fibers. The design at the distal tip of the 2.1 μm holmium:YAG laser handpiece provides a metal notch in which the fiber is recessed. This design protects the fiber tip from mechanical damage and provides appropriate spacing from the tissue for cutting.

Aiming the laser fiber while it is positioned at right angles to the tissue is the most efficient method of handling the fiber (Fig. 3-4). Firing tangentially or parallel to the tissue is useful, such as when smoothing the fluff from chondromalacia. Power densities change when such elongated spots are formed on tissue because of firing at an angle, which minimizes ablation of stable articular cartilage.

Free beam or noncontact fibers provide the option of cutting when placing the fiber near the tissue and then sculpting when backed up 2 to 3 mm. By contrast, contact-type fibers and probes can be used only by directly touching the tissue.

Suggested Reading

Absten GT (1992) Fundamentals of electrosurgery. Advanced Laser Services Corporation, Columbus OH

Absten GT and Joffe SN (1989) Lasers in medicine: an introductory guide. Second edition. Chapman and Hall Ltd., London

Apfelberg D (1987) Evaluation and installation of surgical laser systems. Springer-Verlag, New York, NY

Einstein A (1961) Relativity. Bonanza Books, New York, NY

Goldman L (1981) The biomedical laser: technology and clinical applications. Springer-Verlag, New York, NY

Hallmark C (1979) Lasers, the light fantastic. Tab Books, Blue Ridge Summit, PA

Hecht J (1988) Understanding lasers. Howard W. Sams & Co./Macmillan, New York, NY

Laser Focus. In: 1992 Medical Laser Buyers Guide, Penwell Publications, Littleton, MA

Minton JP and Absten GT (1987) Surgical lasers and how they work. American College of Surgeons Bulletin

4

Surgeon's Evaluation of the Ablation Efficiency of Arthroscopic Laser Systems

Allen T. Brillhart

Parameters that measure the energy output and subsequent tissue effects are usually static (Boulnois, 1986; Walsh and Deutsch, 1988, 1989; Nishioka et al., 1989; Nishioka and Domankevitz 1990; Trauner et al., 1990; Cummings et al., 1993; Shi et al., 1993). They are measures of laser performance that mean more to the engineers than they do to the surgeon. Once a patient is involved however, testing dynamic effects as applied in vivo is essential (Brillhart, 1992). Dynamic effects refer to the results of the surgeon's moving the laser probe (Fig. 4-1).

It is not necessary to evaluate the ablation efficiency of the continuous wave mode of the 10.6 μm CO_2 laser because it is understood that this wavelength is excellent for tissue ablation (Walsh and Deutsch, 1988; Smith et al., 1989; Brillhart 1991b; Vangsness et al., 1991). Similarly, it is not necessary to measure the ablation efficiency of the free beam 1.06 μm neodymium:YAG laser because its wavelength is not efficient for ablating nonpigmented tissue such as meniscal tissue and hyaline cartilage (O'Brien and Miller 1990; Brillhart, 1991d; Vangsness et al., 1991). However, there is still debate about the best parameters for other arthroscopic laser systems (Walsh and Deutsch 1988; 1989; Nishioka et al., 1989; Nishioka and Domankevitz 1990; Trauner 1990; Brillhart 1991a; 1992; Cummings et al., 1993; Shi et al., 1993). Ideally, ablation efficiency is determined in the laboratory before use on a patient (Brillhart, 1992).

Materials and Methods

The most important variables are as follows:

Laser device, including wavelength properties
Laser delivery system
Energy settings
Total energy in joules
Tissue type
Medium in which the work is done
Human factor (surgeon and technique)

The ability of the entire system to ablate tissue using set values of these seven parameters is easily calculated. With different parameters there are different efficiencies. Laser efficiency as it applies to tissue ablation can be measured in kilojoules per gram. This parameter is referred to as *ablation efficiency* (*AE*) (Brillhart, 1992).

The parameters for ablating portions of meniscus, synovium, or unstable hyaline cartilage with a given laser system are determined by repeating a simple experiment. Each experiment's data are saved and compared. to similar data when using alternative, new, or more powerful systems. The experiment is as follows:

1. Human meniscal tissue and hyaline cartilage are best for experimenting in the laboratory. Chicken breast fibrocartilage is a readily obtainable model tissue as an alternative. It has an ablation efficiency approximately 50% more kilojoules per gram than human meniscal tissue, and is good for approximating the relative ablation efficiency for human meniscal tissue.
2. Ten small specimens are weighed before and after lasing. The energy (kilojoules) is recorded before and after. Total energy (kilojoules) for the experiment is recorded, including any energy used for calibration. The surgeon uses the technique in the selected medium. The type of device, energy settings, and delivery system are recorded.
3. The amount of tissue that was ablated is converted from grains to grams by dividing by 15.43 (1 gram = 15.43 grains). The energy (kilojoules) used to ablate

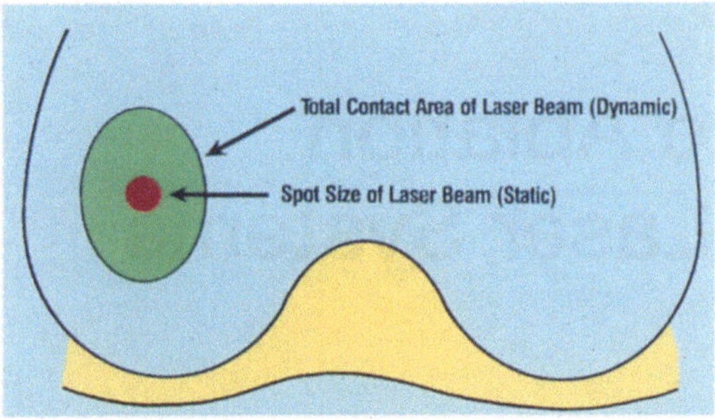

Figure 4-1. Dynamic effects refer to results obtained with a given amount of laser energy when the probe is moved. This is in contrast to a static effect when the probe is held in place. (From Brillhart AT, Arthroscopic laser surgery, first of four articles. *Am J Arthrosc* 1(1):5–12, 1991. With permission.)

Table 4-1. Experiment 1 data.

Specimen no.	Weight of meniscal portion before lasing (grains)	Weight after lasing (grains)	Reading (kJ)	
			Before	After
1	6.00	4.45	0.29	1.15
2	5.30	4.37	1.27	1.95
3	3.95	2.30	2.05	2.90
4	2.62	1.40	3.00	4.26
5	5.20	3.00	4.44	6.08
6	2.75	1.90	6.18	7.46
7	3.10	1.80	7.66	8.50
8	3.30	3.00	8.68	9.15
9	1.56	0.90	9.30	10.09
10	8.25	5.60	10.15	12.22

that volume is divided by the grams ablated, which gives the kilojoules per gram for each of the 10 specimens. An average is then determined for the final ablation efficiency.

4. The surgeon's ablative technique should be similar to what is used on patients. An oscillating technique, with the probe 0 to 1 mm away from the tissue, is standard. Pressure should not be applied to the tip to prevent photomechanical damage.
5. Different ablation efficiencies can be compared using different parameters. This method allows an evaluation of the system in vitro in a way that resembles in vivo use. It produces relative results for comparison purposes. However, the results of this method vary significantly with each surgeon and specimen.

The following experiments were performed to illustrate how to determine the ablation efficiency.

The parameters for experiment 1 are as follows:

Laser device	Coherent Versapulse 3000 2.1 μm holmium:YAG
Delivery system	prototype 500 μm fiber straight handpiece
Energy settings	2 joules per pulse; 16 Hz; 32 watts
Total energy	12.22 kJ (includes calibration)
Tissue type	fresh human menisci; 60-year-old male
Medium	tap water
Surgeon and technique	author; oscillating with probe 0 to 1 mm away

The data and results obtained for experiment 1 are in Tables 4-1 and 4-2, respectively.

Table 4-2. Experiment 1 results.

Specimen no.	Tissue ablated (grams[a])	kJ used	*AE* (kJ/g)
1	0.10	0.86	8.60
2	0.06	0.68	11.33
3	0.11	0.85	7.73
4	0.08	1.26	15.75
5	0.14	1.64	11.71
6	0.06	1.28	21.33
7	0.08	0.84	10.50
8	0.02	0.47	23.50
9	0.04	0.79	19.75
10	0.17	2.07	12.18
Average			14.24

[a] 1 gram = 15.43 grains

The parameters for experiment 2 are as follows:

Laser device	Coherent Versapulse 3000 2.1 μm holmium:YAG
Delivery system	Infratome straight probe 450 μm fiber
Energy settings	2 joules per pulse; 16 Hz; 32 watts
Total energy	12.22 kJ (includes calibration)
Tissue type	Fresh human menisci; 60-year-old male
Medium	Tap water
Surgeon and technique	author; oscillating with probe 0 to 1 mm away

The data and results obtained for experiment 2 are in Tables 4-3 and 4-4, respectively.

Table 4-3. Experiment 2 data.

Specimen no.	Weight of meniscal portion before lasing (grains)	Weight after lasing (grains)	Reading (kJ) Before	Reading (kJ) After
1	4.44	3.10	0.27	1.14
2	3.12	1.37	1.29	2.62
3	5.75	4.25	2.73	3.35
4	4.25	2.87	3.47	5.23
5	4.55	2.00	5.34	7.27
6	4.00	2.30	7.40	9.47
7	4.37	2.12	9.60	10.82
8	2.50	1.45	11.12	11.77
9	1.62	0.90	11.89	12.50
10	3.75	2.37	12.69	13.82

Table 4-4. Experiment 2 results.

Specimen no.	Tissue ablated (grams[a])	kJ used	*AE* (kJ/g)
1	0.09	0.87	9.67
2	0.11	1.33	12.09
3	0.10	0.62	6.20
4	0.09	1.76	19.56
5	0.17	1.93	11.35
6	0.11	2.07	18.82
7	0.15	1.22	8.13
8	0.07	0.65	9.29
9	0.05	0.61	12.20
10	0.09	1.13	12.56
Average			11.99

[a]1 gram = 15.43 grains

The parameters for experiment 3 are as follows:

Laser device	Zeiss 1.44 μm neodymium: YAG
Delivery system	600 μm fiber prototype handpiece
Energy settings	2 joules per pulse; 16 Hz; 32 watts
Total energy	30.73 kJ (includes calibration)
Tissue type	chicken breast fibrocartilage
Medium	tap water
Surgeon and technique	author; oscillating at a 0 to 3 mm distance

The data and results obtained for experiment 3 are in Tables 4-5 and 4-6, respectively.

Table 4-5. Experiment 3 data.

Specimen no.	Weight of meniscal portion before lasing (grains)	Weight after lasing (grains)	Reading (kJ) Before	Reading (kJ) After
1	5.8	4.1	0.46	1.87
2	7.5	5.8	1.87	3.40
3	6.9	3.3	3.83	8.02
4	4.7	3.3	8.46	10.14
5	7.7	4.8	10.57	13.68
6	5.6	3.5	14.27	17.72
7	6.1	4.6	18.08	20.56
8	8.2	7.2	20.83	22.10
9	10.9	7.1	22.31	26.24
10	7.6	4.4	26.97	30.73

Table 4-6. Experiment 3 results.

Specimen no.	Tissue ablated (grams[a])	kJ used	*AE* (kJ/g)
1	0.11	1.41	12.82
2	0.11	1.53	13.91
3	0.23	4.19	18.22
4	0.09	1.68	18.67
5	0.19	3.11	16.37
6	0.14	3.45	24.64
7	0.10	2.48	24.80
8	0.06	1.27	21.17
9	0.25	3.93	15.72
10	0.21	3.76	17.90
Average			18.42

[a]1 gram = 15.43 grains

Discussion

When comparing two or more laser systems, the most important variables are the wavelengths (laser device) (Brillhart, 1991a; Black et al., 1992) and energy settings. Next is the energy tolerance of the delivery system (fibers and handpieces). When a single system is evaluated, most variations occur with the energy settings (joules per pulse and pulses per second) and the energy tolerance of the delivery system (fibers and handpieces).

The tolerance of the delivery system is the kilojoules (kJ) that can be used before total failure. This figure usually varies from 10 to 50 kJ, depending on the energy settings. One may finish half the ablation quickly with a high level of joules per pulse but be left with a burned-out probe to finish the second half. Ten kilojoules per fiber is not acceptable when it normally takes 12 to 15 kJ to ablate 1 g of meniscal tissue. However, this dose is acceptable when an indirect technique is used for chondroplasty, for example. A dose of less than 10 kJ is routinely used in such cases.

More joules per pulse causes a significant amount of photomechanical trauma to the quartz fibers. The smaller the fiber, the less energy that is transmitted before failure at these same high pulse energies. If a small fiber is used, it is best to use fewer joules per pulse and a higher repetition rate. Probe failure starts to occur slowly between 6 and 20 kJ. Failure also occurs more rapidly with angled probes. Energy concentrates at the curve of the probe, and this point is damaged more easily. Sudden, complete failure is usually due to a fractured fiber. Moreover, as stated previously, photomechanical shocks affect the fiber life inversely. This problem is significant with the 0.308 μm Excimer laser (Muller et al., 1988).

The surgeon should select a laser device that has the widest range of joules per pulse settings and pulses per second settings, from which can be determined the "best" settings. A balance between high energy settings and fiber tolerances is critical.

Logically, the more joules per pulse, the more volume of tissue is ablated for a single pulse (Nishioka et al., 1989; Cummings et al., 1993). Solid-state lasers do not work in single pulses, however. They currently have varying repetition rates from 5 to 50 Hz per second. Compounding the effects of multiple pulses does not always guarantee the expected results. Photomechanical factors and thermal relaxation times must be considered.

Photomechanical effects increase with more joules per pulse. Photomechanical effects may be paradoxical, however (Frenz et al., 1988; 1989; 1990; 1991a; Weber et al., 1989). Subsurface irregularities can be created by higher energy. Deeper holes with irregular contours trap debris and alter the absorption of subsequent pulses (Boulnois, 1986; Frenz et al., 1988; 1989; 1990; 1991a; 1991b; Zweig et al., 1990). Also, higher energy displaces target tissue. More energy can be absorbed by tissue when several smaller pulses hit the target than when only one of several large pulses hits it. Higher-pulsed energy also generates more debris, clouding the surgical medium and impairing visualization. Larger pulses of energy also result in shock waves that alter tissue and produce undesirable tissue recoil (Hibst, 1992).

To vaporize 1 mm^3 of water-rich tissue requires at least 2.5 J of energy. To make maximum use of the energy available requires that the energy be delivered ideally in a time that is short compared to the thermal relaxation time of the treated volume. Thermal relaxation time is approximately a few tenths of a second for 1 mm^3 water. The thermal relaxation time scales approximately with the volume of tissue heated by the laser beam: the product of its cross-sectional area and absorption length, or its width and depth.

Conduction of heat in soft tissues takes time (Carslaw and Jaeger, 1959; Weber et al., 1989), and the amount of time increases with the square of the distance. The approximate time for substantial heat conduction to occur over a given distance in soft tissue is shown in Figure 4-2.

Overlapping pulses of lesser energy can have a cumulative photothermal effect because of thermal relaxation properties. It is in this way that a pulsed laser can theoretically function in a modulated, almost continuous mode. More charring is observed with longer pulse widths and increased exposure time. As charring occurs, the optical properties of the tissue change. Also, if thermal relaxation times overlap, drying occurs and water absorption decreases. A balance here must also be obtained and measured.

Use of the probe further away from the tissue substantially decreases the energy that reaches the tissue. Figure 4-3 illustrates the inverse relation of increasing the distance of a 2.1 μm holmium:YAG laser probe from the target tissue.

This relation is more obvious in a liquid medium. Not only does it allow for various tissue effects, but it contributes to the safe use of this laser, the 2.1 μm holmium:YAG, and others like it (e.g., the 1.44 μm neodymium:YAG) in an arthroscopic environment.

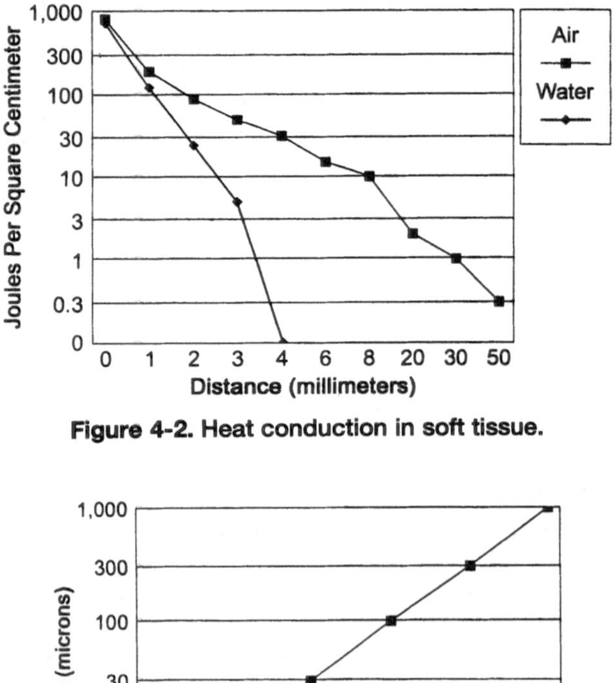

Figure 4-2. Heat conduction in soft tissue.

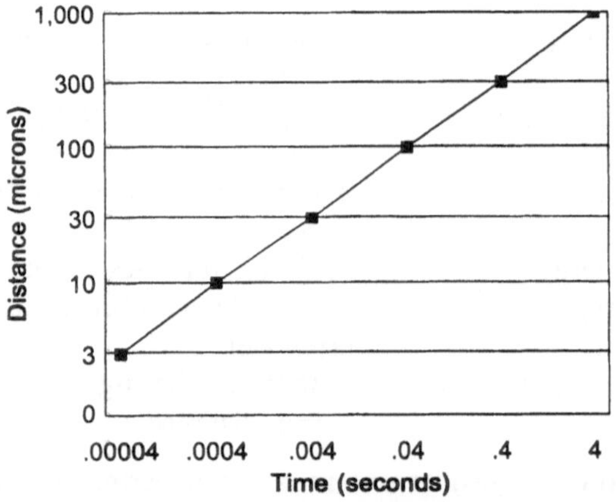

Figure 4-3. A 2.1 μm holmium:YAG laser (1 joule per pulse, 10 Hz).

Conclusion

The potential advantages of higher pulsed energy delivery for arthroscopic laser systems are (1) increased tissue ablation per pulse; (2) faster tissue cutting; and (3) decreased secondary photothermal effects. The potential disadvantages are (1) visual field clouding; (2) increased photomechanical tissue effects; (3) shorter fiber life; and (4) a possible paradoxical decrease in overall ablation efficiency. The paradox of higher pulsed energy must be answered by the arthroscopist. The best energy setting should be determined in the laboratory using the experiments that have been described. The laser system with the widest range of energy settings should be used. Seven major parameters are important for directly evaluating and comparing solid-state laser systems.

Laser device and its wavelength
Delivery system
Energy settings
Total energy used
Tissue type
Arthroscopic medium
Technique of the surgeon

Simple experimentation allows objective comparison and evaluation prior to patient use. In practice, a complete operative report should also mention these variables. This practice will allow future evaluation and comparison of true in vivo tissue effects.

References

Alimpieu S, Artjushenko V et al., (1988) Polycrystalline ir fibers for laser scalpels. Medical Fibers in Medicine III, SPIE vol. 906

Black J, Sherk H, Meller M, et al., (1992) Wavelength selection in laser arthroscopy. Semin Orthop 7:72–76

Boulnois JL (1986) Photophysical processes in recent medical laser developments: a review. Lasers in Medical Science 1:47–66

Brillhart AT (1992) Ablation efficiency determination using the 1.44 μm neodymium:YAG laser. SPIE Proceedings 1880:29–30

Brillhart AT (1991) Arthroscopic laser surgery. First of four articles. American Journal of Arthroscopy 1:5–12

Brillhart AT (1991) Arthroscopic laser surgery: the CO_2 laser and its use. Second of four articles. American Journal of Arthroscopy 1:7–12.

Brillhart AT (1991) Arthroscopic laser surgery: the holmium:YAG laser and its use. Third of four articles. American Journal of Arthroscopy 1:7–11

Brillhart AT (1991) Arthroscopic laser surgery: the contact neodymium:YAG laser. Fourth of four articles. American Journal of Arthroscopy 1:7–10

Carslaw HS and Jaeger JC (1959) Conduction of heat in solids. Oxford: Oxford University Press

Cummings R, Prodoehl J, Rhodes A, et al., (1993) Nd:YAG 1.44 laser ablation of human cartilage. SPIE 1880:34–36

Curcio JA and Petty CC (1951) The near infrared absorption spectrum of liquid water. Journal of the Optical Society of America 41:302–304

Frenz M, Mischler C, Romano V, Forrer M, Muller OM, Weber HP (1991) Effect of mechanical tissue properties on thermal damage in skin after ir-laser ablation. Appl Phys B 52:251–258

Frenz M, Mishcler Greber C, Romano V, Forrer M, Weber HP (1991) Damage induced by pulsed ir-laser radiation at transitions between different tissues. SPIE Laser-Tissue Interaction II, 1427:9–15

Frenz M, Zweig AD, Romano V, Weber HP (1990) Dynamics in laser cutting of soft media. SPIE, Laser-Tissue Interaction, 1202:22–33

Frenz M, Romano V, Zweig AD, Weber HP (1989) Instabilities in laser cutting of soft media. J Appl Phys 66:4496–4503

Frenz M, Mathezloic F, Stoffel MHS, Zweig AD, Romano V, Weber HP (1988) Transport of biologically active material in laser cutting. Lasers in Surg and Med 8:562–566

Hibst R (1992) Mechanical effects of erbium:YAG laser bone ablation. Lasers in Surg and Med 12:125–130

Irvine W, Pollack J (1968) Infrared optical properties of water and ice spheres. Icarus 8:324–360

Mankin HJ, Thrasher AZ (1975) Water content and binding in normal and osteoarthritic human cartilage. J Bone Joint Surg 57A:76–80

Miller DV, O'Brien SJ, Arnoczky SS, Kelly A, Fealy SV, Warren RF (1989) The use of the contact nd:YAG laser in arthroscopic surgery: effects on articular cartilage and meniscal tissue. Arthroscopy: The Journal of Arthroscopic and Related Surgery 5:245–253

Muller G, Kar H, Dorschel K, Ringelhan H (1988) Transmission of short pulsed high power uv laser radiation through fibers depending on pulse length, intensity and long-term behavior. SPIE 906:231–4

Nishioka NS, Domankevitz Y (1990) Comparison of tissue ablation with pulsed holmium and thulium lasers. IEEEJ Quantum Electronics 26:2271–5

Nishioka NS, Domankevitz Y, Flotte TJ, Anderson RR (1989) Ablation of rabbit liver, stomach, and colon with a pulsed holmium laser. Gastroenterology 96:831–837

O'Brien SJ, Miller DV (1990) The contact neodymium-yttrium aluminum garnet laser: a new approach to arthroscopic laser surgery. Clinical Orthopaedics and Related Research 252:95–100

Romano V, Mischler Greber C, Frenz M, Forrer M, Weber HP (1991) Measurement of temperature distributions after pulsed ir-radiation impact in biological tissue models with fluorescent thin films. SPIE Laser-Tissue Interaction II, 1427:16–26

Romano V, Zweig AD, Frem M, Weber HP (1989) Time-resolved thermal microscopy with fluorescent films. Appl Phys B 49:527–533

Shi W, Vari S, van der Veen MJ, et al., (1993) Effect of varying laser parameters on pulsed ho:YAG ablation of bovine knee joint tissues. Arthroscopy: The Journal of Arthroscopic and Related Surgery 9:96–102

Smith CF, Johansen WE, Vangsness CT, Sutter LV, Marshall GJ (1989) The carbon dioxide laser: a potential tool for orthopedic surgery. Clinical Orthopaedics and Related Research 242:43–50

Trauner K, Nishioka N, Patel D (1990) Pulsed holmium:yttrium-aluminum-garnet (ho:YAG) laser ablation of fibrocartilage and articular cartilage. Am J Sports Med 18:316–320

Vangsness CT, Huang J, Smith CF (1991) Light absorption

characteristics of the human meniscus: applications for laser ablation. SPIE 24:16–19
Walsh Jr. JT, Deutsch TF (1989) Er:YAG laser ablation of tissue: measurement of ablation rates. Lasers Surg Med 9:327–337
Walsh Jr. JT, Deutsch TF (1988) Pulsed CO_2 laser tissue ablation: measurement of the ablation rate. Lasers Surg Med 8:264–275
Weber HP, Zweig AD, Frenz M, Romano V (1989) Interaction of laser radiation with tissue. SPIE 1353 Lasers and Medicine:11–17
Zweig AD, Meierhofer B, Muller OM, Mischler C, Romano V, Frenz M, Weber HP (1990) Lateral thermal damage along pulsed laser incisions. Lasers Surg Med 10:262–274

5

Laser Meniscectomy: Wavelength Analysis by the Spectrophotometer

C. Thomas Vangsness Jr.

As laser light hits tissue it is either reflected backward, transmitted through the tissue, absorbed into the tissue, or after entering the tissue deflected (scattered) in a forward or backward direction. Scattered light can then exit the tissue or be absorbed. Increased absorption of light by tissue allows more concentrated laser heating in the tissue, resulting in an increased ability to vaporize the tissue.

A determination of the absorption coefficients of the human meniscus is critical for laser meniscectomy. Except for the 0.308 μm Excimer laser, not yet approved by the Food and Drug Administration (FDA) in the United States for marketing for arthroscopic use, all currently used arthroscopic laser wavelengths are from the infrared portion of the electromagnetic spectrum. In two previous studies (Vangsness et al., 1992; Schwartz et al., 1993), it was demonstrated that the absorption coefficient of the human meniscus parallels that of water. Figure 5-1 overlaps the water absorption curve with that of the human meniscus. The increased absorption noted in the ultraviolet region at 0.3 μm has been associated with the presence of collagen protein (Deyl et al., 1970; Eyre et al., 1984). Spectroscopy studies were performed on human meniscal specimens of various ages and tissue thicknesses through different planes and different zones of the menisci. No significant absorption variation occurred when these factors were considered. In the first study (Vangsness et al., 1992), the wavelengths analyzed were between 0.3 μm and 3.0 μm. A Cary 2415 spectrophotometer was used. In the more complete study (Schwartz et al., 1993) the spectrum encompassed 0.36 μm to 11 μm.

The most efficient arthroscopic lasers for absorption appeared to be the 2.94 μm erbium:YAG and the 10.6 μm CO_2. The 1.44 μm neodymium:YAG and the 2.1 μm holmium:YAG wavelengths also showed good absorption. The 0.308 μm Excimer laser appeared to work because of the collagen protein absorption peak.

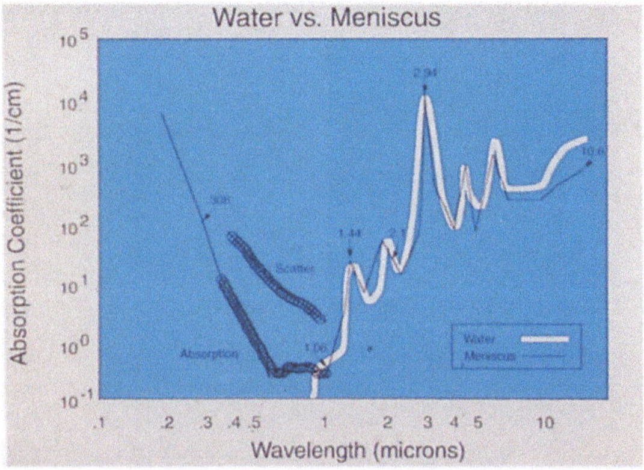

Figure 5-1. Absorption curves for water and the human meniscus.

References

Deyl Z et al., (1970) A fluorescent compound in collagen and its relation to the age of the animal. Exp Gerontol 5:57–26

Eyre D, Koob TJ, van Ness KP, et al. (1984) Quantitation of hydroxypyridinium crosslinks in collagen by high-performance liquid chromatography. Anal Biochem 137:380–388

Schwartz J, Jacques SL, Vangsness CT (1993) Optical properties of the human meniscus. Lasers Surg Med Abstracts, suppl. 5, no. 178, pp. 36–37

Vangsness CT, Huang J, Boll J, Smith CF (1992) The optical properties of the human meniscus. Semin Orthop 7:72–76

6

Thermal Effects of Infrared Laser Systems

Robert S. Cummings Jr., Gregory J. Lane, Har Chi Lau, Jonathan D. Black, and Henry H. Sherk

Laser use in arthroscopy is becoming increasingly common, and the effectiveness and efficiency of numerous systems have been well documented (Sherk et al., 1992). Application of these lasers to intraarticular tissue causes tissue cutting and ablation but can also cause surrounding tissue damage or necrosis. The amount of damage sustained by the tissue is important because the tissue may be permanently damaged and unable to regenerate. This depth of tissue damage depends on the type and specific wavelength of each laser system utilized. We have evaluated various lasers for their effects on meniscal tissue by morphometric and histologic analysis. These lasers have been or are currently being used for arthroscopic knee surgery, and they vary widely in respect to their wavelengths.

Each laser system has its individual wavelength and therefore is absorbed by the meniscal tissue differently, depending on its absorption by water. At a wavelength of 10.6 μm the energy of the CO_2 laser is almost completely absorbed by water and therefore is effective in its cutting and ablating abilities. Black et al. (1992) demonstrated that a free beam and waveguide CO_2 laser produced a 54 μm zone of tissue damage as seen by hexatoxylin and eosin (H&E) staining and a 447 μm zone of damage as seen by trichrome staining (Fig. 6-1). Their values were obtained following 20 watts of continuous wave power. They also tested several other laser systems in a similar manner that have been or are currently used clinically. The 2.1 μm Holmium:YAG laser at 1.3 joules per pulse produced 82 μm of thermal necrosis on H&E staining and 552 μm on trichrome staining (Fig. 6-2). This laser uses pulsed energy that limits the exposure time of the tissue to potential thermal damage. Their evaluation of the 1.06 μm neodymium:YAG laser showed thermal necrosis of 378 μm by H&E staining (Fig. 6-3) and 870 μm as determined by trichrome staining. The laser was used at 30 watts of continuous wave power and as a free beam. We

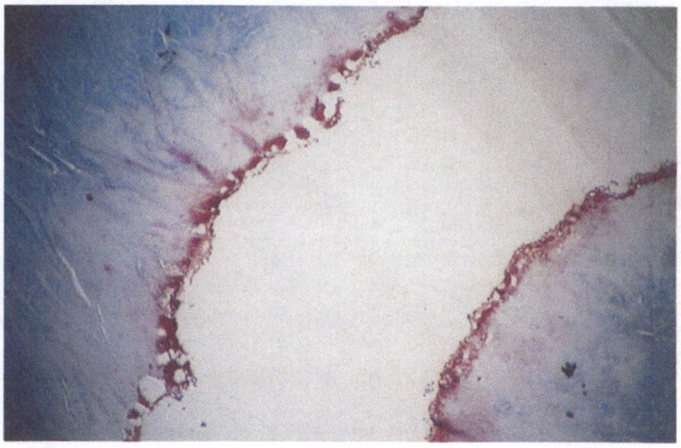

Figure 6-1. Tissue damage produced by the CO_2 laser.

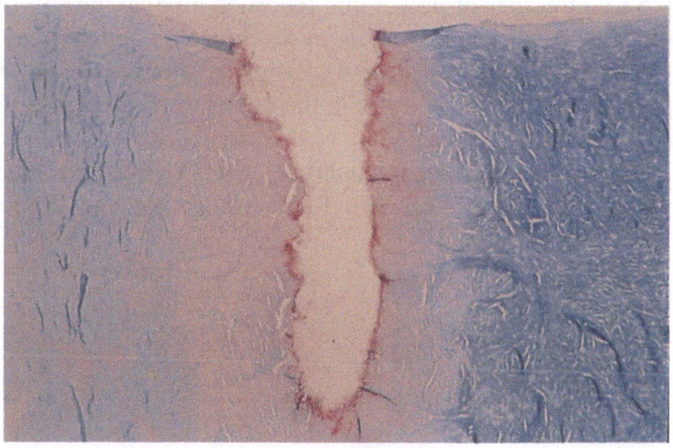

Figure 6-2. Tissue damage produced by a 2.1 μm holmium:YAG laser at 1.3 joules per pulse.

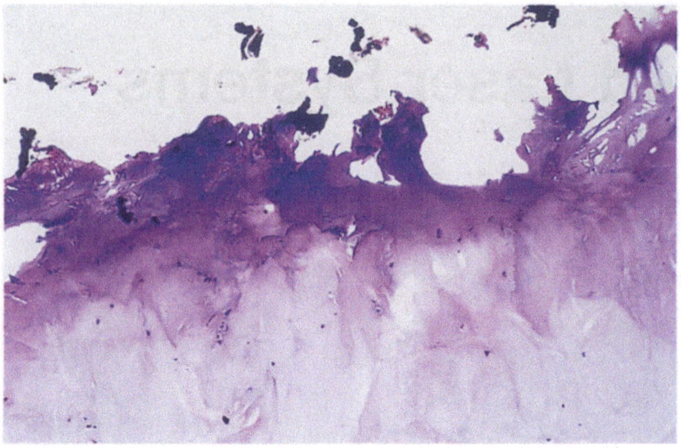

Figure 6.3. Tissue damage produced by a 1.06 μm neodymium:YAG laser.

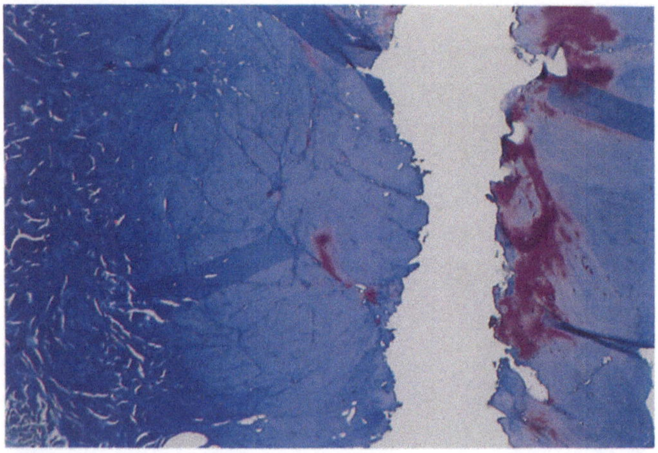

Figure 6-4. Tissue damage produced by a 1.44 μm neodymium: YAG laser at 0.5 to 2.0 joules per pulse.

have performed similar analyses using the same image analysis program (IM Module 2100, Imagemeasure, Federal Way, WA) with a 1.44 μm neodymium:YAG laser at 0.5 to 2.0 joules of power and recorded an average zone of 403 μm of thermal necrosis by trichrome staining (Cummings et al., 1993) (Fig. 6-4). This instrument is a pulsed laser that theoretically limits the exposure time of the tissue to damage.

These various laser systems each are absorbed by water at differing rates and therefore should cut and ablate fibrocartilage at differing rates. In addition, the time the tissue is exposed to the radiation increases the susceptibility to damage. Therefore a pulsed laser should minimize the surrounding depth of thermal necrosis. The comparison completed at our institution shows that the 10.6 μm CO_2 laser produced the least amount of thermal damage to the fibrocartilage, followed by the 1.44 μm neodymium:YAG, the 2.1 μm holmium:YAG, and the 1.06 μm neodymium:YAG laser. Comparable methods and materials were used to evaluate this thermal damage, although different investigators were involved. These results revealed only a slight difference in depth of damage between the 10.6 μm CO_2, the 1.44 μm neodymium:YAG, and the 2.1 μm holmium:YAG lasers. The 10.6 μm CO_2 laser caused the smallest depth of damage but is not widely used arthroscopically because it functions best in a gas medium. The 1.44 μm neodymium:YAG and the 2.1 μm holmium:YAG lasers were close in their respective tissue damage depths. This similarity would be expected as both are pulsed lasers and are nearly identical in their absorption coefficient of water (Irvine and Pollack, 1968). The 1.06 μm neodymium:YAG laser caused a wider depth of damage in the free beam mode. This laser is a continuous beam, and therefore the tissue surrounding the ablation field may absorb more constant energy than the pulsed lasers create.

These comparisons provide relative numbers for the depth of thermal damage created during ablation of fibrocartilage. Further investigation is needed to determine the comparative analysis for articular cartilage. Further study is also needed to determine the long-range effect this thermal necrosis has on fibrocartilage. Whether the full depth partially regenerates or sloughs over time could have long-term implications.

References

Black JD, Sherk HH, Meller M, Divan J, Rhodes A, Lane GJ (1992) Wavelength selection in laser arthroscopy. Sem Orthop vol. 7, no. 2, pp. 72–76

Cummings RS, Prodoehl JA, Rhodes A, Black JD, Sherk HH (1993) Nd:YAG 1.44 laser ablation of human cartilage. SPIE Proceedings vol. 1880, Jan. pp. 34–36

Irvine WM, Pollack JB (1968) Infrared optical properties of water and ice spheres. Icarus vol. 8, pp. 324–360

Sherk HH, Lane GJ, Black JD (1992) Laser arthroscopy. Orthop Rev vol. 9, pp. 1077–1083

7

Effects of Laser Energy on Diarthrodial Joint Tissues: Articular Cartilage and Synovial Cell Metabolism

R. Lane Smith, L. Montgomery, G. Fanton, M. Dillingham, and D. J. Schurman

Laser energy stimulates articular cartilage repair when applied at low energy levels (Schultz et al., 1985; Borovoy et al., 1989). Tissue repair occurs through increased cartilage and synovial cell activity. We review here the organization and function of articular cartilage and summarize effects of laser energy on joint tissue as reported in the literature and from our experimental studies with the 2.1 μm holmium:YAG laser. Our studies showed that human articular cartilage responds to low levels of 2.1 μm holmium:YAG laser energy through cell proliferation (DNA synthesis) and increased proteoglycan synthesis (sulfate incorporation into glycosaminoglycan). At high levels of laser energy, cartilage cell metabolism was inhibited.

Articular Cartilage and Joint Function

Normal function of diarthrodial joints depends on the distribution of relatively large forces across the bony surfaces. The magnitude of the joint forces reaches levels four to seven times body weight; and the forces are dispersed by articular cartilage. Cartilage function occurs via a highly organized extracellular matrix maintaining a fixed charge density and possessing a high affinity for water.

Normal articular cartilage consists of an assembly of large and small proteoglycans, collagens, hyaluronic acid, and glycoproteins (Heinegard and Paulsson, 1987). These matrix macromolecules originate from chondrocytes localized in a nonrandom pattern throughout the cartilage matrix (Aydelotte and Kuettner, 1988). In normal joints, chondrocytes do not proliferate; dividing chondrocytes indicate a change in cartilage homeostasis, either as degeneration or attempted repair (Mankin and Lippiello, 1970).

The cartilage extracellular matrix is composed primarily of proteoglycans and type II collagen (Hascall and Heinegard, 1975). Proteoglycans are hydrophilic and contribute to the tissue water content (70% of the wet weight). The cartilage proteoglycans include the large aggregating proteoglycans, molecules capable of binding to hyaluronate, nonaggregating proteoglycans, and the small proteoglycans biglycan and decorin. The aggregated proteoglycans ($12–20 \times 10^6$ Daltons) imbue cartilage with compressive resilience; and the type II collagen fibrils provide cartilage with tensile strength.

As a class, the large proteoglycans consist of a core protein having a molecular weight of 200 to 350 kDa to which the electronegative, hydrophilic, glycosaminoglycans (GAG) are covalently attached. Chondroitin sulfates and keratan sulfate account for approximately 85% and 13% of the total proteoglycan glycosaminoglycans, respectively, depending on the source and age of the cartilage (Smith et al., 1980). In addition, a number of glycosidically linked oligosaccharides are present on the core protein. Sequence data for human cartilage proteoglycan core protein shows extensive homology with that of the chicken, rat, and cow (Doege et al., 1991).

Degradative events that decrease the proteoglycan content leave cartilage at risk for continued damage. Progressive joint destruction may be accelerated by a reduction of compressive resistance as cartilage proteoglycan is lost (Mow et al., 1991). Without the proteoglycans, normal joint forces denature and disrupt the collagen network, leaving the collagen susceptible to collagenases. Replenishment of the proteoglycan content would represent a positive step toward a reparative process.

Laser Energy Sources and Analysis of Tissue Response

Analyses of the effects of laser energy on joint tissue have used the neodymium-yttrium-aluminum-garnet (1.06 μm neodymium:YAG) laser (Hardie et al., 1989; Miller et al., 1989; O'Brien and Miller, 1990; Bradrick et al., 1992) and the 2.1 μm holmium:YAG laser (Trauner et al., 1990; Collier et al., 1993). The 0.308 μm Excimer laser, the 10.6 μm CO_2 laser (Vangsness et al., 1992; Vangsness and Ghaderi, 1993) and the 0.532 μm KTP laser studies focused on histologic responses, so little is known of the detailed biochemical reactions to these sources of laser energy (Freedland, 1988; Hohlbach et al., 1989; Kroitzch et al., 1989; Gonzales et al., 1990; Raunest and Lohnert, 1990; Dressel et al., 1991; Nixon et al., 1991; Roth et al., 1991).

Laser Energy and Induction of Cartilage Cell Proliferation

Biochemical analyses of the effects of laser energy on stimulation of cartilage cell division have relied on the uptake of ^{3}H-thymidine into chondrocytes either in monolayer culture or in full-thickness tissue explants in organ culture. The 1.06 μm neodymium:YAG laser energy applied to isolated chondrocytes cultured in monolayers in medium containing 15% fetal bovine serum resulted in a twofold elevation in uptake of ^{3}H-thymidine at 72 hours after treatment and a 2.6-fold elevation at 144 hours after treatment. An energy level as low as 1 joule initiated the uptake of thymidine, and levels of 30 and 60 joules were not inhibitory to the laser response (Herman and Khosla, 1988).

Canine cartilage exposed to a low-level of 1.06 μm neodymium:YAG energy (energy density 51 J/cm^2) decreased ^{3}H-thymidine incorporation at 6 days after treatment, whereas increasingly higher levels of energy resulted in an upward trend in the ^{3}H-thymidine uptake, approaching the levels in untreated controls. At 12 days after treatment, ^{3}H-thymidine uptake was not different from that in control cartilage (Spivak et al., 1992).

In our preliminary studies, treatment of full-thickness human cartilage explants using the 2.1 μm holmium:YAG laser showed a significant elevation in cell proliferation (DNA synthesis) at 2 weeks after treatment (Figs. 7-1 and 7-2). The application of laser energy was carried out using a sweeping motion to move the probe uniformly across the synovial surface of the tissue sample. The cartilage samples were obtained during total joint arthroplasty and were visually selected as normal articular cartilage. The total motion consisted of a vertical sweep and a horizontal sweep to ensure complete coverage. The end of the probe was maintained at a distance of 1 mm from the cartilage surface and the angle of the probe at 30 degrees. An energy level of 0.6 joule per pulse proved to be most efficacious for the cartilage proliferative response. The uptake of ^{3}H-thymidine into DNA was characterized as acid-precipitable counts and was normalized to the size of the explants by quantifying the total DNA present.

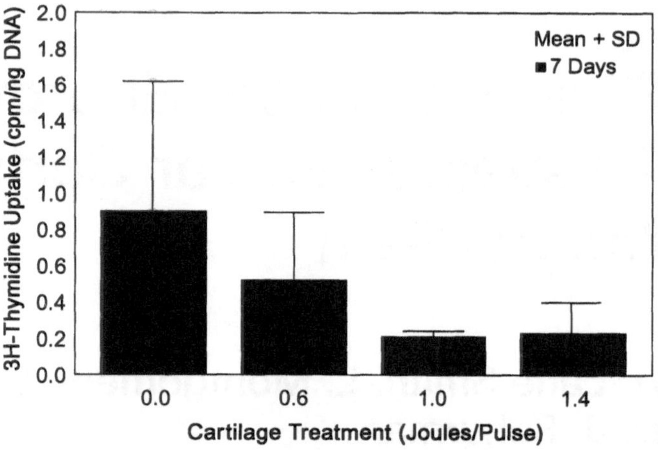

Figure 7-1. Articular cartilage cell proliferation following 2.1 μm holmium:YAG laser treatment: after 7 days of culture. Full-thickness articular cartilage samples were treated with varying levels of laser energy and maintained in Dulbecco's modified Eagle's medium containing 10% (v/v) fetal bovine serum. DNA synthesis was determined using ^{3}H-thymidine uptake into trichloracetic acid-precipitable material. The uptake of ^{3}H-thymidine was normalized to total cartilage DNA values to adjust for variance in the size of the cartilage samples. Each experiment was carried out in quadruplicate for each energy level, and the data represent two replicate cartilage samples. $p < 0.05$ using Student's two-sample t-test.

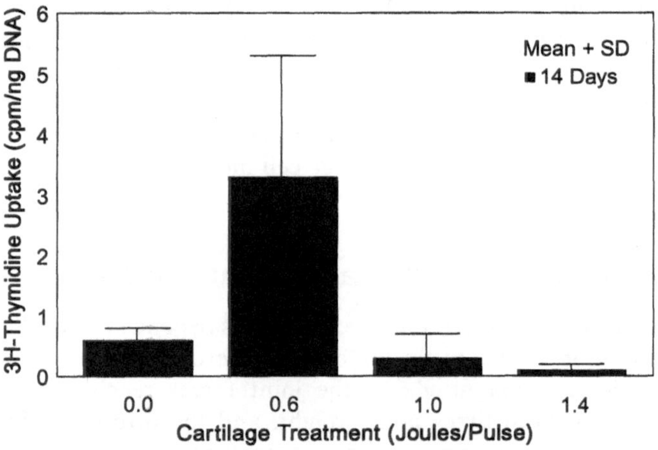

Figure 7-2. Articular cartilage cell proliferation following 2.1 μm holmium:YAG laser treatment: after 14 days of culture.

In our study, articular cartilage explants were maintained in tissue culture medium containing 10% fetal bovine serum to maximize growth. The experiments were carried out in tissue culture medium to mimic the clinical application of laser energy. The experimental methodology brings into question the precise level of energy reaching the cells because of attenuation by the culture medium. Nevertheless, under our conditions of treatment the cartilage was clearly responsive to different energy settings, as demonstrated in Figures 7-1 and 7-2. At higher energy levels (1.0 and 1.4 joules per pulse) the cells were damaged, so DNA synthesis was inhibited relative to untreated control cultures. In these experiments the untreated cartilage was left in the same culture dish as the laser-energy-treated cartilage to control for indirect effects due to exposure of the culture medium to laser energy; an excess volume of culture medium (30 ml) was present during laser treatment of the cartilage, and the temperature of the culture medium remained unchanged.

Studies on the effects of 2.1 μm holmium:YAG laser energy on cartilage defects created in equine cartilage showed that the application of laser energy at 0.16 (127.4 J/cm^2) and 0.20 (159.2 J/cm^2) stimulated defect healing through cell proliferation (Collier et al., 1993).

Laser Energy and Cartilage Proteoglycan Metabolism

The question of cartilage recovery and repair following laser treatment requires quantification of proteoglycan synthesis and accumulation in an extracellular matrix. The biochemical index of proteoglycan synthesis is most often the uptake of $^{35}SO_4$ into the glycosaminoglycan component of the proteoglycan molecule. Several studies have been carried out using this approach with the 1.06 μm neodymium:YAG and the 2.1 μm holmium:YAG lasers.

The 1.06 μm neodymium:YAG laser energy applied to bovine cartilage explants using Q switching showed decreased levels of sulfate incorporation into glycosaminoglycan, whereas use of pulsed laser energy stimulated uptake of sulfate up to a level of 100 joules. The effect of 1.06 μm neodymium:YAG energy was stimulatory over a period of 96 hours, with levels of 200 joules of pulsed energy abolishing any stimulation of cartilage metabolism (Herman and Khosla, 1988).

Studies on the effects of 1.06 μm neodymium:YAG laser energy on canine cartilage proteoglycan synthesis under conditions of low serum exposure showed that low energy levels (energy densities of 51 and 127 J/cm^2) increased sulfate incorporation at 6 days after treatment (Spivak et al., 1992). The treatment was carried out for 5 seconds, applying the laser beam under conditions in which a heat sink grid was present and a 0.632 μm helium-neon laser was the spotting beam. As the energy levels were increased, positive effects on sulfate incorporation were decreased; at the highest energy level tested (1.019 J/cm^2) sulfate incorporation was decreased by 57% relative to the nontreated controls.

Companion studies carried out by the same investigators using bovine cartilage showed that sulfate incorporation was increased by low levels of laser energy (51 and 254 J/cm^2), analogous to that observed for the canine cartilage. At the highest energy level, sulfate incorporation was significantly decreased. By 12 days after treatment, the treated cartilage samples displayed incorporation identical to that in the control tissue. Controls ruled out direct effects of the spotting beam on cartilage metabolism.

In our preliminary investigation of the effects of the 2.1 μm holmium:YAG laser energy on proteoglycan synthesis in human articular cartilage, sulfate incorporation was observed to increase at low energy levels and to be completely abolished at levels that were inhibitory to ^{3}H-thymidine uptake (Figs. 7-3 and 7-4). Human cartilage maintained in explant culture in 10% fetal calf serum

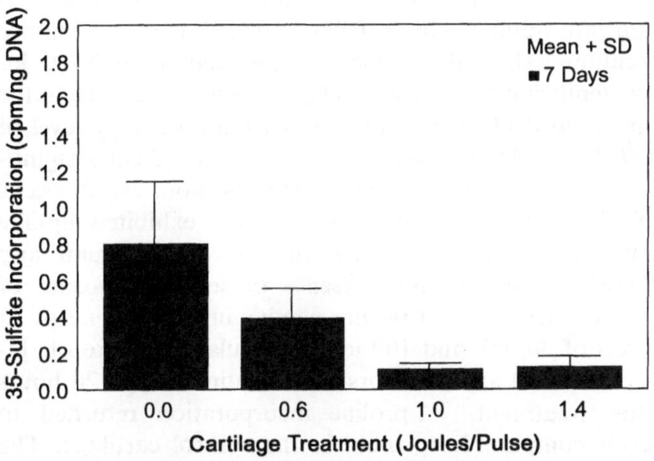

Figure 7-3. Articular cartilage glycosaminoglycan synthesis following 2.1 μm holmium:YAG laser treatment: after 7 days of culture. Full-thickness articular cartilage samples were treated with varying levels of laser energy and maintained in Dulbecco's modified Eagle's medium containing 10% (v/v) fetal bovine serum. Glycosaminoglycan synthesis was determined using uptake of $^{35}SO_4$ into cetylpyridinium chloride-precipitable material. The uptake of radioactivity was normalized to the amount of DNA present in the cartilage samples to adjust for variance in the cartilage samples. Each experiment was carried out in quadruplicate for each energy level, and the data represent two replicate cartilage samples. $p < 0.05$ using Student's two-sample t-test.

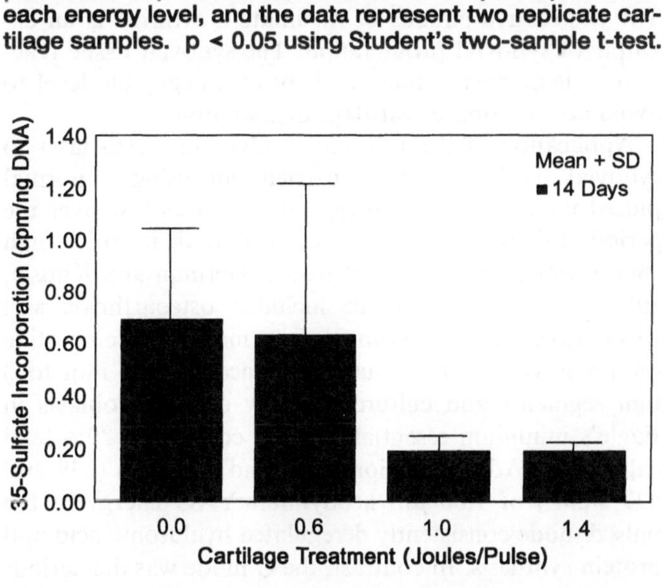

Figure 7-4. Articular cartilage glycosaminoglycan synthesis following 2.1 μm holmium:YAG laser treatment: after 14 days of culture.

showed a return to control levels of incorporation at 14 days after treatment at an energy density of 0.6 joule per pulse. Higher levels of energy prevented the recovery of sulfate incorporation in cartilage.

Laser Energy and Cartilage Collagen Synthesis

Analysis of collagen synthesis using ^{3}H-proline incorporation into adult bovine cartilage under low serum culture conditions showed that the 1.06 μm neodymium:YAG laser significantly increased collagen synthesis relative to the untreated controls at days 7 and 10 at an energy level of 127 J/cm^2. Higher levels of energy (762 J/cm^2) significantly decreased ^{3}H-proline incorporation. By 2 weeks after treatment, the cartilage samples exhibited uptake levels comparable to those in controls (Herman and Khosla, 1988). In the presence of serum, exposure of bovine cartilage to 1.06 μm neodymium:YAG energy at levels of 30, 60, and 100 joules stimulated uptake of ^{3}H-proline at 24 and 72 hours after treatment. By 120 hours after treatment, ^{3}H-proline incorporation returned to levels comparable to those in the control cartilage. The distribution of ^{3}H-proline into collagenous and noncollagenous proteins was not determined.

Laser Energy and Synovial Tissue

Diarthrodial joints are maintained, in part, through normal synovial cell metabolism. With inflammation, the synovial membrane is infiltrated by cells and vascularized. The destructive pannus of rheumatoid arthritis is an example of synovial proliferation. The synovial tissue reaction to laser energy must be kept at a negligible level to avoid acceleration of cartilage degradation.

Application of the 1.06 μm neodymium:YAG laser to synovial tissues has been carried out using a normal pulsed mode in which energy intensity was low over the period of delivery and the Q switched mode in which high energy was applied in short pulses (Herman and Khosla, 1989). The synovial tissue included osteoarthritic and rheumatoid arthritis synovium or mature porcine stifle joint synovium. The tissue was minced into 2 mm to 3 mm segments and cultured directly or as fibroblasts in Eagle's minimum essential medium containing 20% fetal calf serum. Administration of 30 and 60 joules (239 and 477 J/cm^2) of 1.06 μm neodymium:YAG energy in the pulsed mode consistently deregulated hyaluronic acid and protein synthesis. In contrast, the Q mode was deleterious to synovial cell metabolism. Under the conditions used in this study, the laser energy has no significant effect on synovial cell proliferation.

Laser Energy and Enzyme Turnover of Cartilage Matrix

Articular cartilage can be the source of degradative enzymes capable of degrading extracellular matrix (Williams et al., 1991). These enzymes include the lysosomal proteases and the cathepsins, active at acidic pH, and the metalloproteases, active at neutral pH. Although lysosomal enzyme levels are elevated in osteoarthritic cartilage, the extreme pH optimum of these enzymes likely mandates intracellular activity. The chondrocyte derived neutral metalloproteases are potential candidates for causing breakdown of extracellular matrix proteins. Chondrocytes synthesize two neutral metalloproteases: collagenase and stromelysin. Collagenase may function as a key factor in the long-term stability of the cartilage matrix owing to its ability to initiate degradation of the interstitial type II collagen. Activation of stromelysin may represent a regulatory step in cartilage homeostasis owing to its role in activating collagenase.

Evidence that cartilage degradation could be decreased by laser energy was observed by Herman and Khosla (1988). They quantified the release of $^{35}SO_4$ from prelabeled cartilage maintained in organ culture after exposure to pulsed 1.06 μm neodymium:YAG radiation. Levels of 30 and 60 joules were equally effective in decreasing proteoglycan release from viable cartilage explants after 48 hours in culture when compared to the release from nontreated control cartilage.

Discussion and Conclusions

The data from published studies show that laser energy from the 1.06 μm neodymium:YAG laser and the 2.1 μm holmium:YAG laser stimulates cartilage metabolism under defined test conditions. In our preliminary study with the 2.1 μm holmium:YAG laser, human articular cells recovered from laser treatment and exhibited increased cell proliferation 2 weeks after treatment. Extracellular matrix synthesis, although initially depressed, rebounded to levels comparable to untreated, serum-stimulated cartilage at the time cell proliferation was observed. Our study suggests that articular cartilage repair may be induced by low levels of applied 2.1 μm holmium:YAG laser energy. Further investigations on the use of laser energy are needed to define cellular mechanisms underlying the induction of joint tissue repair and regeneration.

References

Aydelotte MB and Kuettner KE (1988) Differences between subpopulations of cultured bovine articular chondrocytes. I Morphology and Cartilage Matrix Production, Connect Tissue Res 18:205–222

Borovoy M, Zirkin RM, Elson LM, Borovoy MA (1989) Healing of laser-induced defects of articular cartilage: preliminary studies. Journal of Foot Surgery 28:95–99

Bradrick JP, Eckhauser ML, Indresano AT (1992) Early response of canine temporomandibular joint tissues to arthroscopically guided neodymium:YAG laser wounds. Journal of Oral and Maxillofacial Surgery 50:835–42

Collier MA, Haugland LM, Bellamy J, et al. (1993) Effects of holmium:YAG laser on equine articular cartilage and subchondral bone adjacent to traumatic lesions: a histopathological assessment. Arthroscopy 9:536–545

Doege KJ, Sasaki M, Kimura T, Yamada Y (1991) Complete coding sequence and deduced primary structure of the human cartilage large aggregating proteoglycan, aggrecan. J Biol Chem 266:894–902

Dressel M, Jahn R, Neu W, Jungbluth KH (1991) Studies in fiber guided excimer laser surgery for cutting and drilling bone and meniscus. Lasers in Surgery and Medicine 11: 569–79

Freedland Y (1988) Use of the excimer laser in fibrocartilaginous excision from adjacent bony stroma: a preliminary investigation. Journal of Foot Surgery 27:303–305

Gonzalez C, van de Merwe WP, Smith M, Reinisch L (1990) Comparison of the erbium-yttrium aluminum garnet and carbon dioxide lasers for in vitro bone and cartilage ablation. Laryngoscope 100:14–7

Hardie EM, Carlson CS, Richardson DC (1989) Effect of Nd:YAG laser energy on articular cartilage healing in the dog. Lasers in Surgery and Medicine 9:595–601

Hascall VC, Heinegard D (1975) The structure of cartilage proteoglycans. In: Extracellular Matrix Influences on Gene Expression, Slavkin HC (ed), Academic Press, New York, p. 423

Heinegard D, Paulsson M (1987) Cartilage In: Methods in Enzymology, Academic Press, Inc., 145: 336–363

Herman JH and Khosla RC (1988) In vitro effects of nd:YAG laser radiation on cartilage metabolism. Journal of Rheumatology 15:1818–1826

Herman JH and Khosla RC (1989) Nd:YAG laser modulation of synovial tissue metabolism. Clin Exp Rheum 7:505–512

Hohlbach G, Moller KO, Schramm U, Baretton G (1989) Experimental results of cartilage abrasion with an excimer laser. histologic and electron microscopy studies. Zeitschrift fur Orthopadie und Ihre Grenzgebiete 127:216–221

Kroitzsch U, Laufer G, Egkher E, Wollenek G, Horvath R (1989) Experimental photoablation of meniscus cartilage by excimer laser energy. a new aspect in meniscus surgery. Archives of Orthopaedic and Traumatic Surgery 108:44–48

Mankin HJ and Lippiello L (1970) Biochemical and metabolic abnormalities in articular cartilage from osteo-arthritic human hips. J Bone Joint Surg 52A:424–434

Miller DV, O'Brien SJ, Arnoczky SS, Kelly A, Fealy SV, Warren RF (1989) The use of the contact nd:YAG laser in arthroscopic surgery: effects on articular cartilage and meniscal tissue. Arthroscopy 5:245–53

Mow VC, Zhu W, Ratcliffe A (1991) Structure and function of articular cartilage and meniscus. In: Basic Orthopaedic Biomechanics, Mow VC and Hayes WC (eds), Raven Press Ltd., New York, p 143

Nixon AJ, Krook LP, Roth JE, King JM (1991) Pulsed carbon dioxide laser for cartilage vaporization and subchondral bone perforation in horses. part ii: morphologic and histochemical reactions. Veterinary Surgery 20:200–8

O'Brien SJ and Miller DV (1990) The contact neodymium-yttrium aluminum garnet laser: a new approach to arthroscopic laser surgery. Clinical Orthopaedics and Related Research 252:95–100

Raunest J and Lohnert J (1990) Arthroscopic cartilage debridement by excimer laser in chondromalacia of the knee joint. a prospective randomized clinical study. Archives of Orthopaedic and Traumatic Surgery 109:155–9

Roth JE, Nixon AJ, Gantz VA, Meyer D, Mohammed H (1991) Pulsed carbon dioxide laser for cartilage vaporization and subchondral bone perforation in horses. part i: technique and clinical results. Veterinary Surgery 20:190–9

Schultz RJ, Krishnamurthy S, Thelmo W, Rodriguez JE, Harvey G (1985) Effects of varying intensities of laser energy on articular cartilage: a preliminary study. Lasers in Surgery and Medicine 5:577–588

Smith RL, Gilkerson E, Kohatsu N, Merchant T, Schurman DJ (1980) Quantitative microanalysis of synovial fluid and articular cartilage glycosaminoglycans. Analytical Biochemistry 103:191–200

Spivak JM, Grande DA, Ben-Yishay A, Menche DS, Pitman MI (1992) The effect of low-level nd:YAG laser energy on adult articular cartilage in vitro. Arthroscopy 8:36–43

Trauner K, Nishioka N, Patel D (1990) Pulsed holmium:yttrium-aluminum-garnet (ho:YAG) laser ablation of fibrocartilage and articular cartilage. American Journal of Sports Medicine 18:316–20

Vangsness CT, Ghaderi B (1993) A literature review of lasers and articular cartilage. Orthopedics 16:593–598

Vangsness CT, Smith CF et al., (1992) Pulsed carbon dioxide laser for cartilage vaporization of articular cartilage. Semin Orthop 7:83–85

Williams RJ, Smith RL, Schurman DJ (1991) Purified staphylococcal culture medium stimulates neutral metalloprotease secretion from human articular cartilage. J Orthop Res 9:258–265

8

Fibrocartilaginous Repair Following 2.1 μm Holmium:YAG Laser Irradiation of Human Degenerative Hyaline Cartilage: Case Report

Allen T. Brillhart

The literature regarding biostimulation is surveyed in other chapters of this text. The following is the first known published case report in the world literature of fibrocartilaginous repair by laser irradiated degenerative hyaline cartilage in a human patient.

Case Report

This was a 53-year-old woman who suffered from chronic left knee patellofemoral arthritis. She had undergone an arthrotomy for realignment of her patellofemoral joint prior to being seen by me. She was first seen for a fracture of the tibial plateau of the left knee in 1987. She underwent an arthroscopic assisted reduction and internal fixation with a percutaneously placed screw for that fracture. In 1988 a third operation was performed to remove the screw and to perform an arthroscopic chondroplasty. At that time she was noted to have grade III changes of the medial femoral condyle and grade IV degenerative changes of the trochlea and patella. Mechanical shaving of unstable cartilage was carried out, but pain in the patellofemoral joint persisted. In December 1990, because of pain, swelling, giving way, and failure of conservative care, another arthroscopy was performed. At that time, grade III degenerative changes of the medial femoral condyle (Fig. 8-1) and grade IV changes of the patellofemoral joint (Fig. 8-2) were noted. The lateral compartment of the knee was also arthritic as a result of the previous fracture.

Using the 2.1 μm holmium:YAG laser at settings of 1 joule per pulse and 15 Hz, an arthroscopic chondroplasty was carried out. The probe was held 1 to 2 mm away from the surface of the defect in the medial femoral condyle. The subchondral plate was not destroyed. The total energy delivered to all surfaces, including the trochlea and patella, was less than 10 kJ. The medium was Ringer's

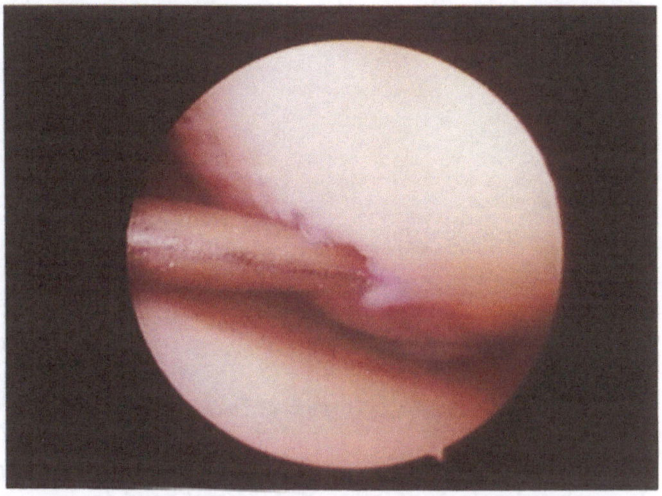

Figure 8-1. Arthritis of the medial femoral condyle.

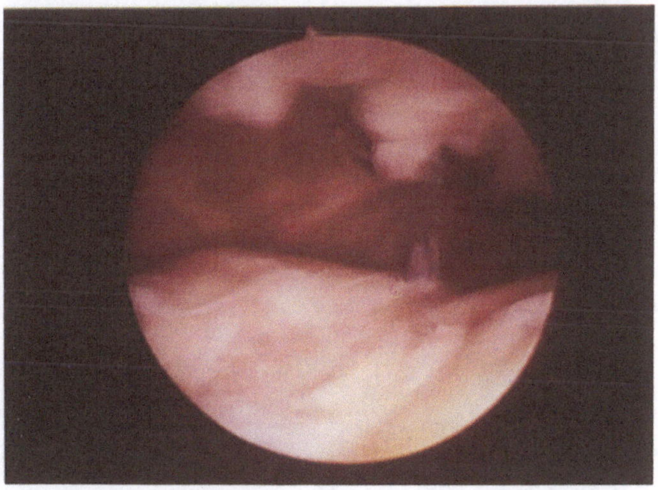

Figure 8-2. Arthritis of the patellofemoral joint.

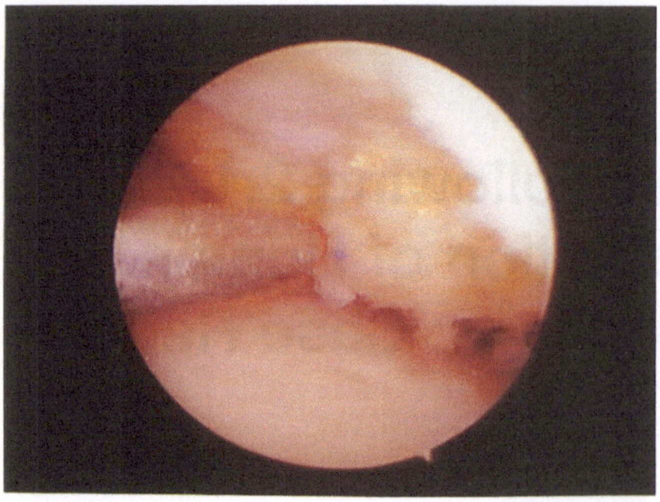

Figure 8-3. 2.1 μm Holmium:YAG laser chondroplasty in progress.

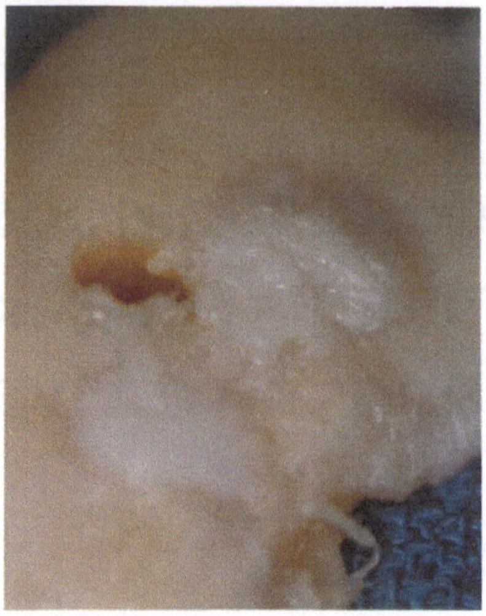

Figure 8-6. Late results of the 2.1 μm Holmium:YAG laser chondroplasty of the medial femoral condyle.

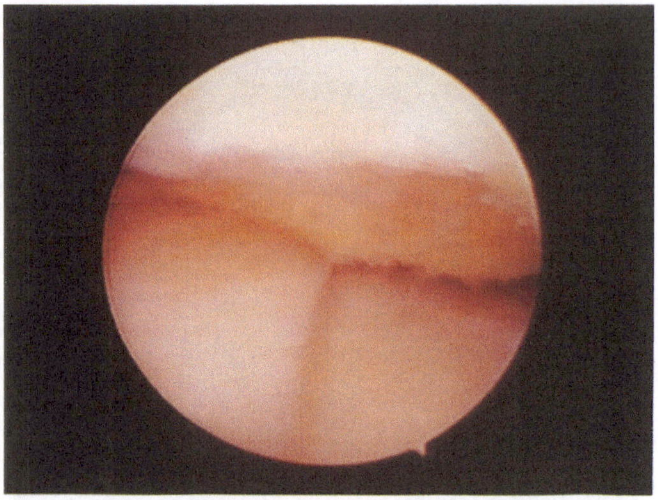

Figure 8-4. Immediate results of the 2.1 μm Holmium:YAG laser chondroplasty of the medial femoral condyle.

Figure 8-7. Histopathology of reparative fibrocartilage created by the 2.1 μm Holmium:YAG laser chondroplasty of the medial femoral condyle.

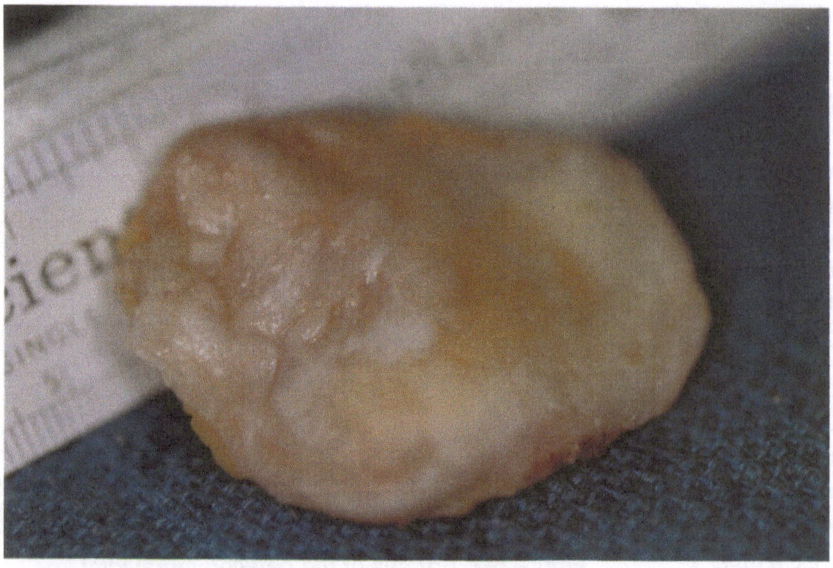

Figure 8-5. Late results of the 2.1 μm Holmium:YAG laser chondroplasty of the undersurface of the patella.

lactate. The laser device was a 15 watt Coherent 2.1 holmium:YAG laser. A 30 degree angled probe, Infratome handpiece, was used. The pulse width was 350 μs, and the fiber size was 450 μm. The exact amount of energy delivered to the medial condyle was not recorded. Figure 8-3 illustrates the procedure, and Figure 8-4 shows the resulting defect after vaporization of the unstable flaps of hyaline cartilage from the medial femoral condyle.

Conservative care was continued in the form of analgesics, antiinflammatory agents, and physical therapy until May 1993. At that time, the patient had begun to experience severe activity limitations and intermittent, painful effusions. A custom-made, noncemented, total knee arthroplasty was elected. The undersurface of the patella is shown in Figure 8-5, revealing grade IV chondromalacia that had been previously irradiated with 2.1 μm holmium:YAG laser energy. Figure 8-6 shows the medial femoral condyle, showing reparative fibrocartilage from grade III degenerative hyaline cartilage previously irradiated by 2.1 μm holmium:YAG laser energy. Figure 8-7 demonstrates the histopathology of the gross specimen of white reparative fibrocartilage seen in Figure 8-6.

Conclusions

This case indicates the potential of grade III degenerative human hyaline cartilage to repair itself with fibrocartilage after 2.1 μm holmium:YAG laser irradiation. It also reveals the failure of arthroscopic mechanical shaving to produce this same result (Mankin, 1982). This case suggests that 2.1 μm holmium:YAG laser chondroplasty does not change the ultimate clinical outcome when grade IV degenerative arthritis is present over large surface areas. Based on a single case report, these conclusions should serve only as evidence that more clinical research is needed. My conclusions are only opinions at this stage and do not represent confirmed medical facts. Long-term studies are needed. The arthroscopist should realize that the 2.1 μm holmium:YAG laser is approved by the U.S. Food and Drug Administration for marketing for debridement of chondromalacia.

Suggested Reading

Collier MA, Haughland LM, Bellamy J, et al. (1993) Effects of holmium:YAG laser on equine articular cartilage and subchondral bone adjacent to traumatic lesions: a histopathological assessment. Arthroscopy 9:536–545

Mankin HJ (1982) The response of articular cartilage to mechanical injury. J Bone Joint Surg 64A:460–465

9

Arthroscopic Laser Chondroplasty

Neil D. Glossop and Robert W. Jackson

As our understanding of the mechanisms of osteoarthritis increases, so too does the prospect of developing better methods of treatment. More than 37 million people are currently afflicted with arthritis in the United States alone. Almost everyone over the age of 60 suffers from osteoarthritis to some extent. Orthopaedists and rheumatologists now treat patients aggressively with nonsteroidal antiinflammatory drugs (NSAIDs), total joint arthroplasty, physiotherapy, arthroscopic lavage, and chondral debridement (chondroplasty). This last treatment, a minimally invasive procedure, is performed routinely on thousands of patients every year and produces mostly favorable results in the short term. It is suitable for young patients who are not candidates for joint replacement and older patients who are at risk from major surgery.

Just why the seemingly inconsequential process of removing fibrillated cartilage is so effective in relieving pain has been the subject of much speculation (Kim et al., 1991). Debridement can be traced to the early 1940s when Magnuson (1941) advocated the procedure for relief of pain associated with degenerative joint disease. He had the opinion that "often repeated small trauma" is the major source of degenerative joint disease, an idea based on the work of Bauer and Bennet (1936), who believed that degenerative joint disease was the result of the wear and tear of increasing age. They maintained that it was not the result of an inflammatory process, metabolic disturbance, or an endocrine dysfunction. By reducing friction through smoothing an irregular surface, these early investigators hoped to reduce pain and slow the progression of the disease. This rationale still holds (Ewing, 1990) even though our understanding of the disease has evolved significantly since the 1940s.

Since Magnuson's time, chondral debridement has undergone major improvements from the open procedure that was first described. Arthroscopic debridement was first performed by O'Connor during the early 1970s (Shahriaree, 1984) and since then has been promoted by several investigators (Jackson and Dandy, 1976; Sprague, 1981; Ewing, 1990). Patients report "fair to good" results (based primarily on pain relief) up to 80% of the time (Sprague, 1981).

In terms of our modern understanding of the mechanisms of osteoarthritis, the pathway of pain relief is not as intuitive and has not been addressed. Debridement certainly does not stop arthritis. Practitioners simply do not know why or how this treatment works, or the best way to apply it. Animal studies are also lacking (Ewing, 1990). Whatever the mechanisms of debridement, it is clear that the procedure is an effective, albeit palliative, treatment. It is also interesting that the process of lavage itself seems to have a significant effect on the pain associated with osteoarthritis, again with little plausible explanation.

The methods available for arthroscopic debridement vary widely in cost and efficacy. The use of laser treatments is growing rapidly. The increased popularity of these treatments has largely been driven by consumer "high tech" demands, instead of clear scientific evidence of superiority. Little research has been done on the effects of these devices, and although laser treatment may be superior (as is commonly claimed), it remains to be proven.

Laser Use in Orthopaedics

In the search for improved treatment of osteoarthritis, orthopaedic surgeons have been particularly keen to embrace laser technology and are enthusiastically applying this instrumentation for chondroplasty. The laser is perceived as an "instrument of the future" by patients and physicians alike and is sometimes endowed with almost supernatural powers. The name alone is such a powerful marketing force, that laser treatments have been accepted much more readily than almost any other therapy.

The estimated number of lasers in use in orthopaedics across the United States is in the thousands. Despite their popularity, at least one orthopaedic task force in the United States (American Academy of Orthopaedic Surgeons, 1992) has urged caution when applying this technology. They have warned surgeons against the use of lasers in orthopaedics until the effects were clearly understood, and they recommended continued research in the field.

To understand their motives in making this statement, it is sufficient to examine some of the effects of laser interaction with tissue. The laser is more than a simple cutting tool; it can act in an almost drug-like fashion, with many side effects that may have systemic repercussions. Lasers are not regarded as a drug by the appropriate regulation agencies but are generally treated as devices. This designation eliminates much of the pertinent biologic testing that arguably should be required. Furthermore, published scientific work on these effects has not kept pace with the use of lasers.

To be sure, some procedures do seem promising and exciting. The initial appearance of some laser-debrided cartilage is superior to what can be obtained with electrocautery or mechanical instruments. Some lasers can smooth fibrillated cartilage with only minor damage to the underlying matrix, apparently sealing the surface. There has also been evidence of cartilage regeneration occurring with some lasers. Other applications of the lasers have not been so successful. It is difficult to justify the expense and risk for procedures such as plica removal or partial meniscectomy. With some exceptions, these operations can be easily and efficiently handled using blades, shavers, and electrocautery.

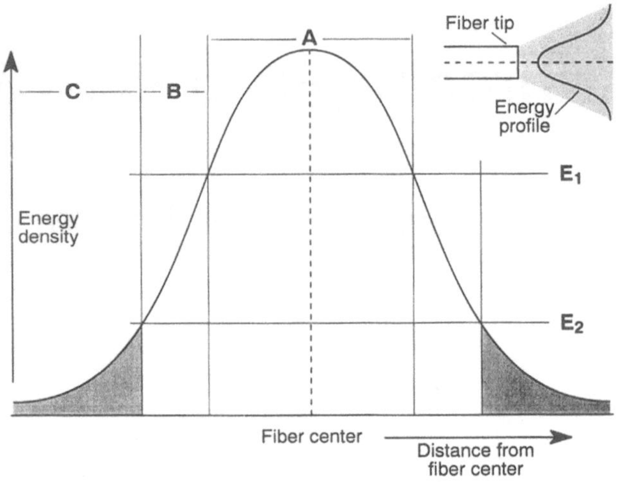

Figure 9-1. Idealized diagram of the emitted energy profile of an optical fiber sampled at a fixed distance from the fiber tip. The energy delivered by the fiber (i.e., the brightness) diminishes with increasing distance from the center of the fiber. In region A, the light is intense enough to cause tissue ablation. In region B, ablation does not occur, but cytolysis does. In region C, cells are exposed to a nonlethal dose of radiation.

Laser–Tissue Interactions

Numerous superimposed phenomena hinder attempts to study and understand the extent and nature of laser–tissue interactions. This point is particularly true with articular cartilage, which can be difficult to investigate properly outside the organism. Most of the laser-precipitated effects occur with all lasers, and some occur as well with other forms of nonmechanical treatment, such as electrocautery. All living tissues illuminated by the laser are affected even when they are not the intended target. It is also possible that many tissues not directly irradiated may be influenced owing to beam reflections and transmissions.

Many investigations characterize laser-tissue interactions by what happens to the tissue when the incident energy is enough to bake, boil, or otherwise kill cells and disrupt the matrix proteins. Clearly, during any laser surgery large populations of cells are exposed to sublethal doses of radiation. We believe that the most important effects result from the irradiation of cells that ultimately survive. Nonlethal doses of laser energy are typically (though not exclusively) delivered near the periphery of optical fibers, as shown in Figure 9-1. Actual "far field" energy distribution patterns differ from the idealized shape shown in Figure 9-1 owing to effects such as modal interference and fiber tip variations.

The precise source of the cellular response is not as clear as might initially be assumed. Much of it is a direct result of the incident light beam, its reflections, and its transmissions. Secondary light results from fluorescent, incandescent, or other emissions. The secondary light generally is not at the same wavelength, intensity, duration, or direction as the incident energy, thereby confounding the interaction. It can also be intense enough to warrant concern.

The transmitted, reflected, or scattered laser light also may influence the situation. Depending on the tissue and wavelength (Black et al., 1992; Vangsness et al., 1992a) this light may continue to propagate deep into the tissue. Moreover, different durations, dosages, and energy densities of laser light may affect the irradiated cells or matrix in different manners.

Debris formed by laser interaction with tissue is of several varieties. Particulate debris probably predominates. This effluvium consists of small lumps of tissue and cells that are expelled from the surface. Other debris is more intimidating and may be punctuated by free ions, cell fragments, and various chemical species, which may or may not react with the surrounding tissue and the fluid circulating in the joint. This material is also mobile and

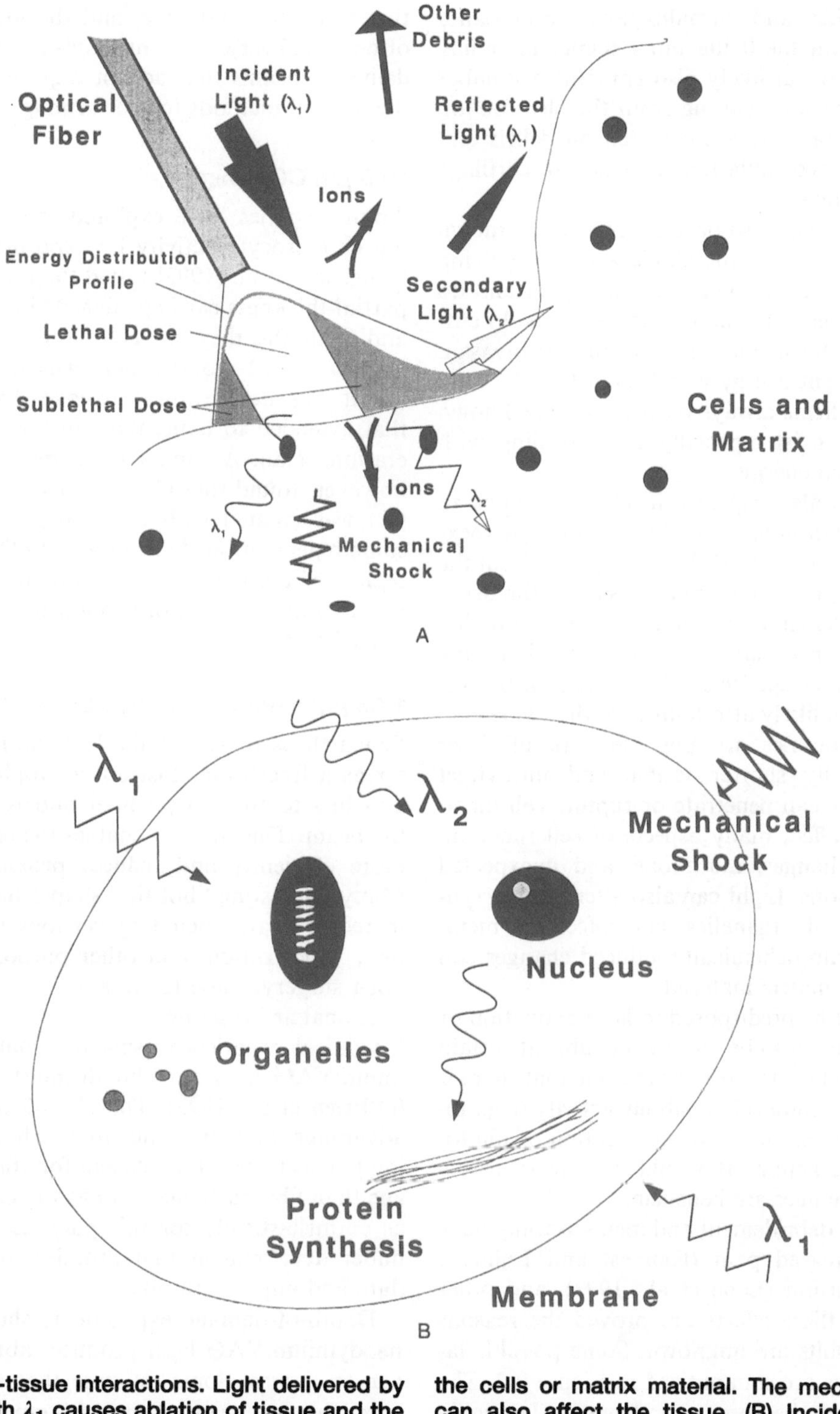

Figure 9-2. (A) Laser–tissue interactions. Light delivered by the fiber at wavelength λ_1 causes ablation of tissue and the formation of debris and ions. Some of the light is transformed by nonlinear and other effects into secondary light at wavelength λ_2. The scattered, reflected, and transmitted light penetrates the tissue where it can cause reactions in the cells or matrix material. The mechanical shock wave can also affect the tissue. (B) Incident light, secondary light, ions, and the shock wave can disrupt the cell membrane, protein synthesis, or organelles within the membrane.

may travel throughout the body. It is certain that myriad chemical debris are formed. The 10.6 μm CO_2 and 1.06 μm neodymium:YAG lasers, for example, are known to produce several noxious chemical by-products when ablating bovine liver tissue in air (Kokosa and Doyle, 1988), including benzene and other polycyclic aromatic hydrocarbons. By-products of 10.6 μm CO_2 laser ablation of polymethylmethacrylate (PMMA) include hydrogen cyanide, carbon monoxide, and formalin (Sherk and Lane, 1989). The debris from the 0.308 μm Excimer laser has not yet been analyzed but likely also contains a number of quenched ionic species resulting from the electron/ion plasma. No studies have been conducted on debris created during arthroscopic ablation of articular cartilage either in or out of saline.

Thermal injury to tissue also occurs. It has been known for years that heat alters the metabolic activity of living cells, tissues, and organisms. Thermal effects can and do occur near the peripheries of the beams of even cold cutting lasers such as the 0.308 μm Excimer (Srinivasan, 1986). When insufficient energy is delivered to ablate the tissue, temperature effects always occur. We have known this phenomenon to exist especially when dealing with fiberoptically delivered energy.

Short-pulsed lasers also impart a mechanical shock to the target. Tissue ablation has been likened to a microexplosion by some investigators. Debris is expelled from the surface at high speed, leading to compression of the tissue and formation of "cavitation bubbles." The outgoing shock wave is so intense that it is capable of shattering the fiber tip (Glossop et al., 1992). An intense local pressure wave of this type likely also influences the tissue.

Photochemical processes are possible with all laser wavelengths, especially shorter visible and ultraviolet wavelengths. Photons can penetrate or rupture cell membranes and directly affect many aspects of cell function, causing metabolic changes, mutations, and unexpected photochemical reactions. Light can also alter protein synthesis, affect individual organelles, and affect the membranes themselves. Photochemically induced changes can occur in intercellular matrix material.

Certain cells might be predisposed to laser activation or deactivation. Cells may also be more vulnerable at certain stages in their division cycles. It is worrisome that there is clear evidence of laser-induced metabolic activity (e.g., regeneration) with most lasers—a demonstration of photobiologic processes in action. It would be unwise to assume that all such changes are beneficial.

Arthroscopic laser debridement and meniscectomy have been linked to decreased pain (Raunest and Lohnert, 1990), decreased effusion (Lane et al., 1992), and other beneficial effects. If these effects are proven the reasons for the enhanced results are unknown. Some possible laser–tissue interactions are summarized in Figure 9-2. The effects shown here may be absent, or they may be highly important depending on the precise laser wavelength and properties.

Laser Chondroplasty

The techniques and results of laser chondroplasty vary drastically with the laser used. The results are dictated not only by the wavelength but by the energy density (radiant exposure used, the pulse duration and energy, the repetition rate, the total dose, and the method and technique of beam delivery. Current trends are toward fiberoptically delivered beams that do not require major alterations in the normal methods for performing arthroscopy.

10.6 μm CO_2 Laser

Animal studies have explored the prospect of stimulating chondrocyte activity by exposing tissue to the laser. Vangsness et al. (1992b) used the laser to create deep and partial-thickness cartilage defects in rabbit cartilage. At 3 and 6 months, they observed no healing or evidence of ingrowth; by 12 months there was some connective tissue but it was not hyaline cartilage. Even with the lesions that extended to bone, they observed no cartilage regeneration at all. A similar experiment by Borovoy (1989), however, found that about 25% of rabbits in which a defect was created with the 10.6 μm CO_2 laser exhibited some regeneration. Lane et al., (1992) found only a slight region of thermal necrosis with the 10.6 μm CO_2 laser, just 54 μm. Thermal disruption of the cells, however, extended to 442 μm.

1.06 μm Neodymium:YAG Laser Chondroplasty

Few arthroscopists use the 1.06 μm neodymium:YAG laser as a free beam. Instead, a sapphire or ceramic tip is attached to the optical fiber and is used to concentrate the beam. This method enables the energy to be delivered more efficiently and reduces proximate tissue damage. Many interesting "hot tip" shapes have become available in recent years, including versions for coagulation, cutting, vaporization, and other purposes. Widely used for open surgery, these lasers are now being applied to conventional arthroscopy.

Clinical experience using the contact 1.06 μm neodymium:YAG laser for chondroplasty has been favorable (O'Brien et al., 1992). They found that the laser has the advantage of being able to reach remote areas of the joint. This laser is less efficient for ablating articular cartilage than fibrocartilage and has therefore not been applied as enthusiastically for this purpose. New tip shapes are under development that promise to simplify the procedure and improve results.

Depth-of-damage experiments show that the 1.06 μm neodymium:YAG laser produces abundant thermal damage to tissues. Some estimate that the damage resulting from the free beam of the 1.06 μm neodymium:YAG laser ranges from 2 to 3 mm, only not; and although this distance is reduced for contact tips, it is still large. Miller et al. (1992) found that damage depths in articular cartilage ranged from 100 to 1,200 μm, depending on the pressure and power used. Raunest (1991) has shown that free beam 1.06 μm radiation at levels high enough to produce an immediately visible clinical effect, causes severe degenerative arthritis in laboratory animals.

Using different levels of free beam energy, various experiments have been carried out to discover more about the apparent regenerative effect of 1.06 μm radiation on hyaline tissue and fibrocartilage (Schultz et al., 1985; Miller et al., 1989; Lane et al., 1991). Miller et al. (1989) applied a contact tip 1.06 μm neodymium:YAG laser to rabbit articular cartilage. (It should be noted that a small percentage of free beam radiation escapes from the contact tip of this laser.) They observed a vigorous healing response to defects created with this device when compared to similar, unlased scalpel cuts. In another study, Schultz et al., (1985) noted that partial-thickness cuts in some guinea pig articular cartilage underwent reparative processes when exposed to the laser. They found that the amount of regeneration varied significantly with the applied laser dose. The replacement cartilage was identified to be fibrocartilage and not hyaline cartilage.

Lane et al. (1991) also discovered that exposure to 1.06 μm radiation had a stimulatory effect on the healing of full- and partial-thickness defects in canine articular cartilage. They exposed scalpel incisions in the femoral condyles to various laser doses; ranging from 13 to 87 joules, and immobilized the legs. The dogs were killed at 2, 4, and 6 weeks after surgery. The healing response was most pronounced at 6 weeks in animals irradiated with a total dose of 25 joules.

Spivak et al. (1992) investigated the effects of low-level noncontact, free beam 1.06 μm neodymium:YAG irradiation of cultured bovine and canine cartilage in vitro. Although their study does not duplicate all arthroscopic conditions (free beam, air exposure of moist sample), the results are likely still relevant. Spivak et al. also found a healing response that was dose-dependent and ranged from reducing collagen synthesis to nearly doubling it. The effects of the laser, however, seemed to last only a few days after the treatment.

Most complications that have been reported for the 1.06 μm neodymium:YAG laser have resulted from fracture of the sapphire tips in the joint. Retrieving these transparent nonmagnetic objects can be challenging. Current technology makes use of integrated ceramic tips, which are thought to be more rugged. Such complications are addressed elsewhere in this text (see Chapter 14).

The thermal damage zone is significantly larger with the 1.06 μm neodymium:YAG than with any other laser (Metcalf and Dixon, 1984). This large zone may lead to iatrogenic damage to the joint due to the heating effect alone. It is also difficult to control the ablation depth.

Although the 1.06 μm neodymium:YAG laser is probably less effective for arthroscopic debridement than some other lasers, the possible metabolic effects of subclinical doses deserve serious consideration. As these effects occur within a window of energy densities and doses, it will be a challenge for researchers to determine the optimal parameters and mechanism for laser action. The existence and repercussions of other possible laser-tissue interactions must also be investigated with some diligence.

2.1 μm Holmium:YAG Laser Chondroplasty

Chondroplasty with the 2.1 μm holmium:YAG laser requires few adaptations from conventional arthroscopic techniques. Fiberoptic probes are available that provide different angulations. The laser can also be used efficiently in fluids, making it compatible with standard arthroscopic practices. Fibers are offered as disposable instruments but would probably endure several operations. No special fiber tips are required, unlike for the 1.06 μm neodymium:YAG procedures. Despite the lower ablation rate of articular cartilage compared to that for the meniscus, the 2.1 μm holmium:YAG lasers usually deliver enough energy to debride degenerative cartilage easily.

Fanton and Dillingham (1992) suggested that the laser should be used in a defocused manner to ablate grade III chondromalacia. It allows the surface to be contoured to a smooth, firm base.

Because of the elimination of moving jaws or sharp surfaces, advocates of the 2.1 μm holmium:YAG laser claim that the laser produces fewer iatrogenic effects. This statement is probably true of all fiber-delivered lasers, however, and is not limited to the 2.1 μm holmium:YAG laser. Because of the thin fiber required by the 2.1 μm holmium:YAG (0.4 mm for many systems), the laser delivers a large amount of energy and permits access to even the most restricted joint spaces. Unlike the 10.6 μm CO_2 device, which must be "scrubbed" of carbon residue following ablation, there is no cleanup required for the 2.1 μm holmium:YAG laser.

There is little direct evidence of biostimulation with the 2.1 μm holmium:YAG laser. Again, although desirable, such effects are worrying because they suggest cellular involvement that extends far beyond the simple killing and removal of cells and matrix.

The all-round clinical results with 2.1 μm holmium:YAG lasers have been superior to results obtained with any of the other lasers on the market. The 2.1 μm holmium:YAG devices deliver enough energy that they are capable of ablating a significant quantity of tissue over a short period. This advantage is not significant when considering only the action of smoothing compared to motorized shavers. According to one account (Fanton and Dillingham, 1992) these lasers produce "as good or better results than mechanical chondroplasty."

A scanning electron micrograph of the effects of 2.1 μm holmium:YAG laser irradiation of articular cartilage is shown in Figure 9-3. We are not aware of any previously published in vivo animal studies on the effect of the 2.1 μm holmium:YAG laser on animal articular cartilage. However, Collier et al. (1993) demonstrated some positive effects so long as the subchondral plate is not intentionally destroyed by laser energy and low levels of radiation are used.

There are few complications associated with 2.1 μm

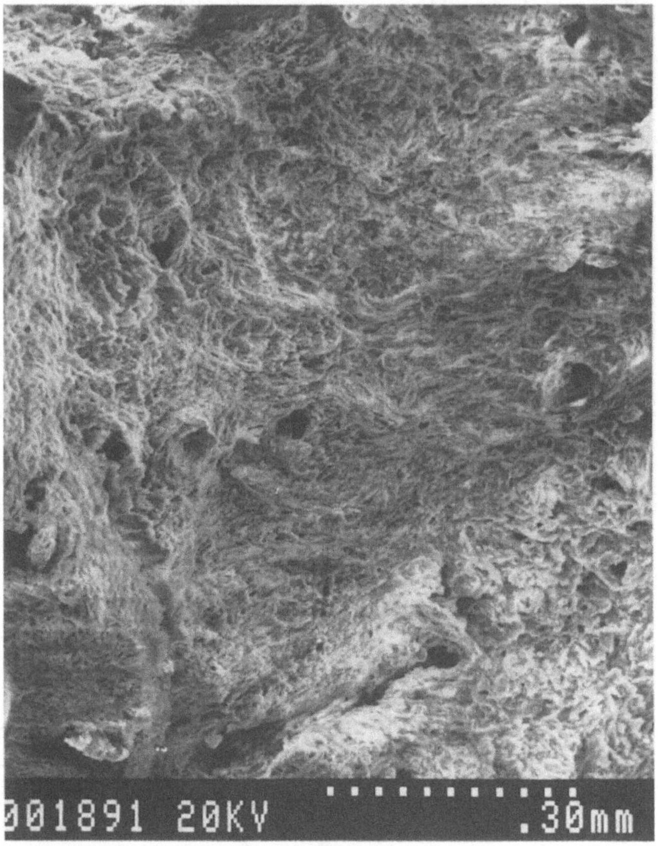

Figure 9-3. Scanning election micrograph of human articular cartilage following debridement by the 2.1 μm holmium:YAG laser.

Table 9-1. Thermal injury in articular cartilage resulting from different lasers.

Type of laser	Thermal injury depth in articular cartilage (μm)
10.6 μm CO_2	442[a]; 450[b]
1.06 μm neodymium: YAG	2000–3000[c]; 100–1200[d]
2.1 μm holmium: YAG	552[a]; 450–500[c]
0.308 μm XeCl Excimer	16[e]
Electrocautery	700–1800[d]

[a] Lane et al. (1992).
[b] Fanton and Dillingham (1992).
[c] Trauner et al. (1990).
[d] Miller et al. (1989).
[e] Vari et al. (1991).

holmium:YAG laser chondroplasty. The threshold radiant exposure for 2.1 μm holmium:YAG ablation of bovine cartilage was determined by Trauner et al. (1990) to be about 50 J/cm², compared with 11 J/cm² for fibrocartilage. Chondroplasty is therefore slower than meniscal procedures.

The 2.1 μm holmium:YAG does offer advantages over the other lasers. There is less thermal damage to the cartilage with the 2.1 μm holmium:YAG compared with the 1.06 μm neodymium:YAG laser. Furthermore, the 2.1 μm holmium:YAG lasers do not suffer from problems related to tip breakages that have occurred with 1.06 μm neodymium:YAG lasers.

The 2.1 μm holmium:YAG is the most promising laser currently available for chondroplasty. Early results with the procedure are favorable. Again, long-term animal studies are required to investigate some of the laser–tissue effects.

0.308 μm XeCl Excimer Chondroplasty

Results obtained with the 0.308 μm XeCl Excimer laser have been encouraging, especially for cartilage debridement. The zone of thermal disruption is insignificant (Table 9-1), and the laser is able to shape articular surfaces precisely. These properties, along with its ability to be delivered fiberoptically, make it ideally suited for the debridement and sculpting of condylar surfaces. Although the 0.308 μm XeCl Excimer has yet to be approved for use in the United States, it has been successfully used in many other countries including Germany and Canada.

The method of application of the 0.308 μm Excimer laser is similar to that of the 2.1 μm holmium:YAG laser. The fiber is usually encased in a hollow tube attached to a handpiece. The tube can be used to provide a concentric flow of saline by connecting an irrigation port to an arthroscopy pump. This apparatus assists in the removal of ablated debris, although it is not always necessary. There is no need to cool the 0.308 μm Excimer fiber, as almost no heat is created.

Fiber bundles are now also available for the 0.308 μm Excimer laser that allow the tip to be bent up to 45 degrees. Unlike the original single-core fibers, which were rigid, these bundles are flexible and deliver almost as much energy to the target.

The fiber (or bundle) functions best when held a few millimeters from the cartilage surface. Using it in this way allows it to remove an area of a few square millimeters at a time. The 0.308 μm Excimer ablates hyaline cartilage in a way that has been compared to the melting of an ice block with a torch. Fibrillations are dissolved by the beam, and debrided surfaces appear to regain their elastic properties. These maneuvers can be controlled with extraordinary precision, making it possible to remove fibrillation with almost no loss in cartilage thickness.

Patients undergoing 0.308 μm Excimer chondroplasty appear to fare better than those undergoing conventional treatment. Raunest and Lohnert's study (1990) discovered a statistically significant decrease in pain reported by the laser group compared to the control (mechanical debridement) group. There was also less effusion in the laser group, with 55% experiencing no effusion compared with 35% in the nonlaser group. Similar functional outcomes were noted for the two groups.

A smaller study by Cinats and Jackson (1989) showed similar results, with a statistically significant increase in Lysholm score in the laser-treated group. The physical ex-

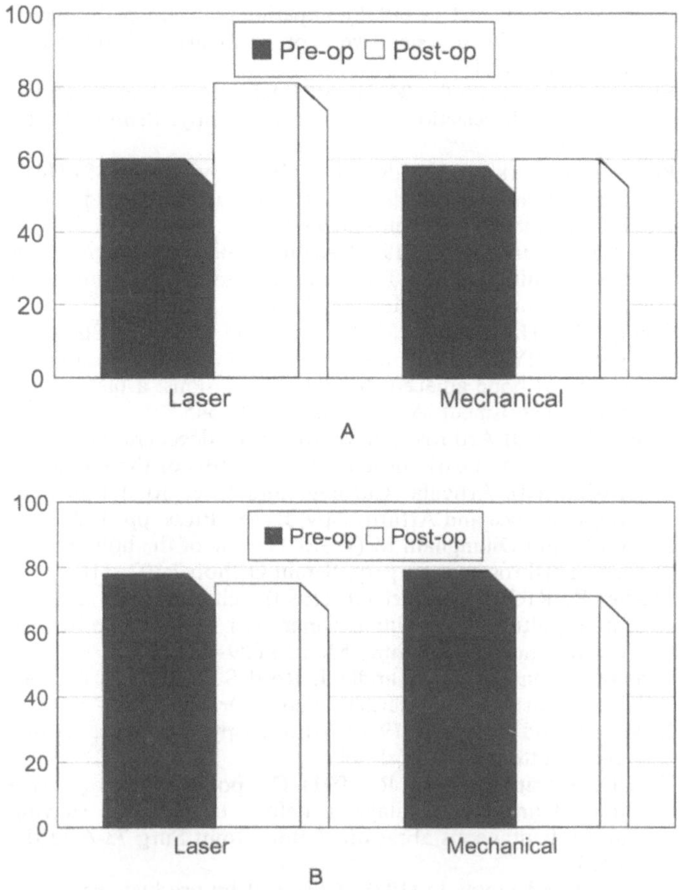

Figure 9-4. (A) Lysholm scores after chondromalacia debridement ($n = 15$), according to Cinats and Jackson (1989). The differences between the laser and mechanical groups were significant ($p < 0.01$). (B) Physical examination scores from the study in (A).

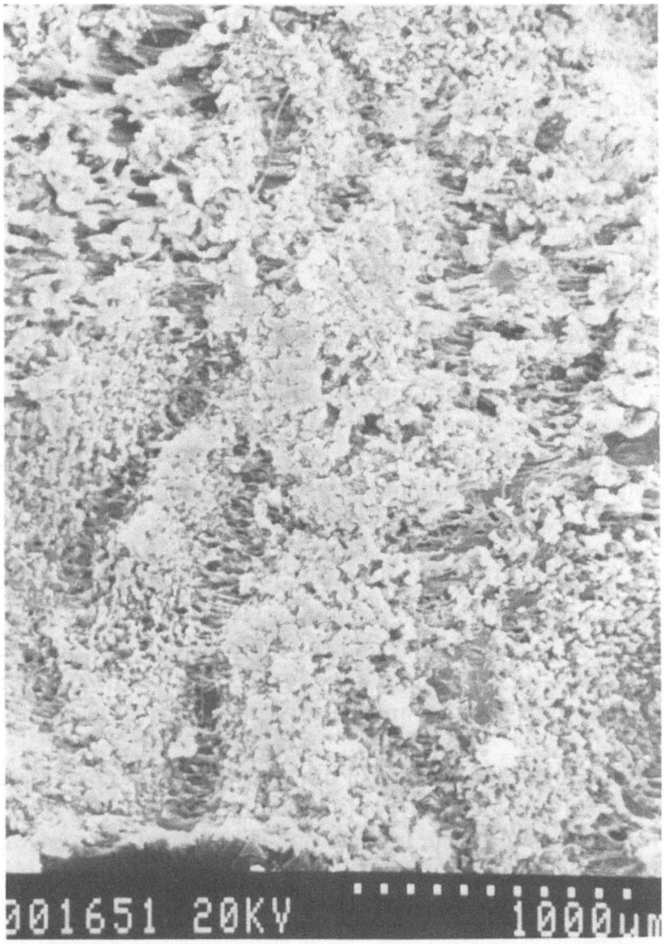

Figure 9-5. Scanning electron micrograph of human articular cartilage following debridement by the 0.308 μm XeCl Excimer. The magnification is approximately three times higher than that in Figure 9-3.

aminations revealed almost identical results, as shown in Figure 9-4.

A scanning electron micrograph showing the effect of 0.308 μm Excimer laser irradiation of articular cartilage is shown in Figure 9-5. Additional photographs of 0.308 μm Excimer debrided cartilage are presented in Chapter 35.

In vitro studies have examined the ablation rate of articular cartilage and other orthopaedic tissues using the 0.308 μm Excimer. Damage depths (Vari et al., 1991) have been measured and range from 16 to 35 μm depending on the energy density, 2–8 J/cm^2. Fischer et al. (1993) have published different results, however.

Animal studies have been undertaken to discover details of the short- to middle-term metabolic effects of the 0.308 μm Excimer laser on articular cartilage. In one study (Reed et al., 1994) a rabbit model of arthritis was created and chondroplasty performed. In another (manuscript in preparation), articular cartilage containing partial-thickness defects was lased and examined for evidence of cartilage regeneration. Although lased cartilage appeared smoother, no permanent effects were observed in either study, nor were there any increases in proteoglycan synthesis. It has not been discounted that some effects may be observed by applying different doses or energy densities.

Initial difficulties with fiberoptic tip fracture have largely been resolved. Improved fibers and handpieces and the new fiber bundles have virtually eliminated this problem. Disadvantages of 0.308 μm Excimer debridement are the cost of the laser and the complexity of the unit itself. Uncertainty about the mutagenic effects of 308 nm exposure is also a concern at this stage.

As more experience is gained with this laser, it will likely be approved for arthroscopic use. The results obtained so far for chondroplasty surpass those of other lasers. With more animal data and technical advances, this laser will likely become a popular alternative to mechanical instruments.

Alternative Wavelengths for Chondroplasty

Other devices currently being considered for use in arthroscopic orthopaedic applications include the 2.94 μm erbium:YAG laser, the 0.532 μm KTP laser, and the 0.488 μm argon-ion laser. One nonlaser alternative is the "ball electrode" electrocautery device, to remove fibrillations. It is simple and inexpensive. Second-look arthroscopies exhibit good results. It may ultimately be shown that many of the same outcomes can be achieved using electrocautery as result from using most lasers.

The 2.94 μm erbium:YAG laser has much potential, especially for chondroplasty. It is an infrared device that produces light at 2.94 μm. Like the 0.308 μm Excimer, this laser has been demonstrated to ablate tissue with almost no adjacent tissue damage. The form of the 2.94 μm erbium:YAG pulse is unique, consisting of a 200 μs burst of 1 μs "spikes." The short micropulse length accounts for some of the interesting properties of this laser. The 2.94 μm erbium:YAG laser can be delivered in water, although the zirconium fluoride glass fibers used to deliver the beam are fragile and degenerate quickly (Vari et al., 1991).

The green 0.532 μm KTP and 0.488 μm argon lasers are likely to find less application for debridement. They function best when interacting with pigmented tissues, and much of their energy is lost when attempting to ablate the mostly white structures of the knee.

Conclusion

It should be emphasized that this survey has dealt only with chondroplasty. Some lasers are not well suited to this application and they are better suited to other common arthroscopic procedures such as meniscectomy or lateral release. Of the lasers that have been applied to chondroplasty, the 2.1 μm holmium:YAG laser appears to be the best commercially available device. This situation is expected to change, however, when the 0.308 μm XeCl Excimer and possibly the 2.94 μm erbium:YAG lasers reach the market.

Laser debridement is an evolving form of treatment. It is difficult to say at this early stage if laser debridement will replace mechanical chondroplasty. It is clear that significant advantages over existing treatment methods must be demonstrated before the cost of lasers can be justified. For chondroplasty, this justification may take the form of slowing or reversal of degenerative changes in cartilage. Much work is still required to establish the side effects that may occur with laser use.

References

American Academy of Orthopaedic Surgeons (1992) Advisory statement: lasers in orthopaedic surgery. Park Ridge, IL, May

Bauer W and Bennet G (1936) Experimental and pathological studies in the degenerative type of arthritis. J Bone and Joint Surg 18:1–18

Black J, Sherk H, Meller M, Divan J, Rhodes A, Lane G (1992) Wavelength selection in laser arthroscopy. Semin Orthop 7:72–76

Borovoy M, Zirkin RM, Elson LM, Borovoy MA (1989) Healing of laser induced defects of articular cartilage: preliminary studies. J Foot Surg 28:95–99

Cinats J and Jackson R (1989) Arthroscopic laser surgery in a fluid medium. Poster Presentation, Canadian Orthopaedic Association Annual Meeting, Toronto, June

Collier MA, Haughland LM, Bellamy J, et al. (1993) Effects of holmium:YAG laser on equine articular cartilage and subchondral bone adjacent to traumatic lesions: a histopathological assessment. Arthroscopy 9:536–545

Ewing W (1990) Arthroscopic treatment of degenerative meniscal lesions and early degenerative arthritis of the knee. *In* J Ewing (ed): Articular Cartilage and Knee Joint Function: Basic Science and Arthroscopy, Raven Press, pp. 137–145

Fanton G and Dillingham M (1992) The use of the holmium laser in arthroscopic surgery. Semin Orthop 7:102–116

Fischer R, Krebs R, Scharf HP (1993) Cell vitality in cartilage tissue culture. Following excimer laser radiation an in vitro examination, Lasers Sung Med 13:629–637

Glossop N, Jackson R, Randle J, Reed S (1992) The excimer laser in arthroscopic surgery. Semin Orthop, 7:125–130

Jackson R and Dandy D (1976) Arthroscopy of the knee. Grune and Stratton, New York, NY

Kim H, Moran M, Salter R (1991) The potential for regeneration of articular cartilage in defects by chondral shaving and subcutaneous abrasion. J Bone Joint Surg 73-A:1301–1315

Kokosa J and Doyle D (1988) Chemical by-products produced by CO_2 and Nd:YAG laser interaction with tissue. SPIE 908:51–53

Lane G, Sherk H, Mooar P, Lee S, Black J (1992) Holmium:Yttrium-Aluminum-Garnet laser versus carbon dioxide laser versus mechanical arthroscopic debridement. Semin Orthop 7:95–100

Lane G, Sherk H, Kollmer C, Uppal G, Rhodes A, Sazy J, Black J, Lee S (1991) Stimulatory effects of Nd:YAG lasers on canine articular cartilage. *In* O'Brien S, Dedrich D, Wigdor H, and Trent A (ed): Proceedings of Lasers in Orthopaedics, Dental and Veterinary Medicine, SPIE 1424:7, Los Angeles, California, 23–24 January

Magnuson P (1941) Joint debridement: surgical treatment of degenerative arthritis. Surg Gynecol Obstet 43:1–9

Metcalf R and Dixon J (1984) Use of lasers for arthroscopic meniscectomy: a preliminary report on laboratory investigations. Lasers Surg Med 3:305–309

Miller D, O'Brien S, Arnosczky S, Kelly A, Fealy S, Warren R (1989) The use of the contact Nd:YAG laser in arthroscopic surgery: effects on articular cartilage and meniscal tissue. J Arthroscopy 5:245–253

O'Brien S, Fealy S, and Miller D (1992) Neodymium:Yttrium-Aluminum-Garnet contact laser arthroscopy. Semin Orthop 7:117–124

Raunest J (1991) Third International Symposium on Lasers in Orthopaedics, Hannover, Germany, Sept.

Raunest J and Lohnert J (1990) Arthroscopic cartilage debridement by excimer laser in chondromalacia of the knee joint: a prospective randomized clinical study. Arch Orth and Trauma Surg 109:155–159

Reed S, Jackson R, Glossop N, Randle J (1994) An in vivo study of the effects of excimer laser irradiation on degenerative rabbit articular cartilage. Arthroscopy 10(1):78–84

Schultz R, Krishnamurthy S, Thelmo W, Rodriguez J, Harvey G (1985) Effects of varying intensities of laser energy on articular cartilage: a preliminary study. Lasers in Medicine and Surgery 5:577–588

Shahriaree H (1984) O'Connor's textbook of arthroscopic surgery. JB Lippincott Co., Philadelphia, PA

Sherk H and Lane G (1989) Clinical uses of lasers in orthopaedics. Medical College of Pennsylvania, Course Notes

Spivak J, Grande D, Ben-Yishay A, Mench DS, Pitman MI (1992) The effect of low level Nd:YAG laser energy on adult articular cartilage in vitro. Arthroscopy 8:36–43

Sprague N (1981) Arthroscopic debridement for degenerative knee joint disease. Clinical Orthopaedics and Related Research no. 160, pp. 118–123

Srinivasan R (1986) Ablation of polymers and biological tissue by ultraviolet lasers. Science 234:559–565

Trauner K, Nishioka N, Patel D (1990) Pulsed holmium: yttrium-aluminum-garnet (Ho:YAG) laser ablation of fibrocartilage and articular cartilage. Am J Sports Med 18:316–320

Vangsness C, Akl Y, Neson S, Liaw L, Smith C, Marshall G (1992) An in vitro analysis of partial human meniscectomy by five different laser systems. Semin Orthop 7:77–80

Vangsness C, Smith C, Marshall G, Sweeney J, Johansen E (1992) CO_2 laser vaporization of articular cartilage. Semin Orthop, 7:83–89

Vari S, Shi W, van der Veen M, Fishbein M, Miller J, Papaioannou T, Grundfest W (1991) Comparative study of excimer and erbium:YAG lasers for ablation of structural components of the knee. *In* O'Brien S, Dedrich D, Wigdor H, and Trent A (ed): Proceedings of Lasers in Orthopaedics, Dental and Veterinary Medicine, SPIE 1424:33, Los Angeles, California, 23–24 January

10

Tissue Repair Using Lasers: Arthroscopic Applications*

Douglas K. Dew, Larry Supik, and Clement R. Darrow II

Numerous attempts have been made to use heating to effect an anastomotic union of severed tissue edges. Improvements in electrocautery and lasers have made experimental tissue anastomosis feasible; but clinical application of tissue welding has undergone only limited clinical trials. Using heat to anastomose tissue is fraught with complications. The technique's limitations and the factors that lead to successful tissue welding are reviewed.

For laser tissue repair, the underlying anastomosis is heated in such a manner as to cause coagulation and sealing with minimal tissue necrosis at the apposed tissue edges, a sometimes difficult task. Laser radiation has a wide range of effects on tissue (Hall et al., 1971). It is through the regulation of heat distribution in tissue (and sometimes the resulting mechanical effects) that lasers can produce controlled physical effects such as drilling, trimming, welding, and ablating. For instance, when tissue is heated to 60° to 70°C, protein coagulation (denaturation with shrinkage) occurs (Stryer, 1981; Gorisch and Boergen, 1982). In practice, "underexposure" or "overexposure" with laser irradiation can change clinical results significantly. A good example of incorrect laser exposure is the formation of a false aneurysm during laser-assisted vessel anastomosis (Quigley et al., 1986).

The three most important processes determining the pattern of heating in tissue are laser irradiation absorption (wavelength-dependent), length of exposure at a specific power level and beam geometry, and operating conditions (Arndt et al., 1981; Dew and Lo, 1983a). Assuming that one does not change the tissue types (each tissue shrinks at a slightly different temperature) (Gorisch and Boergen, 1982), based on the collagen architecture, tissue volume, or operating conditions under which the surgeon is working, the following parameters of laser irradiation are needed to determine the amount of absorption and heat diffusion (and therefore the heat distribution pattern) within the tissue:

1. Wavelength: the distance between two points in a periodic wave; determines the beam's tissue penetration depth
2. Spot Size: size of an area exposed to the beam; determines the diameter or area to be exposed to laser radiation (for tissue welding, it is often desirous to have the smallest possible area of tissue exposure)
3. Power (radiant flux): rate at which energy is delivered to the tissue; determines the amount of available radiation to be absorbed in the tissue
4. Time Exposure: length of time tissue is exposed to the laser radiation; determines the amount of radiation to be absorbed in the tissue
5. Beam Mode: beam geometry, which is a description of the distribution of power over the spot size; determines the direction and distribution the radiation travels after passing through the surface tissue.

Laser radiation should be readjusted for every tissue type and thickness or volume of tissue in order to yield the desired physical effect on each target tissue (Gorisch and Boergen, 1982).

The third factor, operating conditions, is important for predicting the effect of laser energy on tissue in a clinical environment. Laser wavelengths vary greatly in their absorption profiles of blood and water. In a bloody operating field, for example, the radiation of the 0.488 μm argon, the frequency-doubled YAG, and the 1.06 μm neodymium:YAG lasers is absorbed in the surface blood with

*Reprinted in part by permission from *Orthopedics* 16:581–587, 1993.

an often unpredictable effect on the underlying tissue based on how much hemoglobin is present over the surface of the tissue or even in the subsurface of the tissue. In a wet operating field, CO_2 laser energy at the fundamental 10.6 μm wavelength is highly absorbed in the surface water (whether in saline or blood) with an unpredictable effect on the underlying tissue if water is present. Thus wavelength selection becomes critical to ensure repeatable tissue sealing results under changing operating conditions, or operating conditions must be kept constant in order to have no variations based on wavelength specificity.

Report of Prior Investigations

Heat application for thermal vascular anastomosis was described during the early 1960s (Sigel and Acevedo, 1963; Sigel and Dunn, 1965). The importance of precise application of specific temperatures to the anastomosis was reported using wire loop forceps for thermal vascular anastomosis. This report demonstrated that the best results were obtained only with proper heating of the tissue with no shrinkage that could occlude the vessel lumen (Wintermantel, 1981).

In vitro studies of the use of the laser energy for tissue reconstruction was first carried out by Yahr and Strully in New York with the intention of achieving vascular anastomosis without interrupting blood flow (Yahr et al., 1964; Yahr and Strully, 1966). In 1978 the first in vivo feasibility studies were conducted by Jain and Gorisch in Munich, using a continuous wave 1.06 μm neodymium:YAG laser for repair of small incisions in rat arteries with diameters ranging from 0.3 to 1.1 mm (Jain and Gorisch, 1979a,b; Jain, 1980, 1984). Histological studies indicated fusion of the collagen in the vessel wall, and no aneurysm or disruption of the vessel wall was seen.

Following these initial reports by Jain and Gorisch, other investigators reported on the repair of nerve, tendon, fallopian tube, vas deferens, intestine, pleura, cartilage, and skin (Dew et al., 1982; Gomes et al., 1983; Rosemberg et al., 1985; LoCicero et al., 1985; Dew, 1986,b; White et al., 1986).

Laser-assisted vessel anastomosis using the 0.488 μm argon laser is now being clinically tested by White and a preliminary report has been published (White et al., 1989). Use of the 1.3 μm neodymium:YAG laser for laser tissue sealing was reported by Dew (1983a, b, and c). The 1.3 μm neodymium:YAG laser has been in clinical use since June 1988 under two individual device exemptions, both for vas deferens repair and skin closure (Dew et al., 1986). Initial results show viable sperm in a high percentage of patients with clinical follow-up (Dew, 1990). Initial clinical studies for skin closure have had mixed cosmetic results and have been disappointing, but no dehiscence has been reported (Johnson, 1993).

Meniscal Cartilage Repair: Feasibility Study

The purpose of this study on meniscal cartilage repair was to evaluate the effectiveness of laser welding of meniscal tissue using a 1.3 μm neodymium:YAG laser in a large animal, i.e., minipigs (Dew et al., 1993). The laser was used to close scalpel-induced full-thickness meniscal wounds. The pig model was chosen because of its similarity in size to a human meniscus. Controls include the ipsilateral opposite meniscal wound closed with an outside-inside full-thickness PDS suture. Effectiveness was judged on the basis of wound dehiscence, infection, unusual healing results, and consistency of results.

Methods

After adequate anesthesia was achieved, the medial and lateral aspect of the right knee was clipped with animal hair clippers. The area was then shaved with a razor blade, avoiding any inadvertent cuts or abrasions of the skin. The medial and lateral menisci of one knee were alternated in various animals between the laser and suture groups. The menisci were approached through two incisions parallel to the joint line. After adequate exposure was achieved, longitudinal full-thickness cuts, 5 to 6 mm, were made with a No. 15 scalpel blade in both the medial and lateral menisci in the outer one-third of the menisci. The control meniscal defect was closed with a 3-0 PDS suture placed at the center of the wound in an outside-inside manner to approximate the wound edges. Experimental wounds were approximated with mechanical manipulation using a Keith needle until even apposition of the wound edge was achieved. Once evenly aligned, the edges were welded using mechanical exposures of 1.3 μm wavelength radiation.

Using a 400 μm diameter fiber, the optical fiber was held at a fixed working distance (2 mm) from the tissue surface. Thermal denaturation of tissue protein and resulting seal of the tissue edges was achieved with the laser using a power of less than 2 watts. The laser was operated in continuous wave multimode fashion at 1.3 μm gated by a mechanical shutter. Surgical approximation of wound edges and laser application was carried out without use of magnification. Ten to fifteen single exposures were required on each 0.5 cm of the incision to effect a complete weld. The area was not dried of blood or water, wetted, or stained using a 1.3 μm laser other than that needed to visualize the operative site adequately. Welding, using the laser, was accomplished with multiple gated exposures by depressing the footswitch and overlapping the spots until the entire length of the incision was covered. Postoperatively, the lower extremity was kept in extension in a modified Thomas splint for 2 weeks with the animal fully weight-bearing. The study was broken into five groups.

Day 0: medial menisci laser, lateral menisci suture
Day 1: medial menisci suture, lateral menisci laser
Day 10: medial menisci suture, lateral menisci laser
Day 30: medial menisci laser, lateral menisci suture
Day 60: medial menisci suture, lateral menisci laser

Photographs were taken at follow-up in each group to document the visual absence or presence of abnormal wound healing or dehiscence. Each of the pigs were sacrificed at the various follow-up dates, and specimens were collected for histological analysis.

Results

No dehiscence, infection, or other unusual healing result was noted in any group throughout the 60-day follow-up period. The operative time for the entire procedure per laser group was less than 1 minute. The operative time for suture repair was 5 minutes once the meniscal incision was made. The laser-closed wounds remained approximated throughout the follow-up period at all time intervals. There was no dehiscence, and the previous wound edges were completely smooth. The 60-day suture-closed specimens evidenced some buckling owing to poor wound approximation. There was a small step-off in the day 0 suture-closed specimens as well, also due to poor wound edge approximation. No dehiscence in any of the suture-controlled wounds was seen, and all wounds healed via a fiberblastic scar response.

Conclusions

This animal study in the pig model demonstrated effective closure of meniscal scalpel-induced wounds using the laser. Laser closures were effected without the need for fixation sutures or staples. It has been shown that a 1.3 μm neodymium:YAG laser system may be used to weld stable meniscal wounds. All wounds, including those closed with a laser, clinically appeared to heal similarly and fairly consistently with no evidence of wound dehiscence, infection, or unusual healing result. No significant clinical wound healing difference was apparent by gross inspection when comparing the laser wound closures to the suture controls other than a small step-off noted in some of the suture-approximated specimens. In general, the suture-closed specimens were better approximated at the superior surface of the meniscal wound, and these wounds healed from a superior to an inferior direction as noted on histologic evaluation and documented in follow-up photographs. Meniscal closure using the 1.3 μm neodymium:YAG laser was successfully achieved by heat-induced denaturation tissue components under laboratory conditions similar to those seen in the operating room. Laser welding of cartilage was nontactile (minimizing manipulation and resultant tissue trauma that was seen as a prominent inflammatory response along the suture tract). It required no foreign material in the wound (i.e., suture material) in this model. It must be pointed out that no charring of the tissue took place in our animal studies. We were not searing the tissue together (resulting in charring), as has been seen in other laser wound closure and anastomosis studies. Wound edge approximation is the primary consideration when achieving effective laser welding. For this relatively simple meniscal laceration model in the pig, the approximation was easily accomplished with a Keith needle or spinal needle. Unstable complex tears may require stay sutures for approximation of meniscal edges.

Further studies are under way to determine the long-term effect of laser cartilage repair in the pig. These techniques also must be tested through a strictly arthroscopic approach to be clinically useful. Arthroscopic laser-assisted techniques should be feasible.

Discussion

After a review of the current literature on tissue sealing, we concluded that other investigators have had confusing results when comparing laser types and different parameters of even a single wavelength of laser. The results of these various investigators were often confusing, inconsistent, and difficult to reproduce because of the multitude of factors involved in laser tissue repair. For example: What type of laser was used? What was the beam geometry? How stable was the laser system? What were the operating conditions? What tissue was involved? What was the exact thickness and zone of tissue necrosis in the horizontal and vertical directions? How accurate were the investigator's measurement of time exposure, spot size, and power level? How did the surgical technique differ? What was the delivery system of the laser beam? Were blood, water, or "dyes" used to couple the laser energy to a specific area? Did these same variables change from experiment to experiment? Most importantly, what was the heating "endpoint" in each study? Was it charring, boiling, "browning," shrinkage, or almost no reaction? Thus it was difficult to compare prior studies using a single laser type from one investigator to the next.

These inconsistencies point out the variability of results with changes in wavelength-dependent absorption, power density, time exposure, beam mode, and tissue type. Furthermore, we have found that variation in surgical technique and operating conditions (wet or bloody character of the surgical site) is just as important as adjusting the structure. The laser system must be stable and calibrated correctly from laser to laser and fiber to fiber.

Conclusion

Early attempts at laser tissue fusion were centered on microvascular anastomosis, and studies have been extended to include most soft tissues in addition to cartilage. Animal studies have revealed that the process of healing after laser wound closure is similar in most tissues, with an inflammatory response to the initial injury and a progression similar to that found with conventional tissue closure techniques. The greatest difference between laser tissue repair and mechanical tissue repair is the tissue's response to the foreign body (i.e., the suture) that creates the anastomosis in conventional mechanical closures.

In the laboratory the 1.32 μm neodymium:YAG laser was found to be the most useful for tissue fusion. Stokes et al. (1981) demonstrated that 1.32 μm neodymium:YAG laser wavelength is transmitted much more strongly through whole human blood than is the 1.06 μm neodymium:YAG wavelength or the 0.488/0.514 μm wavelength of the argon laser. The penetration depths in blood were reported as relative values of 11.3, 4.2, and 1.0, respectively. Furthermore, Stokes et al. demonstrated that although the absorption coefficient for the 1.3 μm wavelength in 0.7% saline solution was higher than for the 1.06 μm wavelength (0.73 reciprocal centimeters and 0.065 reciprocal centimeters, respectively), the absorption of both wavelengths was low enough to be negligible during normal surgery. Stokes et al. concluded that "typical amounts of saline encountered in a clinical procedure will not alter the absorption of (either 1.3 or 1.06 wavelength) significantly." This wavelength is not highly absorbed by either blood or water, and thus surface fluids do not alter or stop the laser beam's penetration along the entire depth of the anastomotic site. It also provided more uniform heating of tissue under several operating conditions including a dry field, as well as having a thin layer of blood or saline in the tissue surface.

The conclusions of this study are that lasers offer a potential advantage over other instruments of tissue closure. Current lasers are too large, too expensive, and too unstable to be considered replacements for sutures and staples. At this point in laser hardware development, flash lamp pumped lasers should not be used for clinical tissue welding, as the waste heat and inherent instability of this type of laser provides power level and beam geometry fluxes that are unacceptable for the close tolerances required for reproducible clinical application of tissue welding. Semiconductor-type lasers (i.e., laser diodes) may provide the answer for clinical application of laser tissue anastomosis. These lasers are small, relatively stable, and provide little waste heat. Unfortunately, they can be expensive, but their prices are dropping rapidly as diode lasers find nonmedical industrial uses.

References

Arndt KA, Noe JM, Northam DBC, Itzkan T (1981) Laser therapy: basic concepts and nomenclature. Journal of the American Academy of Dermatology 5:649–654

Dew DK (1983c) Nd:YAG and CO_2 laser closure of rat skin incisions. Lasers in Surgery and Medicine 3:109

Dew DK (1983b) Laser microsurgical repair of soft tissue: an update and review. Lasers in Surgery and Medicine 3:134

Dew DK (1986b) Review and status report on laser tissue fusion. Lasers in Medicine, SPIE 712:255–257

Dew DK, Verdeja JC, Shebert R et al., (1982) Carbon dioxide laser is successful in the repair of the transected rat sciatic nerves. Neurology 32:132

Dew DK, Hsu LS, Halpern SJ, et al. (1986a) Development of a software driven medical laser system for tissue fusion at 1.32 μm. International Society of Optical Engineering, SPIE 712:32–33

Dew DK, Supik L, Darrow CR, Price GF (1993) Tissue repair using lasers: a review. Orthopaedics 16:581–587

Dew DK (1990) Review and status report on laser tissue sealing. International Society of Optical Engineering SPIE 1200:38–49

Dew DK, Lo HK (1983a) Carbon dioxide laser microsurgical repair of soft tissue: preliminary observations. Transactions of the American Society for Laser Medicine and Surgery, New Orleans, LA, Jan. 10–12

Gomes OM, Macrus R, Armelin et al., (1983) Vascular anastomosis by argon laser beam. Texas Heart Institute Journal 10:145

Gorisch W, Boergen KP (1982) Heat-induced contraction of blood vessels. Lasers in Surg and Med 2:1–13

Hall RR, Beach AD, Baker E, Morison PCA (1971) Incision of tissue by carbon dioxide laser. Nature 232:131–132

Jain KK (1984) Sutureless microvascular extra-intracranial anastomosis with nd:YAG laser. Lasers in Surgery and Medicine 3:322

Jain KK (1980) Sutureless microvascular anastomosis using a neodymium:YAG laser. Journal of Microsurgery 1:436–688

Jain KK and Gorisch W (1979) Repair of small blood vessels with the neodymium-YAG laser: a preliminary report. Surgery 85:684

Jain KK and Gorisch W (1979) Microvascular repair with neodymium:YAG laser. Acta Neurochir (Wien) 28 (suppl.):260

Johnson DL (1993) Personal communication. Lake Mary, FL

LoCicero J, Frederikson JW, Hartz RS, Kaufman MW, Michaelis LL (1985) Experimental air leaks in lung sealed by low-energy carbon dioxide laser irradiation. Chest 87: 820–822

Quigley MR, Bailes JE, Kwaan HC, Cerullo LJ, Brown JT (1986) Aneurysm formation after low power carbon dioxide laser assisted vascular anastomosis. Neurosurgery 18:292–299

Rosemberg SK, Elson L, Nathan LE (1985) Carbon dioxide laser microsurgical vasovasostomy . Urology 25:53–56

Sigel B and Acevedo FJ (1963) Electrocoaptive union of blood vessels: a preliminary study. J Surg Res 3:90–96

Sigel B and Dunn MR (1965) The mechanism of blood vessel closure by high frequency electrocoagulation. Surgery, Obstetrics and Gynecology 121:823–831

Stokes LS, Auth DC, Tanaka D, Gray JL, Gulacsik C (1981) Biomedical utility of 1.3 micrometer nd:YAG laser radiation. IEEE Trans Biomedical Engineering 28:287–299

Stryer L (1981) Biochemistry. Second Edition, WH Freeman & Co., p. 191

White RA, Kopchok G, Donayre C, Abergel RP, Lyons R, Klein SR, Dwyer RM, Uitto J (1986) Comparison of laser-welded and sutured arteriotomies. Arch Surg 121:1133–1135

White RA, White GH, Fujitani RM, et al. (1989) Initial human evaluation of argon laser assisted vascular anastomoses. Journal of Vascular Surgery 9:542–547

Wintermantel E (1981) The thermic vascular anastomosis (tva). Acta Nurochirurgica 56:5–24

Yahr WZ, Strully KJ, Hurwill ES (1964) Non-occlusive small arterial anastomosis with neodymium laser. Surgical Forum 15:224–226

Yahr WZ and Strully KJ (1966) Blood vessel anastomosis by laser and other biomedical applications. Journal of the Assoc. Adv. in Medical Instrumentation 1:28

11

Indications for Arthroscopic Laser Systems Use

Allen T. Brillhart

In the United States the Food and Drug Administration (FDA) determines the safety of specific arthroscopic laser devices and delivery systems and approves their marketing for specific procedures on specific tissues (US Department of Health and Human Services, 1988). The FDA states it does not approve the lasers but does approve the *marketing* of the lasers. Each manufacturer is required to go through an approval process that includes limited, controlled clinical trials. A 510(k) Approval can be obtained by competitive manufacturers if the FDA determines that the competitive manufacturer's device is essentially similar to an already approved device. Each manufacturer has a list of procedures and tissues for which their arthroscopic laser systems are approved. The surgeon must be aware of these specific indications prior to use. Use of arthroscopic laser systems outside the United States obviously requires a different approval process relative to the specific country in question. Each surgeon must be referred to his or her specific governmental regulatory body for approval. Beyond U.S. federal approval, state regulatory agencies generally follow federal guidelines (US Department of Health and Human Services, 1983). Nevertheless, they should be contacted before arthroscopic lasers can be considered approved for marketing. The specific hospital or outpatient surgical center in which the arthroscopic laser system is to be used usually has the most stringent controls beyond the FDA. The hospital administration, the laser safety committee, and the operating room committee must approve the use of the arthroscopic laser systems for arthroscopy (Ball, 1990; Brillhart, 1991). From a medicolegal tort standpoint, the orthopaedic community ultimately determines whether arthroscopic laser system use is acceptable. In the United States the American Academy of Orthopaedic Surgeons has issued a revised advisory statement in this regard. From a criminal justice standpoint, the FDA is responsible for the enforcement of laws that apply to the improper use of laser systems. Each surgeon should obviously consult with these entities and an attorney if questions arise.

Current Indications for Arthroscopic Laser System Use

It is the current opinion of the author that there are two general indications for use of FDA market-approved arthroscopic laser systems (Brillhart, 1992):

1. When, in the judgment of the surgeon, conventional instruments cannot cut, coagulate, or ablate tissue as safely or as well as the arthroscopic laser
2. When, in the judgment of the surgeon, the patient's outcome, immediate or long-term, will be better than when conventional instruments are used

Based on these two general indications, it is obvious that some surgeons justify arthroscopic laser use for virtually every operative arthroscopy they perform. At the other extreme, some arthroscopic surgeons are never able to justify the use of arthroscopic laser systems in their practice. As with the use of any other FDA market-approved arthroscopic instrument, the final decision to use that device rests with the judgment of the surgeon.

Definition of Inappropriate Arthroscopic Laser System Use

"Inappropriate" arthroscopic laser use should not be misconstrued to mean an absolute medical contraindication. What is inappropriate under most circumstances is not a contraindication in all circumstances. "Inappropriate" in this context means that I would not recommend use of the arthroscopic laser system under the given circumstance.

In my opinion there are 11 circumstances in which use of arthroscopic laser systems should be considered inappropriate.

1. Use of a laser system that is not FDA market-approved, or an untested arthroscopic laser system, device, or probe, used in other than an approved research setting
2. Use of an arthroscopic laser system by an unauthorized individual or a surgeon untrained or noncredentialed for the specific arthroscopic laser system, except under qualified supervision for approved training purposes
3. Use of a faulty arthroscopic laser system, including reusing nonreusable disposable probes
4. Use of an arthroscopic laser system by a surgeon who does not comply with established rules and regulations
5. Use of an arthroscopic laser system in an unapproved or unsafe environment, especially in an unprepared office environment
6. Use of an arthroscopic laser for purposes of financial gain only and no patient benefit
7. Use of an arthroscopic laser for an instrument in an untested procedure other than in an approved research setting
8. Use of an arthroscopic laser without consideration to resultant pathology created from inadvertent tissue damage, including effects not desired because of unacceptable depth of penetration and delayed effects.
9. Use of an arthroscopic laser system for surgery on an uninformed patient (Fig. 11-1).
10. Use of an arthroscopic laser system with a guarantee to the patient of unrealistic or "larger than life" results
11. Use of an arthroscopic laser system by a physician

Laser Informed Consent

1. I, ______________________________, voluntarily consent to the use of the ______________________ laser for the following procedure:
(Laser Type)
____

2. I understand that the final decision whether or not to use the laser will be made at the time of surgery.

3. I have been informed of other possible treatment methods that are available to me. My physician has answered all my questions concerning this form of treatment and its potential complications for this condition.

4. I understand that the risks of laser treatment include the possibility of unintentional surface burns if the laser is misdirected or if the energy beam is unintentionally reflected off a shiny object. There is also a risk of surface burns of the eye if I am not wearing protective glasses. Other risks of laser treatment will be those risks associated with the procedure itself and anesthesia.

5. I understand that the use of the ______________________ laser for my condition is new
(Laser Type)
but not experimental. Although previous research and clinical evidence on the use of lasers indicates that the laser is safe and effective, complete data has not been collected over a long time. Possible benefits of laser use may include a more satisfactory treatment of my condition with a lower likelihood of return of this disorder. However, I understand that there are no guarantees that laser treatment will definitely improve my condition or that it might not worsen my condition. Similarly, I understand that the long-term effects of laser light on human tissue are not known.

6. My questions about this form of treatment have been answered to my satisfaction at this time. I understand that I may make any other inquiries I desire concerning this procedure at any time.

I hereby voluntarily consent to surgery with the assistance of the ______________________ laser.
(Laser Type)

Signature:______________________ Date:______________________

Witnessed by:

Physician:______________________ Second Witness:______________________

Figure 11-1. Example of laser informed consent.

who is not skilled in arthroscopy (especially gas arthroscopy and the use of the 10.6 μm CO_2 laser), except under supervision for training purposes

Agencies currently involved in establishing regulations, guidelines, or advisory statements of laser use in the United States are as follows (US Department of Health and Human Services, 1983, 1988; American National Standards Institute, 1988; Ball, 1990; Brillhart, 1991; Sliney and Trokel, 1993):

American Academy of Orthopaedic Surgeons
6300 North River Road
Rosemont, IL 60018-4262
(708) 823-7186

American National Standards Institute (ANSI)
1430 Broadway
New York, NY 10018
(212) 354-3300

American Society for Laser Medicine and Surgery (ASLMS)
813 Second Street, Suite 200
Wausau, WI 54401
(715) 845-9283

Association of Operating Room Nurses (AORN)
10170 E. Mississippi Avenue
Denver, CO 80231
(303) 755-6300

Food and Drug Administration (FDA)
Center for Devices and Radiological Health (CDRH)
1390 Piccard Drive
Rockville, MD 20850
(301) 427-1307

Joint Commissions of Hospital Accreditation Organization (JCHAO)
1 Renaissance Boulevard
Oak Brook Terrace, IL 60181
(708) 916-5600

Occupational Safety and Health Administration (OSHA)
200 Constitution Avenue NW Rtr N3647
Washington, DC 28210-0001
(202) 523-6148

United States Department of Health and Human Services
200 Independence Avenue SW
Washington, DC 20201-0000
(202) 475-0257

References

American National Standards Institute, Inc. (1988) American national standard for the safe use of lasers in health care facilities. ANSI Z136.d, New York, p. 4

Ball KA (1990) Lasers: the perioperative challenge. CA Mosby Co., St. Louis, MO

Brillhart AT (1991) Arthroscopic laser surgery. American Journal of Arthroscopy vol. 1, no. 1, Mar, pp. 5–12

Brillhart AT (1992) Contraindications of laser use. Presented at the American Academy of Orthopaedic Surgeons Continuing Medical Education Course, Lasers in Orthopaedics. Richmond, Virginia, October

Sliney DH and Trokel SL (1993) Medical lasers and their safe use. Springer-Verlag New York Inc., New York, NY

U.S. Department of Health and Human Services (1983) Suggested state regulations for the control of radiation. vol. II, Nonionizing Radiation, Lasers

U.S. Department of Health and Human Services (1988) HHS Publication FDA 88-8035: Regulations for the administration and enforcement of the radiation control for health and safety act of 1968, Part 1040, sections 1040.10 and 1040.11, April

12

Potential Hazards of Arthroscopic Laser Surgery

David H. Sliney

With the increasing variety of laser wavelengths being employed for arthroscopy, laser safety issues become more complex and more important to address prior to surgery (Sliney and Trokel, 1992). Laser surgeons must be concerned with protecting the patient and the operating room staff as well as themselves. Patient safety is ensured by limiting needless tissue exposure, by avoiding fire, and by protecting the eyes. Safety of the laser surgeon and assistants requires concern for both system safety design and methods to limit potentially hazardous reflections and optical fiber breakage. Environmental hazards from the smoke produced by vaporizing tissue must be minimized by local exhaust ventilation or fume extractors. The pathogenicity and chemical toxicity of vaporized tissue has been the subject of a number of investigations. Safety standards for medical laser applications have been issued that consider all of these potential hazards and their control measures (Sliney and Wolbarsht, 1980; IRPA, 1985; ANSI, 1988, 1993; Sliney and Trokel, 1992; ACGIH, 1993; IEC, 1993).

As with other electrical or electronic equipment, lasers in the surgical environment pose electrical safety problems. The potential for electrical shock exists, thus requiring appropriate grounding and other electrical safety precautions. Biomedical engineers and medical electronics technicians familiar with safe installation of electrical and electronic equipment in hospital and health care environments should have no difficulty providing guidance for safe grounding and installation of laser equipment. Operating room personnel should not attempt to repair these lasers. Electrical shock can result.

As when using electrosurgery or cutting bone with a saw, a laser can produce potentially hazardous tissue particulates and vaporized tissue. Vaporized tissue in sufficient quantities must receive special attention, and fume extraction with local exhaust ventilation generally is required.

The hazard unique to the laser and that requires special attention is that resulting from the laser beam itself—the optical radiation hazard. Unlike other light sources, if the laser beam were to be collimated and directed over some distance, the area of potential hazard could extend far from the immediate surgical site. Fortunately, during arthroscopy the laser beam is normally contained within a closed fiber delivery system, and the beam emanating from a fiber tip or waveguide rapidly diverges. Nevertheless, a zone of hazardous laser radiation still exists, and protective measures are essential. Unwarranted fears often accompany the introduction of lasers for the first time into the clinical environment. Therefore proper appreciation of the real laser beam hazard is necessary for each member of the surgical staff so realistic safety precautions are followed.

Laser hazards depend on the laser in use, the environment, and the personnel involved with the laser operation (the operator, ancillary personnel, and patient). The laser hazard is roughly defined by the hazard classification (classes 1–4), whereas the other factors must be analyzed in each situation. A basic understanding of laser biologic effects and hazards is necessary to intelligently assess laser hazards in the surgical environment. Once the hazards are understood, the safety measures are obvious.

Eye Sensitivity

The special optical properties of the human eye cause it to be the organ most vulnerable to laser light. Aside from the oral mucosa, the only living tissues exposed to the environment are the cornea and conjunctiva. Without the comparative protective features of the stratum corneum of the

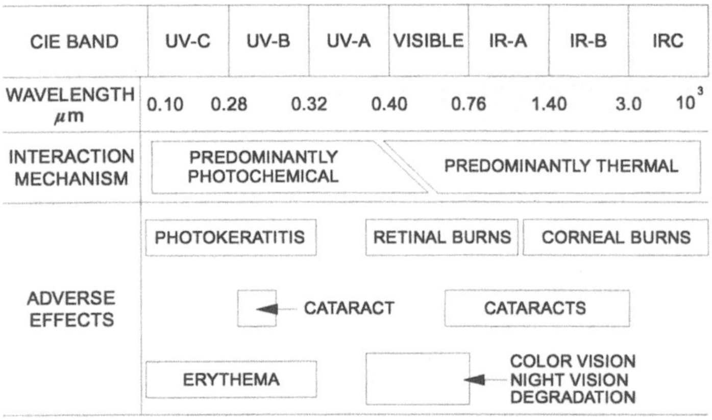

CIE BAND
UV-C
UV-B
UV-A
VISIBLE
IR-A
IR-B
IRC
WAVELENGTH μm
0.10
0.28
0.32
0.40
0.76
1.40
3.0
10^3
INTERACTION MECHANISM
PREDOMINANTLY PHOTOCHEMICAL
PREDOMINANTLY THERMAL
ADVERSE EFFECTS
PHOTOKERATITIS
RETINAL BURNS
CORNEAL BURNS
CATARACT
CATARACTS
ERYTHEMA
COLOR VISION
NIGHT VISION
DEGRADATION

Figure 12-1. CIE (Commission International de l'Eclairage) separates the optical spectrum into seven bands for discussing photobiologic effects of optical radiation on the eye and skin. They depend on the absorption properties, which in turn depend on the spectral region.

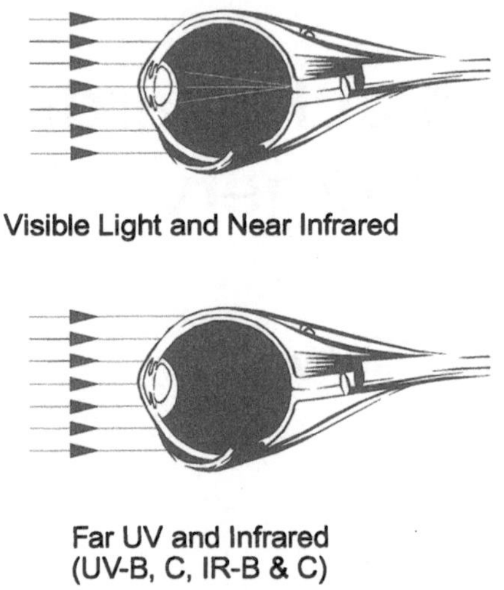

Figure 12-2. Absorption properties of the eye. The focusing effect of the cornea and lens in the visible and near-infrared (0.4–1.4 μm, i.e., 400–1,400 nm) renders the retina particularly vulnerable to laser injury.

skin, the eye is exposed directly to the environment. The lid reflex limits the exposure to the cornea to intense heat from infrared radiation and protects the retina against exposure to intense visible light. However, some laser beam intensities are so great that injury can occur faster than the protective action of the lid reflex, which occurs between 0.20 and 0.25 second (Sliney and Wolbarsht, 1980; Sliney and Trokel, 1992). (Lasers capable of causing injury to the eye within the blink reflex are in safety class 3; if they are also capable of causing severe skin injury they are in class 4.)

The biologic effects of laser radiation on the eye and skin depend mostly on wavelength, as shown in Figure 12-1. When discussing photobiologic effects, it is convenient to divide optical radiation (ultraviolet, visible, infrared) into different spectral bands (Fig. 12-1). Optical energy cannot damage tissue unless the energy is able to penetrate to and be absorbed by that tissue layer. For this reason, rays in the visible and near infrared (visible and IR-A bands), which can be transmitted through clear ocular media and be absorbed in the retina, can in sufficient intensity damage the retina. The high collimation of a laser beam permits the rays to be focused to a small spot on the retina (Fig. 12-2). The image size of such a point at the retina is approximately 10 to 20 μm (smaller than the diameter of a human hair). For this reason, lasers operating between 400 and 1,400 nm are particularly dangerous to the retina. This spectral region is often referred to as the retinal hazard region, as there is an approximately 10^5 increase in the concentration of light after it enters the eye and falls on the retina. Hence a collimated beam of 1 watt/cm^2 at the cornea focuses to a small spot with an irradiance of about 100 kW/cm^2. Although damage to such a small region of the retina may seem insignificant at first, it is important to remember that the central retina—the macula and particularly the fovea (center of the macula)—are small areas responsible for critically important, high-acuity vision. If these areas are injured by laser radiation, substantial loss of vision can result (Sliney and Wolbarsht, 1980).

The image area alone may not be the only site of damage; as a result of heat flow and mechanical (acoustic) transients the tissue surrounding the image site may also be injured, leading to more severe consequences regarding visual function. For example, it has not been uncommon for an individual to lose almost total function in an eye exposed to a small amount of energy (several hundred microjoules) when a Q-switched laser is accidentally imaged on the fovea. Instead of normal visual acuity of 20/20, the visual acuity in such accidental situations has often been recorded as 20/200 following the accident. Such low vision would be considered legally blind in most states. Fortunately, with most accidents only one eye is exposed to a collimated beam. There is normally little recovery of vision, as the neural tissue of the retina has little ability to repair itself. Although visual recovery can take place, the loss, for the most part, is permanent (Sliney and Wolbarsht, 1980; Hirsch et al., 1992; Sliney and Trokel, 1992).

At wavelengths outside the retinal hazard region, in both the ultraviolet and far-infrared regions of the spectrum, injury to the anterior segment of the eye is possible. As shown in Figure 12-1, certain spectral bands may injure the lens (notably at wavelengths of 295–320 nm and 1–2 μm). Injury to the cornea is possible from a wide range of wavelengths in the ultraviolet and most of the infrared regions at wavelengths beyond 1,400 nm. With the 10.6 μm CO_2 laser wavelength, threshold injury to the cornea would be expected to be superficial, involving only the corneal epithelium; and given the cornea's high metabolic rate, corneal repair occurs within a day or two, with eventual total recovery of vision. However, if significant injury occurs in the deep corneal layers in the stroma or endothelium and in the germinative layers of the cornea (as would be more readily possible with the 2.1 μm holmium:YAG wavelength), corneal scars can result, leading to permanent loss of vision unless a corneal transplant can be effected.

Excimer lasers operating in the ultraviolet are now entering the surgical arena. These lasers pose a particular hazard to the cornea, and the 0.308 μm Excimer laser can be considered additionally dangerous as it can produce an immediate cataract of the lens. The argon [0.488 μm (blue), 0.515 μm (green)], krypton [0.647 μm (red), 0.568 μm (yellow), 0.531 μm (green)], copper vapor [0.577 μm (yellow), 0.510 μm (green)], 0.632 μm gold vapor, 0.632 μm helium-neon (HeNe), and 1.06 μm neodymium:YAG lasers are all potentially hazardous to the retina. The 2.94 μm erbium:YAG or erbium:YLF, 2.06 μm holmium:YAG, 2.7-3.0 μm hydrogen:fluoride, and 10.6 μm CO_2 lasers are all potentially hazardous to the cornea because wavelengths that cause corneal damage are not reconcentrated by the eye as are wavelengths in the retinal hazard region. The thresholds for injury of the cornea are generally much higher than those that may injure the retina. Table 12-1 lists some representative maximum permissible exposure (MPE) limits for some commonly used surgical lasers (International Electrotechnical Commission, 1984; IRPA, 1985; ANSI, 1988, 1993; ACGIH, 1993). The safest practice is for laser specific protective eyewear to be used by all personnel and the patient. It goes without saying that the surgeon should not directly view the area through the unprotected (unfiltered) arthroscopic eyepiece if any of the arthroscopic lasers are to be used simultaneously.

Table 12-1. Some selected maximum permissible exposure limits.

Type of laser	Principal wavelength(s) (nm)[a]	Exposure limit
Argon fluoride	193	3.0 mJ/cm^2 over 8 hours
Xenon chloride	308	40 mJ/cm^2 over 8 hours
Argon ion	488,514.5	3.2 mW/cm^2 for 0.1 second
Copper vapor	510,578	2.5 mW/cm^2 for 0.25 second
Helium–neon	632.8	1.8 mW/cm^2 for 1.0 second
Gold vapor	628	1.0 mW/cm^2 for 10 seconds
Krypton ion	568,647	
Neodymium: YAG	1064	5.0 μJ/cm^2 for 1 nanosecond to 50 microseconds; no MPE for t < 1 nanosecond
	1334	5 mW/cm^2 for 10 seconds
CO_2	10.6 μm	100 mW/cm^2 for 10 seconds to 8 hours, limited area
Carbon monoxide	~5 μm	10 mW/cm^2 for > 10 seconds for most of body

All standards/guidelines have maximum permissible exposure limits (MPEs) at other wavelengths and exposure durations.
Note: to convert MPEs in milliwatts per square centimeter to millijoules per square centimeter, multiply by exposure time in seconds (e.g., the He-Ne or argon MPE at 0.1 second is 0.32 mJ/cm^2.
[a] Sources: ANSI Standard Z-136.1—1993; ACGIH TLVs (1993) and IRPA.

Skin Sensitivity

The skin is less sensitive to injury than the eye. However, it should be remembered that the probability of direct exposure to some part of the skin from a laser beam is far greater than to the small area occupied by the eye. Injury to the skin can occur from either photochemical damage mechanisms (predominant in the ultraviolet end of the spectrum) or by thermal mechanisms (predominant in the infrared end of the spectrum). For example, erythema ("sunburn") results from injury to the epidermis—and to some extent the dermis as well—and originates from a photochemically initiated event. First, second, and third degree skin burns can be induced by visible and infrared laser beam exposure, producing thermal injury.

The severity of the injury depends on the length of exposure and the penetration depth of the laser radiation. Generally, if the exposure lasts one second or more a pain response elicits a reflex movement to move the exposed tissue away from the laser beam, thereby limiting the exposure duration to 1 second or less. High power laser beam exposure does not result in a deep tissue burn at 10.6 μm CO_2 wavelengths if the exposure time is extremely short, as the penetration depth of the 10.6 μm CO_2 laser beam is shallow (~20 μm) and, in fact, does not penetrate the normal thickness of the stratum corneum. Injury to the epidermis from the 10.6 μm CO_2 laser is by heat conduction from the stratum corneum to deeper layers. However, short-pulsed exposure to 1.06 μm neodymium:YAG laser radiation, which penetrates several millimeters into tissue, can cause a deep, severe burn at a radiant exposure just above burn threshold, albeit at a much higher threshold than for a 10.6 μm CO_2 laser burn. A 2.1 μm holmium:YAG laser and a 0.532 μm KTP (doubled YAG) or an argon (0.488 and 0.514 μm) laser would produce a burn depth intermediate between that incurred by the 10.6 μm CO_2 and 1.06 μm neodymium:YAG lasers.

Clearly, the focal spot of a focused surgical laser or the concentrated beam irradiance at the tip of an optical fiber is designed to ablate or vaporize tissue and is hazardous to skin if located near the focal spot. Significant skin injuries from accidental exposure to industrial or medical lasers rarely occur (at least they are rarely reported). Actual thresholds of injury to the skin are normally of the order of a few joules per square centimeter, and this level of exposure does not occur outside the focal zone of a surgical laser. One of the most serious complications of any surgery is an operating room fire. Because of the photothermal effects of arthroscopic laser beams associated with their concentrated energy levels the possibility exists of inadvertently igniting drapes, endotracheal tubes, flammable liquids, sponges, and clothing. Severe burns, respiratory

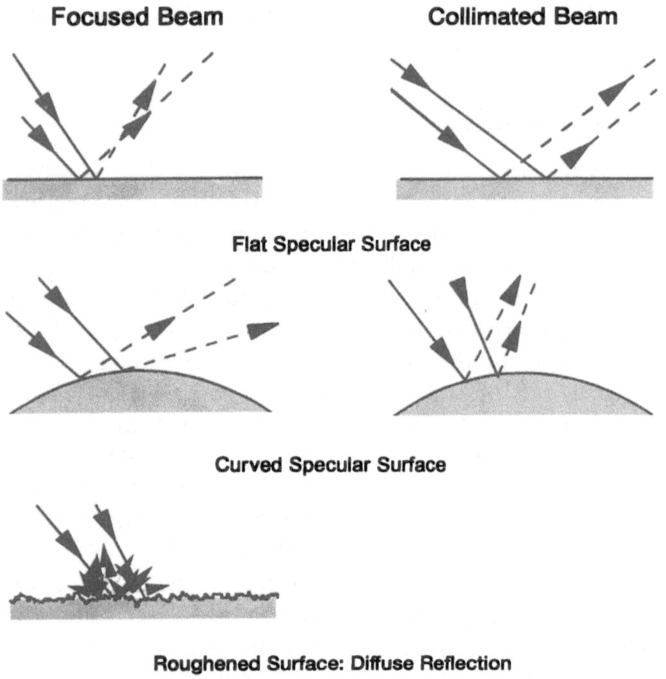

Figure 12-3. Examples of reflections of laser radiation from specular (mirror-like) surfaces (e.g., shiny metallic instrument surfaces).

damage, and even death could possibly result. Moist sponges, moist drapes, and flame retardant materials should be used. A basin of water should be available to extinguish in the rare event of a fire when lasers are used (AT Brillhart, 1991). Precautions are outlined in Chapter 13.

Risks of Inadvertent Exposure During Arthroscopy

During most arthroscopic procedures the beam is enclosed within an optical waveguide or fiber, and exposure is limited. During an operation hazardous exposure occurs when the beam leaves the delivery system, or there is a break in the delivery system. Accidental firing of the laser represents the greatest hazard. This can result in a drape or clothing fire, a direct skin burn, inadvertent tissue damage, or eye injury. When one examines the records of accidental eye injuries due to lasers used in industry, science, and medicine, it becomes apparent that the source of ocular exposure is most frequently a reflected beam. Figure 12-3 illustrates mirror-like (specular) laser beam reflections from the flat or curved surfaces characteristic of metallic instruments used during some surgical procedures. At first thought it appears that a collimated beam would pose the most hazardous exposure condition, but at close range a diverging beam may have a greater likelihood of striking the eye (Sliney and Wolbarsht, 1980). In arthroscopy, avoiding direct viewing into the eyepiece decreases this risk. Inadvertent exposure of a nonreflected beam is more likely to cause a skin burn or fire.

A number of steps can be taken to minimize the potential hazards to both the patient and surgical staff. Preventive measures depend on the type of laser. The most common type of laser employed in the past for surgical applications has been the 10.6 μm CO_2 laser. Because the CO_2 laser wavelength of 10.6 μms is in the far-infrared spectral region—and invisible—the presence of hazardous secondary beams could go unnoticed. This added hazard resulting from an infrared laser beam's lack of visibility is common to other infrared lasers as well, such as the 2.1 μm holmium:YAG and 1.06 μm neodymium:YAG lasers. Because there have been a number of serious retinal injuries caused by improper attention to safety with neodymium:YAG lasers, the use of the 1.06 μm neodymium:YAG laser must be approached with even greater caution than the 10.6 μm CO_2 laser. By contrast, the 0.488 μm and 0.515 μm argon lasers and the 0.532 μm second-harmonic neodymium:YAG (sometimes referred to as the KTP) laser emit highly visible, blue-green beams and in some ways pose less potential hazard. **The reader is referred to Chapter 13 for laser specific precautions.**

Pulsed Versus Continuous Mode Lasers

Some surgical lasers (e.g., the 10.6 μm CO_2, 1.06 μm neodymium:YAG, and 0.488 and 0.515 μm argon lasers) are continuous wave instruments, or nearly so. The 2.1 μm holmium:YAG and the 1.44 μm neodymium:YAG arthroscopic lasers are pulsed. The biologic effects and potential hazards from high-peak power pulsed lasers are different from those of continuous wave lasers, particularly the lasers operating in the *retinal hazard region of the visible* (400 to 760 nm) and near-infrared (760-1,400 nm) spectrum, as shown in Figure 12-2. The severity of retinal lesions caused by a visible or near-infrared continuous wave laser are normally considered to be far less than from a Q-switched laser.

Nominal Hazard Zone

Another major factor that influences the potential hazard is the degree of beam collimation. Almost all surgical lasers are focused, thereby limiting the hazardous area (referred to as the nominal hazard zone) (ANSI, 1988, 1993; Sliney and Trokel, 1992). An exception is the highly collimated beam that can be emitted from most laser systems when the beam delivery system has been removed (which may occur during servicing). A collimated beam can remain hazardous at some distance from the instrument (Sliney and Mainster, 1987; Sliney and Trokel, 1992; Wood and Sliney, 1992). Eye protectors should be worn

Figure 12-4. Beam irradiance of a laser beam as a function of distance from an open laser fiber or contact tip. Note the rapid decrease of beam irradiance beyond the focal point.

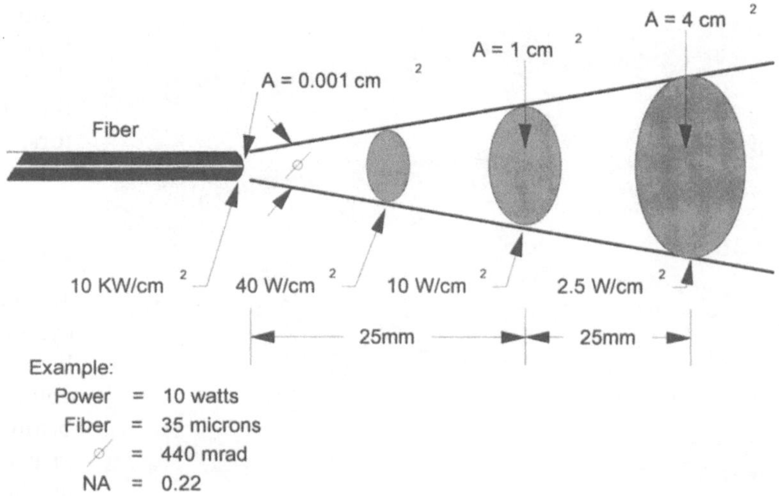

within the nominal hazard zone and strict safety rules applied.

Once the laser beam leaves the delivery system, it rapidly diverges from a contact tip (or if it is a focused beam, it comes rapidly to a focus and then diverges again). If emerging from a broken or disconnected, open fiber, it also rapidly diverges. The nominal hazard zone is normally limited to an area of 1 to 2 meters around the emission point from a fiber. Typical nominal hazard zones are about 30 to 60 cm from a 2.06 μm holmium:YAG laser, 2 meters from a 10.6 μm CO_2 laser, and 10 meters from a 1.06 μm neodymium:YAG laser.

Surface Reflection Hazards

Reflections are of greatest concern if originating from flat mirror-like (specular) surfaces, characteristic of many metallic surgical instruments. Reflections are also a problem when performing arthroscopy for a total joint replacement. Obviously, free beam laser use should be avoided in these cases.

Many surgical instruments used during open surgery have black "anodized" or sand-blasted, roughened surfaces to reduce (but not eliminate) potentially hazardous reflections. The surface roughening is generally more effective than the black (ebonized) surface, as the beam is diffused. Combining a black polymer surface with roughening has been shown to offer the greatest protection (Sliney and Mainster, 1987).

The surface finish and reflectance seen in the visible spectrum do *not* indicate those qualities in the invisible far-infrared spectrum. A roughened surface that appears dull and diffuse at short, visible, or near-infrared wavelengths, is always much more specular at far-infrared wavelengths (e.g., at 10.6 μms). This behavior results from the fact that the relative size of the microscopic structure of the surface relative to the incident wavelength determines whether the beam is reflected as a specular or a diffuse reflection.

A specularly reflected beam with only 1% of the initial beam's power can still be hazardous. Hence the rougher the surface of an instrument likely to intercept the beam, the safer is the reflection. For example, even a 1% reflection of a 40 watt laser beam is 400 mW. It is somewhat surprising that there have been few cases reported of eye injuries to residents and other persons observing 1.06 μm neodymium:YAG laser surgery without eye protectors. Hazardous specular reflections from a laser beam emerging from an endoscopic optical fiber are limited in extent because the beam rapidly diverges, as shown in Figure 12-4.

Aiming Beam Hazards

Most invisible-beam surgical lasers have a visible alignment beam. Infrared lasers most often make use of a low-power coaxial 0.632 μm helium-neon red laser. It is desirable where feasible for this alignment beam to be 1 mW or less, as the maximum continuous wave, visible laser beam power that can safely enter the eye within the aversion response (i.e., within the blink reflex of 0.25 second) is 1 mW. **The aiming beam should not be directed into the eye.**

Patient's Hazards

Current laser safety regulations do not limit the exposure of the patient at the target site for surgery. Accidental exposure to the patient from misdirection of the laser beam should be of concern. This can result in injury of eye and skin (Sliney and Trokel, 1992). This point is of particular concern when lasers are used in or near the eye and when exposure of the eye itself is not intended. Particular hazards of gas arthroscopy exist, including rare reports of gas emboli and neurologic sequelae, pneumopericardium, pneumothoraces, and even death. These rare complications are not due to the laser but to the gas medium and are addressed in Chapter 14. Specific precautions for patient safety are outlined in Chapter 13.

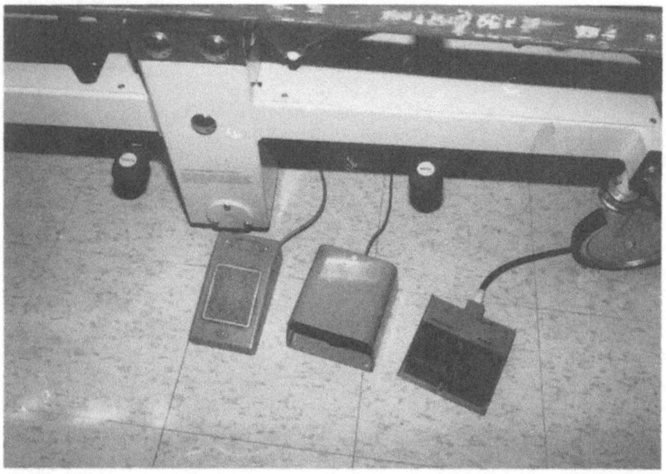

Figure 12-5. Foot pedals used to switch on and off operating microscope lights and other instruments may be mistaken for the laser footswitch. The laser footswitch should always be shielded and be clearly identified to avoid accidental laser emission.

Surgeon's Hazards

The eyes of the surgeon or laser operator are normally protected from injury due to the design of the laser and video camera. The surgeon should view the target tissue through television monitor and not directly through the optics of the arthroscope. Despite this, use of laser wavelength—specific eyewear is still the best safety practice. Also, with hand-held laser delivery systems, one should remember that the surgeon's hand is the closest to the hand piece and therefore it is most vulnerable to potentially hazardous laser burns. This can happen if the fiber breaks or the laser is inadvertently fired.

Surgical Staff's Hazards

Nurses, other surgical assistants, and operating room staff may be exposed to misdirected laser beams. Lasers have been accidentally initiated when the beam delivery system was directed other than at the patient, a foot switch was accidentally pressed, or similar errors have occurred, and the beam was directed at a person. Figure 12-5 shows multiple foot switches positioned below an operating room table. Assistants are potentially exposed to secondary reflections from open-beam laser surgical devices. Again, eye injury, skin burns, or clothing fires are of concern.

Bystanders' Hazards

Bystanders in the surgical facility or outpatient laser facility who are present to observe or calm the patient (e.g., a patient's relative) may be susceptible to exposure from laser beams in the same manner that a surgical assistant or nurse may be susceptible. In addition, because of lack of training or knowledge about the laser surgical procedure, bystanders may be at greater risk by inadvertently placing themselves in a dangerous position. Individuals observing the operation should be provided with laser eye protectors, even if they are located outside the nominal hazard zone.

Hazards During Service

A number of laser service technicians have sustained laser eye injuries. For example, at least two serious eye injuries have occurred to service personnel exposed to secondary, collimated, invisible 1.06 μm neodymium:YAG laser beams when they gained access to the laser cavity. Service personnel are particularly susceptible to laser injury as they often gain access to collimate laser beams from the laser cavity itself or by opening up the beam delivery optics and gaining access to collimated laser beams prior to the beam focusing optics or fiberoptic beam delivery system. Frequently, the hazardous beam is a specular reflection from a turning mirror or Brewster window in the laser console. To protect bystanders from a beam emitted from the laser cabinet when the service person gains access, a temporary laser controlled area should be established and unprotected persons denied access to the area.

Occupational Exposure Limits

Relevant exposure limits for lasers of interest are given in Table 12-1 and are calculated or measured at the cornea. If the laser beam is less than 7 mm in diameter, it is assumed that the entire beam could enter the dark-adapted pupil, and one can express the maximal safe power or energy in the beam (in the 0.4 to 1.4 μm retinal hazard region); it is the exposure limit multiplied by the area of a 7 mm pupil (i.e., 0.4 cm^2). For example, for the visible continuous wave lasers, an exposure limited by the natural aversion response of 0.25 second is 2.5 mW/cm^2, and this exposure limit multiplied by 0.4 cm^2 results in the limiting power of 1 mW. This 1 mW value has a special significance in laser safety standards, as it is the accessible emission limit (AEL) of class 2 (i.e., the dividing line between two laser safety hazard classifications: class 2 and class 3).

Laser Hazard Classification

As mentioned, the continuous wave visible laser (400–700 nm) that has an output power of less than 1 mW is termed a class 2 (low risk) laser, and could be considered more or less equivalent in risk with staring at the sun, at a tungsten-halogen spotlight, or at other bright lights that can cause photic maculopathy (central retinal injury). Only if individuals force themselves to overcome their natural aversion response to bright light, can a class 2 laser pose a real ocular hazard. An aiming beam or alignment laser operating at a total power above 1 mW would fall into hazard class 3 and could be hazardous even if viewed momentarily within the aversion response time. A subcategory of class 3, termed class 3a, comprises lasers of 1 to 5 mW in power; and these lasers pose a moderate ocular hazard under viewing conditions where most of the beam enters the eye. Class 3b is then the subcategory that comprises, certain pulsed lasers and all continuous wave visible lasers that emit 5 to 500 mW. Even momentary viewing of class 3b lasers is potentially hazardous to the eye (Hirsch et al., 1992; ACGIH, 1993).

Only lasers that are totally enclosed or that emit extremely low output powers fall into class 1 and are safe to view. Any continuous wave laser with an output power above 0.5 watt (500 mW) falls into class 4. Class 4 lasers are considered to pose skin or fire hazards as well as eye hazards if not properly used. The purpose of assigning hazard classes to laser products is to simplify the determination of adequate safety measures; that is, class 3a measures are more stringent than class 2 measures, and class 4 measures are more stringent than class 3b measures. Virtually all surgical lasers fall into class 4.

Laser Eye Protectors

In the operating room laser eye protectors provide the principal means to ensure against ocular injury from the direct or reflected laser beams. In this regard, ordinary optical glass protects against all wavelengths shorter than 300 nm and longer than 2,700 nm only. Laser protective filters may be obtained for endoscopes and other viewing optics for the spectral region between these two spectral bands. However, from a practical standpoint, these are seldom used. Eye protectors are available as spectacles, wraparound lenses, goggles, and related forms of eyewear. It is important that the eyewear be marked with the wavelengths and optical densities at those wavelengths. The markings should be understood by the operating room staff. Clear plastic safety glasses with side shields known to be made of polycarbonate are suitable for use with the 10.6 μm CO^2 laser but should be marked by the Laser Safety Officer with "OD = 4 at CO_2 wavelength 10.6 μm." Eyewear for one laser wavelength cannot be routinely assumed to work for another wavelength.

Airborne Contaminants

One of the more perplexing safety issues related to laser surgery is not an optical radiation hazard but the potential hazard from breathing vaporized tissue: Both the chemical toxicity and the pathogenicity of the airborne contaminants are of concern. At the high temperatures in the laser ablation zone it is difficult to imagine that viable tissue could be present in the "plume." Nevertheless, Garden et al. (1988) demonstrated the presence of viral particles in vaporized tissue, and Baggish et al. (1991) showed that fragments of human immunodeficiency virus (HIV) DNA could be present in the laser plume. Local exhaust ventilation is therefore important. This is essential for gas arthroscopy with the laser.

Arthroscopic Damage

Damage to the arthroscope itself can occur by either directly firing the laser into the lens and destroying it or by heating the metal cover, causing the cement that secures the lens to melt, thereby allowing water vapor to leak inside the arthroscope. Obviously, surgeons should not touch the arthroscope in any way with the laser beam (Brillhart, 1992).

Conclusions

The potential hazardous exposure levels to the eye and skin from *scattered* laser radiation from most surgical laser applications are substantially below threshold. The *direct beam* or *specular reflections* are of concern. Precautions to prevent inadvertent exposure to the eye, skin, and flammable material should be taken (**see Chapter 13**). Smoke evacuation is needed for gas arthroscopy with the laser. Only with ultraviolet lasers should one be seriously concerned with chronic exposure and delayed effects. Nevertheless, the surgical laser user can be assured that today a consensus exists almost worldwide (IRPA, 1985; ACGIH, 1993; ANSI, 1988, 1993; IEC, 1993) regarding the appropriate laser safety measures to preclude injury from acute or chronic effects.

References

ACGIH (1993) TLV's threshold limit values and biological exposure indices for 1990–1991. American Conference of Governmental Industrial Hygienists, Cincinnati, OH

ANSI (1988) Safe use of lasers in health care facilities. Standard Z-136.3-1988. American National Standards Institute, Laser Institute of America, Orlando, FL

ANSI (1993) Safe use of lasers. Standard Z-136.1-1993, American National Standards Institute, Laser Institute of America, Orlando, FL

Baggish MS, Poiesz BJ, Joret D, Williamson P, Refai A (1991) Presence of human immunodeficiency virus DNA in laser smoke. Laser Surg Med vol. 11, pp. 197–203

Brillhart AT (1991) Arthroscopic laser surgery. Am J Arthroscopy 1:5–12

Brillhart AT (1992) Technical problems of laser arthroscopy. Abstracts Arthroscopy: The Journal of Arthroscopic and Related Surgery vol. 8, no. 3, pp. 403–4

Garden JM, O'Banion MK, Shelnitz LS, Pinski KS, Bakus AD, Reichman ME, Sundberg JP (1988) Papillomavirus in the vapor of carbon dioxide laser-treated verrucae. JAMA vol. 259, pp. 1199–1202

Hirsch DR, Booth DG, Schocket S, Sliney DH (1992) Recovery from pulsed-dye laser retinal injury. Arch Ophthalmol, 110:1688

IEC, International Electrotechnical Commission (1993) Radiation safety of laser products. Equipment Classification and User's Guide, Document WS 825-1, IEC, Geneva

IRPA, International Non-Ionizing Radiation Committee (1985) Guidelines for limits of human exposure to laser radiation. Health Physics vol. 49, no. 5, pp. 341–359

Sliney DH, Wolbarsht ML (1980) Safety with lasers and other optical sources. Plenum Publishing Corp, New York

Sliney DH, Mainster MA (1987) Potential laser hazards to the clinician during photocoagulation. Amer J Ophthalmol vol. 103, pp. 758–760

Sliney DH, Trokel SL (1992) Medical lasers and their safe use. Springer-Verlag, New York

Wood RL, Sliney DH, Basye RA (1992) Laser reflections from surgical instruments. Lasers Surg Med, 12:675–678

13

Safety and Institutional Controls

Allen T. Brillhart and Michele Cook

The institution in which a laser is used is responsible for regulating its use and ensuring the safety of the patients and personnel involved. It includes the control and monitoring of manufacturers' representatives, vendors, and rental agents when they are in the institution. The following are outlines of example policies used for these purposes.

Composition of the Laser Safety Committee

The committee should be composed of, but not limited to, the following members:

Chief of medical advisory board or designee
Director of nursing
Laser safety officer
Chief of anesthesia or designee
Biomedical engineer
Administration or financial representative
Surgeon from each department utilizing a laser

Duties of the Laser Safety Committee

The duties of the Laser Safety Committee should be as follows:

1. To review, no less often than annually, laser safety policies and standards of practice.
2. To be responsible for coordinating ongoing activity as to the laser(s) in the center (i.e., credentialing, education requirements, maintenance, reviewing of standards to ensure they are current).
3. To ensure that (a) the standards address, as a minimum, restriction of those allowed to use the laser clinically; and (b) they have attended a laser workshop with a minimum of 4 hours CME-approved credit. The workshop should include hands-on experience, laser basic sciences, laser safety, and equipment operation (must submit course outline).
4. To ensure that each physician requiring laser privileges has the necessary credentials that are wavelength- and procedure-specific. This physician must be credentialed in the basic laser procedures, but this certification does not credential the surgeon for similar procedures that do not require use of the laser.
5. To ensure that the credentialed surgeons be reviewed by the Laser Safety Committee at the time of recredentialing for continued use of the laser. (Credentialed individuals who have not used the laser or attended an updated hands-on workshop between review periods require proctoring until the laser safety committee deems the reinstatement application appropriate.)
6. To assist in the final decision as to the model purchased when a new laser is required.
7. To review and act on all incidents and accidents.
8. To meet no less than quarterly and maintain a permanent record of its proceedings, actions, reports, findings, and recommendations to the credentialing and risk management committees. A quorum of at least 50% of the members must be present.

Laser Safety Officer

The laser safety officer, under the general direction of the director of nursing, directs, organizes, and coordinates all activities of the laser program. The laser safety officer functions as facilitator of nursing practice for quality patient care. The following is a list of typical responsibilities of the laser safety officer:

1. Supervises and evaluates, during training, the staff of the laser program
2. Assesses and evaluates the quality of care delivered

Any use of the material from *Medical Lasers and Their Safe Use* (1992) by David H. Sliney and Steven L. Trohel is by permission of Springer-Verlag. The author would also like to acknowledge the importance of the work of K.A. Ball, *Lasers:* The Perioperative Challenge.

and determines action to be taken in regard to staffing patterns and staff development needs; maintains, evaluates, and reports quality ensurance indicators
3. Coordinates the activities of the laser program within the operating room
4. Collaborates with director of nursing and the schedule coordinator to meet the needs of the physician, patient, and institution
5. Identifies learning needs of the staff; plans, develops, coordinates, implements, and evaluates teaching tools for individual and group education and support
6. Initiates and recommends policies and procedures necessary to achieve safe and appropriate use of the laser and the objectives of the laser program
7. Serves on the laser committee and functions as the laser resource person to physicians and staff members
8. Reviews, reports, and evaluates laser statistics to note trends as requested
9. Assists with laser procedures as needed
10. Remains current in the field of laser surgery
11. Ensures the appropriate medical surveillance of all workers, including eye examinations
12. Ensures that all workers are adequately trained
13. Maintains the laser log

Laser Safety Policy

The following rules and regulations must be observed by all physicians utilizing a laser and by all employees and any other individuals present during the demonstration or utilization of laser equipment. A copy of the rules and regulations should be issued to each individual directly or indirectly involved in the use of the laser.

1. When the laser is in use, the operating room staff directly involved in the procedure must wear a gown, gloves, laser mask, and protective eyewear. Laser-specific protective eyewear must be worn by all personnel within the room. Patients who are awake must wear a laser mask to eliminate contact with the smoke plume.
2. Patients undergoing laser procedures on the head and neck must have their eyes lubricated with a water-based artificial tear solution, taped closed, and covered with a moist eye pad or proper, specific eyewear. Eye pads should be kept moist throughout the procedure. Patients with local or regional block anesthesia must wear eyewear specific to the laser being used.
3. The laser is not used in the presence of flammables or explosives [i.e., anesthetics, preparation solutions, degreasing agents, combustible drying agents, or methane (intestinal gas)].
4. The master control key for the laser is retained by the laser safety officer(s) or designee who shall limit access to only those personnel qualified to use or operate the laser. The key is removed from the laser when it is not in use and is kept in the locked operating room medication room key cabinet.
5. A sign is posted on each operating room door leading into the room when the laser is in use. The sign states the type and class of laser, its maximum output, and the aiming beam and its output. Appropriate eye glasses are put with the sign on each door.
6. All physicians desiring to use the laser clinically must have been granted privileges by the institution's credentialing committee. A list of credentialed physicians is maintained at the surgical schedule desk along with the surgeons' privileges files.
7. The laser safety officer(s) or designee must be present whenever the laser is in operation. The laser safety officer/designee has full authority to supervise and control the laser. The laser safety officer/designee functions only as the laser operator during a procedure. Circulating duties are delegated to a registered nurse. The laser safety officer must be an institution employee.
8. The laser machine remains off when not in use.
9. During the laser operation, the machine is placed on Standby when adjusting the power meter or when using other instrumentation (i.e., cautery, bipolar, or dissection). A verbal exchange must be undertaken between the laser surgeon and the laser operator at all times when there is a change in settings or power and regarding all other machine adjustments.
10. The operating surgeon controls the laser foot pedal with *no other* foot pedal(s) to operate.
11. All instrumentation and contiguous tissue are covered with moist sponges, towels, or cottonoids.
12. Those instruments that cannot be covered are brushed-finish or ebonized if laser beam reflectance is a danger.
13. During oral, nasopharyngeal, or laryngotracheal surgery, the endotracheal tube, if used, must be a special laser-shielded tube. Cuffs are inflated with dyed saline and padded with moist cottonoids. **(CAUTION: Laser-shielded tubes can be used only when the laser is in pulsed mode and under 20 watts of power.)** Any visible reflective surface shall be covered with moist cottonoids. **A polyvinylchloride tube must never be used.**
14. Suction tubing to evacuate smoke and fluid from the operative site is attached to a suction canister in conjunction with a smoke evacuator or in-line filter.
15. Specifically manufactured laser facial masks should be worn by all personnel during laser operations to prevent inhalation of laser plumes.
16. Only medical grade gases are purchased for use with the laser. The supplying company must provide written assurance of the purity of the gas and assume responsibility for any laser tube damage resulting from impure gases.
17. The laser safety officer, schedule coordinator, or director of nursing has the authority to shut down the

laser in event of malfunction of the laser or associated equipment or noncompliance with the institution's policy and procedures for laser use.

18. Procedure- and wavelength-specific precautions must be observed.
19. A baseline funduscopic eye examination, including a macular evaluation, is required of all laser personnel and physicians.

10.6 μm CO_2 Laser Policy

WARNING: The 10.6 μm CO_2 laser is potentially hazardous if not properly used. The emergent beam can burn the skin or eyes or ignite clothing of the operator, bystanders, or patient. Do not use volatile sterilizing agents in the operative field, as a flash fire may occur. Heat generated by the laser may cause the glass to fragment. Eye protection is usually required, and adequate venting of vaporized tissue is essential to avoid exposure to potential toxic agents produced in the plume.

Use of the 10.6 μm CO_2 laser is restricted to physicians and staff members properly trained or credentialed. The purpose of these limits is to provide for patient safety during the use of the laser, personnel safety during use of the laser, and proper care and handling of the laser.

1. Only personnel qualified to use and operate the laser should have access to the laser key. The key is removed when the laser is not in operation and is kept locked in the operating room medication room key cabinet.
2. The laser safety officer or designee, trained in the proper care and handling of the laser, is assigned to each case.
3. The laser operator is responsible for documenting, on the operating room/laser record, the type of laser used.
4. A log is maintained and kept at the operating room control desk. The laser operator is responsible for recording the following information on each case.
   a. Patient information (label)
   b. Physician performing laser treatment
   c. Type of procedure
   d. Wattage, seconds, and mode used
   e. Microscope/lens used, if applicable
5. Preoperative, intraoperative, and postoperative safety checklists are completed by the nurse for each procedure and maintained in the laser logbook.
6. All personnel, including the anesthesiologist, should wear laser safety eye protection with appropriate wavelength and optical density. Contact lenses, half-glasses, and sunglasses are not sufficient. Protective eyewear is not necessary for physicians using the microscope.
7. Additional goggles are kept at ready access outside the laser surgery room for personnel entering the laser area.
8. The patient's eyes should be covered with moist eye pads, which are kept moist throughout the procedure. When performing surgery under local or regional block anesthesia, the patient should wear protective eyewear.
9. Signs are posted on all doors entering the room, stating, "Laser surgery in progress."
10. The laser beam should not be aimed at any personnel, and personnel should not look directly into the 10.6 μm CO_2 or 0.632 μm helium-neon light source.
11. When the laser is not in use, the laser safety officer/designee switches the laser to Standby mode. If the laser is not in use for a substantial length of time, it should be turned off.
12. The laser should not be used in the presence of flammable anesthetics.
13. Alcohol solutions should not be used as a preparatory agent.
14. Whenever the laser is used near the area of the endotracheal tube special precautions must be observed: The laser endotracheal tube must be used as per the manufacturer's instructions.
15. All sponges on the field are moistened when the laser is used. Drapes close to the surgical site are covered with moist lap pads or moist towels.
16. Guard against the laser beam coming in contact with reflective instruments.
17. Extra suction should be available for the plume of smoke from vaporization of tissue. The suction bottle port exiting to the wall vacuum should be connected with a filter, available from the suction canister manufacturer. A heavy-duty smoke evacuator may be necessary for vaporization of large areas. Laser masks should be worn when the laser is in use.
18. The rectum must be packed with wet sponges when laser surgery is performed in the perineal area: Methane gas is flammable, and a burn could occur.
19. The laser team is responsible for the cleaning, maintenance, and storage of laser instruments and equipment. After the operation is completed, return the arm to its proper position and secure the arm in its holder.
20. Surgical consent must be obtained from the patient, specifying the laser surgery to be performed.
21. Comply with the institution's policy for laser safety at all times.
22. Direct the laser beam at a target board to ensure location and quality of the focal spot. Use the built-in calibrations, if available. Check to ensure that connectors in the articulated arm are properly attached and secure.
23. Use the focusing head that has the shortest focal length applicable for each procedure. This practice minimizes any specular (mirror-like) reflections, because the reflected beam diverges more rapidly.
24. Do not use cautery with this laser.

25. Wear flame-retardant surgical clothing. Check that laundering does not change flammability characteristics. (Fabric softener is known to impair flame-retardation treatments.)
26. Maintain the plume exhaust nozzle within 10 cm of the site of laser vaporization at all times; surgical masks must be worn.
27. Biomedical engineering representatives should be called if technical difficulties arise.
28. The surgeon and anesthesiologist should be aware of the risk of a gas embolus, and know how to recognize and treat it.
29. When gas insufflation is used, all operators must be trained on proper technique.
30. The gas insufflation device must be in proper working order before use. The biomedical engineer must inspect this device periodically.

1.06 μm Neodymium:YAG Laser Policy

WARNING: The 1.06 μm neodymium:YAG laser is potentially hazardous if not properly used. The emergent beam can burn the skin or eyes or ignite clothing of the operator, bystanders, or the patient. Do not use volatile sterilizing agents in the operative field, as a flash fire may occur. Heat generated by the laser may cause the glass to fragment. Eye protection is usually required and adequate venting of vaporized tissue is essential to avoid exposure to potential toxic agents produced in the plume.

Follow these precautions to minimize the hazards to the eyes of bystanders from the direct and reflected beams of this laser.

1. If patient is not positioned in the beam path, the beam should be directed toward the wall. Reflected beams should strike a nearby wall behind the laser operator.
2. Do not allow persons without eye protection behind or at the side of the laser operator during laser treatment.
3. One or more pairs of eye protection (optical density of at least 5 at 1.06 μm) should be readily available at all times.
4. To avoid unauthorized use of a laser not in use, remove and secure the keyswitch master control key.
5. Only authorized persons knowledgeable in the use of the laser should operate the laser.
6. Post a laser warning sign at the closed door during laser operation.
7. If technical difficulties arise, contact the biomedical engineering representative.
8. Only contact lenses approved by the chief of service should be used with the laser.

1.44 μm Neodymium:YAG Laser Policy

WARNING: The 1.44 μm neodymium:YAG laser can be potentially hazardous if not properly used. The emergent beam can burn the skin or eyes or ignite the clothing of the operator, bystanders, or patient. Do not use volatile sterilizing agents in the operative field, as a flash fire may occur. Heat generated by the laser may cause the glass to fragment. Eye protection is usually required, and adequate venting of vaporized tissue is essential to avoid exposure to potential toxic agents produced in the plume.

Follow these precautions to minimize the hazards to the eyes of bystanders, from the direct and reflected beams of this laser.

1. If patient is not positioned in the beam path, the beam should be directed toward the wall. Reflected beams should strike a nearby wall behind the laser operator.
2. Do not allow persons without eye protection behind or at the side of the laser operator during laser treatment.
3. One or more pairs of eye protection (optical density of at least 5 at 1.44 μm) should be readily available at all times.
4. To avoid unauthorized use of a laser that is not in use, remove and secure the keyswitch master control key.
5. Only authorized persons knowledgeable in the use of the laser should operate the laser.
6. Post a laser warning sign at the closed door during laser operation.
7. If technical difficulties arise, contact the biomedical engineering representative.
8. Only contact lenses approved by the chief of service should be used with the laser.

0.532 μm KTP Laser Policy

WARNING: The 0.532 μm KTP laser is potentially hazardous if not properly used. The emergent beam can burn the skin or eyes or ignite clothing of the operator, bystanders, or patient. Do not use volatile sterilizing agents in the operative field, as a flash fire may occur. Heat generated by the laser may cause the glass to fragment. Eye protection is required, and adequate venting of vaporized tissue is essential to avoid exposure to potential toxic agents produced in the plume.

Follow the precautions noted below to minimize the hazards. Use of the 1.06 μm neodymium:YAG laser is not the same as that for the 0.532 μm KTP laser. The purpose of these precautions is to ensure safe and proper use of the 0.532 μm KTP (frequency-doubled 1.06 μm neodymium:YAG) laser system with fiberoptic delivery system, to provide safe conditions for the patient and operating room staff, and to provide optimum usage of the laser equipment.

1. Only personnel qualified to use and operate the laser should have access to the laser key. The key should be removed when the laser is not in operation and kept locked in the operating room medication key cabinet.
2. Before inserting the optical fiber into the endoscopic delivery system:
   a. Ensure that the laser is in the Off or Standby mode;

inspect the tip for cleanliness with a magnifying loupe.
b. Insert the fiber into the laser power monitor, turn on the laser, and adjust and calibrate the output power.
3. Ensure that the fiber cannot easily slip out of the endoscope. If a short endoscopic device is used, secure the fiber to the device to prevent accidental escape of the fiber.
4. One or more pairs of eye protection (optical density of at least 5 at 0.532 μm) should be readily available at all times. Eye protection should be worn by all persons within 60 cm of the fiber tip at any time the optical fiber has been intentionally removed from the endoscope and is not clamped in the power monitor.
5. Post a laser warning sign at the closed door during laser operation.

0.632 μm Helium-Neon Aiming Beam Laser Policy

WARNING: The 0.632 μm helium-neon aiming beam is not entirely safe.

1. Only authorized, trained personnel may operate the laser.
2. Do not direct the laser beam at the eye or at any reflective surfaces.
3. Secure the laser when not in use.
4. When directing the beam near the patient's face, secure eye protection over the patient's eyes.

2.1 μm Holmium:YAG Laser Policy

WARNING: The 2.1 μm holmium:YAG surgical laser is potentially hazardous to the operator, bystanders, or patient if not properly used. The emergent beam can burn the skin or eyes and ignite clothing.

Precautions must be followed to to minimize the potential hazard. The material below delineates proper use of the 2.1 μm holmium:YAG laser according to safety rules and regulations established by the institution's medical advisory board.

1. Obtain laser key, equipment, and laser.
2. Move equipment to the room in which the laser will be used.
3. Post "Holmium laser in use" signs on all doors; secure additional safety eyewear on each door entering the room; and cover all windows in the room.
4. Keep operating room door closed.
5. Position the laser and plug into a 220-volt outlet.
6. Put on safety glasses specific for the 2.1 μm holmium:YAG laser. All personnel and the patient in the operating room must wear laser safety glasses or goggles with a minimum optical density of 4.0 at 2.1 μm to prevent accidental eye damage.
7. Open sterile items and place in the sterile field. For the sterile fiber delivery system, have a spare handpiece of the same degree available at all times.
8. Insert fiber delivery system into the fiberoptic receptacle; ensure a proper connection.
9. Turn key on. Warm up laser 30 minutes before the first case.
10. Select desired energy by depressing the energy/pulse increase or decrease button.
11. Select the rate by depressing the increase or decrease button.
12. Select aiming beam intensity.
13. Place the foot pedal near the surgeon's foot. *Only one foot pedal at a time is to be near the surgeon's foot.*
14. Press the Ready mode when the surgeon states that he or she is ready to deliver the treatment beam. Always return to Standby mode when the laser is not in use.
15. Turn key off at the end of the procedure and record the energy settings and total energy utilized in the operating room laser record.
16. Comply with the institution's policy for laser safety at all times.

Laser Credentialing of Physicians

A written policy is established for those who wish to use lasers within the institution, requiring the physician to obtain the necessary training and experience in the safe and appropriate use of lasers.

1. The physician seeking laser credentials must have staff privileges in good standing at the institution.
2. The physician must send a copy of the certificate of attendance for a laser course (4 hours CME credit, to include safety, basic science, hands-on, and equipment operation training) to the chairman of the laser safety committee. The certificate should state the types of lasers involved and the number of contact hours given. Special consideration is given by the laser committee to physicians who undergo laser coursework and have gained experience during their residency or fellowship training. Appropriate documentation must be submitted to verify this experience. Clinical requirements are issued for each laser type and are not transferable to another laser.
3. Laser coursework or education programs are reviewed by the laser committee for approval of appropriateness, including those on safety, basic science, hands-on, and equipment operation.
4. The laser committee chairman contacts the physicians seeking laser credentialing to communicate that the coursework has been approved.
5. Applicants are required to meet with the laser safety officer for familiarization with the institution's lasers and equipment. They are also required to have a practice session before using the laser on patients. A preceptorship should be required.

6. The physician seeking laser credentials must contact a physician already credentialed in using that particular wavelength to precept the laser procedure (oversee the safe and appropriate use of the laser and complete a preceptor form). The laser safety officer delivers the completed form to the laser committee chairman.
7. The laser committee chairman submits the copy of the laser coursework and the preceptor form(s) to the director of administrative services for filing in the physician's folder. The specialty department chairman is notified to process the physician's request for privileges, and the credentials committee is told to make recommendations on which the governing board can act at their next scheduled meeting.
8. The credentials committee/medical advisory board action is forwarded to the governing board for final approval. The physician receives a written communication from the executive director as to the status of the laser credentialing approval. A copy of this letter is kept in the physician's file in the administrator's office.
9. The laser credentialing status is documented in the laser credentialing file of the institution by the laser committee chairman.
10. Preceptors are credentialed, experienced, laser surgeons who observe, guide, and certify the applicant's acceptable performance. They report their findings, good or bad, to the laser safety committee. They have the authority to stop laser usage at any time during the preceptorship.

Investigational Requirements

To use a laser that is not market-approved by the U.S. Food and Drug Administration (FDA) for a specific procedure, the laser-credentialed physician must provide the institutional review board (IRB) of the institution consent for the procedure. The IRB reviews and grants approval to perform the procedure if all of the specified criteria have been met. The IRB routinely monitors the status of each investigational protocol to continue the investigation.

Physician Annual Credentialing Review Policy

The purpose of the annual physician review is to provide a means of reviewing physician laser utilization and to monitor laser credentialing status on an annual basis.

1. Each laser-credentialed physician's utilization is noted based on statistics for the previous fiscal year.
2. Physicians with fewer than three laser procedures recorded are designated "low users." The laser committee then contacts each physician to determine the reason for the low utilization.
3. The laser committee reviews the analysis and recommends corrective measures to increase utilization and to help physicians who are "low users" to remain proficient in the laser's use.

Forms Used

Laser Privilege Form

Requirements of the laser safety committee for the credentialing of laser privileges:

The applicant must have received minimum laser surgery training from a recognized 4 hour CME, including laser basic science, laser safety, hands-on experience, and equipment operation. This training may be waived based on documentation of residency training or previous experience and proficiency with appropriate credentialing at another institution [attach documentation].

Applicant: I understand and have reviewed the policies and safety procedures for the laser surgery privileges for which I now apply.

Name: ______________________
(Please Print)

Office Address ______________________

____

____

Signature ____________ Date ____________

Certification of Laser Education

Laser course [attach CME certification copy and course outline]

Name ______________________

Program Director ______________________

Location ______________________

Date ______________________

I have read all safety rules of the institution and will follow them.

____
Signature

Preceptor Form

A separate preceptor form is required for each laser type requested. In specialties in which adjunctive instrumentation for therapy is required, certification of training and documentation of experience with such instruments must be provided.

Wavelength: ☐ 10.6 μm CO_2 ☐ 2.1 μm holmium:YAG ☐ 1.06 μm neodymium:YAG ☐ 1.44 μm neodymium:YAG

Specfic Procedure ______________________

____________ Signed ____________
Date Applicant

____________ ____________
Date Laser Section Representative

____________ ____________
Date Laser Safety Chairman

Having satisfied above requirement, the applicant must demonstrate to his/her department chairman, in a minimum of three (3) procedures, his/her ability to operate in a safe and effective manner.

____________ ____________
Date of 1st Preceptor Signature

____________ ____________
Date of 2nd Preceptor Signature

____________ ____________
Date of 3rd Preceptor Signature

I believe this applicant has demonstrated adequate proficiency in this procedure and so recommend unrestricted privileges.

Final approval

____________ Approved ____________
Preceptor for Last Procedure Laser Section Representative

____________ ____________
Date Laser Safety Chairman

____________ ____________
Date Medical Advisory Board Chairman

____________ ____________
Date Governing Board Chairman

Sample Laser Intraoperative Record

CO_2 Laser Log # ______________ □N/A ______________ (Other Laser Type) Log # ________ □N/A

Date: ______________ Laser Tested By: ______________________ Time: ______________

CO_2 Laser Settings □N/A

Watts	Seconds	Cont.	S.P.1	S.P.2	Time On	Time off	Total Time

______________ (Other Laser Type) Laser Settings □N/A

Energy Pulse Joules	Pulse/Sec	Avg Power/Watts		Total Energy Kilojoules	Time On	Time Off	Total Time

Personal Safety

Warning Signs Posted On Doors	□Yes	□No
Involved Personnel Wear Appropriate Safety Glasses	□Yes	□No
H_2O Basin in Room	□Yes	□No
Safety Eyewear Placed in Hallway	□Yes	□No
Windows Covered	□Yes	□No

Patient Safety

Eye Protection	□Goggles	□Moist gauze	□Covered with moist towel	
Operative Area Drapes	□Dispos.	□Cloth	□Combin.	□None
Prep Soln. Dried	□Yes	□N/A		
Moist Sponges On Field	□Yes	□N/A		
E.T. Tube Protected	□Yes	□N/A	Type ________	

Laser Accessories

In Line Laser Plume Filter □Yes □N/A Smoke Evacuator □Yes □N/A

□Microscope □Endoscope Type ______________ □Free Hand

□Fiber Lot # ______________________________ □N/A

Regulation of Vendors

Vendors, rental agents, and manufacturing representatives should obviously not be allowed to perform arthroscopic laser surgery on patients. Their exact role depends on many factors, but it must be defined by the rules and regulations for laser use of the institution. The ultimate responsibility for their action and safety rests with the institution. The institution must not believe that the vendor is justified in assuming responsibility. Granting privileges is an established responsibility of the hospitals and ambulatory surgical centers.

Conclusion

Institutions should adapt or modify the policies and procedures outlined. Constant revision, updating, and additions to these policies must occur as laser technology and laser surgical practices evolve.

References

ACGIH (1993) TLV's threshold limit values and biological exposure indices for 1990–1991. American Conference of Governmental Industrial Hygienists, Cincinnati, OH

ANSI (1988) Safe use of lasers in health care facilities. Standard Z-136.3-1988. American National Standards Institute, Laser Institute of America, Orlando, FL

ANSI (1993) Safe use of lasers. Standard Z-136.1-1993, American National Standards Institute, Laser Institute of America, Orlando, FL

Baggish MS, Poiesz BJ, Joret D, Williamson P, Refai A (1991) Presence of human immunodeficiency virus DNA in laser smoke. Laser Surg Med 11:197–203

Ball KA (1990) Lasers. The perioperative challenge. C.V. Mosby Company, St. Louis, MO

Brillhart AT (1992) Technical problems of laser arthroscopy. Abstracts Arthroscopy: The Journal of Arthroscopic and Related Surgery 8:403–4

Garden JM, O'Banion MK, Shelnitz LS, Pinski KS, Bakus AD, Reichman ME, Sundberg JP (1988) Papillomavirus in the vapor of carbon dioxide laser-treated verrucae. JAMA 259:1199-1202

Hirsch DR, Booth DG, Schocket S, Sliney DH (1992) Recovery from pulsed-dye laser retinal injury. Arch Ophthalmol 110:1688

IEC, International Electrotechnical Commission (1993) Radiation safety of laser products. Equipment Classification and User's Guide, Document WS 825-1, IEC, Geneva

IRPA, International Non-Ionizing Radiation Committee (1985) Guidelines for limits of human exposure to laser radiation. Health Physics 49:341–359

Sliney DH, Wolbarsht ML (1980) Safety with lasers and other optical sources. Plenum Publishing Corp, New York

Sliney DH, Mainster MA (1987) Potential laser hazards to the clinician during photocoagulation. Amer J Ophthalmol 103:758-760

Sliney DH, Trokel SL (1992) Medical lasers and their safe use. Springer-Verlag, New York

Wood RL, Sliney DH, Basye RA (1992) Laser reflections from surgical instruments. Lasers Surg Med 12:675–678

14

Technical Problems of First Generation Arthroscopic Laser Surgery

Allen T. Brillhart

The enthusiasm of laser arthroscopy is accompanied by technical problems that should be viewed by all arthroscopists. First generation 10.6 μm CO_2 lasers have been the most cumbersome systems. The dual gas and liquid mediums they require have been burdensome (Brillhart 1991b, 1992). The large waveguides and associated defocused laser beams used with the first generation 10.6 μm CO_2 laser systems made them more prone to inadvertent tissue damage when compared to the newer, smaller waveguides. The delivery systems for the 1.06 μm neodymium:YAG and first generation 2.1 μm holmium:YAG lasers were more user friendly but were associated with probe failures and tip breakages (Brillhart l991c, d, 1992). The angles of the probes and the probe tip designs were not suited ideally for all arthroscopic procedures. Arthroscopists must be aware that some of these problems have yet to be eliminated. Surgeons should familiarize themselves with associated potential technical problems and be prepared to deal with them. The latest generation laser systems should be considered for use.

Materials and Methods

The first 100 laser-assisted arthroscopic procedures I performed have been reviewed: Ten were done using the 10.6 μm CO_2 laser, 10 with the contact 1.06 μm neodymium:YAG laser, and 80 with the 2.1 μm holmium:YAG laser using a 15-watt system. There were 4 shoulder procedures and 96 knee procedures. Technical problems not noted by me but reported by surgeons at scientific meetings are included in this chapter (Marquez and Nelson, 1990; Massam and Crowgey, 1990; Abelow, 1991; Garrick, 1991a; Miller, 1991; O'Brien and Miller, 1991; O'Brien, 1991; Sherk et al., 1990; Siebert, 1991; Smith, 1991). Because of the small number of cases and because they were early cases during which the number of technical problems were expected to be high, no statistical analysis was performed. The problems are divided into those that were avoidable and those that were unavoidable. Avoidable problems were those the surgeon could have avoided with experience. Unavoidable problems were those that required improved laser systems, primarily the responsibility of the laser manufacturers.

Results

Avoidable problems common to all three laser systems included: inadvertent tissue damage, inadvertent laser firing, improper portal selection, probe contamination, failure to comply with eyewear rules, fogging of laser goggles, slow ablation, slow cutting or coagulation, failure to obey other laser safety rules, and failure to record energy levels used.

The most prevalent avoidable 10.6 μm CO_2 laser systems technical problems included: cumbersome articulating arms, loss of mirror alignment, need for dual gas and liquid mediums, running out of CO_2 gas, too much insufflation, fluid behind the lens, abundant laser plume, improper portal selection, debris clouding vision, damaged arthroscopic scope lens, inadvertent firing of the laser, fogging of laser goggles, failure to comply with eyewear rules, and breakage of the disposable waveguides at their attachment.

Avoidable problems prevalent with the first generation contact 1.06 μm neodymium:YAG laser system included: failure to test-fire and properly set up the laser device, probe contamination, ceramic tip breakage, failure to perform cutting or coagulation, cable breakage, and failure to comply with eyewear rules.

Avoidable problems associated with first generation 2.1 μm holmium:YAG laser arthroscopy included: failure to connect the cable to the laser device properly, failure to test-fire the laser device, intraoperative failure of the laser device, eyestrain, failure to obey laser safety rules, fracture of probe tips, inadvertent tissue damage, failure to record energy levels used, inadvertent firing of the laser, fogging of laser goggles, and failure to comply with eyewear rules.

Unavoidable first generation 10.6 μm CO_2 laser technical problems included: loss of mirror alignment, cumbersome articulating arm, dual medium of liquid and gas, need for irrigation and debridement of char, and a need for backup disposable waveguides. Unavoidable contact 1.06 μm neodymium:YAG laser technical problems included: ceramic tip burnout, improper probe tip angle, inadequate tissue ablation, and need for backup probes. Unavoidable first generation 2.1 μm holmium:YAG laser technical problems included: burnout of fiber tips, need for backup probes, and slow ablation, and coagulation.

Discussion

First Generation 10.6 μm CO_2 Laser Systems

There are several models of the 10.6 μm CO_2 laser device from various manufacturers that are applicable to arthroscopic laser surgery. They fit into two categories: (1) conventional devices with articulating arms; and (2) small, low wattage, portable units with a hand-held resonator (Brillhart, 1991b, 1992).

Conventional units have articulating arms that are believed by many to be cumbersome. The mirror systems that reflect the beam through this delivery system can become misaligned and render this device inoperable. The waveguide system that attaches to the articulating arm may not be entirely reliable on a case by case basis.

Switching from a liquid to a CO_2 medium, and back and forth again, can be technically demanding. A Y switching device has been devised for this maneuver, but it does not guarantee a smooth transition from one medium to another. Many surgeons have developed their own multiple tubing setup. If the CO_2 and the fluid are not switched properly, the fluid backs up into the probe on the permanent probe model and blocks the laser beam. Sufficient CO_2 should be available, especially for multiple procedures.

The CO_2 medium must not be insufflated beyond 1.5 pounds per square inch or excessive tissue absorption results. Even a tourniquet may not guarantee the possibility of gas emboli, though it is helpful. Gas emboli may result in airway emergencies, pneumopericardium, pneumoperitoneum, and cerebral or spinal infarction that may be fatal or result in permanent neurologic damage (Abelow, 1991). Use of gas arthroscopy in cases with open vascular beds, especially with large intraarticular fractures, may result in air emboli and death. The surgeon must be aware of these medical complications and know how to minimize, recognize, and treat them. The surgeon is referred to the anesthesia literature for a review of this subject.

Ambient air pressure is advocated, rather than gas insufflation (Garrick, 1991a,b), although, visualization may be compromised when this low pressure is used. Theoretically, this technique does not guarantee that emboli will never occur. A tourniquet should be used and the patient must be informed of these remote possibilities before surgery. Fortunately, I have never seen these problems nor heard of them occurring with the ambient air technique. Gas distention in the shoulder, spine, and temporomandibular joint is contraindicated because pneumothoraces and air emboli are common. To circumvent this problem in the shoulder, the "bubbling" technique, or "Moses" effect, has been developed. It allows the experienced surgeon to operate through a gas bubble inside a liquid medium (Smith, 1991; Smith et al., 1992). This technique is difficult to learn and is not completely reliable, especially for a beginner (Marquez and Nelson, 1990; Massam and Crowgey, 1990).

Problems with permanent probes or the disposable waveguides are sometimes aggravating. If liquid accumulates behind the laser lens attached to the permanent probe, the aiming beam and the laser beam are rendered ineffective. With the disposable waveguide system, the apparatus may break while being attached and the beam is ineffective. At least two disposable probes should always be available (Brillhart, 1991b, 1992).

Because of the debris and char produced, the arthroscopic lens frequently is covered during the procedure. It is often necessary to clean the lens by rubbing it against the synovium (Marquez and Nelson, 1990; Massam and Crowgey, 1990). If the laser beam strikes a lens, the scope is damaged and must be replaced. A backup scope should be available (Massam and Crowgey, 1990).

If the laser foot pedal is placed next to the shaver foot pedal, inadvertent firing of the laser beam may ensue. For this reason, only one foot pedal should be allowed in the field at a time. The laser probe should not be rested on the patient or on the drapes as burns or a fire may result. The standby mode must be used whenever the laser device is not actively utilized. Instruments that reflect highly may direct the 10.6 μm CO_2 beam to areas of the joint that are unsuspected, and inadvertent tissue damage may occur. Nonbrushed or blackened instruments are preferred.

Fogging of safety glasses and goggles does occur when the humidity in the room and the room temperature are not ideal. The surgeon must resist the temptation to remove the protective eyewear. Even though the patient's eyes are closed during general anesthesia, protective eyewear must be worn by the patient, as a misdirected beam may theoretically cause corneal damage.

Evacuation systems and laser masks are needed to prevent unacceptable inhaling of the plume. This point is especially important when viral spread is a concern, but even these devices are not technically guaranteed to work. If the laser device fails to work during the case, mechanical instruments should be available to take over. The patient must be forewarned of this possibility. Second laser devices are not usually readily available for backup.

First Generation Contact 1.06 μm Neodymium:YAG Laser Systems

The contact 1.06 μm neodymium:YAG arthroscopic delivery laser system was developed to adapt contact tip technology for use in arthroscopic surgery. Because of the less favorable thermal shock characteristics and reported intraoperative probe tip breakage, the conventional sapphire tips are not to be used for arthroscopy (Brillhart, 1991b, 1992). The ceramic contact laser scalpel was developed to compensate for the thermal shock encountered when a hot probe tip is introduced into a cool liquid environment. The ceramic tip works best with liquid cooling, but it can be used in a gas environment (Brillhart, 1991b, 1992; Miller, 1991; O'Brien, 1991; O'Brien and Miller, 1991). Because of the thermal characteristics, the hot ceramic tip can burn out if it is not used properly or if it is used for an excessively long time. Less than 15 minutes of continuous "on" time is usually what this probe can tolerate (Fig. 14-1). The current laser devices do not provide a time-clock and the "on" time should be clocked manually. If a longer time is needed, another probe should be used, which adds to the expense (Miller, 1991). Levering or probing with a handpiece using firm pressure can fracture the tip of the probe (Fig. 14-2). If fracture occurs, retrieval efforts may be impossible (Johnson, 1991).

Inadvertent firing is avoided by taking foot pedal precautions and using the standby mode when appropriate. The handpieces should not be rested on the patient or on the drapes. If the cable of the delivery system is broken by such things as a towel clip, a free beam risks serious eye damage (O'Brien, 1991). All personnel, especially patients, are required to wear eyewear in many hospitals, although many surgeons choose not to wear it because of its inconvenience. The laser device should be turned on and tested prior to the patient being placed under anesthesia. This maneuver prevents an unnecessary anesthetic if the laser devices fail to work properly.

Probe tip failures and fractures such as the ones seen in Figures 14-1 and 14-2 have occurred with different arthroscopic 1.06 μm neodymium:YAG systems. Although I have not directly evaluated these systems, similar technical problems have been reported by other surgeons (Abelow, 1991; Garrick, 1991b; Johnson, 1991; Smith, 1991). Mechanical instruments should be available.

First Generation 2.1 μm Holmium:YAG Laser Systems

The 2.1 μm holmium:YAG laser is a free beam laser that is believed by many to be safe for use without protective eyewear so long as one maintains a distance of at least 60 inches from the tip of the probe. Many surgeons choose not to wear goggles or glasses because of the eyestrain as-

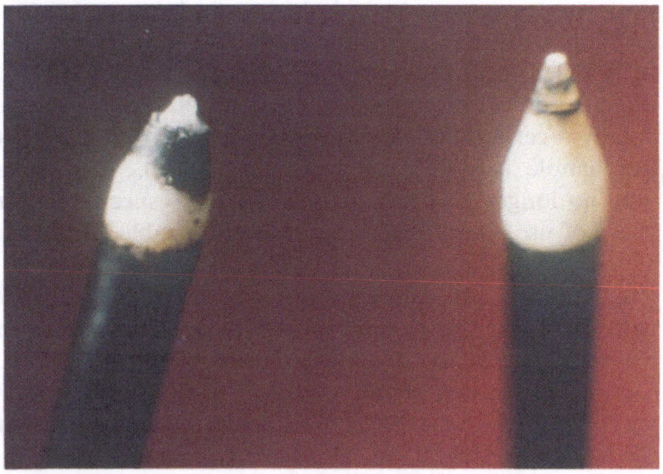

Figure 14-1. At left, the ceramic tip of a contact 1.06 μm neodymium:YAG probe has burned out. At right, is a used tip that did not burn out.

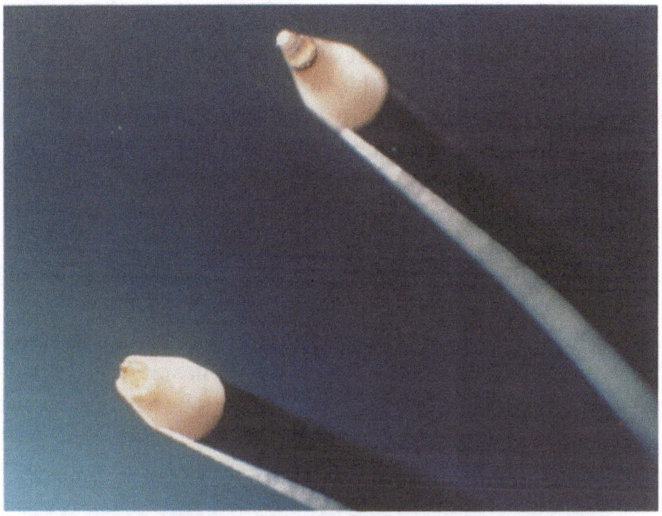

Figure 14-2. Broken ceramic tip of a contact 1.06 μm neodymium:YAG probe (bottom) compared to one after normal use (top).

sociated with them and their fogging. Various hospitals have different policies regarding the use of eyewear, which is confusing at best. A decision should be made prior to the operating procedure by the laser committee, and it should not be an ongoing topic during the procedure (Brillhart, 1991a, 1992). New standards require eyewear use, and I believe eyewear should be used.

The laser device is easy to turn on and off, similar to using any piece of electrically powered equipment. The temptation is to not test-fire the laser prior to placing the patient under anesthesia. However, it is possible that the laser device does not work, and an awkward situation may develop if the patient has been placed under anesthesia. Backup laser devices are too expensive for this practical step to be overlooked. Mechanical means of performing arthroscopic surgery must be available to back up a failed laser attempt. The patient should be told of this possibility beforehand. As with any laser fiber, there is only a certain amount of continuous "on" time that it can handle before burning out (Fig. 14-3). The probe may no longer be effective with overuse, especially after 20 kJ of use. Other probes should be available (Brillhart, 1991c, 1992).

Attempts to use the device for coagulation may be met with disappointing results. Vessels larger than 2 mm in diameter present too much of a challenge for this device. Use of 2.1 μm holmium:YAG laser for arthroscopic surgery of the shoulder to debride bursal tissue and to cut the coracoacromial ligament is a slow process.

Fiber tips break when the 30 degree angle probe is improperly inserted into the joint. Currently the manufacturer recommends that the 30 degree probe be inserted with a disposable cannula system. Better protected fiber tips should be considered (Fig. 14-4). If the fiberoptic cable is pulled or twisted with any force, it may break at the junction between the handpiece and the cable, resulting in a burn to the patient or to the surgeon's hand. Care must be taken to avoid this maneuver. A laser beam that strikes the lens of the arthroscope will damage it, and this can result in loose fragments in the joint (Fig. 14-5).

Conclusions

First generation arthroscopic laser systems have been used successfully by many surgeons. With increased experience, the technical problems encountered have become decreasingly significant and have been deemphasized. Nevertheless, most arthroscopic surgeons have chosen not to use first generation lasers in their practice. The learning curve required to overcome most of these technical problems is discouraging, especially when most arthroscopic surgeons have been comfortable with mechanical techniques. Nevertheless, manufacturers have continued to work with those surgeons who have a commitment to the advancement of laser arthroscopy to correct these problems. Hence there is wider use of the newer generation arthroscopic laser systems. Many of these better second, third, fourth, and fifth generation systems are discussed elsewhere in this text.

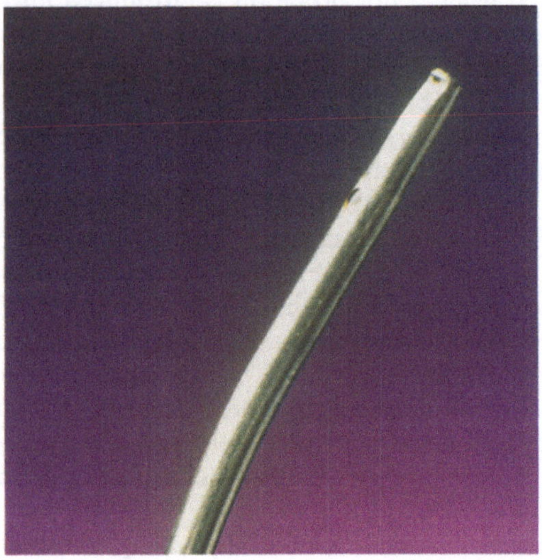

Figure 14-4. Fully protected 2.1 μm holmium:YAG fiber tip, or ring tip design, prevents breakage on insertion.

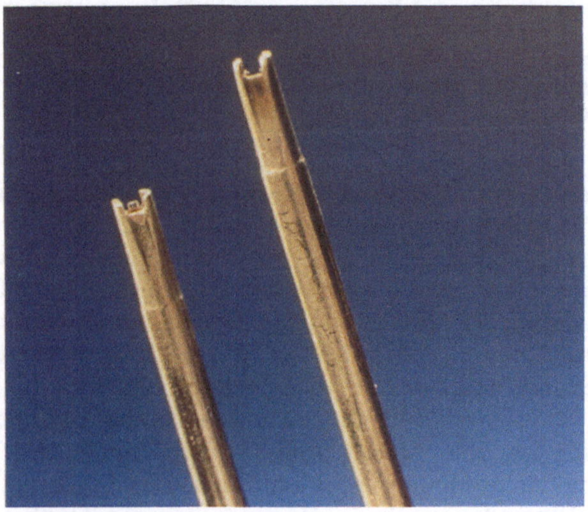

Figure 14-3. At right is the burned out fiber tip of a 2.1 μm holmium:YAG probe after 20 kJ of use. At left is the normal appearance of the fiber tip.

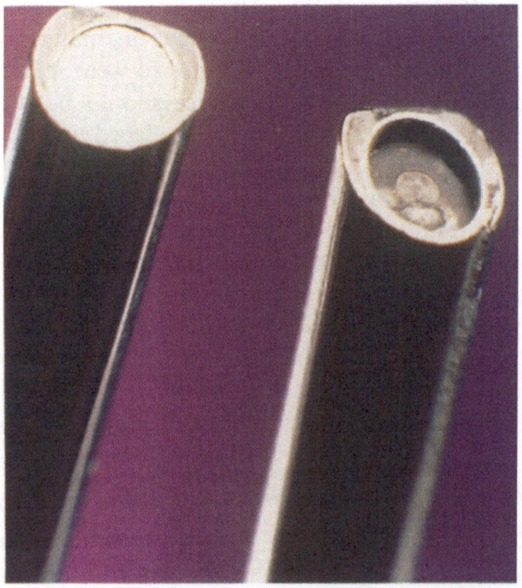

Figure 14-5. Damage to the arthroscopic lens on the right was caused by the free beam of a 2.1 μm holmium:YAG laser. (From Brillhart, 1991b. With permission.)

References

Abelow SP (1991) Use of lasers in orthopaedic surgery. Lasers in Orthopaedic Surgery: 16:551–556

Brillhart AT (1992) Technical problems of laser arthroscopy. Abstracts Arthroscopy: The Journal of Arthroscopic and Related Surgery 8:403–404

Brillhart AT (1991a) Arthroscopic laser surgery: the CO_2 laser and its use. Am J Arthroscopy 1:7–12

Brillhart AT (1991b) Arthroscopic laser surgery: the holmium:YAG laser and its use. Am J Arthroscopy 1:7–12

Brillhart AT (1991c) Arthroscopic laser surgery: the neodymium:YAG laser and its use. Am J Arthroscopy 1:7–10

Brillhart AT (1991d) Arthroscopic laser surgery: basic sciences and safety. Am J Arthroscopy 1:5–12

Garrick JG (1991a) The future of lasers. Laser Instructional Course for Orthopaedic Surgeons, Philadelphia, October

Garrick JG, Kadel N (1991b) The CO_2 laser in arthroscopy: potential problems and solutions. Arthroscopy 7:129–137

Johnson GK (1991) Letter to the editor: risk of laser tip breaking inside joint. Am J Arthroscopy 1:32

Marquez R and Nelson JS (1990) CO_2 laser in arthroscopic surgery. Educational Workshop Chicago, September

Massam R and Crowgey S (1990) CO_2 laser in arthroscopic surgery. Educational Workshop, Miami, December

Miller DV (1991) The use of the contact neodymium:YAG laser in arthroscopy. Twenty-eighth international MAPFRE traumatology-orthopaedics symposium, Madrid, Spain, November

O'Brien SJ (1991) The contact neodymium:YAG laser in arthroscopic surgery. Laser Instructional Course for Orthopaedic Surgeons, Philadelphia, October

O'Brien SJ and Miller DV (1991) The contact neodymium:YAG laser in arthroscopic surgery. Surgical Laser Technologies Symposium, Anaheim, California, March

Sherk HH, Mooar P, Matthews T (1990) Advanced laser workshop: holmium:YAG and CO_2 lasers in arthroscopic surgery. Educational Workshop, Oakland Park, Florida, July

Siebert WE (1991) Lasers in orthopaedics in Europe. Lasers in Orthopaedics: Third International Congress, Hannover, Germany, September

Smith CF, Johansen EL, Vangsness CT, Marshall GJ, Sutter LV, Bonavalet T (1992) "Gas bubble" technique in laser arthroscopic surgery. Semin Orthop 7:86–89

Smith CF (1991) CO_2 laser arthroscopy. Laser Instructional Course for Orthopaedic Surgeons, Philadelphia, October

15

Arthroscopic Laser Surgery Using the Coherent VersaPulse Select Holmium Laser

Ed Reed and Sandra Abbott

Since its introduction and U.S. Food and Drug Administration (FDA) approval for marketing in 1990, the VersaPulse laser has proved to be a powerful new tool for arthroscopic surgeons.

1. Its pulsed 2.1 μm holmium:YAG wavelength is strongly absorbed by water, so its effect on tissue is localized. The laser energy is fully absorbed in 0.5 mm of tissue.
2. Because water is the absorbing medium, it produces the same effect, independent of tissue pigmentation or type.
3. High pulse energy and peak power enables the VersaPulse to remove tissue and cartilage more efficiently than previous laser technologies (Trauner et al., 1990). This capability is rapidly improving and is expected to surpass the tissue removal efficiency of mechanical shavers.
4. The 2.1 μm holmium:YAG wavelength is highly transmitted by optical fibers. It is the fiber delivery of this wavelength in a water environment that makes it particularly useful for arthroscopic surgery. The VersaPulse laser and its fiber delivery systems offer several improvements over existing conventional techniques, including better access to difficult-to-reach areas (e.g., the posterior horn of the meniscus), more precise control of tissue removal and smoothing, and less bleeding. VersaPulse fiber delivery systems are as small as 0.68 mm in diameter (approximately three to four times smaller than conventional arthroscopic tools).

The current version of the VersaPulse, the VersaPulse Select, is shown in Figure 15-1. The VersaPulse Select consists of a laser console, which houses the laser assembly, cooling system, power supplies, and control electronics; a touchscreen control panel where the treatment parameters are set and adjusted; a footswitch that activates the laser energy; and a fiberoptic delivery system that transmits the laser energy to the target tissue.

Control Panel

The touchscreen control panel, which provides all the displays and controls normally used to monitor and regulate treatment levels, is located on the top of the laser console. Selections are made by touching the display. As settings are changed, the system beeps to alert the user. An optional remote control unit is also available, which can be placed within the sterile field, allowing the surgeon to alter treatment parameters directly. The remote control has an 18 foot (5.6 meter) power cable that plugs into a receptacle on the side of the laser. The VersaPulse Select control panel is shown in detail in Figure 15-2.

A keyswitch ensures that the instrument is used only by authorized personnel. The system power keyswitch is a spring-loaded, three-position lock switch which controls the power to the laser system. The laser can only be turned on with the proper key, and the laser is not operable with the key removed. When the VersaPulse Select is turned on, the Power On indicator illuminates.

The Aim/Beam pushbutton activates and adjusts the aiming beam. Because the 2.1 μm treatment beam is invisible, a red 0.650 μm diode laser beam, coaxial with the treatment beam, is used as an aiming device. Once a delivery system has been properly attached, the aiming beam is available to the user. The aiming beam is disabled when the delivery system fiberoptic cable is removed. Depressing the Aim/Beam Increase pushbutton once turns the aiming beam on at its minimum, or low, setting. The "low" indicator illuminates on the control panel. To increase to medium intensity, depress the Aim/Beam In-

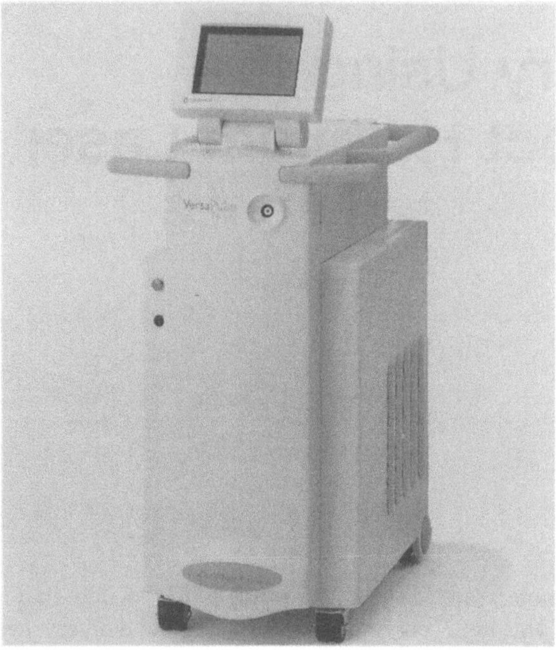

Figure 15-1. The VersaPulse Select laser.

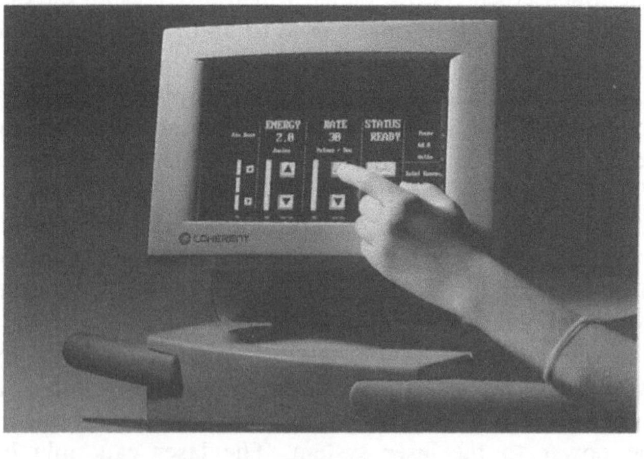

Figure 15-2. VersaPulse Select control panel.

crease pushbutton again. The "low" indicator then changes to "medium." Depressing the Increase pushbutton a third time sets the aiming beam to "high" intensity. To lower the intensity of the aiming beam or to turn it off, depress the Aim/Beam Decrease pushbutton until the desired setting illuminates on the control panel.

The Energy/Pulse display indicates the selected laser energy per pulse, expressed in joules. The energy per pulse may be set to one of the system's available settings using the Increase and Decrease pushbuttons. The settings available depend on the model of the laser.

The Rate display indicates the selected number of laser treatment pulses per second (hertz). Use the Increase or Decrease pushbuttons accordingly to attain the desired setting.

Depressing the system status pushbuttons places the system in either Ready or Standby mode. The system status indicators illuminate to show the selected mode. In Ready mode, the laser and footswitch are enabled. When the footswitch is depressed, the safety shutter opens and the laser treatment beam is delivered to the target tissue. As the treatment beam is delivered, the Treatment indicator illuminates. As a safety feature, a treatment exposure is delivered only when the system is in Ready mode. In Standby mode, the footswitch is disabled and the safety shutter is closed; no treatment beam is available. After a procedure has been completed and before removing a delivery device, the laser should be placed in Standby mode.

The system status indicators illuminate to show the present operating state of the laser system. The Treatment indicator illuminates as the treatment laser beam is delivered to the treatment site. The system must be in Ready mode. Ready and Standby illuminate to show the selected operating mode. At system start-up, Self Test illuminates to show that the system is performing a self test sequence. To verify that all control panel lights are operational, various control panel indicators and displays illuminate simultaneously. The self test sequence lasts approximately 5 seconds.

The Average Power display shows the average power of the laser treatment beam, expressed in watts. The average power is the product of energy per pulse (joules) and the repetition rate (pulses per second).

Warning indicators alert the user to important system status information; for instance, Attach Fiber illuminates to tell the user that the delivery device is not yet connected. In some cases, accompanying error codes may also appear in the Average Power display. The system cannot be placed in the Ready mode if a fault indicator is illuminated.

The Total Energy display shows the cumulative delivered energy, expressed in kilojoules. The Total Energy display may be reset to zero in two ways: when the system is restarted and the Ready pushbutton is initially pressed, and when the Standby button is depressed for 2 seconds. The display does not reset to zero when the system is turned off. Should hospital personnel forget to record the total energy value before turning off the system, the value is displayed upon system start-up.

Depressing the Emergency Off pushbutton deenergizes the laser system. To restart the system, turn the keyswitch to the start position and hold for 1 second. This pushbutton may also be used to turn the system off in nonemergency situations.

Footswitch

The footswitch plugs into a receptacle on the back of the laser console. The VersaPulse Select footswitch has an entirely waterproof enclosure, providing safety in an arthroscopic environment. The footswitch, like the laser system itself, has been designed and approved to UL544, FDA, TUV, IEC, and other international electrical and regulatory standards.

Delivery Systems

Unlike 10.6 μm CO_2 lasers, which typically use an articulated arm to transport the laser beam from the laser cavity to the treatment site, the 2.1 μm holmium:YAG laser can be delivered via fiberoptic cables. Although more fragile than an articulated arm, fiberoptic delivery devices are easier to use and less cumbersome when trying to access a difficult-to-reach treatment site. In addition, surgeons need not be concerned about the beam alignment issues typically associated with CO_2.

As for mechanical instrumentation, there are a wide variety of fiberoptic laser delivery systems available, specific to a surgical application. There are more than 20 handpiece designs presently available for the VersaPulse, and the list continues to grow. Although most of the variations are dimensional or due to differences in tip configuration, there are essentially three basic types of VersaPulse delivery systems: single-use handpieces, single-use handpieces with viewing optics and flexible tip, and multiple-use delivery devices.

Single-Use Handpieces

The Coherent single-use delivery devices all share some basic components. Figure 15-3 is an illustration of the InfraTome handpiece, outlining the basic elements.

InfraTome delivery systems consist of a fiberoptic cable, connector, handpiece, and fiber tip. The fiberoptic cable transmits the laser aiming and treatment beams from the laser console to the treatment site. The connector secures the fiberoptic cable to the laser console. The handpiece is designed to feel like a conventional surgical instrument to facilitate manipulation at the treatment site. The laser beam exits the delivery system at the fiber tip.

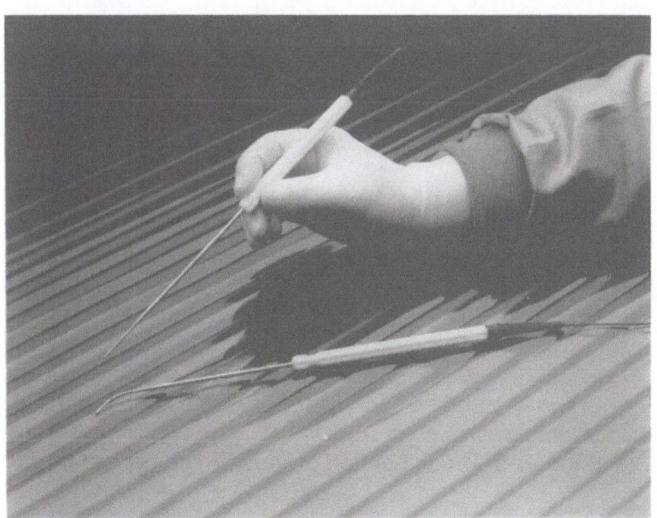

Figure 15-3. InfraTome handpiece.

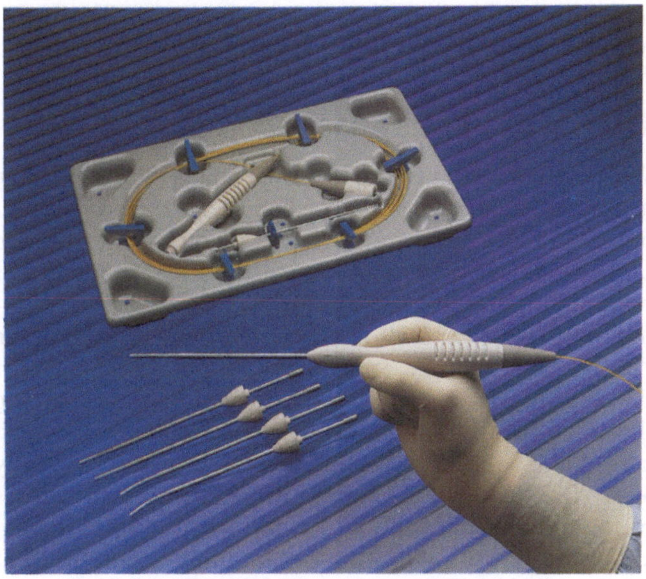

Figure 15-4. VersaLink handpiece.

The VersaLink™ Delivery Device

The reusable VersaLink delivery device has all of the components of the single-use InfraTome but, in addition, is reusable. The VersaLink is used in conjunction with a detachable VersaTip™, which locks into the VersaLink handpiece. The VersaTip probe tip can be used either as a single-use, disposable device, or it can be resterilized. Resterilization allows the VersaLink to be used on multiple cases, reducing overall patient cost. Also, with the VersaLink, multiple tip configurations can be used during a single, difficult case. A VersaLink handpiece is shown in Figure 15-4.

Connecting and Using the Delivery System

In general, fiberoptic delivery devices are easy to connect and use. On the VersaPulse Select laser the fiberoptic receptacle is on the front of the unit. To connect a delivery system, finger-tighten the fiberoptic connector into the fiberoptic receptacle. When the delivery system fiberoptic connector is properly seated and tightly screwed into the fiberoptic receptacle, the Attach Fiber indicator extinguishes on the control panel. A contact sensor in the receptacle verifies that the fiberoptic cable is properly seated. The indicator does not extinguish and the system does not deliver a treatment beam unless the delivery system fiberoptic is properly connected. Once treatment parameters are set, the delivery system is ready to use.

Theory of VersaPulse Operation

With a solid-state laser such as the VersaPulse the lasing medium is a pure crystal that has been "doped," or impregnated, with an impurity element during the growth process. (These crystals are synthetic; they do not occur naturally.) In the VersaPulse the laser crystal is a rod 4 mm in diameter and 89 mm long. The pure crystal is the "host" and simply provides the environment for the impure atoms to carry on the business of making the laser light. In the case of the VersaPulse the host crystal is YAG (yttrium-aluminum-garnet, chemically $Y_3A_{15}O_{12}$), and the laser light is produced by the atoms of the holmium dopant. To be precise, the YAG crystal is also doped with chromium and thulium; but the function of these atoms is simply to assist in getting the energy into the upper energy level of the 2.1 μm holmium:YAG. Generally speaking, we refer to the VersaPulse laser simply as a 2.1 μm holmium:YAG laser, referring to its holmium-doped crystal of yttrium-aluminum-garnet.

The energy source that excites the crystal is a high intensity flashlamp. The laser is driven, or "pumped," with flashlamp, driven by an electrical current pulse of 600 μs duration. This spectrally broad energy is first absorbed by the broad absorption bands of chromium. Figure 15-5 shows the rather complex pumping scheme. The energy undergoes a radiationless transfer to the thulium and then to the holmium, where lasing occurs at a wavelength of 2.1 μm. Because the lower laser level is near the ground state, it is significantly populated at room temperature, which decreases the efficiency of the laser. The efficiency (the ratio of laser output energy to the electrical input energy) can be improved by cooling the laser crystal with chilled water.

For optical pumping, the crystal rod and flashlamp are arranged inside a diffusely reflecting pump cavity, and precisely aligned mirrors are positioned at each end of the rod. One of these mirrors is highly reflective at 2.1 μm, whereas the other reflects only a prescribed portion of the light and allows a certain percentage to pass through. This percentage of light that passes through the mirror is, in fact, the usable output of the laser.

Specifications* for the Coherent VersaPulse Select 2.1 μm Holmium: YAG Laser

Wavelength: 2.1 μm
Energy per pulse delivered to tissue (varies by model): 0.5 to 2.8 joules
Lamp input energy: up to 150 joules
Pulse repetition rates: 5 to 40Hz
Pulse width: 300 μs
Maximum average power delivered to tissue: up to 80 watts

Delivery System Mechanics

Although some laser wavelengths are not suitable for fiber delivery (e.g., that of the 10.6 μm CO_2, which uses mirrors in an articulated arm), the 2.1 μm holmium:YAG wavelength can be delivered to the treatment site via a quartz optical fiber. A cross section of the optical fiber is shown in Figure 15-6. It has a quartz core, quartz cladding, silicone buffer, and nylon jacket. A variety of optical fiber diameters are used, with 400 mm being the most common. The laser light is guided down the fiber by the core

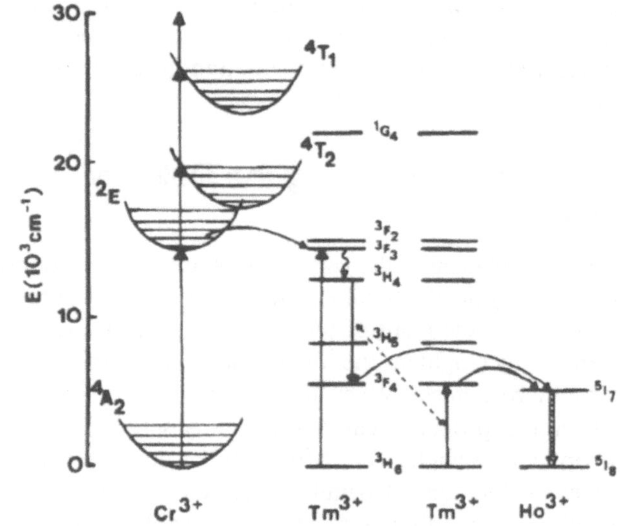

Figure 15-5. VersaPulse pumping scheme. Chromium, Thulium, and Holmium are needed.

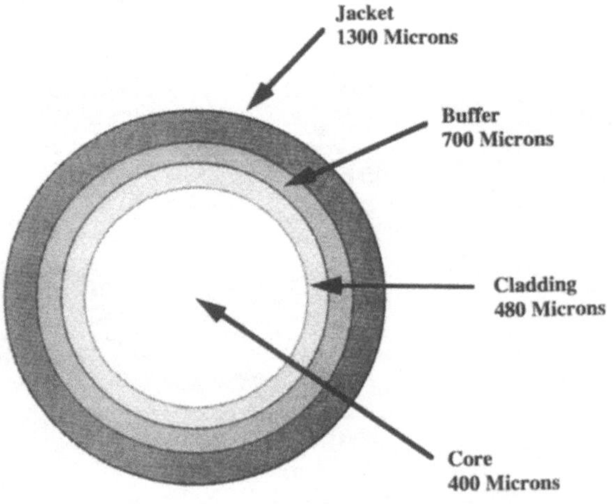

Figure 15-6. Cross section of VersaPulse optical fiber.

*These specifications, established as of February 1993, are subject to change.

and cladding layers, and the buffer and jacket serve as outer protection. At the interface of the core and cladding, the light undergoes what is termed a total internal reflection process in order to make its way down the core and out the fiber tip.

Optically, total internal reflection occurs at the interface of two optical media and can occur when light travels from a medium of high refractive index to a medium of lower index. This reflection process is efficient when the core and cladding materials are highly transparent at the light's wavelength and when the interface has few imperfections. The specially manufactured quartz material has a low water content so absorption is minimized (about 2% per meter). The power transmission of a typical VersaPulse Select delivery system, including the reflection losses at each end, is approximately 88%.

To launch the 2.1 μm holmium:YAG laser beam into the fiber, the beam is focused to a spot size smaller than 400 μm (the diameter of the core) on the proximal end of the fiber. After traversing the length of the fiber, the light exits the distal end of the fiber tip in a cone of light with an angle of divergence similar to the divergence angle of the beam that was launched into the fiber.

Laser–Tissue Interaction

The absorption length in water and tissue of the 2.1 μm holmium:YAG laser is approximately 400 μm, so that the minimum amount of thermal damage surrounding tissue that has been vaporized is around 0.5 millimeter. For comparison, the absorption length of the 0.532 μm KTP laser in nonpigmented tissue is more than 4 mm, which means that regardless of any other surgical parameter the surrounding thermal effect cannot be less than 4 mm.

The 2.1 μm holmium:YAG laser, with its absorption length of 400 μm, vaporizes and cuts efficiently, yet provides hemostasis. This trait, combined with its suitability to fiberoptic delivery in a water environment, make it particularly adaptable to arthroscopic surgery.

The practical surgical effect of the VersaPulse Select laser on tissue is determined by a combination of energy per pulse, spot size, and the amount of time the energy is applied to the tissue. These basic principles apply to light delivered via a fiber (e.g., 2.1 μm holmium:YAG laser) or to light delivered as a free beam (e.g., 10.6 μm CO_2 laser).

VersaPulse Select Energy Density Calculations

Referring to the calculations in Chapter 3 [E/A = energy (in the spot) ÷ area (of the spot)], we can make the following energy density calculations for the VersaPulse. The VersaPulse beam is delivered through a 0.4 mm (400 μm) diameter fiber and exits in a cone of rays whose full angle is about 23 degrees. The area of the beam at the fiber tip is approximately 0.13 mm^2 and at 1 mm from the tip the area is about 0.5 mm^2. Given the 2.1 μm holmium:YAG absorption length of 0.4 mm, the calculated absorbing tissue volumes are then 0.05 mm^3 at the tip of the fiber and 0.2 mm^3 1 mm away from tissue. The VersaPulse Select has an available energy per pulse of 2.8 joules, which is enough energy to easily vaporize the volumes of target tissue calculated above. (Remember that vaporizing 1 mm^3 of tissue requires at least 2.4 joules of energy.) In addition, the VersaPulse Select pulse duration is short enough, (300 μs) to prevent conduction and resulting thermal damage to surrounding tissue.

Moses Effect

The VersaPulse works through the Moses Effect (van Leeuwen et al., 1991), depicted in Figure 15-7. The initial part of each laser pulse (approximately 10–20% of it) vaporizes a small portion of the water, creating a bubble. This bubble then serves to "part the water" for the remainder of the pulse, providing a "dry" path for the remaining 80% to reach to the target tissue.

Clinical Application

VersaPulse lasers are approved for marketing by the FDA** for use in arthroscopic procedures involving soft tissue ablation, excision, and coagulation in various joints.

Orthopaedics

Listed below are some of the arthroscopic procedures for which surgeons have found the VersaPulse effective.

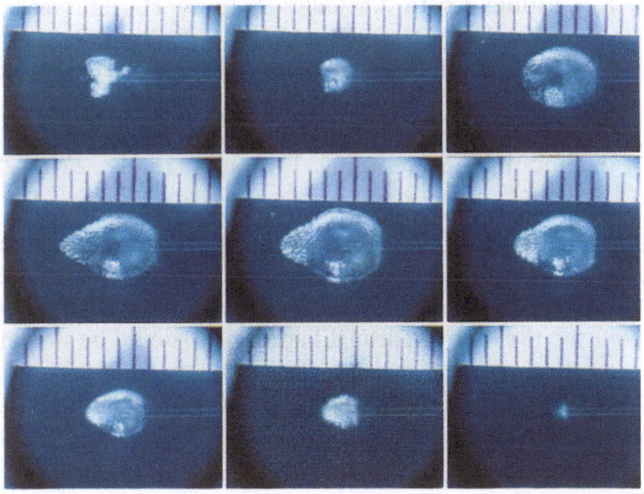

Figure 15-7. Moses effect. Pulse energy is 1.5 joules; ruler divisions are in millimeters.

**The use of a laser instrument for an application is at the surgeon's discretion except in cases where the indication has been contraindicated. The FDA requires that the surgeon apply sound medical judgment in the application of the laser to any particular indication.

Ankle: osteochondral fracture debridement, removal of osteophytes impinging on tibia/talus, synovectomy
Elbow: debridement of extensor tendon, removal of loose body, synovectomy
Knee: chondroplasty, excision of meniscal cyst, lateral release, meniscectomy, plica removal, resection of anterior cruciate ligament, synovectomy
Shoulder: acromioplasty, biceps tendon tear debridement, capsular release, labral tear resection, lesions, loose body removal, removal of scar tissue, rotator cuff debridement, subacromial bursal resection, subacromial decompression
Wrist: debridement of torn triangular fibrocartilage complex, osteochondral fracture debridement, synovectomy

Clinical Parameters

Typical VersaPulse Select energy and repetition rates for various applications are as follows.

1. Soft tissue, such as degenerative tissue where chondromalacia is diagnosed
   a. Cutting: 1.6 joules (energy), 10 Hz (pulses), 16 watts (average power)
   b. Ablation/debridement: 1.8 joules, 10 Hz, 18 watts
   c. Coagulation: . 8 joules, 16 Hz, 12.8 watts
   d. Smoothing/contouring, 1.4 joules, 16 Hz, 22.4 watts
2. Dense tissue, such as meniscus, retinaculum, synovium, cartilage, osteophytes
   a. Cutting: 1.6 to 2.8 joules, 8 to 24 Hz, 60 watts - maximum system power
   b. Ablation/debridement: 2 to 2.8 joules, 8 to 30 Hz, 60 watts - maximum system power
   c. Coagulation: 1 joules, 18 Hz, 18 watts
   d. Smoothing/contouring: 1.4 joules, 16 Hz, 22 to 28 watts

Power settings should be determined by the surgeon upon careful monitoring of tissue effect during the procedure. Tissue effects vary with the distance of the handpiece from the tissue. For cutting, handpieces should be in contact with tissue; for ablation, the probe tip should be 1 to 2 mm from the tissue; and for coagulation, it should be 2 to 3 mm from the tissue.

Tissue Effect

VersaPulse surgical lasers have proved to be clinically effective for coagulation of blood vessels without damaging surrounding or nontarget tissues. Coagulation can be effected by reducing the power density incident on vascularized tissue in three ways. When the tip of the handpiece or fiber is in direct contact with the target tissue, the energy and repetition rate setting on the control panel may be reduced. The physician may also elect to defocus the beam by moving the tip of the handpiece away from the target tissue approximately 2 to 5 mm without the need to change the system controls.

Eye Protection

The laser safety eyewear recommended for use with the VersaPulse lasers should have an optical density of 2.0 to 3.0 at 2.1 μm. However, laser safety eyewear may be considered optional with 2.1 μm holmium:YAG laser systems. The local laser safety officer should determine if laser safety eyewear is required.

David Sliney (see Chapter 12), physicist and chairman of the American National Standards Institute (ANSI) subcommittee on Hazard Analysis, evaluated the potential optical radiation hazard of the 2.1 μm holmium:YAG laser as compared to visible wavelength lasers and determined the following: For the 2.1 μm holmium:YAG laser the nominal hazard zone, as defined by ANSI Standard Z136.1–1986 and measured from the fiber output, is 12 inches for exposures of less than 1 second and 24 inches for exposures longer than 10 seconds. These figures compare with a nominal hazard zone of 13 feet for a 20-watt, visible, green-wavelength laser. For medical applications, the nominal hazard zone of 12 inches is most applicable, as an exposure longer than 10 seconds is unlikely and would require deliberate, prolonged viewing.

Laser safety eyewear is routinely required with most lasers. However, because of its small nominal hazard zone and because the 2.1 μm holmium:YAG laser is used primarily endoscopically, laser safety eyewear may be considered optional. This determination should be made by the local laser safety officer. If the officer is satisfied that operating procedures eliminate the possibility of the laser being discharged outside the nominal hazard zone, the need for laser safety eyewear may be waived. **EDITOR'S CAUTION: Even though many sugeons feel no need to wear 2.1 μm wavelength specific eyewear, the editor does not agree with this practice. This laser beam will damage the eye if exposed.** If laser safety eyewear is deemed necessary within the operating environment, laser safety eyewear with an optical density of 2.0 to 3.0 at 2.1 μm is recommended to prevent accidental eye damage. To avoid possible eye damage, never look directly into the laser aperture or fiberoptic tip when power is applied, even with laser safety eyewear in place.

Smooth objects reflect the laser beam, and the potential hazards and exposure limits are the same as for an unreflected beam. Reflection hazards can exist within 24 inches of the distal end of the delivery system fib although practically speaking for most medical applications these hazards would occur within 12 inches.

Avoid directing the laser beam at unintended objects. The beam will damage the scope lens and may fracture it. Regardless of the color of a surface, reflection is a potential hazard when the laser strikes a nonabsorbing surface, such as a metallic surgical instrument. Use low or nonreflecting instruments whenever possible. Two types of reflection can occur: specular and diffuse. *Specular (mirror-like)* reflection occurs when the size of surface irregularities is less than the wavelength of the incident radiation. In this instance the laser beam reflects at the same angle as the angle of incidence. Should a concentrated beam of laser light accidentally strike unintended tissue, it could cause significant thermal damage.

Diffuse reflection occurs when surface irregularities are randomly oriented and are much greater than the wavelength of the incident light. In this instance the reflected laser beam is disorganized and scatters in many directions. The laser light may still strike an unintended target surface, but the energy density is reduced to a degree that causes minimal, if any, thermal effect.

Surgical instruments that are be used in proximity to the laser beam should be dulled so they reflect diffusely. A smooth, blackened surface still specularly reflects the laser beam, however. Plastic instrumentation may melt when hit by the laser beam, possibly resulting in chemical burns.

Operating Room Setup Requirements

There are no specific size or operating room setup requirements for the VersaPulse Select laser, except that, as for any medical instrument, there should be enough room for the operating room personnel to work comfortably with it. Positioning the equipment is a matter of surgical preference. The laser console may be positioned anywhere within the reach of the power cable (of variable length, specified by the operating room at time of installation) and the fiberoptic delivery system. When the laser system is on, position the laser console at least 18 inches (45.7 cm) away from walls, furniture, or other equipment to allow proper air circulation for system cooling. The laser console is 27.4 inches (69.6 cm) wide, by 48 inches (122 cm) long, by 49.5 inches (126 cm) high.

VersaPulse Select Electrical Requirements

Electrical power should be supplied from a 200 to 240 voltz alternating current (VAC), single phase, 50/60 Hz, 30 ampere (A) outlet with ground. A dedicated electrical service line with a single phase switch in the room and a 30 ampere circuit breaker are required (Fig. 15-8). All VersaPulse Select systems can be installed with a removable wall plug with ground or can be hard-wired.

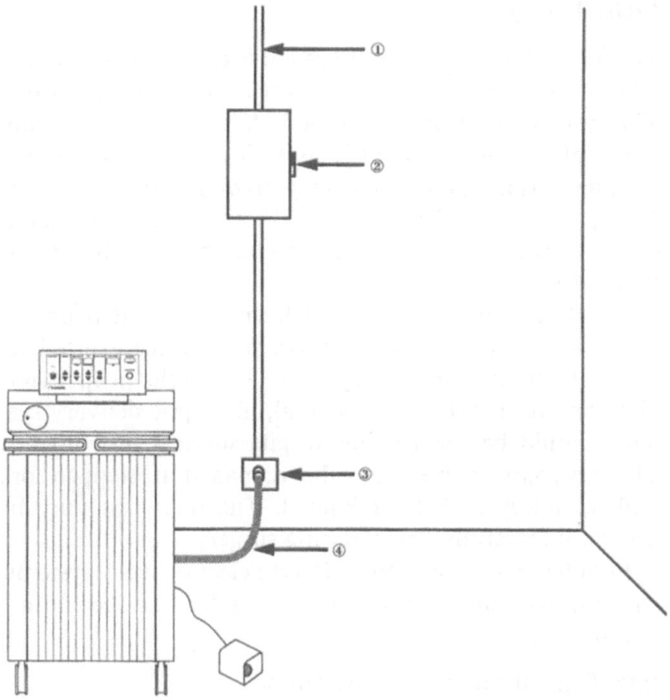

Figure 15-8. Typical VersaPulse electrical scheme. 1 = 200- to 240-volt electrical service from fused distribution panel; 2 = electrical service disconnect; 3 = three-pronged power receptacle; 4 = power cable with three-pronged plug.

Plumbing Requirements

VersaPulse Select lasers utilize a self-contained cooling system. No special water utilities are required.

Maintenance

There is no required user maintenance of the *laser console*, and no recommended maintenance, except the cleaning routinely required for operating room equipment. To clean the external surface of the laser console, wipe using a cloth dampened with a noncaustic cleaning solution, such as soap and water, isopropyl alcohol, or a "hospitalgrade" disinfectant. Do not spray or pour cleaning agents directly on the system. Dry with a clean, dry cloth or allow to air-dry. Do not clean while the laser is in use.

Each VersaPulse single-use, disposable delivery system is shipped sterile from the factory, making it maintenance-free for the user. The VersaLink and VersaTip may be cleaned using a laboratory cleaner (e.g., Microsoap in a solution of 2.5 ounces to 1 gallon of warm tap water. The VersaLink may be steam-sterilized. The VersaTip can be sterilized only with ethyl alcohol.

Durability

The VersaPulse Select laser system is designed and manufactured to withstand the harshest rigors of hospital use. The systems meet or exceed the U.S. manufacturing standards of UL-544 and ETL, as well as the international manufacturing and regulatory requirements of IEC 601.1, ISO 9000, BSI, and TUV. Coherent Medical is one of only 500 companies in the United States that is certified to ISO 9001.

The durability of fiberoptic delivery systems depends on a number of factors: total energy used, force exerted on the probe tip during surgery, and, if reusable, proper sterilization and handling. In general, fiberoptic delivery systems should be regarded as fragile surgical instruments. The fiberoptic cables may be damaged if stepped on, pulled, tightly coiled, or kinked. The fiber tips may be broken if forcefully flexed during surgery.

Following are some VersaPulse Select delivery systems, showing maximum power settings and other specific use parameters.

InfraTome 0°: maximum system power
InfraTome 15°: maximum system power
InfraTome 30°: maximum system power
InfraTome 15°: maximum system power
InfraTome TIR 70°: maximum system power
VersaLink: maximum system power
(Use of a cannula or sheath strongly advised to prevent possible damage to the probe tip during introduction into a joint; handpiece must not be operated in air; for use in fluid only.)

Editor's Cautions

1. **Even though many surgeons believe there is no need to wear 2.1 μm wavelength-specific protective eyewear, I do not agree. The 2.1 μm holmium:YAG is a class IV laser, and its wavelength can damage the eye.**
2. **These fibers should be used in a standard liquid arthroscopic environment. Use in a gas environment is not recommended.**
3. **Each fiber is fragile and can fracture if not fully protected. Forcing, levering, or using the "probe" as a mechanical probe will likely result in a fracture and an intraarticular foreign body.**
4. **All fibers have a definitive life-span. Optimal, satisfactory use of this system requires some experience. It is best to start in the laboratory, not with patients. The best techniques, energy settings, and probe selections can be preliminarily determined in this way. The reader is referred to Chapter 4, on ablation efficiency.**
5. **Mechanical instruments should be available at all times during arthroscopic laser surgery.**
6. **This chapter is only an introduction to this arthroscopic laser system. The reader is encouraged to study this entire text, follow acceptable training and credentialing procedures, as well as research the subject at hand for additional information and changes before undertaking this arthroscopic laser system's use.**

Suggested Reading

Sagi A, Avidor-Zehavi A, Shitzer A, Gerstmann M, Akselrod S, Katzir A (1992) Heating of biological tissue by laser irradiation: temperature distribution during laser ablation. Optical Engineering 31:1425–1431

Sagi A, Shitzer A, Katzir A, Akselrod S (1992) Heating of biological tissue by laser irradiation: theoretical model. Optical Engineering 31:1417–1424

Trauner K, Nishioka N, Patel D (1990) Pulsed holmium: yttrium-aluminum-garnet (ho:YAG) laser ablation of fibrocartilage and articular cartilage. The American Journal of Sports Medicine 18: 316–320

van Gemert MJC and Welch AJ (1989) Time constants in thermal laser medicine. Lasers in Surgery and Medicine 9:405–421

van Leeuwen T, van der Veen M, Verdaasdonk R, Borst C (1991) Noncontact tissue ablation by holmium: YSGG laser pulses in blood. Lasers in Surgery and Medicine 11:26–34

Welch AJ (1984) The thermal response of laser irradiated tissue. IEEE JQE 20:1471-1481

16

Eclipse 3200 2.1 μm Holmium:YAG Laser System for Arthroscopic Laser Surgery

Douglas R. Murphy-Chutorian

The Eclipse 3200 is a class IV pulsed solid-state 2.1 μm holmium:YAG laser system (Fig. 16-1). The laser system is indicated for arthroscopic and surgical applications in joints, including meniscectomy, cutting or ablation of soft tissue including fibrous tissue, adhesions, treatment of chondromalacia, and cutting or ablation of diseased cartilage. The specifications for the device are as follows.

Model: Eclipse 3200
Laser Type: pulsed, solid-state holmium:YAG (Ho:YAG)
Wavelength: 2.1 μm, mid-infrared
Energy/pulse: 3.2 joules maximum upgradable to 5 joules
Power: 40 watts upgradable to 60 watts
Pulse length: 250 μs
Pulse rate: 5 to 32 Hz upgradable to 44 Hz
Aiming beam: 7 mW helium-neon laser
Electrical service: 200, 208, or 220 volts alternating current (VAC), 50 to 60 Hz, 30 amperes, single phase
Cooling: internal, no running water required
Dimensions: 29 × 23 × 44 inches (length/width/height), portable on wheels
Weight: 420 pounds (approximately)
Classification: class IV device in accordance with 21 CFR 1040.10(8)
Delivery systems: hand-held fiberoptic attachments

Laser System

The major internal and external components of the laser system include the following:

Laser head
Laser control and power supply
Laser emission aperture
Chiller system
Control console
System control
Power meter with input aperture
Foot pedal

The laser head consists of the 2.1 μm holmium:YAG crystal, flashlamp, optics, and interlocked laser safety shutters. The crystal receives electrical power from the laser control module, fed by the power supply module, and transforms this energy into laser energy. The laser energy then exits the system through the laser emission aperture. Cooling for the system is handled by an internal chiller system, which requires no running water or water hoses.

The operator is able to control the amount of laser energy released, as well as other operations of the laser, by means of the control console (Fig. 16-2). The control console is located on the top front of the system, just above the laser emission aperture. It features an on/off keyswitch, an emergency off button, and Ready and Standby mode displays and buttons. Red-light-emitting diode (LED) displays and controls allow the operator to adjust the pulse repetition rate (in pulses per second) and energy per pulse settings (in tenths of joules). LED displays also accrue and read out the total pauses and total energy delivered in real time; they may be reset to zero at any time.

All internal and external functions of the laser are centrally controlled by the system controller, which is comprised of both hardware and software. In addition to providing instructions to the various components, the system controller evaluates functional input and returns feedback instructions. This practice allows the system to monitor its own performance and eliminates the need for user maintenance.

Power output is monitored in this fashion by the system controller with the aid of an integrated, internal power meter. Without interrupting the emitted laser energy, the power meter periodically "picks off," or samples, the la-

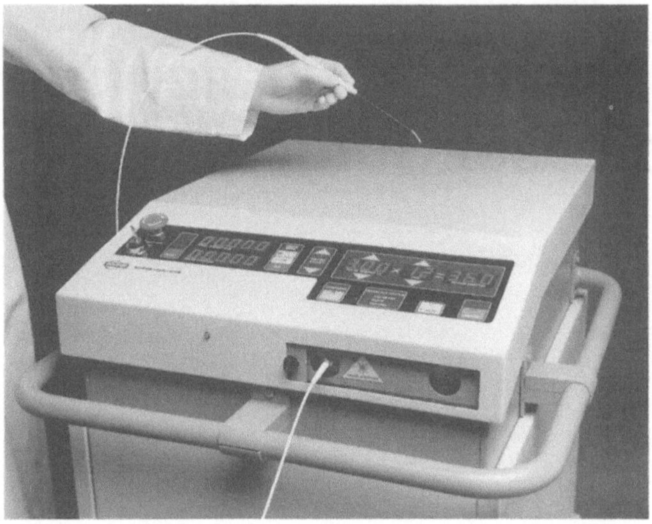

Figure 16-1. Eclipse 3200 2.1 μm holmium:YAG laser system. This portable self-contained unit measures 23 × 29 × 44 inches (width/length/height), weighs approximately 420 pounds, and can be readily moved by one person. The system requires standard 220 volt, 30 ampere, single-phase electrical service and is internally cooled so no external water service is required.

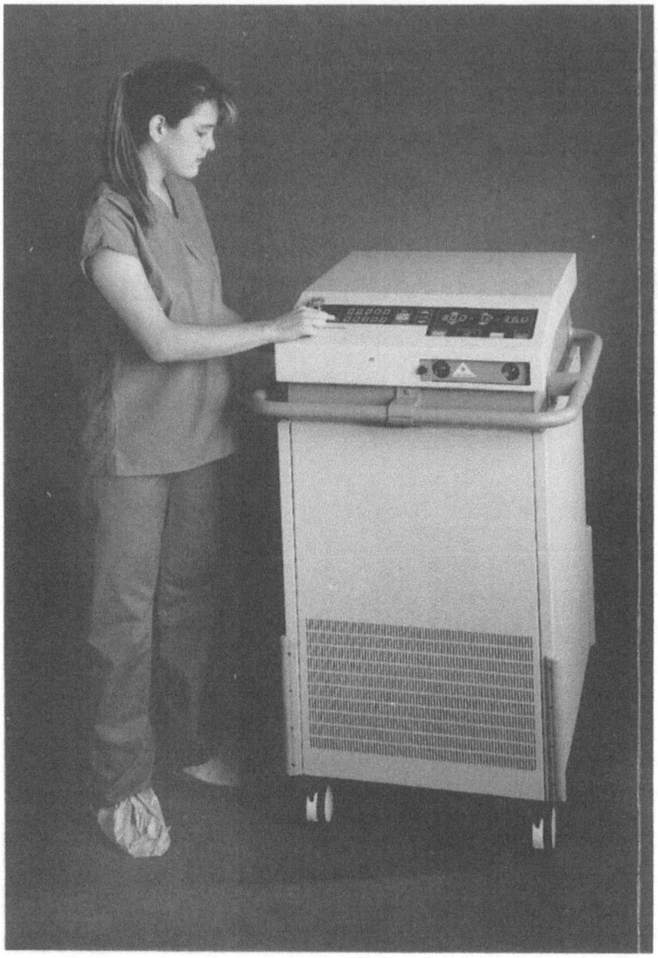

Figure 16-2. Eclipse 3200 system control console. Pushbutton controls for energy per pulse (0.1-joule increments) and pulse repetition rate (in pulses per second) illuminate red LED displays. Other controls include aiming beam, power test, and standby/ready. The laser emission aperture is located on the front of the system near the control console.

ser energy being emitted and then delivers it to the system controller, which compares these actual measurements to the desired power settings on the user control console. In addition to these internal audits, the power meter has an input aperture that allows the user to check the laser power output being emitted from the currently attached fiberoptic probe.

Fiberoptic Laser Delivery Systems

The fiberoptic attachment (probe) is an essential element to the clinical use of the laser system. This removable device is utilized to deliver the laser energy from the laser emission aperture of the laser system to the site of clinical application within the body.

The Eclipse PowerSculptor probes are flexible and feature a plastic handle and stainless steel shaft at their proximal end. To satisfy varying clinical applications and anatomic differences, a variety of probe designs are available that vary in the length and diameter of the metal shaft as well as the angulation and design of the probe tip.

The probe consists of a single 500 μm diameter core silica optical fiber that is 3 meters in length. The proximal and distal ends of the optical fiber are prepared utilizing proprietary processes intended to enhance laser energy transmission and delivery. A standard screw-in subminiature adaptor (SMA) laser coupling adaptor is mounted to the proximal end of the device to move laser energy into the optical fiber.

The length of the fiber is encased in a flexible protective white polyethylene jacket to increase the durability of the probe. A 4 or 5 inch long white plastic handle is mounted near the distal end of the probe with a 4, 5, or 8 inch long stainless steel shaft emerging from the handle and comprising the most distal portion of the device. The probe shafts are offered in either low profile (1.7 mm) or standard profile (3.0 mm) diameters. All probe tips are 1.7 mm in diameter and are available in either straight, 8 degree, 20 degree, or 30 degree tip angulations. In addition, a straight probe tip that delivers laser energy in a CrossFire pattern is also available.

Operation of the Device

The machine is simple to operate. Place the key into the keyswitch, and turn it on. The Eclipse 3200 system starts up and performs a self-test for 30 seconds. Once this test has been completed, the system is ready to use.

To perform an arthroscopic surgical procedure with the laser, the proximal end of the laser probe is installed into the laser aperture. The pulse energy and repetition rate (PPS) controls are set as desired by the surgeon, and the power display indicates the wattage that will be delivered at the chosen settings. When the probe has been positioned in the intraarticular space using standard arthroscopic procedure, the laser system is placed in Ready mode. Laser energy is delivered when the foot pedal is depressed and stops when the foot pedal is released.

The laser head is the component within the system where the laser energy is produced. When the foot pedal is depressed, the system controller instructs the laser control module to release electrical energy to the laser head. The flashlamp utilizes this energy to turn on, releasing light that is absorbed by the elements in the 2.1 μm holmium:YAG crystal. The absorption of this light causes the atoms in the crystal to enter an excited state and as these atoms return to their ground state they spontaneously release extra energy by emitting photons. The key to laser energy is the potential of these photons to stimulate other excited atoms to emit photons. As this happens, a chain reaction ensues, and the light is amplified with the help of specially arranged optics within the laser head. Some of these photons are released in a directed stream of laser light (in the mid-infrared range of the spectrum), which exits the laser through the laser emission aperture.

Application

The Eclipse 32002.1 μm holmium:YAG laser system and PowerSculptor fiberoptic arthroscopic surgical probes have received 510(k) clearance from the U.S. Food and Drug Administration (FDA) for marketing for use in arthroscopic surgery of all joints, including meniscectomy, cutting or ablation of soft and fibrous tissue, adhesions, treatment of chondromalacia, and the cutting or ablation of diseased cartilage.

Prior to conducting any procedures, surgeons are instructed to attend a certified training course on laser use and, more specifically, on the use of lasers in arthroscopic procedures; and they must then obtain hospital laser privileges. During the procedure it is advisable that surgeons carefully assess the target and surrounding tissue to determine the appropriate power and pulse repetition rate of the laser.

During energy delivery, the distal tip of the probe should be in contact with or within 1 mm of the tissue. Direct tissue contact is necessary to cut with the laser. When the laser is fired at the diseased tissue, it vaporizes the material with which it comes into contact. The 2.1 μm holmium:YAG laser energy can also coagulate tissue and thus control bleeding. A variety of cutting, ablating, and smoothing effects can be achieved by varying laser energies, pulse repetition rates, distance of laser probe tip to tissue, and speed of probe movement over tissue.

Safety Requirements

Adequate and proper eye protection is the most important safety concern in the use of any laser. The 2.1 μm holmium:YAG laser can cause retinal damage to the eye under certain conditions; however, adherence to proper laser safety procedures can virtually eliminate any risk. Important guidelines include the following:

1. All personnel in the procedure room, including the patient, must always have protective eyewear (laser goggles or laser spectacles) whenever the laser is in use. Different wavelength lasers require laser goggles with different optical filtration characteristics; hence eyewear that protects the eye from damage with one wavelength may not protect from damage with another. The Eclipse 3200 operates at a wavelength between 2.0 and 2.2 μm, and the minimum optical density for the eyewear should be 3.0.
2. Never look directly into any laser beam. Protective eyewear is intended to protect from reflected or stray laser light, not a direct laser beam. Even properly filtered eyewear does not protect eyes from direct laser energy. Likewise, a person should never look directly into the distal end of an optical fiber or probe that has been installed into the laser emissions aperture of a laser system. The laser should never be directed into the scope. Its beam will damage and/or fracture the lens.

The Eclipse 3200 system meets or exceeds all mandated safety requirements, which include several main safety interlock systems that are intended to avoid inadvertent or unwanted emission of laser energy. The interlock systems are described below.

For laser energy to be emitted from the system, four conditions must exist simultaneously:

1. The system must be plugged in and turned on.
2. Because it is not possible to emit laser energy from the laser emission aperture directly into the room, a fiberoptic probe must be correctly installed in the laser emission aperture. A built-in mechanical detector is integrated into the laser emission aperture, which senses the absence or presence of the probe coupler. Laser energy cannot be emitted unless the probe is present and correctly installed.
3. The laser system must be taken off Standby mode and placed in Ready mode by the user by pressing the Ready button on the user control console. Laser energy cannot be emitted unless the laser system is in Ready mode.
4. The foot pedal must be depressed. Unless conditions 1, 2, and 3, above are met, pressing the foot pedal does not cause emission of laser energy. *Note*: If the foot

pedal itself is not correctly installed into the appropriate socket on the rear of the laser system, an error message is displayed on the user control console and the user is unable to place the system in the Ready mode.

The laser system features two additional safety interlock systems.

1. Covers: Light-tight metal panels (covers) fully encase the outside of the laser system. Should these panels be ajar or removed, the covers interlock LED illuminates on the user control console, and the laser system cannot be placed in Ready mode.
2. Remote interlock: A remote interlock socket is present on the back of the laser that allows a remote interlock to be placed on the procedure room door in order to automatically terminate emission of the laser energy in the event the door is opened. Use of the remote interlock is optional and infrequent.

Installation Requirements

The Eclipse 3200 requires 208, 220, or 240 VAC, 50/60 Hz, 30 ampere, single-phase electrical service. Because the system contains an internal refrigeration chiller subsystem, no other utility service (e.g., running water or water drainage access) is required. Owing to the portability and rapid setup of the laser system, multiple operating rooms may be equipped with the required electrical service, allowing serial use of a single laser system in several rooms if desired.

Maintenance Requirements

The Eclipse 3200 requires no user maintenance. Periodic preventive maintenance of the system performed once or twice a year by trained engineers includes flashlamp, chiller water, and air filter replacements. The flashlamp has a lifetime of approximately 4 million pulses, and chiller water and air filters should be replaced on an annual basis. The expected lifetime of the fiberoptic probes is approximately 50 kJ of energy transmission, with a typical single arthroscopic procedure involving 15 kJ.

Editor's Cautions

1. **Even though many surgeons believe there is no need to wear 2.1 μm wavelength-specific protective eyewear, I do not agree. The 2.1 μm holmium:YAG is a class IV laser, and its wavelength can damage the eye.**
2. **These fibers should be used in a standard liquid arthroscopic environment. Use in a gas environment is not recommended.**
3. **Each fiber is fragile and can fracture if not fully protected. Forcing, levering, or using the "probe" as a mechanical probe will likely result in a fracture and an intraarticular foreign body.**
4. **All fibers have a definitive life-span. Optimal, satisfactory use of this system requires some experience. It is best to start in the laboratory, not with patients. The best techniques, energy settings, and probe selections can be preliminarily determined in this way. The reader is referred to Chapter 4, on ablation efficiency.**
5. **Mechanical instruments should be available at all times during arthroscopic laser surgery.**
6. **This chapter is only an introduction to this arthroscopic laser system. The reader is encouraged to study this entire text, follow acceptable training and credentialing procedures, as well as research the subject at hand for additional information and changes before undertaking this arthroscopic laser system's use.**

Suggested Reading

Quinn J (1992) TMJ arthroscopic surgery—new laser use. LDA Journal, vol. 51, no. 4

Stein E, Dedlacek T, Fabian RL, Nishioka NS (1990) Acute and chronic effect of bone ablation with pulsed holmium laser. Lasers Surg Med, vol. 10, pp. 384–388

Trauner K et al. (1990) Pulsed holmium:YAG (ho:YAG) laser ablation of fibrocartilage and articular cartilage. Am J Sports Med, 18:316–320

17

Laser Photonics ML210 Holmium Surgical Laser System for Arthroscopic Laser Surgery

C. Darrow II, W. Williams, T. Shea, and B. Smith

The Laser Photonics (LPI) ML210 Holmium Surgical Laser System is a pulsed flashlamp-pumped, solid-state laser operating at a fundamental wavelength of 2.1 μm (Fig. 17-1). This laser system is manufactured by Laser Photonics and is distributed on an exclusive basis by Surgilase. The Laser Photonics ML210 Holmium Laser System can be used in many endoscopic procedures including orthopaedic arthroscopic applications such as synovectomy, lateral release, meniscectomy, and chondroplasty.

Description

The Laser Photonics ML210 Holmium Surgical Laser System has the following components:

Laser optics module
Power supply system
Cooling system
System control electronics module
Cabinet and appurtenances
Optical fiber delivery system

Laser Optics Module

The laser optics module consists of resonator mirrors, optics for alignment, the laser rod and pump enclosure with laser rod and laser pump (in this case a xenon flashlamp), an energy monitor, helium-neon laser, and a fiberoptic coupler. This module, where the laser beam is generated and maintained, is located in the top of the laser cabinet.

The ML210 emits laser irradiation on two discrete wavelengths. The treatment beam, which is generated by the flashlamp-pumped CTH:YAG (chromium-thulium-holmium doped yttrium-aluminum-garnet) laser rod, has a wavelength of 2.1 μm, which is in the infrared range of the electromagnetic spectrum and is invisible to the unaided human eye. The pulse energy-to-tissue is 0.4 to 5.0 joules with a pulse width of 550 μs and repetition rates of 4 to 10 pulses per second.

The term "holmium laser" is somewhat generic, as it has been used to encompass lasers that employ crystalline rods using the rare earth metal holmium (Ho) ions as the active lasing medium. However, as with the Laser Photonics ML210 Holmium Surgical Laser, the rod may contain other elements to facilitate transfer of flashlamp-pumped energy to the holmium ions.

The CTH:YAG laser is often referred to as a THC:YAG laser in the medical literature, although the convention is to indicate, in the acronym, the direction of energy flow. In this case the flashlamp-pumped energy is transferred to chromium ions to the thulium ions to the holmium ions to laser light.

The 5 mW helium-neon laser that is integral to the laser optics module emits the visible beam used for aiming. The wavelength of 0.594 μm is in the yellow portion of the visible spectrum.

The configuration of the laser optics module has been designed to provide the ruggedness necessary so that transporting the system does not require "on site" realignment while at the same time minimizing the size of the unit. This assembly configures the beam for optimal coupling into the fiberoptic delivery system and provides for simultaneous monitoring of laser beam energy. The helium-neon laser beam is optically aligned to be coaxial with the 2.1 μm holmium:YAG laser treatment beam.

The fiberoptic coupler, a female sub miniature adaptor (SMA) connector, launches the laser beams into the optical fiber delivery system. The fiberoptic coupler has a safety interlock shutter that prevents energy transmission until the male SMA connector of the fiberoptic delivery system is attached properly.

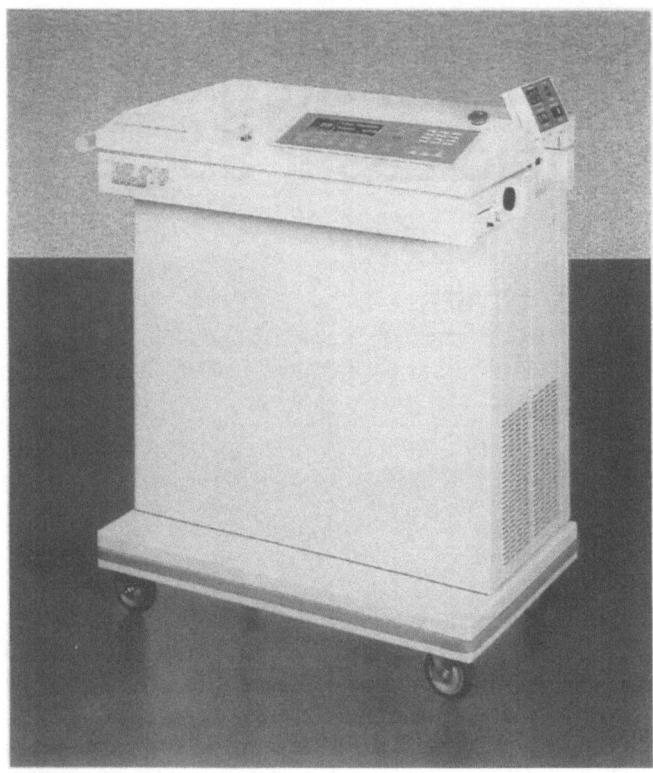

Figure 17-1. LPI ML210 Holmium Surgical Laser System.

Power Supply Unit

The power supply unit houses the lamp trigger and simmer source, the switching converter, the pulse forming network and high voltage control electronics, and the transformer to supply power to the laser optics module. The power supply unit is in the main body of the laser cabinet and requires a 220 volt alternating current (VAC) ± 10%, 30 ampere, single-phase, 60 Hz electrical service.

Cooling System

The cooling system consists of a closed cycle refrigeration unit, pump, reservoir and filter, temperature sensors, and a deionizing cartridge for the internal cooling system. The deionized coolant is pumped from the chiller assembly through the channels in the laser head to maintain the rod at the proper temperature for consistent laser operation. The chiller assembly is located in the main body of the laser cabinet. No external water or drain connections are necessary.

System Control Electronics Module

The system control electronics module consists of the "soft touch" control panel located on the top cover of the laser cabinet, microprocessor with system controls, sensors, safety interlocks, passive remote LED display located above the laser output connector, and a multifunction footswitch.

When the laser is first turned on, the microprocessor executes an internal calibration protocol (initialization procedures) to ensure that the laser is operating within program-defined test limits as well as to determine that all systems are functioning. The system microprocessor ensures flexibility in function and ease in operation. It interfaces with the "soft touch" control panel to allow the operator to input the exposure parameters of pulse energy, exposure limit for a specific time interval during timed exposures, and pulse repetition rate (pulses per second). The microprocessor provides the control and interface systems for the three available operating modes: continuous exposure, timed exposure, and pulse accelerator.

During use, the microprocessor employs software known as "dynamic calibration technology." This program monitors all functions and operations of the laser, holmium resonator, and security and safety systems. Included is an extensive surveillance system for detecting malfunctions. Alerts and warnings are displayed on the main LED control panel. This program provides procedures to ensure optimal performance and compensates for resonator aging, optical aging, or misalignments.

Cabinet and Dimensions

The baked enamel laser cabinet is 40 inches high, 33 inches wide and 23 inches deep and is mounted on 4 inch diameter easy rolling castors. The system weighs 390 pounds. Because of its relatively compact size and weight, the Laser Photonics ML210 is easily maneuverable. The Laser Photonics ML210 Holmium Surgical Laser has a "footprint" of less than 6 square feet. Figure 17-2 depicts the laser cabinet layout.

Controls and Switches

All of the controls with the exception of the footswitch are located on the front right-hand side of the cabinet top cover (Fig. 17-2B). The controls include the keyed on/off switch, the emergency stop switch, and the 48-character alphanumeric control panel with LED laser energy meter, laser emission indicator, LED alphanumeric display, and "soft touch" numeric keypad and function keys (Fig. 17-3).

Control Panel

The control panel comprises the following components:

Laser energy meter: displays the selected power settings.

Alphanumeric display: displays the parameter selection, prompts operator selections, system status, system error messages, and warnings.

Laser emission indicator: illuminates when the system is in

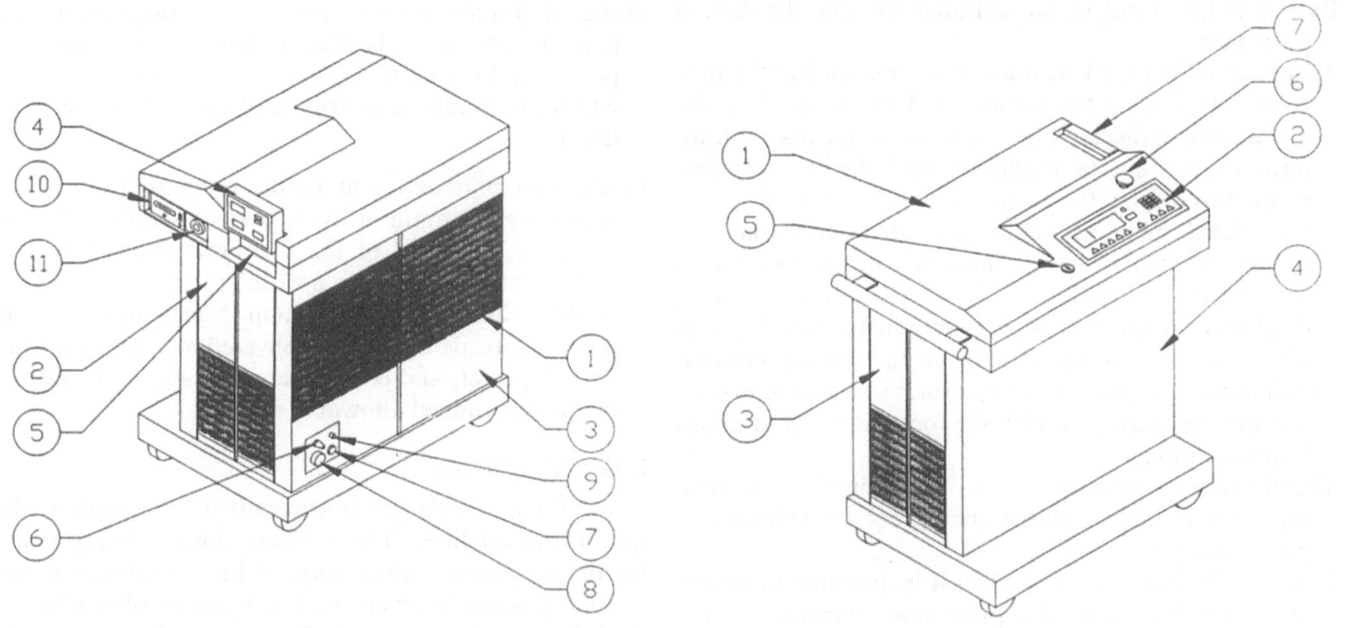

Figure 17-2. LPI ML210 Holmium Surgical Laser System. (A) Rear view. 1 = cooling system vent; 2 = right side panel; 3 = rear panel; 4 = remote display (open); 5 = fiber connection (standard 905 SMA); 6 = remote door interlock; 7 = footswitch connection; 8 = power cable and strain relief; 9 = CO_2 gas port; 10 = on-board printer; 11 = calibration port. (B) Front view. 1 = system top (interlocked); 2 = control panel; 3 = left side cover; 4 = front cover; 5 = on/off keyswitch; 6 = emergency shutdown switch; 7 = remote display (closed).

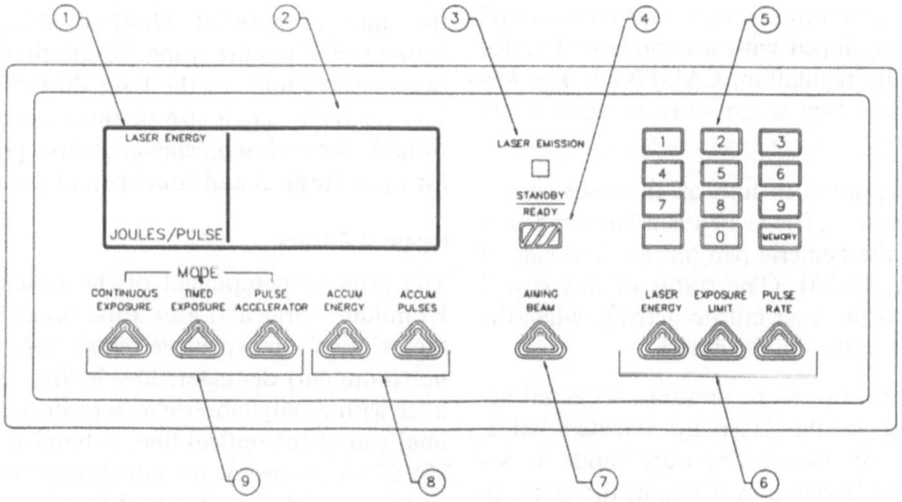

Figure 17-3. Control panel of the LPI ML210 Holmium Surgical Laser. 1 = laser energy meter; 2 = alphanumeric display; 3 = laser emission indicator; 4 = standby/ready key; 5 = numeric keypad; 6 = mode data entry keys; 7 = aiming beam key; 8 = accumulated display/average power keys; 9 = laser mode keys.

Ready mode, the footswitch is depressed, and laser energy is being emitted to the delivery system.

Standby/Ready key: toggles the system status from Standby to Ready to Standby, and so on.

Numeric keypad: for entering numeric lasing parameters.

Aiming beam key: actuates the aiming beam. For safety, the aiming beam is off when the system is turned on; this key must be pressed to activate (turn on) the aiming beam.

Laser energy key: must be pressed after the desired laser energy has been entered via the numeric keypad.

Exposure limit key: must be pressed if the length of laser exposure is to be limited, i.e., when the laser is in the Timed Exposure mode.

Pulse rate key: must be pressed after entering the desired pulse rate.

Accumulated energy key: used, as desired during the procedure, to display the accumulated energy used on the alphanumeric display (these data are displayed continuously on the remote display panel). This key may also be used to display the average power being used.

Accumulated pulses key: used, as desired during the procedure, to display the accumulated number of pulses used on the alphanumeric display (these data are also displayed on the remote display panel). This key can also be used to display the average power being utilized.

Continuous exposure key: used when it is desirable to control the exposure time with the footswitch (Continuous Exposure mode).

Timed exposure key: used when it is desirable to control the exposure time with the microprocessor (Timed Exposure mode).

Pulse accelerator key: used when it is desirable to manually control or vary the pulse rate. Pressure on the footswitch increases the pulse rate to the maximum previously selected or to preprogrammed limits. This Pulse Accelerator mode is a feature that is unique (exclusive) to the Laser Photonics ML210 Holmium Surgical Laser.

Other Controls

On/Off keyswitch: used to turn the laser system on and off (Fig. 17-2B). It is equipped with a removable key for safety as required by regulation. **CAUTION: The key should be removed and kept secure when the laser is not in use.**

Emergency switch: depressed to turn off the laser system in case of an emergency. The switch is a large red button directly above the numeric pad on the right side of the top cover (Fig. 17-2B). (The status of this switch should be checked if the laser fails to activate when the keyswitch is turned to the On position.)

Footswitch/accelerator: covered to prevent accidental activation; connected to the laser by shielded cable. When Continuous or Timed Exposure mode is selected, the footswitch/accelerator activates the laser. In the Pulse Accelerator mode, increasing pressure accelerates the pulse repetition rate up to the specified limits.

Other Features

Remote display panel: located above the fiberoptic coupler, where it is readily visible to the surgeon during the procedure. The panel displays the standby/ready status of the laser system, the selected pulse energy, and the "real time" accumulated energy and accumulated pulses that may be critical to the procedure in progress. This panel folds down to cover the fiberoptic coupler when the laser is not in use.

Onboard printer: on the right side of the laser cabinet (Fig. 17-2A); records fiber output power, number of pulses, pulse duration, and pulse energy (in joules, which are totaled and printed at the end of the procedure).

Calibration port: adjacent to the onboard printer; calibrates the fiberoptic delivery system should it become necessary. The end of the fiberoptic cable is inserted into a sterile calibration port adapter, which is placed in the calibration port. Within 3 seconds the microprocessor reads the power delivered, compares it to the desired power, and compensates for any variance from the predetermined allowable ranges.

Delivery Systems

The 2.1 μm wavelength is transmissible through a silica quartz optical fiber. The recommended delivery system for the ML210 Holmium Surgical Laser System is a component system of a single-use low hydroxy silica silica optical fiber and separate disposable handpiece (reusable handpieces are available). The advantage of such a system is that some procedures require two or more handpieces of somewhat different configuration. Being able to remove one handpiece and replace it with another on the same fiber can result in reduced expenditures of time and money. Because the handpiece exchange can be accomplished in the sterile field, risk of inadvertent contamination may be reduced. Unitized fiber/handpiece delivery systems may require using, connecting, and disconnecting two or three units to the laser during a single procedure. The relatively small size of this delivery system makes it suitable for endoscopic/arthroscopic procedures as well as for open surgical and some percutaneous applications.

Optical Fibers

The primary component of the Laser Photonics ML210 Holmium Surgical Laser Fiberoptic Delivery System is the relatively inexpensive, single-use, 4 meter long, 400 μm (nominal) diameter, low hydroxy silica silica optical fiber with a polyfluorethylene protective jacket. The proximal end of the optical fiber is bonded to a standard male 905 SMA connector for attachment to the laser fiberoptic coupler, which is a standard female 905 SMA connector. The SMA connector has been machined for precise centering of the fiber. The distal (treatment) end of the fiber has a polished, flat tip. The optical fibers are sterilized by ethylene oxide gas and are supplied to the user in packs of five.

Occasionally it is necessary to repair the tip of the optical fiber during a procedure. Reusable, gas-sterilizable fiber strippers and cleavers are available for that purpose.

Handpieces

The ML210 Holmium Surgical Laser System has several indications for use in orthopaedic surgery. These indications may have varying operating conditions depending on the nature, location, and extent of the problem as well as the size, weight, and muscular development of the patient (e.g., shoulder arthrotomy on a 75 pound Little League pitcher would have somewhat different instrument requirements than the same procedure on a 350 pound weight lifter). To provide for these contingencies, Laser Photonics has available a variety of handpiece configurations for the ML210 Optical Fiber Delivery System. Sterile disposable (single-use) handpieces have molded plastic handles and malleable or rigid stainless steel tubing cannulas. (Reusable, steam-sterilizable handpieces of all steel construction with rigid stainless steel tubing are available.)

A variety of cannula lengths from 1 to 40 cm with uniform diameter or swaged tips are available. The handpieces with malleable steel can be bent (within certain limits) by the surgeon to fit particular operating circumstances. For most orthopaedic applications, handpieces with rigid steel tubing that may be straight, curved at varying degrees, or offset by angles are more durable and utilitarian. The disposable handpieces are gas-sterilized and supplied in packs of five.

The distal end of the optical fiber is inserted in the handle end of the handpiece and advanced until it protrudes from the metal tubing. The fiber is held in place by the collet in the handle.

System Dynamics

The Laser Photonics ML210 Holmium Surgical Laser is a flashlamp-pumped solid-state laser that is controlled and monitored by an integrated central microprocessing unit. The flashlamp pump is a xenon lamp in the laser head resonator cavity that receives power from the power supply system. The light from the flashlamp impinges on the adjacent "solid state" laser rod. The reference to "solid state" refers to the fact that the lasing media and matrix are crystalline substances (i.e., solid state, rather than a gas (e.g., CO_2 or argon) or a liquid (e.g., the tunable dye lasers).

The active lasing medium of the CTH:YAG laser rod is the Ho^{3+} ion. The Cr^{3+} ions in the laser host serve to enhance the pump light absorption. The absorbed energy is transferred, nonradiatively, from the Cr^{3+} ions to the Tm^{3+} ions, causing an electron excitation state. There is rapid, nonradiative transfer of the excitation energy between the Tm^{3+} and Ho^{3+} ions owing to the closely matched energy gaps between the upper and lower laser levels of the ions of the two elements. This ready transfer of excitation energy is the key to ambient temperature laser operation.

Lasing occurs between the Ho 5I7 upper level and higher stark components of the Ho 5I8 ground state. Boosting the power to the xenon flashlamp increases its irradiance (brilliance), thereby increasing the number of photons released. These photons impinge on the atoms of the lasing medium, causing electrons to move into a higher orbit (i.e., the atoms enter an "excited" state). This "excited" atomic state is unstable, and the electrons tend to seek their original orbit (decay). When the electrons drop from the higher orbit to a lower orbit, light energy (photons) of specific wavelengths (in this case 2.1 μm) are released. Some of these photons collide with adjacent atoms, and others escape into the laser cavity. The interior of the laser head cavity is highly reflective. As the photons are reflected about the laser cavity, some of them pass into the laser rod. Some of this stimulated radiation begins to move through the long axis of the lasing rod and oscillates between the resonator mirrors, with gain occurring with each pass. Light amplification occurs as these photons stimulate the lasing media to emit more wavelength-specific radiation. A portion of the building laser energy passes through the output resonator mirror, which is partially reflective and partially transparent, to the 2.1 μm wavelength laser light. A system of optics focuses this amplified light into the launch mechanism of the optical fiber delivery port, where it passes into the optical fiber.

A sample of the laser beam is obtained by an optical beam splitter in the optical pathway. This sample is used for "real time" monitoring of the laser output and allows the microprocessor to detect and correct any fluctuations as they occur. The Laser Photonics ML210 Holmium Surgical Laser controls the laser output energy to $\pm$ 10% of that specified by the operator.

Laser Operation

A review of the controls of the ML210 Holmium Surgical Laser System (Fig. 17-3) indicates how uncomplicated this laser is to use.

1. The keyswitch is turned to the On position. The laser automatically shows on the display screen the "Initialization in Progress" message and performs the initialization protocol, which generally requires less than 1 minute.
2. Following initialization, the microprocessor displays the "Initialization Completed-Enter Mode" prompt. The operator enters the desired mode by pressing the appropriate key.
3. When the Continuous Exposure mode is selected, the prompt, "Set joules/pls, available range, press LE" appears on the screen (the CPU automatically defines the range of energy settings permitted for the mode setting). Using the numeric keypad, the operator enters the desired numeric energy setting (joules per pulse) and presses the laser energy key.
4. The requested energy setting appears in the laser energy display and the prompt, "Sct pulse rate, range of pulse rates per second available is automatically included in the prompt, Press PR." The numeric value for the desired pulse rate is entered, and the pulse rate (PR) key is pressed.

5. The display now shows the pulse energy selected in joules per pulse, the mode selected, the pulse rate (PR) selected in pulses per second (PPS), and the timed exposure (TE) if appropriate. It also indicates that the laser is at Standby.
6. If operator wishes to use the aiming beam, the aiming beam key is pressed to activate the helium-neon aiming beam laser.
7. The ML210 Holmium Laser "idles" until the operator presses the standby/ready key. The display then changes from Standby to Ready.
8. The ML210 automatically returns to standby if the footswitch is not depressed within 15 seconds. The standby/ready key must be pressed to proceed.
9. The ML210 Holmium Laser will fire when the footswitch is depressed.
10. To change the pulse energy, enter the numeric value at standby and press the laser energy key. The new energy level appears on the display.
11. Pulse rate may be changed by entering the numeric value and pressing the pulse rate key; the new value appears on the display.
12. For each mode, a similar but appropriate prompt/response routine appears.
13. When the procedure is finished or the laser is no longer needed, the operator places the laser in Standby mode and moves the laser away from the table (out of the way). After 5 minutes, the keyswitch can be turned to the off position. Power to the laser head is disrupted immediately, although the cooling pump and chiller may continue to run for a time, to ensure that the laser is not "ridden hard and put away wet."

Delivery System Operation

The ML210 Optical Fiber Delivery System is a passive system in that there are no buttons to push, no "joysticks," no mirrors to adjust. Its function is to transmit the laser beam from the laser to the target tissue. As described above, the male SMA connector on the proximal end of the optical fiber is inserted into the female SMA connector of the laser fiberoptic output coupler, being sure that the connection is tight. The distal end of the fiber is stripped of the protective sheath according to directions included on the package and inserted into the handpiece until the appropriate length protrudes from the end of the handpiece tubing. The fiber is secured by tightening the collet on the handpiece. The nature of the helium-neon aiming beam spot is observed by projecting it onto an opaque surface. If the projected spot is not distinct and circular, the fiber is not transmitting properly and it is necessary to change fibers. The end of the fiber is brought into proximity with the target tissue through the arthroscope port and the introducing trocar or through an incision. For most indications, the end of the fiber is in contact or in near contact with the target tissue.

Indications and Applications

The Laser Photonics ML210 Holmium Surgical Laser System has been cleared by the U.S. Food and Drug Administration (FDA) for marketing for use in general and orthopaedic/arthroscopic surgery procedures for cutting (incision/excision), coagulating, and vaporizing soft tissue and firm cartilage. Applicable surgical procedures include direct, open incisions and endoscopic procedures through both natural body channels and incision/puncture wounds (e.g., arthroscopy and laparoscopy). The soft tissues encountered in orthopaedic surgical procedures under this indication include (but are not limited to) skin, subcutaneous tissue, striated and smooth muscle, cartilage, mucous membranes, lymph vessels and tissue, tendons, ligaments, and connective tissue structures (e.g., synovium and joint capsules).

Use of the Laser Photonics ML210 is suggested for, but not limited to, the following orthopaedic/arthroscopic procedures:

Incision, excision, ablation, and vaporization of cartilage
Meniscectomy
Synovectomy
Bursectomy

Tissue Effects

The results obtained with the ML210 Holmium Surgical Laser System lie between those obtained with the 10.6 μm CO_2 laser and the 1.06 μm neodymium:YAG laser. They are more impressive than results with the 0.488 μm argon laser and the 0.532 μm KTP laser.

The 2.1 μm holmium:YAG laser appears to induce relatively good hemostasis during arthroscopic procedures, which results in few clincial reports of postoperative hemarthrosis.

Studies (Dew et al., 1992) have shown that there is a pulse energy threshold at which cartilaginous tissue is more efficiently ablated by the 2.1 μm holmium:YAG laser. During these studies using human meniscal tissue obtained at total knee arthroplasty, the average total power was maintained at 18 to 20 watts. With pulse energies of 2 joules at 10 Hz (20 watts average total power) and 4 joules at 5 Hz (20 watts average total power), there was some increase in the amount of tissue ablated per pulse. A pulse energy of 3 joules at 7 Hz (21 watts average total power) appeared to be less effective for ablating meniscal tissue. There was clearly visible discoloration (caramelization/carbonization) of the tissue edges. At these lower energy levels, the zone of collateral damage is approximately 400 μm wide. Although a pulse energy of 5 joules at 4 Hz (20 watts average total power) and 5 joules at 5 Hz (25 watts) appeared to ablate more tissue per pulse (Fig. 17-4), there was almost no discoloration of the tissue edges evident, and collateral thermal injury was only 10 to 40 μm in width. Microscopically, the area of thermal necro-

Figure 17-4. Human meniscal cartilage ablation (tissue loss/pulse) using the ML210 Holmium Surgical Laser.

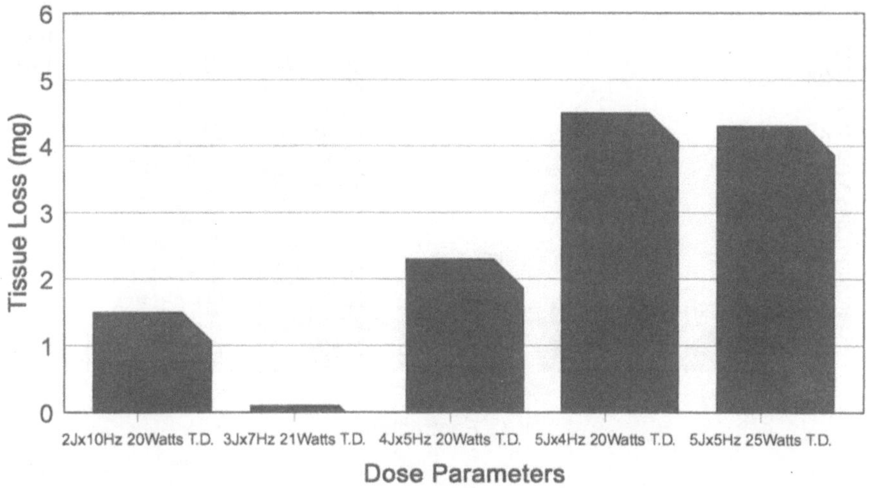

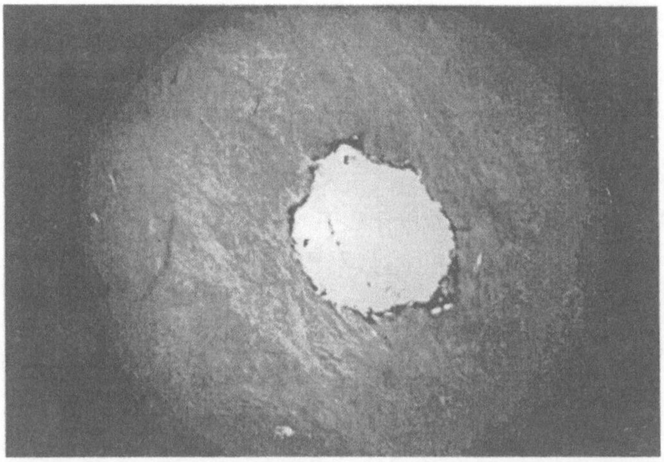

Figure 17-5. Photomicrograph of human meniscal cartilage after 5-joule exposure using the ML210 Holmium Surgical Laser.

sis was discreet, with little if any eosinophilic hyalinization of the adjacent tissue (an indication of thermal injury often seen at lower pulse energy levels) and virtually no carbonization (Fig. 17-5).

A study using bovine meniscal cartilage confirmed these results. The average amount of tissue ablated per pulse showed a linear step increase as the energy setting was raised from 2 joules at 10 Hz (20 watts) to 3 joules at 7 Hz (21 watts) to 4 joules at 5 Hz (20 watts). However, raising the pulse energy to 5 joules resulted in a geometric increase (more than double) in tissue ablated per pulse (Fig. 17-6).

In another study, lesions were mechanically induced in the articular cartilages of rat femoral condyles. In each rat, the lateral condyle of the left leg was not treated and the left medial condyle was treated with a single 3-joule pulse exposure. The right lateral condyle was treated with a 4-joule exposure and the right medial condyle with a 5-joule exposure. The zone of thermal necrosis was similar to that seen in the human and bovine meniscus, that is 10 to 40 μm in the 5-joule condyles and much wider in those where lower energy/pulse was applied. Rats sacrificed 30 days following the procedure had fibrosis and limited range of motion of the left knee (control and 3 joules) and little or no fibrosis with full range of motion of the right knee (4 joules and 5 joules). The control articular cartilage defect was prominent and had irregular borders. The 3-joule treated defect has somewhat smoother edges but was still prominent. The 4-joule treated defects were less prominent with smooth edges; and the 5-joule treated condyles had smooth edges with some new cartilage.

The response of bovine compact cortical bone from the phalanx was similar to that in cartilage (Fig. 17-7). Pulse energies of 2, 3, and 4 joules resulted in a near-linear step increase in bone tissue ablated per pulse. One sample group at 5 joules and 4 Hz yielded minimal mass loss when weighed, although craters left by tissue ablation were clearly visible macroscopically. Because the procedure was done in a waterbath, it was postulated that the bone samples had retained enough water to offset the tissue mass loss. A second set was exposed at 5 joules and 4 Hz, carefully dried, and weighed. The per-pulse tissue mass loss for the 5-joule exposures was double that seen with the lower pulse energies.

Energy Settings

For most soft tissue applications, it is recommended that the surgeon start with low pulse energy and rate settings. These settings should be changed only as necessary while directly or indirectly observing (e.g., with a video during endoscopy or arthroscopy) the tissue and tissue reactions.

The tissue effect of 2.1 μm holmium:YAG laser energy depends on the location of the optical fiber tip in relation to the target tissue. For fine incisions the fiber tip is in direct contact with the tissue and is moved slowly along the tissue plane. The 2.1 μm holmium:YAG is a pulsed laser, not a continuous wave laser; therefore the exposure sites

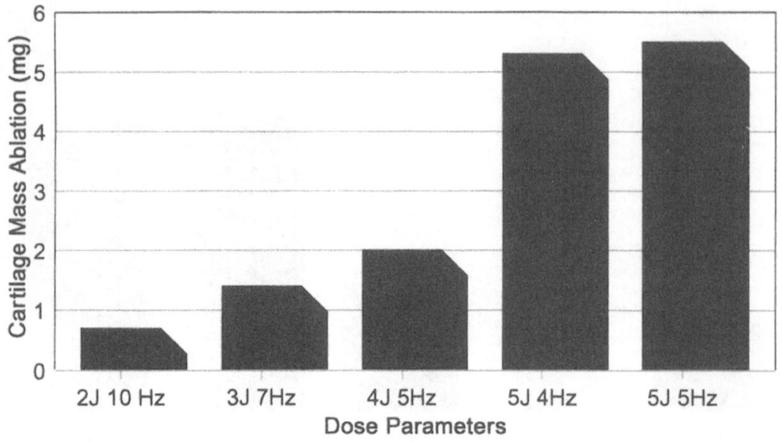

Figure 17-6. Bovine meniscal cartilage (tissue loss/pulse) using the ML210 Holmium Surgical Laser.

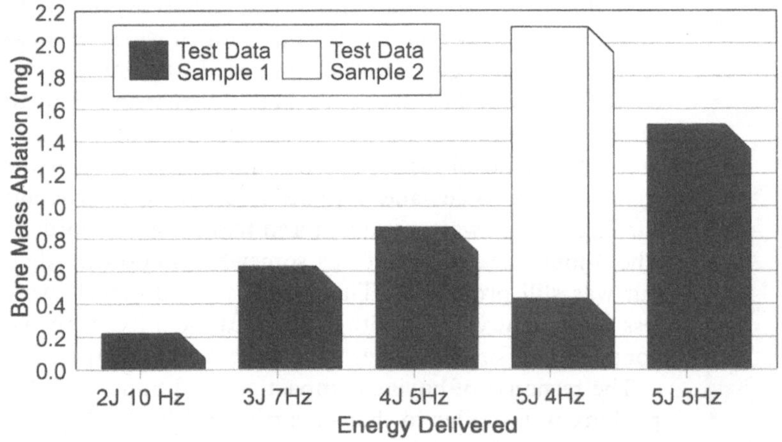

Figure 17-7. Bovine bone ablation (tissue loss/pulse) using the ML210 Holmium Surgical Laser.

should be "overlapped" to ensure a continuous incision. Soft tissue cutting with the fiber tip in contact with target tissue requires 0.2 to 1.5 joules per pulse. The pulse rate may vary according to the site, tissue, and "comfort zone" of the surgeon. When ablating (vaporizing) tissue, the tip of the fiber is positioned 1 to 3 mm from the tissue and methodically moved over the target tissue.

To use the Laser Photonics ML210 Holmium Surgical Laser for coagulating tissue, the tip of the optical fiber is held approximately 5 mm from the tissue, and the target area is slowly "painted." When using the system in air, at higher powers and repetition rates, frequent irrigation should be used to reduce overheating, charring, and "flaring."

The Laser Photonics ML210 Holmium Surgical Laser Optical Fiber may be used in contact or noncontact fashion without compromising the fiber or fiber tip.

Arthroscopic procedures can be performed in a fluid environment, which avoids "plume" formation because the combustion waste and vaporization products dissolve or suspend in the fluid medium and are removed from the joint by flushing. As described above, cartilage is efficiently cut and ablated at a pulse energy of 5 joules and 4 to 5 pulses per second. Specific exposure parameters are provided in more detail in the labeling and professional instructions provided by Laser Photonics with the ML210 Holmium Surgical Laser.

Contraindications

1. An inability to visualize the surgical site clearly at all times during laser application can result in unwanted injury to adjacent tissues.
2. The safety of vaporizing tumors or cancerous tissues using the 2.1 μm holmium:YAG laser has not been proved and may result in an increased risk of metastasis.
3. Patients undergoing radiotherapy may be at an increased risk of tissue perforation during laser exposure and delayed or complicated healing after laser treatment.
4. The 2.1 μm holmium:YAG laser, as with most lasers, should never be used in the presence of explosive or flammable anesthetic gases or other vapors.

5. Although well suited for tissue vaporization with good hemostasis, the hemocoagulative capabilities of the 2.1 μm holmium:YAG laser are not fully documented; therefore use of the laser on patients with impaired clotting is contraindicated.

Hazards

CAUTION: Use of controls or adjustments, or performance of procedures other than those specified herein, may result in hazardous radiation exposure.

CAUTION: This 2.1 μm holmium:YAG laser system is intended for use only by fully trained, qualified physicians.

The Laser Photonics ML210 Holmium Surgical Laser System has been designed to minimize the hazards associated with laser systems in general. Because the laser beam uses a fiberoptic delivery system, the hazards associated with free beam delivery are ameliorated. However, mechanically stressing or sharply bending it may break the fiberoptic cable and could allow free beam emissions, a serious hazard to both eyes and skin. Although the fiber jacket is designed to contain laser energy in the event of a fiber break, the laser beam eventually burns through the jacket if the laser is allowed to continue to run. The laser should be turned off immediately if fiber breakage occurs. The laser nurse or technician should inspect the fiber periodically during the procedure for "leakage" of the yellow helium-neon aiming beam, which shows through the jacket near the point of a break.

The Laser Photonics ML210 Holmium Surgical Laser is an electrical device and has been manufactured to meet or exceed all applicable electrical safety requirements. However, as with any electrical device, exposure to water or other electrically conductive substances or operation with the safety panels removed could result in a harmful or fatal electric shock or fire.

The Laser Photonics ML210 Holmium Surgical Laser emits invisible light at 2.1 μm wavelength, which is in the infrared spectrum. Direct or reflected exposure can result in eye or skin damage.

The laser beam can result in the combustion of flammable surfaces, substances, liquids, and gases, such as drapes, endoscopes, endotracheal tubes, alcohol-based disinfectants, acetone and other flammable solvents, and flammable anesthetic gases. Because an oxygen-rich environment increases the possibility of fire or explosion, the oxygen concentrations should not exceed 20% during laser use.

Once the target tissue has been ablated (vaporized), other tissue directly in line with the axis of the laser beam may be thermally injured if the laser is allowed to continue to pulse beyond the desired surgical endpoint. Adequate visualization of the surgical site, familiarity with the tissue effects of the laser energy, and practiced technique are required to prevent such inadvertent injury.

The helium-neon aiming beam of the ML210 Holmium Surgical Laser is visible yellow (0.594 μm) laser light that may result in retinal damage if directed into the eye.

Smoke generated during open air or gas environment laser surgery (laser plume) may contain viable cells and other substances that represent an inhalation risk to operating room personnel and patients. Pulsed lasers, such as the 2.1 μm holmium:YAG laser, may increase this hazard. Standard surgical masks may not afford adequate protection. Smoke should be quickly evacuated using equipment designed specifically for laser plume removal during surgery.

One advantage of the ML210 Holmium Surgical Laser in arthroscopic procedures is the ability to operate in a fluid environment. In such cases no smoke is produced, and the residue of tissue ablation is dissolved or suspended in the liquid, thereby reducing the laser plume hazard.

As with any laser, use in a gaseous environment in a closed body cavity may increase the risk of gas emboli developing in the circulatory system.

Precautions

Precautions taken to avoid inadvertent injury to the patient include (l) covering the patient's eyes with wavelength-specific protective eyewear and covering uninvolved areas of the body to prevent damage from scatter or accidental exposure; (2) avoiding the use of surgical accessories (e.g., drapes or endotracheal tubes) made of combustible materials; (3) moistening materials that must be used in the procedure (e.g., gauze sponges and cotton swabs for limiting exposure of adjacent tissues); and (4) keeping the oxygen concentration below 20%.

The operating room personnel should wear wavelength-specific protective eyewear and must be familiar with and follow all instructions, precautions, and warnings in the operator's manual provided with the laser system. Serious injury can result to personnel and patients if the surgeon and system operator are not thoroughly familiar with the controls and function of the device.

Physician training should include (1) a thorough review of the relevant literature and attendance at professional symposia where information regarding basic tissue reaction, general use in the specialty field, and specific procedures for the 2.1 μm holmium:YAG laser are presented; (2) attendance and participation in workshops where didactic and hands-on instruction is provided; and (3) thorough familiarity with the Laser Photonics ML210 Holmium Surgical Laser System operator's manual. In addition, the physician should be experienced with endoscopic and arthroscopic procedures.

Installation

Most operating rooms can easily accommodate the relatively compact Laser Photonics ML210 Holmium Surgical Laser System, which requires less than 6 square feet of space (approximately 2 × 3 feet). The ML210 connects to a dedicated single-phase, 220 (±10%) volts, 60 cycle, 30 ampere power circuit, a common electrical service (in the United States), via an abrasion-resistant, insulated electrical cable. The self-contained cooling system means that no external water or drain service is necessary. Remote door interlocks are provided and can be connected, depending on the institution's policy. Windows and door lights, if any, should be covered and laser warning signs posted when the laser is use. Smoke evacuation equipment should be used during open air procedures. There are no other special installation requirements.

Maintenance

The Laser Photonics ML210 Holmium Laser System has been designed around the modular concept and requires limited maintenance by the end user. It is warranted to the original purchaser to be free of defects in material and workmanship, except for consumables, under normal usage for a period of 12 months from the date of shipment.

The optics module has been designed to require virtually no alignment adjustments and has been totally enclosed to shield it from dust and foreign matter. Flashlamps are warranted free of defects in material or workmanship for 5 million shots or 180 days, whichever comes first on a pro-rated basis. The helium-neon aiming system warranty is for 1 year from shipment. The control electronics and microprocessor are easily replaced if necessary.

The cabinet design provides for ready accessibility of the power supply and cooling system if service or replacement is required. The deionizing cartridge should be inspected at 6-month intervals and replaced when the medium becomes discolored. The cartridge is warranted free of defects in materials and workmanship for 90 days. Replacement of the deionizing cartridge necessitates refilling the reservoir. Laser Photonics recommends that service, when necessary, be conducted by authorized service personnel.

The fiberoptic delivery systems recommended for use with the Laser Photonics ML210 Holmium Surgical Laser are single-use, disposable optical fibers and handpieces. Reusable handpieces are available and have 90-day materials and workmanship warranties.

Conclusion

The relatively compact, low maintenance, easy-to-use Laser Photonics ML210 Holmium Surgical Laser System employs single-use disposable fiberoptic delivery systems with interchangeable disposable handpieces adaptable to arthroscopic and endoscopic procedures. The ML210 delivers pulse energy levels of up to 5 joules and repetition rates of 4 to 10 pulses per second to the tissue. When used on dense tissues, such as cartilage, this high pulse energy and slow repetition rate results in increased tissue mass ablation and little collateral tissue thermal damage or necrosis. The Laser Photonics ML210 Holmium Surgical Laser System is destined to become a valuable tool in the orthopaedist's armamentarium.

Editor's Cautions

1. **Even though many surgeons believe there is no need to wear 2.1 μm wavelength-specific protective eyewear, I do not agree. The 2.1 μm holmium:YAG is a class IV laser, and its wavelength can damage the eye.**
2. **These fibers should be used in a standard liquid arthroscopic environment. Use in a gas environment is not recommended.**
3. **Each fiber is fragile and can fracture if not fully protected. Forcing, levering, or using the "probe" as a mechanical probe will likely result in a fracture and an intraarticular foreign body.**
4. **All fibers have a definitive life-span. Optimal, satisfactory use of this system requires some experience. It is best to start in the laboratory, not with patients. The best techniques, energy settings, and probe selections can be preliminarily determined in this way. The reader is referred to Chapter 4, on ablation efficiency.**
5. **Mechanical instruments should be available at all times during arthroscopic laser surgery.**
6. **This chapter is only an introduction to this arthroscopic laser system. The reader is encouraged to study this entire text, follow acceptable training and credentialing procedures, as well as research the subject at hand for additional information and changes before undertaking this arthroscopic laser system's use.**

Suggested Reading

Aretz HT et al (1989) Effects of holmium:YSGG laser irradiation on arterial tissue: preliminary results. SPIE Symposium, Los Angeles, CA

Dew DW et al (1992) Talk given at Am Academy of Orth Surg Laser Workshop, Richmond, VA

Lilge L, Radtke W, and Nishioka N (1989) Pulsed holmium laser ablation of cardiac valves. Lasers in Surgery and Medicine 9:458–464

McKenzie AL (1989) An extension of the three-zone model to predict depth of tissue damage beneath er:YAG and ho:YAG laser excisions. Phys Med Biol 34:107–114 (U.K.)

Nishioka NS, Domankevitz Y, Flotte TJ, Anderson RR (1989) Ablation of rabbit liver, stomach, and colon with a pulsed holmium laser. Gastroenterology 96:831–7

Nuss RC, Fabian RL, Sarkar R, Puliafito CA (1988) Infrared laser bone ablation. Lasers in Surgery and Medicine 8:381–391

Oz MC, Bass LS, Popp HW, et al (1989) In vitro comparison of thulium-holmium-chromium:YAG and argon ion lasers for welding of biliary tissue. Lasers in Surgery and Medicine 9:248–253

Shapshay SM (1989) In vitro comparison of holmium and CO_2 lasers on sinus bone, cartilage, and soft tissue. Lahey Clinic Internal Report, February

Shapshay SM (1989) Holmium laser sinus study. Lahey Clinic Internal Report, February

Shapshay SM et al. Soft tissue effects of the holmium-YSGG laser in the canine trachea. Submitted to Otolaryngology-Head and Neck Surgery

Treat MR, Trokel SL, Reynolds RD, et al. (1988) Preliminary evaluation of a pulsed 2.15 μm laser system for fiberoptic endoscopic surgery. Lasers in Surgery and Medicine 8: 322–326

18

Luxar 10.6 μm CO_2 LX-20 Laser and Luxar Extend Systems for Adaptation to Other 10.6 μm CO_2 Lasers for Arthroscopic Laser Surgery

Kathy Laakmann

The 10.6 μm CO_2 laser is the most prevalent type of laser found in the operating room today. It derives its name from its active medium (i.e., CO_2 gas), but it typically contains other gases as well, including helium, nitrogen, and xenon. Most 10.6 μm CO_2 lasers are excited by a radiofrequency discharge or a direct current discharge. Manufacturers point to advantages of their particular laser tube technology, but for the most part these advantages are not apparent to the user.

Advantages and Disadvantages of 10.6 μm CO_2 Laser Versus Other Lasers

The 10.6 μm CO_2 laser has the following advantages compared to the 1.06 μm neodymium:YAG and 2.1 μm holmium:YAG lasers:

1. Speed and precision: Because of its affinity for water-laden cartilage tissue, the 10.6 μm CO_2 laser is by far the fastest ablating tool among the lasers used for arthroscopy. Because 10.6 μm CO_2 energy is so rapidly absorbed by joint tissues, it has minor thermal penetration in tissue-about 0.5 mm. The basic truism with the 10.6 μm CO_2 laser is "what you see is what you get."
2. Nothing to break in the joint: The 10.6 μm CO_2 laser energy is delivered through narrow stainless steel waveguides. There is no fiber tip that can break and become lost in the joint, whereas both 2.1 μm holmium:YAG and 1.06 μm neodymium:YAG fibers have demonstrated fracture vulnerability within the joint.
3. Noncontact capability: The 10.6 μm CO_2 laser does not require direct contact with tissue to be effective, whereas 1.06 μm neodymium:YAG contact fibers must touch tissue to be effective and the 2.1 μm holmium:YAG laser requires near contact (1–2 mm) to be effective. Noncontact capability allows clinicians to affect tissue in difficult-to-access areas that they cannot physically touch.
4. Most hospitals have a 10.6 μm CO_2 laser that can be adapted for arthroscopic use.

The 10.6 μm CO_2 laser has the following disadvantages compared to the 1.06 μm neodymium:YAG and 2.1 μm holmium:YAG lasers:

1. Inability to work in saline environment.
   a. Because the 10.6 μm CO_2 laser cannot penetrate water, it is necessary to perform 10.6 μm CO_2 laser arthroscopy in a "dry field." For surgeons accustomed to working in a fluid medium, the "dry field" approach requires some readjustment.
   b. The 1.06 μm neodymium:YAG and 2.1 μm holmium:YAG lasers, on the other hand, penetrate adequately through an aqueous medium (which is ironically the very reason they do not ablate tissue efficiently); therefore surgeons can continue to work in a fluid medium with these two lasers.
2. Lack of flexible fiber delivery systems.
   Other than the Luxar LX-20 laser, every other 10.6 μm CO_2 laser has an articulating arm or a hand-held resonator. The 1.06 μm neodymium:YAG and 2.1 μm holmium:YAG lasers, on the other hand, contain silica fibers, providing far more supple delivery than the articulating arms of the 10.6 μm CO_2 laser.

10.6 μm CO_2 LX-20 Laser

The 10.6 μm CO_2 laser systems are available in three configurations, characterized by their delivery systems: (1) a hollow flexible fiber delivery system; (2) articulating arm systems; and (3) hand-held devices. Luxar Corporation is the only company that manufactures a 10.6 μm CO_2 laser with a flexible fiber delivery system. Luxar introduced the

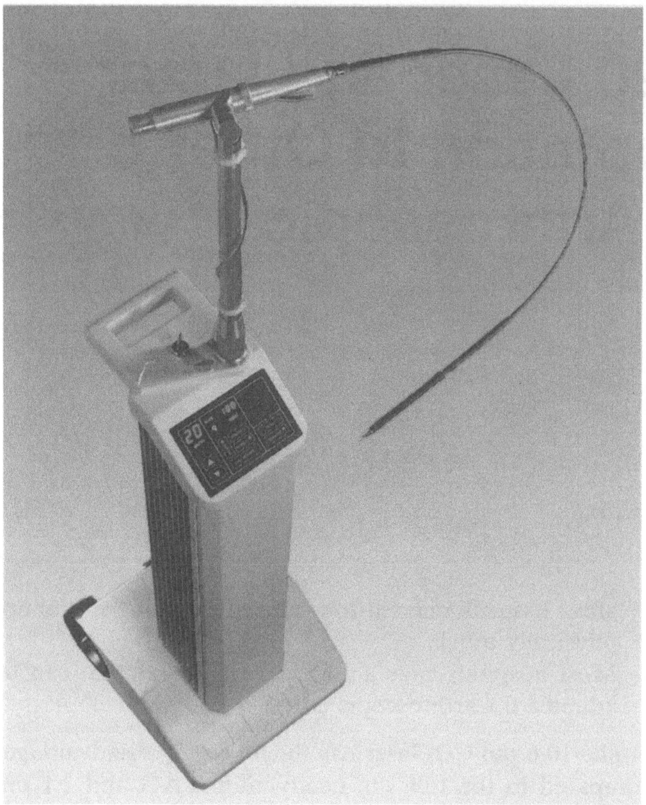

Figure 18-1. LX-20 Laser manufactured by Luxar Corporation.

LX-20 laser (Fig. 18-1) in 1990. This laser delivers 20 watts to tissue and is utilized for both hand-held and endoscopic surgery. The Extend System adapts to this laser. The advantage this laser has over other 10.6 μm CO_2 lasers is the greater flexibility of its delivery system, its small physical size, and its greater versatility. Many surgeons delight in the freedom of movement the Luxar LX-20 provides vis-à-vis the articulating arm systems.

The routine articulating arm systems are produced by a variety of manufacturers, including Sharplan, Laser Engineering, Surgilase, Zeiss, Coherent, and Heraeus. For the reader unfamiliar with an articulating arm it is a hollow, rigid tube with articulated knuckles of typical diameter of about 2 cm. Mirrors within the tube allow the beam to be directed. Most 10.6 μm CO_2 laser systems utilize a seven-knuckle system, as this number has been found to be the lowest that can provide adequate flexibility to the surgeon.

Articulating arms were once the Achilles' heels of 10.6 μm CO_2 laser systems, becoming frequently misaligned and requiring constant service. Today's articulating arms (i.e., systems manufactured during the late 1980s up through today) generally preserve alignment well and should maintain sufficient alignment to use with the Extend System.

Hand-held devices are some manufacturers' answer to the articulating arm. The surgeon holds the entire laser tube, obviating the need for an articulating arm. The major advantage of the hand-held approach is elimination of the substantial portion of the cost of the laser system (i.e., the delivery system). Unfortunately, the weight of these systems (~ 1 pound) makes them difficult to use for extended periods (in excess of several minutes). In addition, the laser power is frequently limited because of the difficulty of adequately removing heat from the laser head.

Luxar Extend Systems

Because most 10.6 μm CO_2 laser systems currently used have articulating arms, Luxar has developed another excellent laser arthroscopy system that adapts most of these devices for arthroscopic use. It does not adapt to the hand-held resonator versions, however.

The Extend CO_2 Laser Delivery System consists of a launch coupler, which attaches to the end of the laser's articulated arm, a waveguide, which delivers the laser energy to tissue, and a protective sheath, which surrounds the waveguide (Figs. 18-2 and 18-3). The entire distal assembly is inserted into the joint through a second puncture cannula.

The Luxar 10.6 μm CO_2 Laser Arthroscopy System consists of the following elements: The Extend Luxar Delivery System components include the ambient air arthroscopy kit, which contains nondisposable sheaths and cannulas (Fig. 18-4), waveguides (Fig. 18-2) (Microguides or Endoguides) that direct the laser energy to tissue, and the Luxar launch coupler appropriate to the laser system being used and that allows the clinician to adapt the arthroscopy kit to most 10.6 μm CO_2 lasers.

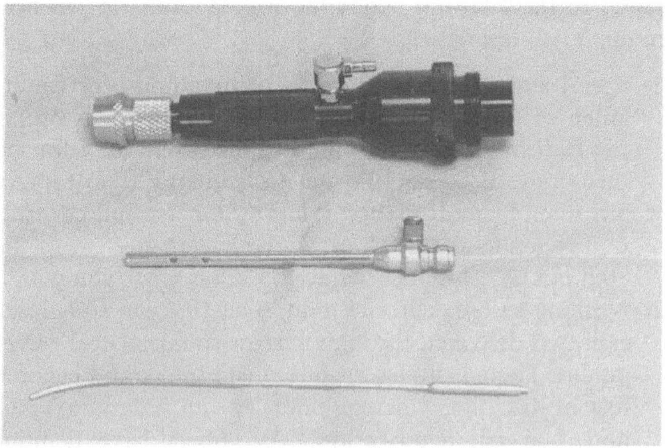

Figure 18-2. Additional Extend System components. To adapt the Extend System to a hospital-based laser requires a launch coupler (black device shown at the top), which attaches directly to the distal end of the articulated arm of most 10.6 μm CO_2 lasers; a waveguide (shown at bottom), which delivers the laser energy to tissue; and a sheath, which surrounds the waveguide for protection (middle). Figure 18-3 shows these components assembled.

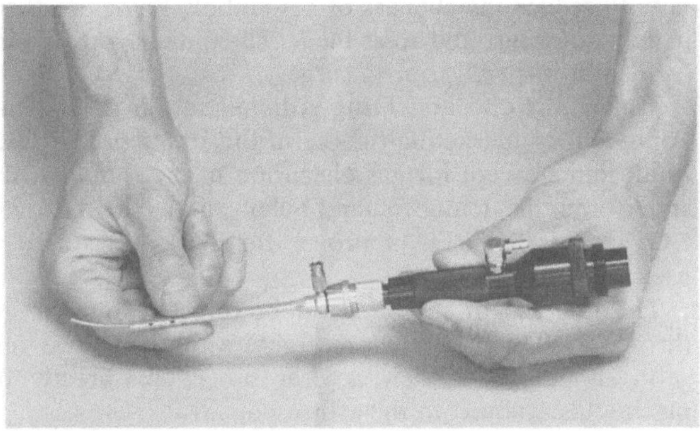

Figure 18-3. Extend System components assembled.

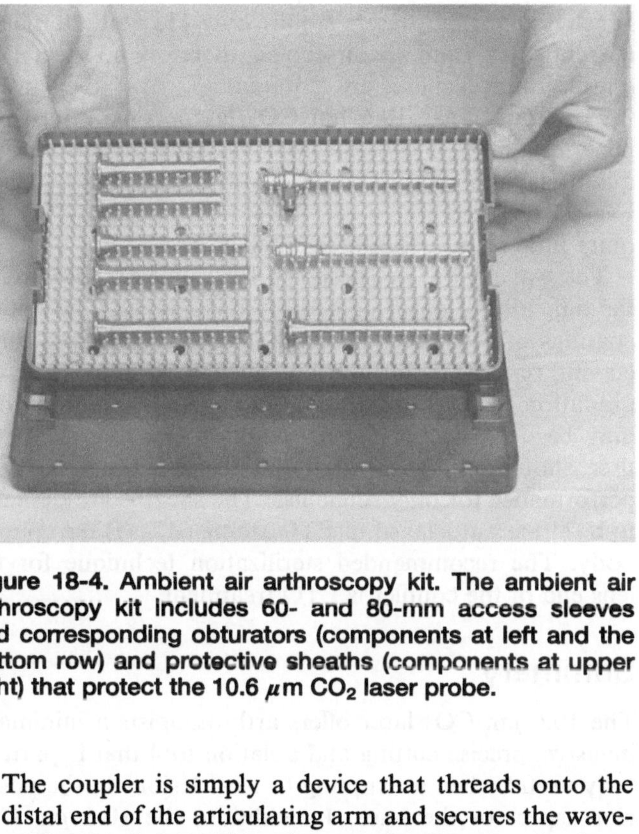

Figure 18-4. Ambient air arthroscopy kit. The ambient air arthroscopy kit includes 60- and 80-mm access sleeves and corresponding obturators (components at left and the bottom row) and protective sheaths (components at upper right) that protect the 10.6 μm CO_2 laser probe.

1. The coupler is simply a device that threads onto the distal end of the articulating arm and secures the waveguides. A lens within the coupler focuses the laser beam exiting the articulating arm into the waveguides. The focal length of the lens is optimized for maximum laser beam transmission through the waveguide and minimum sensitivity to misalignment of the articulating arm. Typically, the beam size at the proximal end of the waveguide is 0.4 mm, compared to a waveguide diameter of about 0.9 mm.
2. The Luxar Endoguides and Microguides are all-metal, with a metal/dielectric layer evaporated onto the inner lumen to provide high reflectivity. The arthroscopic waveguides are rated for 10.6 μm CO_2 laser transmission in excess of 85% for an articulating arm in nominal alignment. If the distal end clogs with debris or the articulating arm is severely misaligned, optical transmission may deteriorate. The users' manual of the Extend System discusses this situation in detail.
3. The Luxar launch coupler (Figs. 18-2 and 18-3) attaches to the distal end of the articulating arm of the 10.6 μm CO_2 laser. As stated, the Luxar coupler attaches to most brands of 10.6 μm CO_2 lasers. The matrix below shows which coupler attaches to which model laser:

LC2001	Zeiss
LC3001	Heraeus/Lasersonics
LC4001	Laser Dynamics
LC5001	Surgilase (compatible with models 25, 40, 45, 55, 60, 80, 100)
LC6001	Coherent (compatible with Xanar XA50, XL40, XL60, Ultrapulse)
LC7001	Sharplan (compatible with models 1020, 1040, 1060, 1100)
LC8001	NIIC
LC9001	Laser Engineering (compatible with models MD30, MD50, MD75)

4. Sheaths (Figs. 18-2, 18-3, and 18-4) perform several functions, including the removal of smoke and provision of additional rigidity to the waveguide to minimize the likelihood of its being inadvertently bent or damaged during surgery. The most widely used sheath is 4.6 mm, which is large enough to accommodate the curved Microguides. The oversize diameter of this sheath, relative to the Microguide, ensures gas egress to maintain the gas pressure within the knee to ambient air pressure.
5. The "waveguides" are truly the heart of the system, as they transmit laser energy from the laser system to the surgical site. The waveguides are available in two standard diameters: 1.6 mm (Microguides) and 3.1 mm (Endoguides). The Microguide is 120 mm long and is available in a curved (Fig. 18-2), straight, or mirrored configuration. The Endoguide is also 120 mm long and is available in straight or mirrored configurations. The advantage of the Endoguide over the Microguide is its greater ruggedness, whereas the Microguide's small diameter and availability in curved configurations greatly enhances its ability to access almost all areas of the knee.
6. The Luxar LXF-l fiber delivery system, the Luxar Flexiguide, the Luxar Microguide, and Luxar Endoguide utilize the same Luxar hollow fiber technology. What differentiates these hollow fibers from one another are the sheathing, the length, and whether they are prebent or straight.
7. The 0.632 μm helium-neon aiming beam is typically stronger with the straight guides, somewhat less with the angled guides, and weakest with the curved guides. On the other hand, particularly with two-punc-

ture techniques, the end of the guide can generally be visualized, mitigating the need to be able to see the aiming beam.

Setting Up the Laser and the Extend System

1. The laser system should be tested for proper operating prior to surgery, in accordance with the operator's manual of the particular laser system in use.
2. The gas purge regulator should be attached to the appropriate CO_2 gas bottle and the regulator tested for proper functioning in accordance with the Extend System operator's manual. Gas pressure should be set for 80 to 100 mm Hg. The flow rate of the CO_2 gas should be set to approximately 0.5 liter per minute.
3. The coupler is attached to the articulating arm, and the tubing for the gas purge is connected from the gas purge system to the coupler, securing the tubing with tape to the arm to prevent drooping on the ground. Drape the arm, the laser, and the coupler.
4. The waveguide is taken from its sterile pack. If a curved guide is to be used, thread the guide through the Extend sheath prior to insertion into the coupler. In accordance with the operator's manual, the guide should be connected to the coupler.
5. Check for proper arm alignment and attachment of the waveguide by burning a small spot onto a wet tongue depressor, as described in the operator's manual. Do not use if the system is not functioning properly.

Safety Requirements

Clear glasses, either plastic or glass, preferably with side shields, should be worn by all operating room personnel. The patient's eyes should also be protected with either wet gauze or safety glasses. To minimize the risk of fire, flammable material must be kept away from the path of the laser beam and a fire extinguisher kept nearby. Drapes should be moistened. Attention must be given to the reflection of the laser beam, and inadvertent stepping on the foot pedal avoided. Special laser masks that filter viral particles are available, and particular care should be paid to have adequate smoke evacuation systems, especially when treating human immunodeficiency virus (HIV)-positive patients.

The ambient air technique reduces the potential hazards associated with gas embolism and subcutaneous emphysema so long as sufficient egress of gas is allowed to avoid the buildup of gas pressure in the knee. Nonetheless, the surgeon should be careful to not position the waveguide in blood vessels, in order to avoid the possibility of embolism. A tourniquet should be used. A large vascular bed, as occurs sometimes with acute fractures is a contraindication to using this technique. The surgeon must understand how to reduce the chances of gas emboli, recognize them if they do occur, and treat them. The patient must be informed of this risk prior to surgery.

The U.S. Food and Drug Administration (FDA) has approved for marketing the use of the 10.6 μm CO_2 laser in all joints except for gas distension in the shoulder, the spine, and the temporomandibular joint. The 10.6 μm CO_2 laser is not FDA-approved for marketing for bone use.

The laser beam should never be directed into the arthroscope. It will damage or fracture the lens. The surgeon should never view a laser procedure directly by placing his eye next to the arthroscope.

Operating Room Requirements/Special Maintenance

Most 10.6 μm CO_2 lasers require only 115 volt alternating current (VAC) and are air-cooled, therefore no special operating room facilities are required.

For flowing-gas 10.6 μm CO_2 lasers, operating room personnel must check the laser gas level to ensure adequate gas supply during surgery. Fortunately, most 10.6 μm CO_2 lasers used today are the sealed-off variety and require little or no periodic maintenance.

The waveguides are designed for single use because of the difficulty of ensuring sterility upon reuse. The optical coatings of the waveguide can generally withstand autoclaving or (ETO) sterilization, but not without some degradation in performance. Users report that autoclaving may be done succesfully as many as five times, but the user should remember that the manufacturer warrants performance for only single use. The sheaths are designed to be either autoclaved or ETO-sterilized, as is the coupler body. The recommended sterilization technique for the lens end of the coupler is ETO treatment.

Summary

The 10.6 μm CO_2 laser offers arthroscopists a minimally invasive, precise cutting and ablation tool that is particularly useful when attempting to treat lesions in the posterior aspect of the knee. In addition, the 10.6 μm CO_2 laser, coupled with the Luxar Extend System, combines the functions of cutting, ablation, sculpting, and hemostasis in a single device, offering the potential of improved operative efficiency (with minimal trauma to normal articular cartilage) compared to that with mechanical instruments. The 10.6 μm CO_2 laser has the most favorable tissue response of the lasers approved for arthroscopy, providing the quickest ablations with the least residual tissue damage. The components necessary to perform the technique can be adapted for most brands of 10.6 μm CO_2 lasers, allowing institutions that already have a 10.6 μm CO_2 laser to maximize utilization of an already acquired asset.

Editor's Cautions

1. **This laser should not be used without 10.6 μm wavelength-specific protective eyewear. Regular glasses or contact lenses are not enough. All personnel in the room, especially the patient, should be protected.**
2. **This laser could start a fire or cause a burn if inadvertently misdirected. Therefore, simultaneous use of flammable substances must be avoided. Foot pedal clutter also must be avoided.**
3. **Any gas technique, including the ambient air and gas bubble or Moses technique, but especially a CO_2 gas distention technique, can result, although rarely, in gas emboli. Emboli, in turn, can result in permanent neurologic sequelae or fatality. Danger exists so long as there is an unfavorable pressure gradient between the gas and the tissues. This situation has never been reported with the ambient air technique, but it is theoretically possible. The surgeon should inform the patient of this rare possibility preoperatively, as well as know how to minimize the potential for it occurring. The surgeon and anesthesiologist should know how to recognize and treat gas emboli. Appropriate pressures should be used—never more than 1.5 pounds per square inch. A tourniquet should be used. Gas distention must not be used in the shoulder, temporomandibular joint, or spine. These techniques must not be used when there are large vascular beds, as is especially seen with intraarticular fractures.**
4. **Gas arthroscopy should be learned prior to using the 10.6 μ CO_2 laser with gas arthroscopy.**
5. **This technique must be used with mechanical instruments available.**
6. **Reflectance is a major factor to consider for safe operation of the 10.6 μm CO_2 laser.**
7. **Char should be debrided or irrigated from the joint.**
8. **Inadvertent tissue damage caused by a misdirected laser beam may result in intraoperative and postoperative complications. Small probes are preferred to large probes.**
9. **Smoke evacuation is essential.**
10. **Optimal, satisfactory use of this system requires some experience. It is best to start in the laboratory, not with patients. The best techniques, energy settings, and probe selections can be preliminarily determined in this way.**
11. **This chapter is only an introduction to this arthroscopic laser system. The reader is encouraged to study this entire text, follow acceptable training and credentialing procedures, as well as research the subject at hand for additional information and changes before undertaking this arthroscopic laser system's use.**

Suggested Reading

Brillhart AT (1991) Arthroscopic laser surgery: the CO_2 laser and its use, second of four articles. American Journal of Arthroscopy 1:7–12

Garrick JG (1992) CO_2 laser arthroscopy using ambient gas pressure. Semin Orthop 7:90–94

Shupak RC, Shuster H, Funch RS (1984) Airway emergency in a patient during CO_2 arthroscopy. Anesthesiology 60:171–172

Smith CF, Johansen WE, Vangsness CT et al (1989) The carbon dioxide laser: a potential tool for orthopedic surgery. Clin Orthop 242:43–50

19

Premier 10.6 μm CO_2 Laser for Arthroscopic Laser Surgery

Colette Cozean

Premier Laser Systems, formerly Pfizer Laser Systems, has U.S. Food and Drug Administration (FDA) approval to market lasers of six wavelengths and a combination system for the orthopaedic market. Beginning with the first arthroscopic clinical trials and first approval to market a portable 10.6 μm CO_2 laser in 1987, Premier has been a leader in providing portable, reliable, cost-effective gas and solid-state lasers to the orthopaedic surgeon.

10.6 μm CO_2 Laser Model 20CH: Description

The model 20CH CO_2 surgical laser system (Fig. 19-1) is a reliable, precise surgical tool that provides the physician with an instrument capable of performing incision, excision, hemostasis, coagulation, ablation and vaporization of living tissue. The system is comprised of a hand-held laser head with an optical attachment coupler and a power supply with built-in laser power meter, 0.632 μm helium-neon laser aiming beam, air source, and pulse control system. The system, fully portable and self-contained with built-in fault and safety monitors, is capable of producing peak laser powers of 20 watts at a user-preset rate of either 20 or 2 pulses per second. The pulse durations can be varied from 5 to 450 ms per pulse and depend on the user-preset pulse rate. The system may also be set to run in a continuous wave (CW) mode of operation. The system is compatible with a series of laser attachments.

The laser head is comprised of a single radiofrequency excited and sealed laser tube that is isolated within nonsubmersible aluminum housing. The laser head also contains a radiofrequency power converter unit that converts the 50-ohm impedance of the radiofrequency input signal to the proper impedance of the laser tube. The output end of the laser head is supplied with a specialized optical coupler that is compatible with various optional optical attachments. The laser head also contains a manual safety shutter and a 0.632 μm helium-neon/10.6 μm CO_2 laser beam combiner. The laser head is connected to the power unit via a flexible, nonsubmersible umbilical cord. A red light on top of the laser head turns on whenever the main power switch on the power supply is turned on.

The power unit is a portable, self-contained system that includes a radiofrequency generator, a 0.632 μm helium-neon laser with fiberoptic coupler, an air source, a laser power meter, a radiofrequency pulse modulator system, and system fault monitors. The front panel of the power unit is illustrated in Figure 19-2. The main power breaker/switch is located on the left side of the front panel. The keyswitch is located on the far bottom left of the front panel of the power unit and acts as a safety delay switch (5 seconds delay from Standby to Ready) as well, with indicator lights located to the left of the keyswitch. At the bottom right of the front panel are the connections for the umbilical cord to the laser head, labeled Laser, RF, and Coolant. To the right of the RF connection to the laser on the front panel is the Footswitch input where the foot switch is connected. To the bottom left of the front panel is the Power Level control, which modulates the radiofrequency signal delivered to the laser so as to control the average laser power. The Power Level control is continuously adjustable by the user. At the bottom center of the front panel are the user-adjustable pulse Duration and pulse Total controls, which adjust the pulse duration and total pulse count, respectively. The Accu/Expand pulse switch is located below the pulse Duration switch and allows the user two modes of operation at either equal to (Accupulse) or ten times (Expand Pulse) the pulse duration setting (which represents 20 or 2 pulses per second, respectively). The laser power meter is located above the Power Level control. When the laser is pushed into the power meter shield, activating a microswitch, and

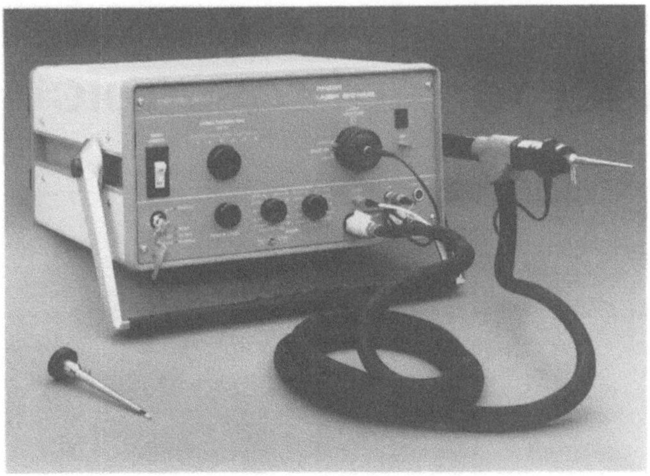

Figure 19-1. 20CH laser system.

the footswitch is simultaneously depressed, the Laser Calibration meter reads out the laser power set by the Power Level control. The air coupler and enable switch are located on the upper right of the front panel of the power unit. The interlock connector is located on the rear panel. This interlock is disabled with either the laser holder connector or a supplied interlock plug.

Specifications of Model 20CH Surgical 10.6 μm CO_2 Laser System

Peak output power: resonator (25 watts maximum; 20 watts nominal; 17 watts minimum)
Mode: resonator: geometric TEM mode with near gaussian intensity distribution at prime focus
Beam diameter/divergence: 5.5 mm/16 mrad nominal
Wavelength: 10.6 μm nominal
Exposure time: continuous or pulsed operation; in pulsed mode:
5.0 to 45.0 ms per gate pulse at 20 pulses/second
50 to 450 ms per gate pulse at 2 pulses/second with 1 to 1000 pulses per activation command
Spot size at focal point: depends on optical attachment
Coolant: distilled water with copper sulfate additive
Gas supply: self-contained, sealed tube
Air pump gas flow: 3 liters per minute (nominal)
Electrical input
110–120 volts alternating current (VAC), 6 amperes at 50/60 Hz
220–240 VAC, 3 amperes at 50/60 Hz
Electrical isolation: less than 100 μA
Weight (nominal): laser head 540 g
Power supply: 18 kg

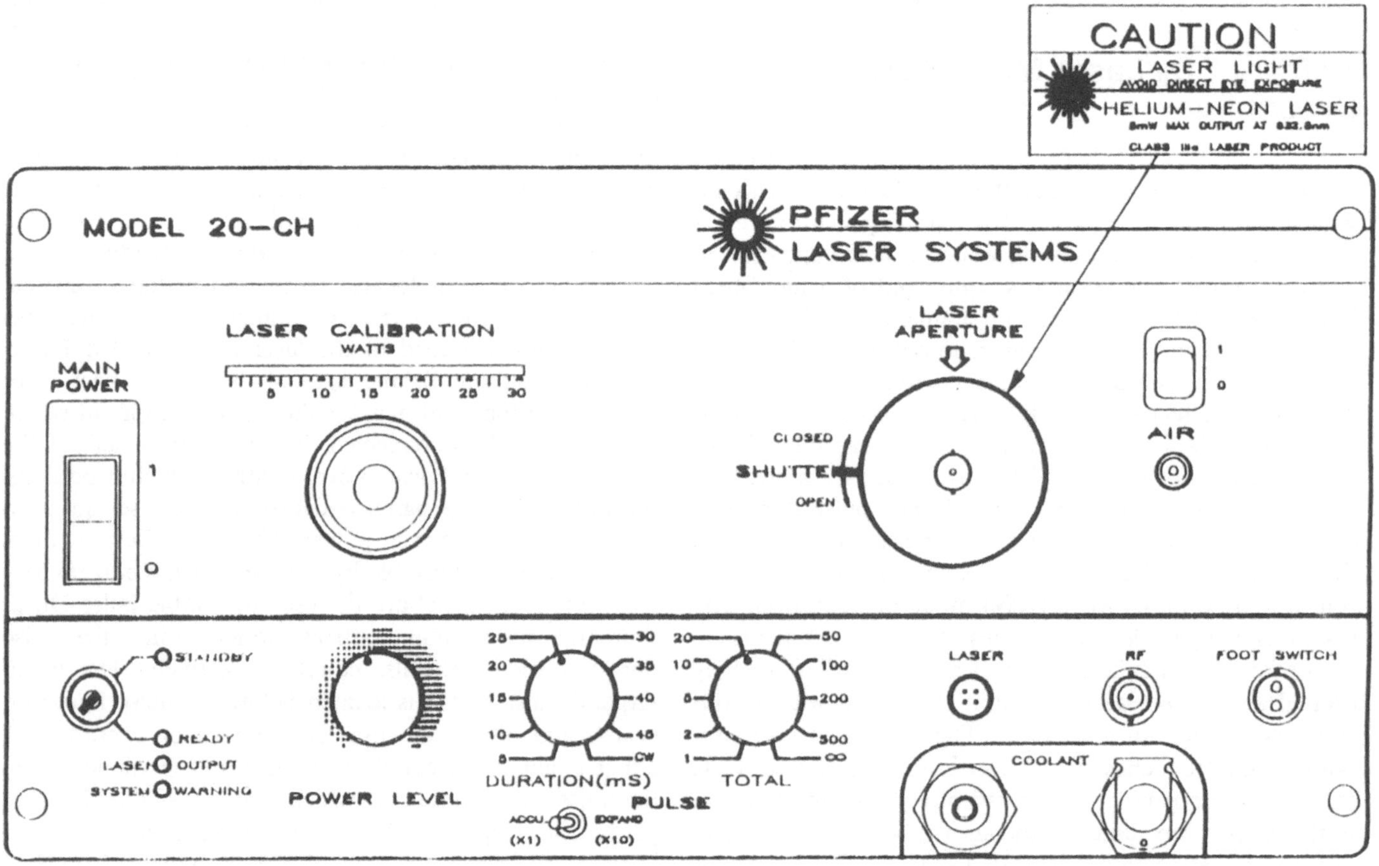

Figure 19-2. Front panel of 20CH power unit.

Delivery System

The AR-10A/U orthopaedic attachment is specifically designed for delivery of CO_2 laser radiation at 10.6 μm wavelength through a series of nontoxic and nondisposable tapered laser inserters for arthroscopic surgical applications. The attachment comes in separable parts and is compatible with the model 20CH system. The AR-10A attachment is supplied with a gas inlet port for inserting CO_2 insufflation gas down the metal inserter tips to (1) prevent charring of the tissue, (2) keep the inserter casements clear of debris, and (3) insufflate the joint. A coaxial helium-neon laser aiming beam at 0.632 μm is supplied through the laser head. The AR-10A/U attachment features a separable "laser inserter" including a 30 degree angled inserter and a straight inserter for directing the laser radiation into the joint area. (Note that 60 and 90 degree inserter tips are also available but optional.)

Premier Laser Systems has plans to introduce a fiberoptic delivery system within the next year that is flexible and should provide even greater access to the joint. This company has provided an Orthopac, which facilitates exchange of fluid and gas. A knee joint can be completely filled with gas in less than 5 minutes using this device.

The 10.6 μm CO_2 laser can also be employed in a fluid environment using the gas bubble technique. With this method, gas flows through the 10.6 μm CO_2 laser, creating a bubble in which to operate. Surgeons must develop their techniques to stay within this bubble.

Principles of Laser Operation

The 10.6 μm CO_2 gas laser system generates a highly intense laser radiation beam in the infrared spectrum that is produced through the stimulated emission of radiation from the CO_2 molecule. The CO_2 molecule is excited to the proper level for stimulated emission via a radiofrequency (27.12 MHz) "electrodeless" electrical discharge whereby the electrical energy is coupled through the wall of the laser tube via capacitive coupling. The high electrical field produced inside the laser tube produces a discharge that excites the CO_2 molecules into states that emit infrared radiation. This radiation is then amplified via precisely aligned mirrors located on each end of the laser tube. Laser power is extracted by making one of the mirrors partially reflecting, thereby coupling out some energy, whereas the reflected energy from the partially reflecting mirror is used to "feed back" into the laser tube, thereby stimulating the CO_2 molecules to continue emitting radiation at a precise frequency and in a coherent (tightly collimated) fashion. The extracted laser energy is then focused to a point (or recollimated with certain attachments to the laser) to produce a highly intense spot of radiation suitable for many surgical applications.

The chief absorber during CO_2 laser surgery is water. It is also absorbed by blood and is known for its ability to vaporize bulk tissues and provide coagulation. These characteristics have made it a workhorse of surgical laser procedures.

Clinical Applications

The FDA has approved the marketing of the 10.6 μm CO_2 laser for excision, incision, vaporization, and hemostasis of joint tissues, and specifically for arthroscopy (e.g., meniscectomy, chondroplasty, chondromalacia, and synovectomy with inclusion of various tissues). The knee joint has the largest percentage of 10.6 μm CO_2 laser usage. Gas distention and simultaneous 10.6 μm CO_2 laser use is not recommended for the shoulder, spine, or temporomandibular joint.

Histopathology/Tissue Response

The 10.6 μm CO_2 laser, because it is highly absorbed by water and absorbed by hemoglobin, is excellent at vaporizing pigmented and nonpigmented tissues with minimal thermal damage. As mentioned above, the 10.6 μm CO_2 laser offers the advantage of being selectively absorbed by degenerative tissue. It is also indicated that use of the 10.6 μm CO_2 laser may promote healing.

Laser Beam Hazards

Because of the frequency and the spectrum where the laser works, it must be understood that the beam, in a large percentage of the lasers being used in medicine today, cannot be seen by the human eye because it operates in an infrared zone. Hence a tracer light or another laser that is visible is added to these powerful lasers in an effort to provide a beam visible to the human eye.

The beam, unlike the sculpted tips and end probes, can extend far beyond the reach of the surgeon's hand. Objects out of reach of the surgeon's hands can still be reached by the laser, which is an advantage or a disadvantage depending on whether the surgeon is aware of, understands, appreciates, and remembers the far-reaching effects of the beam. Nonreflective instruments should be used to reduce this risk.

Laser Effects on Adjacent Tissues

Any inadvertent application of the laser may damage adjacent tissue structures. In addition, the use of power levels or pulse durations significantly higher than surgically indicated may result in thermal damage to adjacent structures.

Plume Hazards

Plume results from vaporization of a tissue substance by a high intensity laser beam. This plume may or may not be visualized in the form of smoke. Because of the extreme

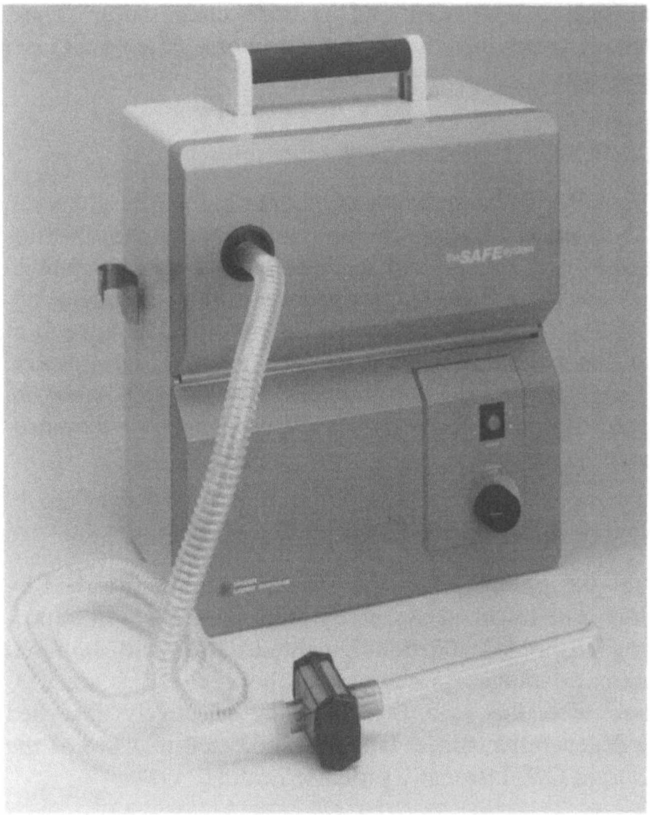

Figure 19-3. Instrument for smoke evacuation.

heat required for the vaporization, an odor may accompany the smoke.

Transmittance of viruses and DNA particles into the air through the plume have been documented in several studies. General safety precautions include appropriate masking as well as evacuation of the plume and smoke using a smoke evacuator. Premier Laser Systems provides a portable smoke evacuator, SAFE, which removes odor, fluid, and particles larger than 2 μm in diameter (Fig. 19-3).

Masks have been used in the operating room since Lister determined that isolating the patient from the surroundings was important. Now we must look at the other side of this coin: vaporization of body parts can cause the inflow of vaporized particles through the surgical mask. Therefore the Occupational Safety and Health Administration (OSHA) has suggested that small-pore masks be used in a surgical setting. Laser-type masks are easily accessible now and are to be the standard in the operating room setting for people within phase one.

No special surgical gowns are required. The evolution of gowns has progressed from cloth to paper, so general precautions must be taken to prevent the laser from igniting a gown (the laser should be in Standby mode whenever it is not in use). An extinguishing device should be part of the safety mechanisms in the operating room.

Precautions

Patients

It is primarily important that the eyes of the patient are protected whether the patient is awake or under anesthesia. If awake, appropriate glasses should be used. With the 10.6 μm CO_2 laser, clear glass acts as an absorptive device and protects the retina and cornea. If the patient is under anesthesia, moist pads must be placed over the eyes.

Draping can be flammable because the modern mode of draping is with paper. General precautions, such as using wet towels around the wound, should be adopted.

Precautions for Operating Room Personnel

Use of reflecting devices can cause scattering of the laser beam, so protective eye glassware is important. The general safety rule states that anyone within the operating arena must have protective glasses as well as side vents. Side shields are not required but are suggested for anyone outside the general operating field. This protection should include the patient.

Barriers of Entry into the Operating Room

It is important in the operating room setting to disclose to the general personnel outside the room the dangers present upon entrance into the room. It is imperative that a sign be posted outside the door of the operating room that the laser may be or is in use. This forewarning allows the person to adopt the proper safety procedures before gaining entry.

Distention of the Joint

Gas insufflation has two purposes. One is to create a medium in which the 10.6 μm CO_2 laser can work effectively. Because of the hydrophilic nature of the 10.6 μm CO_2 laser, a water medium is not acceptable for work in and around the joint when using this instrument. All water must be extracted if the laser is to be used effectively. Overdistention of the joint is usually not a problem because of an autoregulator on the gauge (provided by Premier Laser Systems) that dispenses the gas. There should be constant checks on the regulator and the alarm mechanism. If these devices fail to work properly, gas embolus is a significant risk.

Gas utilization in any operating room setting is by no means new. The same precautions must be taken when using any high pressure tank gas. Turning the gas on and off should be done with a valve regulatory mechanism. It is always a double-valved system, allowing regulation of the gas from the tank to a regulator and from a regulator to the desired device. This process is also used with the 10.6 μm CO_2 laser.

Use of a Tourniquet

With the 10.6 μm CO_2 laser, the joint is entered after insufflation with CO_2; and CO_2 is the medium in which the laser is effective. Because of the permeable nature of the CO_2, it is important that a tourniquet be used in all work on any extremity to prevent extravasation. A tourniquet used on the extremity should be set at approximately 200 mm Hg above the patient's systolic pressure. Generally, this setting creates a pressure of 300 to 350 mm Hg. The anesthesiologist should be constantly aware of the patient's CO_2 level. The use of CO_2 for prolonged periods has been found to increase extravasation, but this complication has been minimized with use of the tourniquet.

Training Requirements

A given amount of knowledge must be ascertained and mastered prior to use of laser devices. A hands-on laser course of 8 to 16 hours is offered by Premier Laser Systems. A certificate verifying that the arthroscopist has mastered and understood all phases of laser operation is awarded upon completion of the course. Most hospitals throughout the United States have set up laser committees that establish the training and safety requirements of that particular institution. The hands-on laser courses demonstrate proper use of the laser and allow the trainee to vary the settings required by the manufacturer for a particular procedure.

The completion of a laser-specific didactic course with a hands-on experience is necessary for laser privileges at most hospitals. Thereafter it is recommended that 7 to 10 cases be undertaken and overseen by surgeons with more experience. This process helps avoid the pitfalls incurred during this learning period.

Installation Requirements

There are no special installation requirements. All laser systems manufactured by Premier can be placed on an ordinary surgical cart. The 10.6 μm CO_2 laser system can be plugged into a standard 110 volt outlet and needs no external cooling. Premier also provides a smoke evacuator, surgical drapes, and disposable tubing systems for the convenience of the hospital.

Maintenance

Premier surgical lasers require maintenance or service on an average of once every 2 years. Gas lasers are refilled with gas and fluid for the cooling system during regular maintenance. Premier guarantees 24-hour service and a "loaner" for any laser under service contract.

Editor's Cautions

1. **This laser should not be used without 10.6 μm wavelength-specific protective eyewear. Regular glasses or contact lenses are not adequate protection. All personnel in the room, especially the patient, should be protected.**
2. **This laser could start a fire or cause a burn if inadvertently misdirected. Simultaneous use of flammable substances must be avoided. Foot pedal clutter must be avoided.**
3. **Any gas technique, including the ambient air and gas bubble (Moses) technique, but especially a CO_2 gas distention technique, can result (though rarely) in gas emboli, which in turn may result in permanent neurologic sequelae or fatality. Danger exists so long as there is an unfavorable pressure gradient between the gas and the tissues. This problem has never been reported with the ambient air technique or the Moses technique, but it is theoretically possible. Surgeons should inform their patients of this rare possibility preoperatively, and know how to minimize the potential for gas emboli. The surgeon and anesthesiologist should know how to recognize and treat gas emboli. Appropriate pressures should be used; never more than 1.5 pounds per square inch. A tourniquet should be used. Gas distention must not be used in the shoulder, temporomandibular joint, or spine. These techniques must not be used when there are large vascular beds, especially with intraarticular fractures.**
4. **Gas arthroscopy should be learned prior to use of the 10.6 μm CO_2 laser with gas arthroscopy.**
5. **This technique must be used with mechanical instruments available.**
6. **Reflectance is a major factor to consider for safe operation of the 10.6 μm CO_2 laser.**
7. **Char should be débrided or irrigated from the joint.**
8. **Inadvertent tissue damage caused by a misdirected laser beam may result in both intraoperative and postoperative complications. Small probes are preferred to large probes.**
9. **Smoke evacuation is essential.**
10. **Optimal, satisfactory use of this system requires some experience. It is best to start in the laboratory, not with patients. The best techniques, energy settings, and probe selections can be preliminarily determined in this way.**
11. **This chapter is only an introduction to this arthroscopic laser system. The reader is encouraged to study this entire text, follow acceptable training and credentialling procedures, as well as research the subject at hand for additional information and changes before undertaking this arthroscopic laser system's use.**

Suggested Reading

Altman RD, Gray R (1983) Diagnostic and therapeutic uses of the arthroscope in rheumatoid arthritis and osteoarthritis. Am J Med 75:50–55

Altman RD, Kates J (1983) Arthroscopy of the knee. Semin Arthritis Rheum 13(7):188–199

Andrews JR, Broussard TS, Carson WG (1985) Arthroscopy of the shoulder in the management of partial tears of the rotator cuff: a preliminary report. Arthroscopy 2:117–122

Andrews JR, Carson WG (1983) Shoulder joint arthroscopy. Orthopedics 6:1157–1162

Andrews JR, Carson WG (1985) Arthroscopy of the elbow. Arthroscopy 1:297–107

Andrews JR, St. Pierre RK, Carson WG (1986) Arthroscopy of the elbow. Clin Sports Med 4:653–662

Andrews JR, Previte WJ, Carson WG (1985) Arthroscopy of the ankle: technique and normal anatomy. Foot Ankle 6:29–33

Aritomi H (1984) Arthroscopic synovectomy of the knee joint with the electric resectoscope. Scand J Haematol Suppl 40 33:249–262

Balduini FC, Peff TC, Torg JS (1985) Application of electrothermal energy in arthroscopy. Arthroscopy 1:259–263

Bentley G, Dowd G (1984) Current concepts of etiology and treatment of chondromalacia patellae. Clin Orthop 189: 209–228

Boe S (1990) Arthroscopy of the ankle joint. Arch Orthop Trauma Surg 105:285–286

Bora FW, Osterman AL, Maitin E, Bednar J (1986) The role of arthroscopy in the treatment of disorders of the wrist. Contemp Orthop 12(4):28–36

Brillhart AT (1991) Arthroscopic laser surgery: the CO_2 laser and its use: second of four articles. Am J Arthrosc 1(2):7–12

Dew DK (1982) Laser assisted microsurgical research. Faculty/ University of Miami Postgraduate Course, New Technology in Orthopaedics and Rehabilitation [with panel discussion on microsurgery and laser], Bal Harbour, FL

Dew DK, Lo HK (1983) Carbon dioxide laser microsurgical repair of soft tissue: preliminary observations. Presented to the American Society for Laser Medicine and Surgery, New Orleans

Dew DK, Verdeia JC (1983) Carbon dioxide laser repair of rat sciatic nerves. Eastern Student Research Forum, Miami

Fox JM, Ferke RD, DelPizzo W, Friedman MJ, Snyder SJ (1984) Electrosurgery in orthopaedics. II. Applications to arthroscopy. Contemp Orthop 8(2):37–44

Hefti F, Morscher E, Koller F (1984) The use of laser beams for operations in haemophilia. Scand J Haematol Suppl 40 33:281–289

Henning CE, Lynch MA, Clark JR (1987) Vascularity for healing of meniscus repairs. Arthroscopy 3:13–18

Herman JH, Khosla RC (1987) Laser (Nd:YAG) induced healing of cartilage. Arthritis Rheum 30:s128

Horoszowski H, Heim M, Seligsohn U, Farine I (1981) Use of the laser scalpel in orthopaedic surgery on the haemophilic patient. In Haemophilia. Castle House Publications, pp 189–193

Johansen WE, Smith CF, Vangsness CT, et al (1986) Comparison of percutaneous laser discectomy with other modalities for the treatment of herniated lumbar discs and cadaveric studies of percutaneous laser discectomy. SPIE Proc 712: 218–221

McKenzie AL (1983) How far does thermal damage extend beneath the surface of CO_2 laser incisions? Phys Med Biol 28:905–912

Miller GK, Drennan DB, Maylahn DJ (1987) The effect of technique on histology of arthroscopic partial meniscectomy with electrosurgery. Arthroscopy 3:36–44

Norton LA (1982) Effects of a pulsed electromagnetic field on a mixed chondroblastic tissue culture III. Basic science and pathology. Clin Orthop 167:280–290

Rand JA, Gaffey TA (1985) Effect of electrocautery of fresh human articular cartilage. Arthroscopy 1:242–246

Schosheim PM, Caspari RB (1986) Evaluation of electrosurgical meniscectomy in rabbits. Arthroscopy 2:71–76

Schultz RJ, Krishnamurthy S, Theimo W, Rodriguez J, Harvey G (1985) Effects of varying intensities of laser energy on articular cartilage. Lasers Surg Med 5:577–588

Smith CF, Johansen WE, Sutter LV, Marshall GJ (1987) Meniscal repair utilizing a hand held carbon dioxide laser. Poster Exhibit presented at Annual Meeting of American Academy of Orthopaedic Surgeons, San Francisco

Smith CF, Johansen WE, Vangsness CT, et al (1986) Does success of arthroscopic laser surgery in the knee joint warrant its extension to "non-knee" joints? SPIE Proc 712:214–217

Smith CF, Marshall GJ, Snyder SJ, et al (1984) Comparisons of tissue effects of a surgical scalpel, an electrocautery apparatus and a carbon dioxide laser system when used for making incisions in to the menisci of New Zealand rabbits. Lasers Surg Med 3:305–369

Verschueren RCJ (1976) Thermal damage in adjoining tissues after using the focused CO_2 laser beam. In: The CO_2 Laser in Tumor Surgery. Van Gorcum, Amsterdam

Verschueren RCJ (1982) Tissue reaction to the CO_2 laser in general. In Microscopic and Endoscopic Surgery with the CO_2 Laser. John Wright, Boston

Whipple TL, Caspari RB, Meyers JF (1982) Arthroscopic meniscectomy by CO_2 laser vaporization in a gas medium. Orthop Trans 6:136

Whipple TL, Caspari R, Meyers JF (1983) Laser energy in arthroscopic meniscectomy. Orthopedics 6:1165–1169

Whipple TL, Caspari RB, Meyers JF (1984a) Laser subtotal meniscectomy in rabbits. Lasers Surg Med 3:297–304

Whipple TL, Caspari RB, Meyers JF (1984b) Synovial response to laser induced carbon ash residue. Lasers Med Surg 3:291–295

Whipple TL, Caspari R, Meyers JF (1985) Arthroscopic laser meniscectomy in a gas medium. Arthroscopy 1:2–7

20

Sharplan 10.6 μm CO_2 Lasers and Waveguides for Arthroscopic Laser Surgery

Michael Slatkine and Douglass Mead

Introduction

The 10.6 μm CO_2 laser has a long history of use in the orthopaedic field, with more than 10 years of experience in arthroscopy and many thousands of procedures performed (Whipple et al., 1983, 1984, 1985; Smith et al., 1989, 1990; Garrick, 1992; Smith, 1992). Advances in the development and production of miniature 10.6 μm CO_2 laser waveguides have paved the way to new possibilities in arthroscopic surgical procedures. The 10.6 μm CO_2 laser with these waveguide delivery systems provides excellent noncontact surface ablation and incision using the free laser beam technique. With these delivery systems, tissue at locations normally inaccessible using mechanical instruments such as biting forceps and shavers are now easily accessible for treatment.

Because waveguides can be classified as "pointing" rather than "grasping" tools, the surgical techniques are easy to learn and safe. Only tissue in near contact with the instrument tip is treated, and forceful manipulation and abrasion of tissue is avoided.

Several wavelengths have been shown to be effective in arthroscopy and other orthopaedic procedures, but Sharplan has committed considerable effort to develop 10.6 μm CO_2 orthopaedic applications for the following reasons:

1. Excellent clinical results can be achieved with these systems by taking advantage of the attributes of the 10.6 μm CO_2 wavelength and refining the skills that maximize its performance. The 10.6 μm CO_2 laser has been used for thousands of arthroscopic procedures with few major complications.
2. The 10.6 μm CO_2 laser is already widely available in most hospitals and is familiar to the operating room staff. Sharplan supports an installed base of almost 6000 of the 10.6 μm CO_2 lasers worldwide (2500 in the United States) that are suitable for arthroscopy. Hence hospitals that already have this laser need not purchase a new laser to use the technique effectively in orthopaedic procedures.
3. The 10.6 μm CO_2 laser has extensive surgical applications in other surgical specialties, allowing hospitals that purchase this laser type to maximize utilization. Also, 10.6 μm CO_2 lasers are much less expensive than the popular 2.1 μm holmium:YAG lasers and are affordable for hospitals and surgicenters.

We present a brief description of the operating principles of Sharplan's 10.6 μm CO_2 lasers with waveguides for orthopaedic surgery. We present information on tissue effects and summarize the applications with these systems. We also discuss some exciting future applications of lasers in orthopaedics.

The Sharplan 10.6 μm CO_2 Arthroscopic Laser System

Sharplan offers at least 10 models of the 10.6 μm CO_2, laser ranging in power from 20 to 100 watts. These 10.6 μm CO_2 lasers rely on CO_2 gas as the lasing medium, which is sealed in the laser tube and excited by a direct-current (DC) electrical field. The wavelength of 10.6 μm is invisible and a 0.632 μm helium-neon (HeNe) laser is introduced in conjunction with the 10.6 μm CO_2 laser beam to allow effective aiming (Fig. 20-1). Because the 10.6 μm CO_2 laser wavelength cannot be transmitted through fiberoptics such as the 1.06 μm neodymium: YAG wavelength, an articulating arm delivers the free beam through a series of mirrors to the final delivery system. Sharplan lasers are equipped with new articulating arms that use lightweight composite materials, spring balancing designs, and fixed mirror alignment technologies

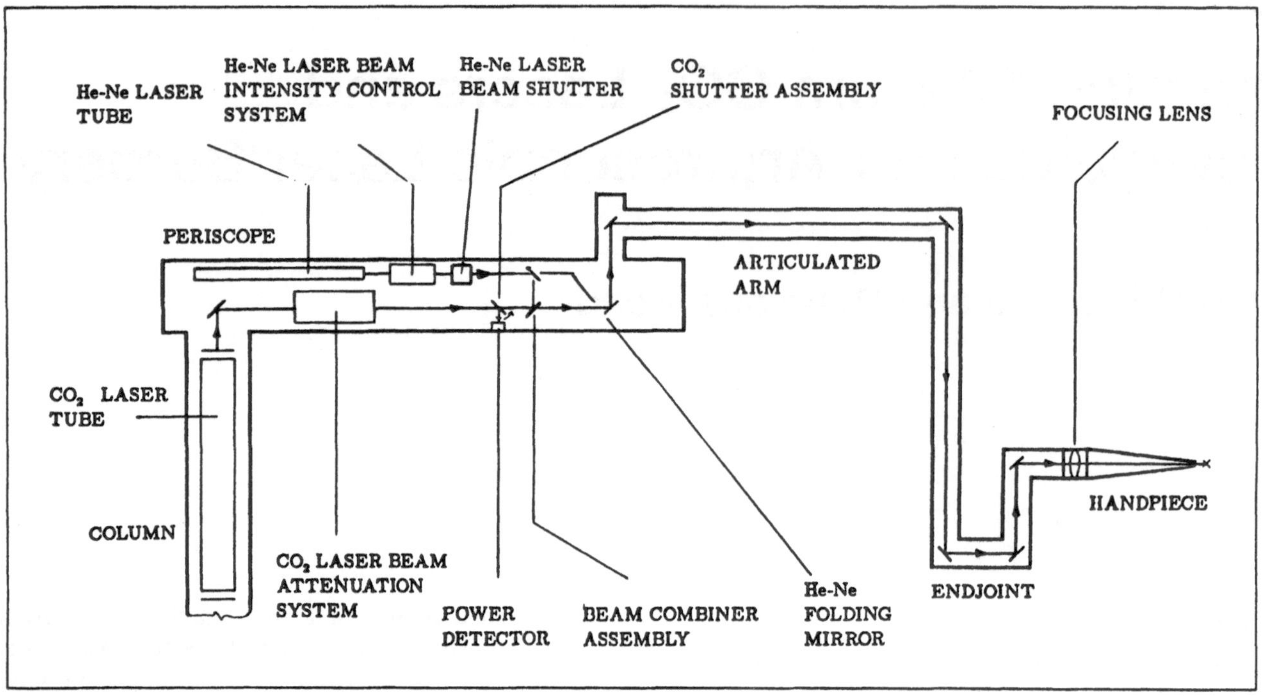

Figure 20-1. The 10.6 μm CO_2 laser tube and articulated arm. The waveguide delivery systems connect at the handpiece.

that have greatly improved the ease of use of the Sharplan 10.6 μm CO_2 lasers compared to other models.

The output of the Sharplan 10.6 μm CO_2 lasers can be delivered as a continuous wave or in a variety of pulsed outputs. The Superpulse mode delivers high peak powers (400–500 watts), and the Sharpulse mode delivers high energy (160 mJ) pulses (Fig. 20-2). These pulse modes improve the vaporization effects of tissue and minimize the residual carbon ash created. Most arthroscopic laser procedures can be performed at 30 watts or less.

Within the Sharplan 10.6 μm CO_2 product line, the Sharplan models 1030, Surgicenter 40 and models 1041S and 1055S are ideally suited for arthroscopy. The 1030 and Surgicenter 40 are 30- and 40-watt sealed tube lasers that are small and lightweight (98 pounds) but with a superpulse mode and features often found only on higher powered 10.6 μm CO_2 lasers (Fig. 20-3). The 1041S and 1055S are 40- and 55-watt lasers, respectively, and are the latest technology for the hospital with both Superpulse and Sharpulse modes (Fig. 20-4).

Features of the Sharplan 10.6 μm CO_2 lasers include the following:

1. Variable-intensity 0.632 μm helium-neon beam with an exclusive Off at Lasing mode so tissue effects are more clearly seen
2. Multiple setup memories for commonly programmed parameters
3. User prompt displays that guide users through setup and operation
4. Continuous, single pulse, repeat pulse, superpulse, and Sharpulse, milliwatt (very low power) ouput modes
5. Smoke evacuation device synchronized to laser activation
6. Self-contained cooling and low power requirements.

Sharplan offers two types of waveguide delivery system for 10.6 μm CO_2 arthroscopy: the rigid Microguide (Luxar Corporation) waveguides in straight, curved, and 90 degree angled versions (Fig. 20-5); and the fully flexible FlexiLase fibers (Fig. 20-6). The Microguide waveguides are 120 mm in length and 1.8 mm in diameter, and they produce a beam diameter of 0.8 mm. The 10.6 μm CO_2 laser radiation is focused with an appropriate lens coupler into the hollow waveguide and reflected internally along its wall. Laser radiation is emitted from the distal end of the waveguide with a divergence angle ranging from 5 to 10 degrees. The Microguides are available as prepackaged, presterilized disposable items for single use and have no total time or energy limit during a single case.

The FlexiLase 10.6 μm CO_2 laser waveguides are hollow plastic tubes coated internally with a metal and dielectric layer. Internal diameters are 1 mm. The length of the flexible waveguide is approximately 1.2 meters and is terminated with a handpiece for introduction into the knee. FlexiLase fibers may be resterilized and reused up to 5 times.

Hollow waveguides transmit the 10.6 μm CO_2 laser beam much like optical fibers. Using CO_2 gas as the trans-

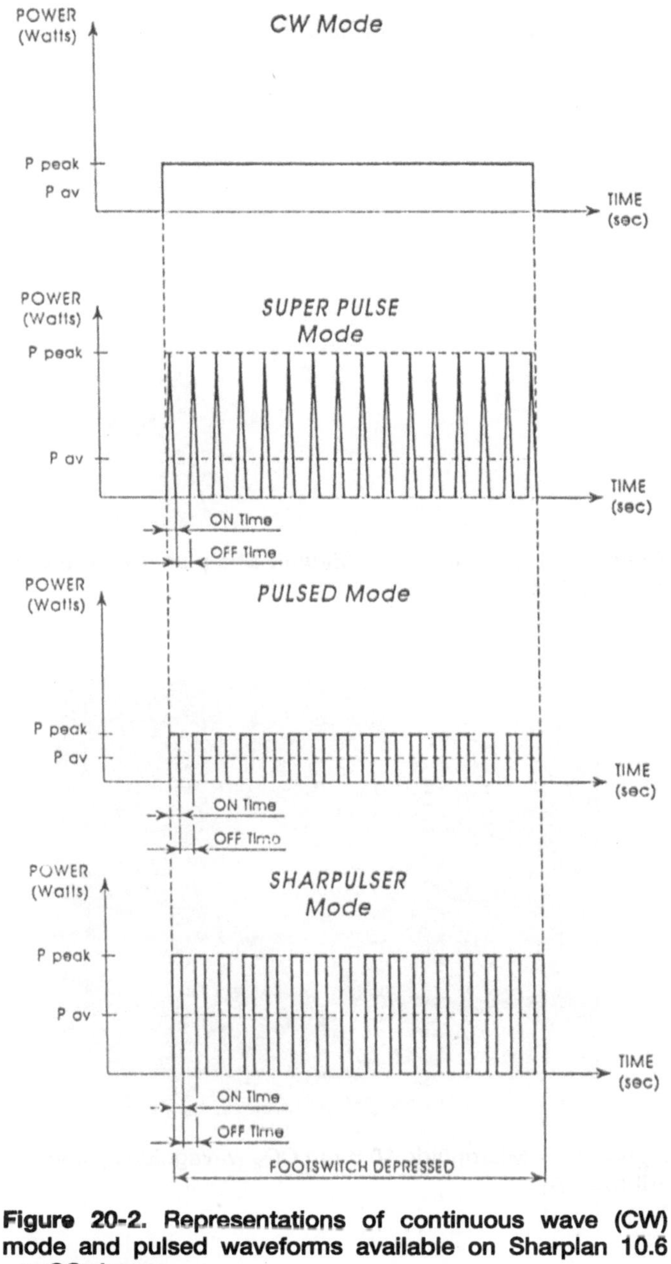

Figure 20-2. Representations of continuous wave (CW) mode and pulsed waveforms available on Sharplan 10.6 μm CO_2 lasers.

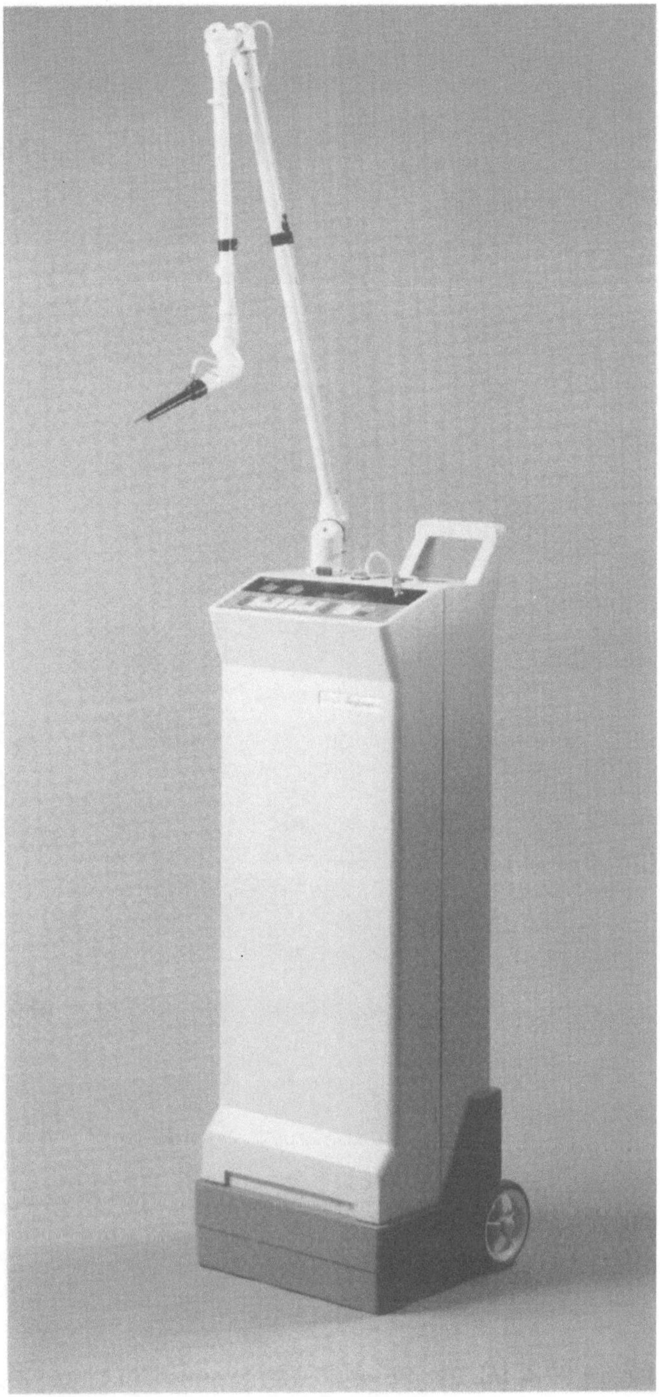

Figure 20-3. Portable 40-watt Sharplan Surgicenter 40 10.6 μm CO_2 laser.

mission medium, the beam is reflected within the internal surfaces of the waveguide, allowing the beam to pass through bends and the angled tips available.

All waveguides must be internally gas-cooled while the laser is on to protect the internal surfaces of the waveguide. It is achieved with a slow background flow of CO_2 gas (1 liter/minute).

The 10.6 μm CO_2 laser wavelength is highly absorbed by water. Therefore the operative site must be dry. Typically, diagnostic arthroscopy is performed in a saline environment, and the knee is then prepared for the 10.6 μm CO2 laser using one of three techniques: CO_2 insufflation, ambient air, gas bubble. The laser delivery system, which consists of an optical coupler, gas purge fitting, and the 10.6 μm CO_2 waveguide, is covered using standard sterile sleeve drapes. Power levels of 10 watts in the Superpulse mode or up to 30 watts in the continuous mode are usually used. The short, 100 μm/second pulses (superpulse or Sharpulse modes) minimize carbon residues. Tissue is most efficiently removed when the tip is held 0.5 to 1.0 mm from the tissue. Shaving is carried out from a greater distance using the 90 degree lateral probe.

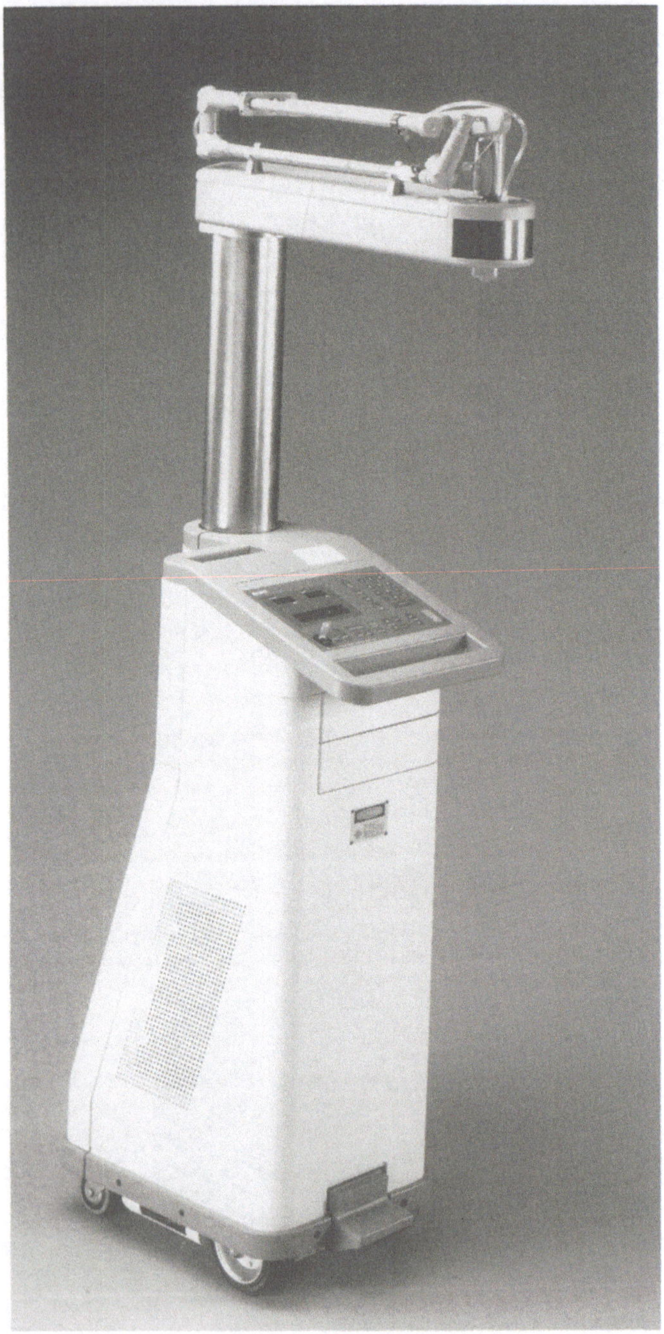

Figure 20-4. (A) The 40- or 55-watt Sharplan 10.6 μm CO_2 laser.

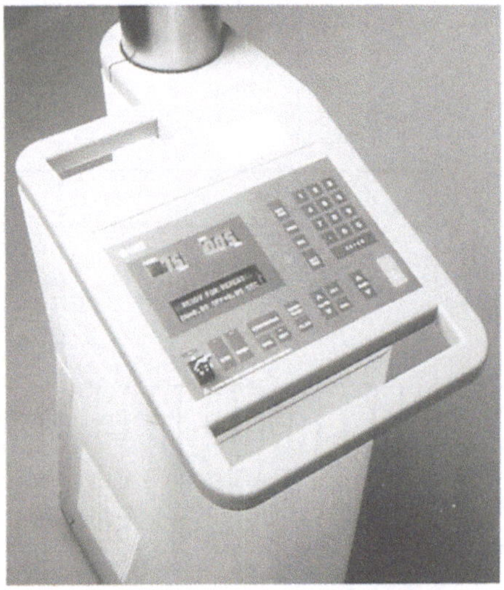

Figure 20-4. (B) The 40- or 55-watt Sharplan 10.6 μm CO_2 laser control panel.

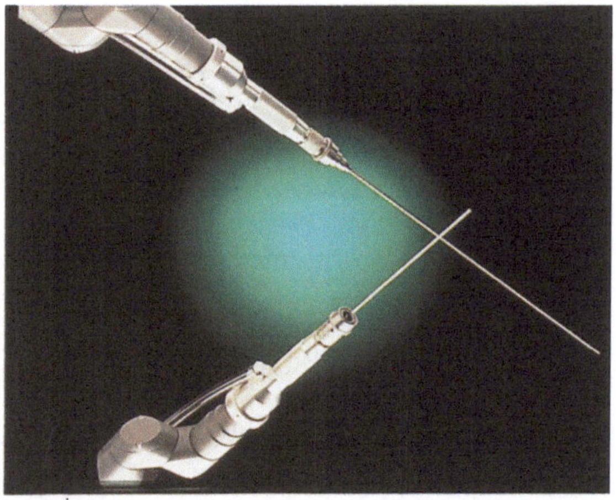

Figure 20-5. Microguide 10.6 μm CO_2 waveguide system for arthroscopy.

Absorption of 10.6 μm CO_2 laser radiation occurs in all body tissues including cartilage and meniscus within less than 50 μm depth. By using the superpulse mode, thermal necrosis around and below the crater does not exceed 0.5 mm (Black et al., 1992).

Although the 10.6 μm CO_2 laser wavelength is widely held to be the best available wavelength for tissue vaporization, a layer of residual carbon ash may remain on the treated surface. This ash can easily be removed by irrigation or gentle manipulation of the treated surface following use of the laser. Removal of the ash has been shown to eliminate the increased risk of synovitis and delayed healing that has been associated with it (Whipple et al., 1984; Smith et al., 1989, 1990).

Several thousand 10.6 μm CO_2 laser arthroscopies have been performed in the United States with rare lasting complications. **EDITOR'S CAUTION: Complications can occur and the reader is urged to study Chapter 14.** Incisions, excisions, and ablation and vaporization of cartilage, chondromalacia, synovium, and loose bodies have been carried out. Because of the gas environment requirement, the 10.6 μm CO_2 laser has been used predominantly in the knee, and research has been conducted to determine its benefits in endoscopic carpal tunnel release.

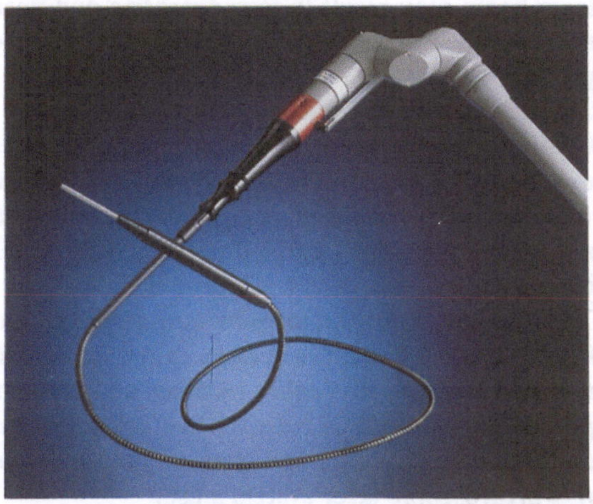

Figure 20-6. FlexiLase flexible waveguide delivery system eliminates the awkwardness associated with the articulated arm.

Laser Safety and Facility Requirements

Hospitals should develop policies and procedures mandated by the Joint Commission for the Accreditation of Healthcare Organizations (JCAHO) and the Occupational Safety and Health Administration (OSHA), as guided by the American National Standards Institute (ANSI) Standard for Safe Use of Lasers in Health Care Facilities (document Z136.3). Such policies should include, as a minimum, restricted access to operating rooms during laser procedures, the use of laser safety goggles (properly labeled with optical density and wavelength) at all times, and a policy ensuring that windows to the operating room are covered with opaque material. Sharplan has assisted many hospitals to establish appropriate policies.

There are no special electrical hazards that concern the operating room staff, although biomedical service technicians need to be aware of high voltage safety precautions when servicing any laser. All Sharplan 10.6 μm CO_2 lasers operate with conventional 115 volts alternating current (VAC) supplies. All currently marketed Sharplan lasers are internally cooled and need no special gas supplies. A low pressure CO_2 regulator is recommended for the waveguide purge gas.

Laser plume (smoke) becomes suspended in liquid irrigant during 1.06 μm Neodymium:YAG arthroscopy, whereas suction of the plume during 10.6 μm CO_2 laser arthroscopy is necessary for improving the operative view. The introducing cannula for the 10.6 μm CO_2 microguide has a suction port for such purposes. A suitable smoke evacuator such as Sharplan XPlume smoke evacuator or a filtered vacuum system should be used.

At any time gas arthroscopy is performed, especially with gas distention, there is a risk of gas emboli so long as a pressure gradient exists between the gas and the vascular system. The surgeon must be aware of this possibility, know how to decrease its chances of happening, and know how to diagnose and treat it.

Gas arthroscopy should not be performed in the shoulder, spine, or temporomandibular joint using distension or in any joint where an open vascular bed is present, especially with an acute fracture.

Gas distension pressures of more than 1.5 pounds per square inch substantially increase the risk of gas emboli. The ambient air technique is preferred. A tourniquet should be used.

Maintenance and Delivery System Considerations

Sharplan recommends a preuse check of the laser and delivery system to avoid the minimal risk of a malfunction during the case. The Sharplan 10.6 μm CO_2 lasers have an integral power meter that constantly monitors output (calibration is automatically set by the laser). However, the laser may be test-fired by directing the beam on a wet wooden tongue blade placed on a wet cloth and metal tray and fired for a 0.1 second single pulse at 10 watts.

The Sharplan 10.6 μm CO_2 lasers are of mature technology, and their reliability has been established over many years. However, Sharplan recommends comprehensive preventive maintenance every 6 months to inspect the water cooling system, power meter, and internal lenses, mirrors, and shutters. This maintenance should be performed only by Sharplan trained and authorized technicians. Sharplan offers several service schools throughout the year for hospital technician training on the service of Sharplan 1.06 μm neodymium:YAG and 10.6 μm CO_2 lasers.

Conclusions

Arthroscopy with the 10.6 μm CO_2 laser has been developed to the point where it now provides unique surgical capabilities beyond what has been available in mechanical instruments. Laser waveguides, which act as pointing tools rather than grasping tools, are easy to use and effective. Used by a properly trained surgeon, they are an important advance in the available tools for performing arthroscopic surgery. Although technically more difficult than other wavelengths that can be used in a fluid environment (e.g., 2.1 μm holmium:YAG, 1.06 μm neodymium:YAG), the 10.6 μm CO_2 laser is probably the most accessible to the orthopaedic surgeon and offers the best vaporizing wavelength available. The real benefit of these tools is improved access to tissue in the smallest spaces in the knee and other joints and the ability to vaporize undesired or diseased tissue rather than having to employ mechanical extraction.

Editor's Cautions

1. **This laser should not be used without 10.6 μm wavelength-specific protective eyewear. Regular glasses or contact lenses are not enough. All personnel in the room, especially the patient, should be protected.**
2. **This laser could start a fire or cause a burn if misdirected. Simultaneous use of flammable substances must be avoided. Foot pedal clutter must be avoided.**
3. **Any gas technique, including the ambient air and gas bubble (Moses) technique, but especially a CO_2 gas distention technique, may potentially result, though rarely, in gas emboli, which in turn may result in permanent neurologic sequelae or fatality. Danger exists so long as there is an unfavorable pressure gradient between the gas and the tissues. This problem has never been reported with the ambient air technique or the Moses technique, but it is theoretically possible. Surgeons should inform their patients of this rare possibility preoperatively, and know how to minimize its potential. The surgeon and anesthesiologist should know how to recognize and treat gas emboli. Appropriate pressures should be used: never more than 1.5 pounds per square inch. A tourniquet should be used. Gas distention must not be used in the shoulder, temporomandibular joint, or spine. These techniques must not be used when there are large vascular beds, especially with intraarticular fractures.**
4. **Gas arthroscopy should be learned prior to use of the 10.6 μm CO_2 laser for gas arthroscopy.**
5. **This technique must be used with mechanical instruments available.**
6. **Reflectance is a major factor to consider for safe operation of the 10.6 μm CO_2 laser.**
7. **Char should be débrided or irrigated from the joint.**
8. **Inadvertent tissue damage caused by a misdirected laser beam may result in intraoperative and postoperative complications. Small probes are preferred to large probes.**
9. **Smoke evacuation is essential.**
10. **Optimal, satisfactory use of this system requires some experience. It is best to start in the laboratory, not with patients. The best techniques, energy settings, and probe selections can be preliminarily determined in this way.**
11. **This chapter is only an introduction to this arthroscopic laser system. The reader is encouraged to study this entire text, follow acceptable training and credentialling procedures, as well as research the subject at hand for additional information and changes before undertaking this arthroscopic laser system's use.**

References

Black J, Sherk HH, Meller M, et al (1992) Wavelength selection in laser arthroscopy. Semin Orthop 7:72–76

Garrick JG (1992) CO_2 laser arthroscopy using ambient gas pressure. Semin Orthop 7:90–94

Smith CF (1992) "Gas bubble" technique in laser arthroscopic surgery. Semin Orthop 7:86–89

Smith CF, Johansen WE, Vangsness CT, et al (1989) The carbon dioxide laser: a potential tool for orthopedic surgery. Clin Orthop 242:43

Smith CF, Johansen WE, Vangsness CT, et al (1990) Arthroscopic surgery with a free beam CO_2 laser. In Sherk HH (ed), Lasers in Orthopaedics, Lippincott, Philadelphia, pp 146–157

Whipple TL, Caspari RB, Meyers JF (1983) Laser energy in arthroscopic meniscectomy. Orthopedics 6:1165–1169

Whipple TL, Caspari RB, Meyers JF (1984) Synovial response to laser induced carbon ash residue. Lasers Surg Med 3:291–295

Whipple TL, Caspari RB, Meyers JF (1985) Arthroscopic meniscectomy in a gas medium. Arthroscopy 1:2–7

21

Sharplan High Power 1.06 μm Neodymium:YAG Lasers and SharpLase Contact Fibers for Arthroscopic Laser Surgery

Michael Slatkine and Douglass Mead

Advances in the development and production of novel optical fiber scalpels and ablators have paved the way to substantial new possibilities in arthroscopic surgical procedures. The 1.06 μm neodymium:YAG laser fibers, in contact with tissue, provide smooth, consistent incision and contact vaporization using the touch technique. With the probe's slim profile, tissue at locations normally inaccessible to mechanical instruments (e.g., biting forceps and shavers) are easily accessible for treatment. Because optical fibers are "pointing" rather than regular "grasping" tools, the surgical techniques are easy to learn and safe. Only tissue in contact or near contact with the instrument tip is treated, and forceful manipulation of tissue is avoided.

Several wavelengths have been shown to be effective for arthroscopy and other orthopaedic procedures, but Sharplan has committed considerable effort to develop 1.06 μm neodymium:YAG lasers for orthopaedic applications for the following reasons.

1. Excellent clinical results can be achieved with these systems by taking advantage of the attributes of the 1.06 μm neodymium:YAG wavelengths and refining the delivery systems that maximize performance and safety. The 1.06 μm neodymium:YAG laser has been used in several hundred orthopaedic procedures with no major complications.
2. The 1.06 μm neodymium:YAG laser is already widely available in most hospitals and is familiar to the operating room staff. Sharplan supports an installed base of almost 600 of the 1.06 μm neodymium:YAG lasers suitable for arthroscopy. The hospitals that have them need not purchase a new laser to effectively use lasers in orthopedic procedures.
3. The 1.06 μm neodymium:YAG laser has extensive surgical applications in other surgical specialties, allowing hospitals who purchase this laser type to maximize its utilization. Also, the Sharplan 1.06 μm neodymium:YAG laser is much less expensive than the popular 2.1 μm holmium:YAG lasers and is affordable for hospitals and surgicenters.

We present here a brief description of the operating principles of Sharplan's 1.06 μm neodymium:YAG laser with SharpLase sculptured fibers for orthopaedic surgery. We present information on tissue effects and summarize the applications that are most suitable for the laser.

Sharplan 1.06 μm Neodymium:YAG Arthroscopic Laser System

The Sharplan model 3000 1.06 μm neodymium:YAG laser (Fig. 21-1) is a mobile, air-cooled solid-state laser that utilizes a yttrium-aluminum-garnet (YAG) crystal doped with the element neodymium. Photons are emitted when an excitation lamp activates electrons in the crystal matrix. These photons are emitted as a collimated, coherent beam at a wavelength of 1.064 μm in the near-infrared region of the electromagnetic spectrum. The laser beam is focused at the proximal end of a quartz optical fiber for transmission to the surgical site. Because this wavelength is invisible, a 5 mW helium-neon (HeNe) laser is also transmitted for aiming and illumination purposes.

Within the laser console lies the 1.06 μm neodymium:YAG laser head, which consists of the optical cavity housing, front and rear mirror resonators, shutter system, internal power meter, stabilizing photodiode and helium-neon laser and intensity control (Fig. 21-2). With microprocessor control, the shutter system first allows calibration of the laser output whenever a power setting change is made and then adjusts for laser delivery to the focusing lens and optical fiber port. The laser fires and

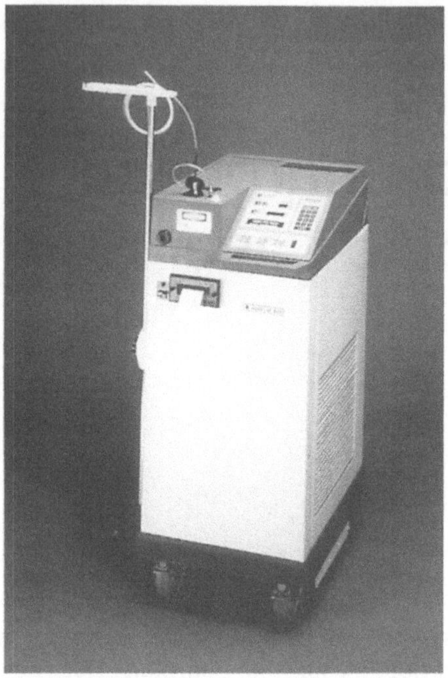

Figure 21-1. The 100-watt Sharplan model 3000 1.06 μm neodymium:YAG laser.

the shutter opens only when the user activates the footswitch control. The power amplifiers and laser head are cooled with internally circulating water and a radiator fan. Thermosensors monitor the circulating water temperature and prevent laser emission if insufficient water flow is detected.

The power range of the Sharplan model 3000 1.06 μm neodymium:YAG laser is from 1 to 100 watts, and the laser can be operated in the continuous mode or a repeat pulse mode with a minimum pulse duration of 0.1 second. For arthroscopy, only the continuous mode is needed. Additional controls are provided for selecting power, repeat pulse time intervals, helium-neon intensity, and total pulses or energy delivered during a procedure (Fig. 21-3). Display messages prompt the user through the start-up procedure and whenever any setting is changed, and they alert the user to alarm conditions. A printer records physician, patient, and date information, setting changes made during a case, and the total energy delivered.

The 1.06 μm neodymium:YAG laser energy is delivered to the surgical site through a fiberoptic delivery system. The free-beam fiber delivery system is used by other surgical specialties for deep coagulation, whereas orthopaedic applications rely on a sculptured fiber tip in contact with tissue for minimal depth of penetration and thermal injury.

For laser arthroscopy, Sharplan has developed specific probes that can be used with its 1.06 μm neodymium:YAG lasers as well as with any other 1.06 μm neodymium:YAG laser that is equipped with SMA-905 proximal fiber connectors. The probe has a 150 mm working length (3 mm diameter) and is available with a 15 degree curved or straight tip (Fig. 21-4).

Other significant features of the SharpLase Arthroscopy Probe include the following.

1. A 1000 μm hemispheric fiber tip that is small enough to access tight spaces within the knee and cut cartilage and soft tissue, yet wide enough to vaporize broader surfaces smoothly.
2. The large fiber extends only 1 mm from the metal cannula tip to give optimal mechanical support while lasing.
3. For increased safety of the fiber tip, a fixed distance retraction mechanism is built into the handpiece. The tip can be easily retracted into the handpiece cannula during insertion and manipulation into the field of view, and the cannula tip can be used with absolute safety as a mechanical probe.

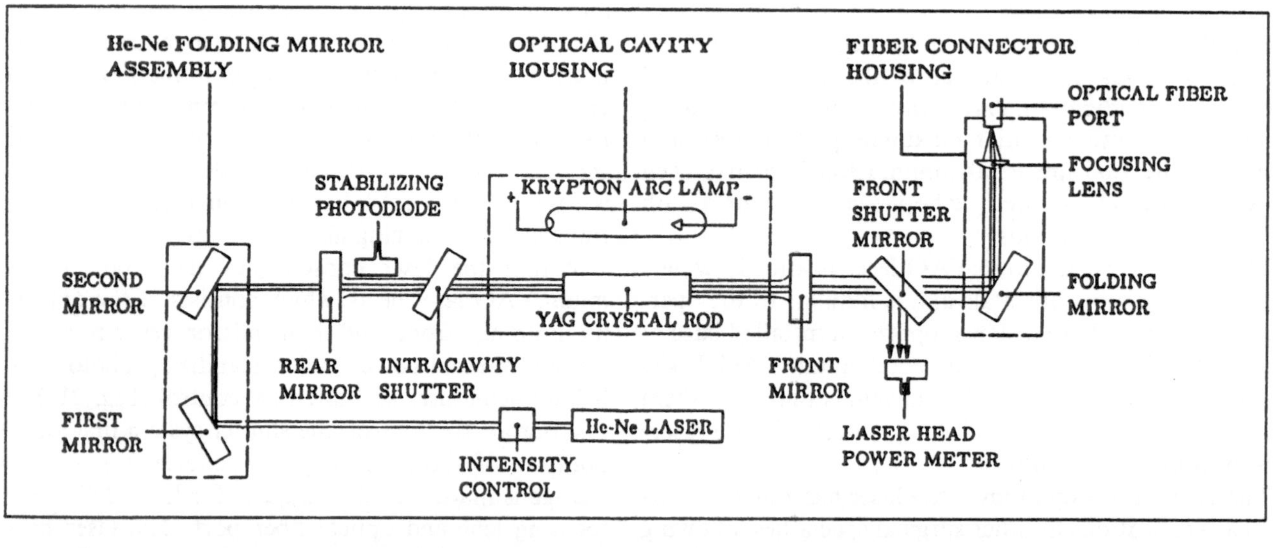

Figure 21-2. The 1.06 μm neodymium:YAG laser head assembly: principles of operation and design.

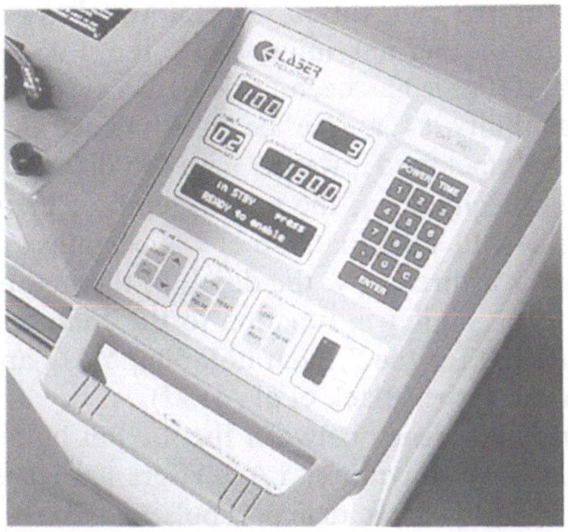

Figure 21-3. Sharplan model 3000 user control panel and displays.

4. The probe is intended to be used in a fluid medium at relatively high powers (e.g., 70–80 watts). Therefore the probe quickly cuts and vaporizes tissue. Depending on the technique and application, the probe can be used for 14 to 30 kJ total energy before the fiber should be replaced, which is more than sufficient power for a single case.

The operating principles of the hemispherical SharpLase fibers are depicted in Figure 21-5. The emerging beam is tightly focused 0.5 mm in front of the lens-shaped hemispherical tip, creating a high intensity focal region and an optical beam of large divergence (>80 degrees). Tissue vaporization can occur only at the focal point where the laser energy is absorbed primarily by tissue proteins. With strong beam divergence and diffuse scattering, the power density of the laser beam is insufficient to cause thermal injury in deeper tissue layers.

Upon contact with tissue and activation of the laser, a second principal effect rules. A fine layer of carbonized tissue instantaneously coats the fiber tip, thereby increasing the absorption of laser energy on the surface of the tip. The tip temperature increases to above 200°C, resulting in vaporization of water in tissue cells; hence the apparatus both cuts and vaporizes—its predominant typical use. Because the percentage of water in bone is low, the probe does *not* effectively cut or vaporize dense bone.

At power levels of about 70 watts, vaporization of cartilage and soft tissue, in contact with the tie, occurs within less than 0.1 second. It thus creates a lesion with a diameter the size of the fiber and leaves a thermal damage zone (absorption depth) less than 0.5 mm thick (Fig. 21-6). Constant motion of the tip across tissue during lasing minimizes the depth of thermal injury. Heat transfer to underlying tissue may result if the probe is held in the same spot for prolonged periods.

Contact vaporization is the basis of all arthroscopic applications. For example, small meniscal tears in the posterior medial meniscus can be easily accessed and vaporized away simply by touching the fiber tip to the torn tissue and "sculpting" the tissue until a smooth surface remains. Because only the meniscus is touched, the articular surfaces can be left unaffected.

When treating degenerative articular cartilage on the femoral condyles, the contact fiber can sculpt this tissue. Surgeons particularly prefer this laser to remove degenerative cartilage because of the rate of tissue vaporization and the tactile feedback given by the contact probe. The SharpLase fiber is especially ideal for hemostatic incision of soft tissue, such as excision of plica, lateral release, and partial synovectomy. Chondromalacia and fibrillated cartilage can be swept away by using the contact fiber with a painting technique in constant motion. The SharpLase fiber has been used in hundreds of cases in the knee and more than 40 cases in the shoulder. Applications in the shoulder include coracoacromial ligament release, syno-

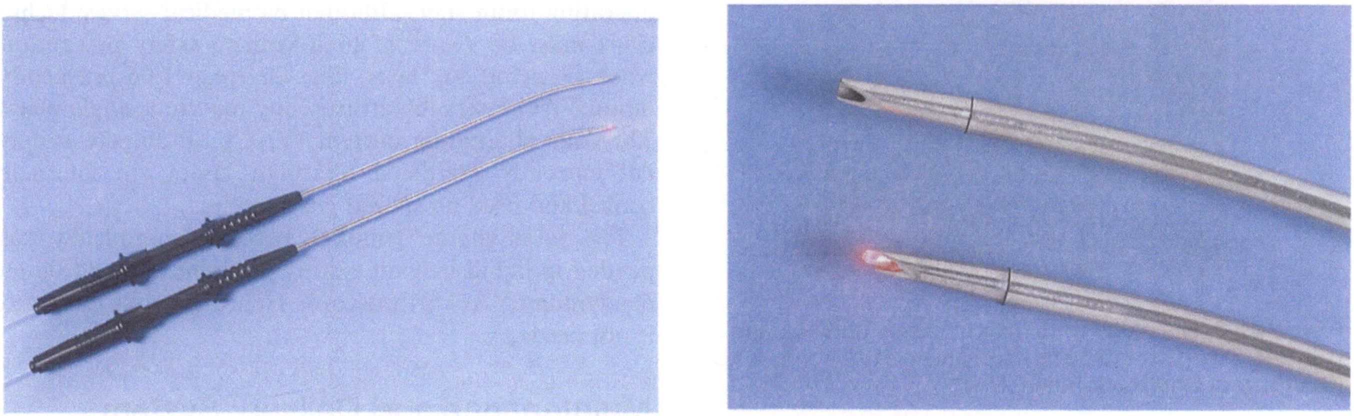

A B

Figure 21-4. (A) SharpLase arthroscopic 15-degree angled handpiece with fiber tip advanced and retracted. (B) Close-up 1000-μm fiber tip advanced and retracted.

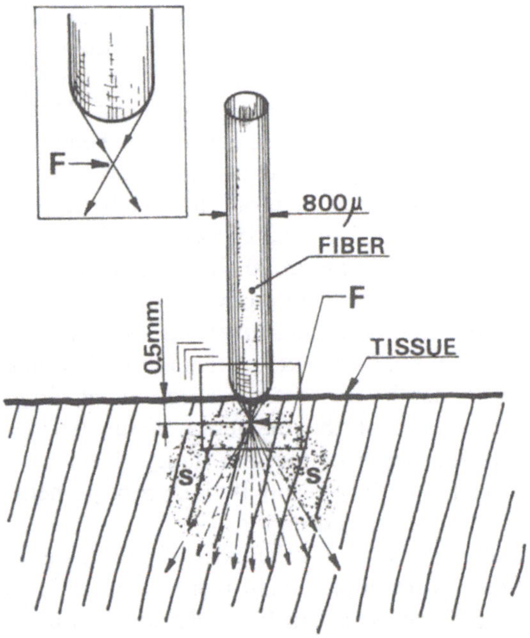

Figure 21-5. Sculpted hemispheric tip focuses the 1.06 μm neodymium:YAG laser beam immediately in front of the fiber. The beam diverges rapidly beyond the focal point. Once in contact with tissue, the fiber tip carbonizes and absorbs the laser energy on the surface of the fiber, causing tissue vaporization.

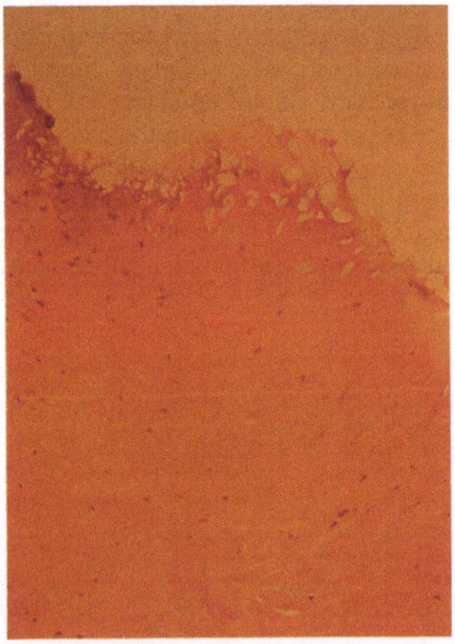

Figure 21-6. Histology of human meniscal cartilage incised with the Sharplan 1.06 μm neodymium:YAG contact fiber. (Courtesy of Chadwick Smith, M.D.)

vectomy, and vaporization and dissection of scar tissue. Applications in the elbow, wrist, and ankle are increasing.

Prior to the innovation of sculptured contact fibers, the depth of thermal injury with the 1.06 μm neodymium:YAG laser has been an issue because of this wavelength's ability as a free beam to penetrate tissue by several millimeters. However, with the different principles of contact technology, the actual depth of thermal injury is much less. In a comparison of wavelengths and delivery systems for arthroscopy, the depth of thermal injury for a sapphire tip, similar in function to the contact fibers, was less than that for the 2.1 μm holmium:YAG and 10.6 μm CO_2 wavelengths (Black et al., 1992).

Another difference between the 2.1 μm holmium:YAG and 1.06 μm neodymium:YAG lasers is that the 2.1 μm holmium:YAG laser delivers pulses of energy with a pulse repetition rate as low as 10 Hz, whereas the 1.06 μm neodymium:YAG laser delivers energy continuously. Thus more uniform cutting and vaporization may occur with the 1.06 μm neodymium:YAG laser contact fibers, especially in soft fibrous tissue. Also, at 70 to 80 watts of power, the 1.06 μm neodymium:YAG contact fibers may cut and ablate more rapidly than the 20- to 30-watt 2.1 μm holmium:YAG laser.

Laser Safety and Facility Requirements

Hospitals should develop policies and procedures mandated by the Joint Commission for the Accreditation of Healthcare Organizations (JCAHO) and the Occupational Safety and Health Administration (OSHA), as guided by the American National Standards Institute (ANSI) Standard for Safe Use of Lasers in Health Care Facilities (Z136.3). These policies should include, as a minimum, restricted access to operating rooms during laser procedures, the use of laser safety goggles (properly labeled with optical density and wavelength) at all times, and a policy that ensures that windows to the operating room are covered with opaque material. Sharplan has assisted many hospitals in establishing appropriate policies.

There are no special electrical hazards that concern the operating room staff, although biomedical service technicians must be aware of high voltage safety precautions when servicing any laser. The Sharplan 1.06 μm neodymium:YAG lasers for arthroscopy require a single-phase, 220 volts alternating current (VAC), 40 ampere supply. All currently marketed Sharplan lasers are internally cooled and need no special gas supplies.

The laser plume (smoke) becomes completely suspended in liquid irrigant exiting the joint during 1.06 μm neodymium:YAG arthroscopy. Hence a smoke evacuator is not needed.

Maintenance and Delivery System Considerations

Sharplan recommends a preuse check of the laser and delivery system to avoid the minimal risk of a malfunction during the case. Calibration of the Sharplan 1.06 μm neodymium:YAG laser may be performed manually with a free beam test fiber and the laser's integral power meter, although it is not necessary (calibration is automatically set by the laser).

The Sharplan 1.06 μm neodymium:YAG lasers are of mature technology, and their reliability has been established over many years. However, Sharplan recommends comprehensive preventive maintenance every 6 months to inspect the water cooling system, power meter, internal lenses and mirrors, the krypton arc lamp, and the procedure data printer. This maintenance should be performed only by Sharplan trained and authorized technicians. Sharplan offers several service schools throughout the year for hospital technician training on the service of Sharplan 1.06 μm neodymium:YAG lasers.

Conclusions

Arthroscopy with the 1.06 μm neodymium:YAG laser has been developed to the point where it now provides unique surgical capabilities beyond what has been available with mechanical instruments. Laser contact fibers act as pointing tools rather than grasping tools, and they are easy to use and effective. When used by a properly trained surgeon, this laser represents an important advance in the available tools for performing arthroscopic surgery. The real benefit of these tools is improved access to tissue in the smallest spaces in the knee and other joints and the ability to vaporize undesired or diseased tissue rather than having to employ mechanical extraction.

Editor's Cautions

1. **The free-beam mode of tissue application for arthroscopic laser surgery of the 1.06 μm neodymium:YAG has been shown by Raunest to cause severe degenerative changes in articular cartilage in laboratory animals. It has also been shown by Bradrick to cause subchondral fibrosis of bone and noncontact hyaline cartilage burns. Noncontact, cleaved, bare, or non sculptured fibers are not recommended for use on these structures. Noncontact tips should also not be used in the posterior popliteal area or near skin when working from within the joint.**
2. **Contact tips do emit some free- beam 1.06 μm neodymium:YAG radiation, especially if they have not been in contact with tissue. Use of any probe emitting 1.06 μm neodymium:YAG radiation on articular cartilage may cause problems problems similar to those mentioned above.**
3. **Probing or levering with any fiber or fiber tip will likely result in fracture of the "probe" and thus an intraarticular foreign body. These tips are fragile and must be handled as such. Forcing a "probe" is not recommended.**
4. **Each fiber has a definite life-span, and the system should not be used without standard mechanical instruments available.**
5. **This laser should *not* be used without 1.06 μm-specific protective eyewear.**
6. **Optimal, satisfactory use of this system requires some experience. It is best to start in the laboratory, not with patients. The best techniques, energy settings, and probe selections can be preliminarily determined in this way. The reader is referred to Chapter 4 for a discussion on ablation efficiency.**
7. **This chapter is only an introduction to this arthroscopic laser system. The reader is encouraged to study this entire text, follow acceptable training and credentialling procedures, as well as research the subject at hand for additional information and changes before undertaking this arthroscopic laser system's use.**

Suggested Reading

Bickerstaff DR, Wyman A, Laing RW, et al (1991) Partial meniscectomy using the neodymium:YAG laser: an in-vitro study. Arthroscopy 7:63–67

Black J, Sherk HH, Meller M, et al (1992) Wavelength selection in laser arthroscopy. Semin Orthop 7:72–76

Brillhart AT (1991) Arthroscopic laser surgery: the contact neodymium:YAG laser; Fourth of four articles. Am J Arthrosc 1(4):7–10

Miller DV, O'Brien SJ, Arnoczky SS, et al (1989) The use of the contact Nd:YAG laser in arthroscopic surgery: effects on articular cartilage and meniscal tissue. Arthroscopy 5: 245–253

22

Sunrise sLASE 210 Surgical Holmium:YAG Laser for Arthroscopic Laser Surgery

Stuart D. Harman and Art Vassiliadis

The sLASE 210 Laser system is a pulsed thulium-holmium-chromium-doped YAG (THC:YAG) solid-state laser that emits energy at a wavelength of 2.1 μm (Fig. 22-1). This wavelength is relatively new as a therapeutic energy source, but because of its unique effects on tissue the 2.1 μm holmium:YAG laser has rapidly developed into a user-friendly clinical tool with a growing number of surgical applications.

The current sLASE 210 product line consists of the sLASE 210 (10 watts), and sLASE 210 PLUS (20 watts). Each of these lasers has different features designed to meet specific clinical requirements. Unlike scientific lasers, the sLASE 210 is a clinical device that includes a highly sophisticated combination of software and hardware elements to ensure reliable, safe operation to the user and patient. Furthermore, because the laser is only one of many sophisticated instruments used in the operating room, it is designed to be as user-friendly as possible.

The design also takes into consideration the rigorous environment of the operating theater and the need for compactness and transportability. The following information provides detailed information about the internal and external components and how the sLASE 210 holmium:YAG laser works.

Internal Systems

The sLASE 210 system utilizes a metal frame design to which internal subassemblies and discrete components are fastened. Despite the numerous mechanical systems incorporated within, the internal design is compact, minimizing the size of the complete laser system as much as possible. Because there is both high voltage and water systems found within, care has been taken to isolate the two conditions, for the unlikely event of a water leak. The major subassemblies of the internal system consist of the laser head assembly, high voltage power supply, cooling system, low voltage power supply, and sLASE 210 control system.

Laser Head Assembly

The laser head assembly includes the 2.1 μm holmium:YAG laser resonator, a 3-mW helium-neon gas laser, a series of optical beam steerers and combiners, mechanical safety shutters and apertures. Because all of the optical components are located here, its precise optical alignments are preserved by isolating the entire assembly from mechanical vibration or shock with a proprietary shock absorber. The laser head assembly is connected to the high voltage network, and because of the tremendous heat generated during the laser excitation process the 2.1 μm holmium:YAG laser head is water-cooled by the internal cooling system.

The helium-neon laser is a small, low power gas laser with a visible wavelength (red: 0.633 μm). This laser's output beam is combined optically with the 2.1 μm holmium:YAG beam path and is delivered concentrically through the delivery system to act as an aiming reference for the surgeon. The helium-neon laser energy is low, so there is no tissue effect caused by the red beam.

Most of the laser head assembly components interface in some manner with the central processor unit as part of the normal operating process and safety protection. In many cases certain monitors are redundant, particularly with respect to safety systems. Parameters that are monitored are the laser head power level, safety shutter position and timing, and many others too numerous to discuss in this chapter. In essence, this complex network ensures that the laser is properly set up for operation, is off when it should be, turns on when it should and at the correct power level, and is delivered to the treatment site

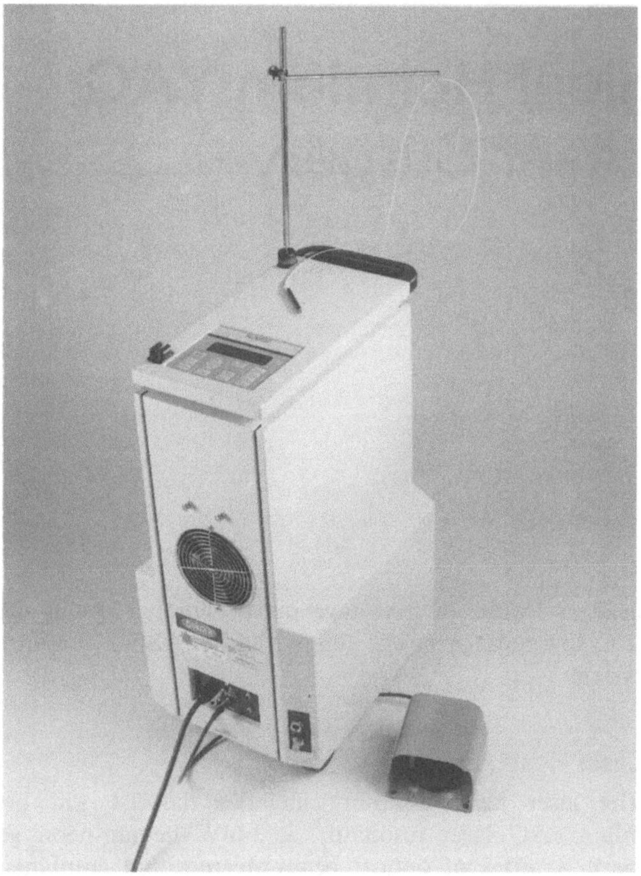

Figure 22-1. sLASE 210 laser system.

for the proper time interval. Any hazardous operating condition detected by the sLASE safety monitors causes immediate disabling of the laser system and instant interruption of all laser energy transmission if lasing is in progress during the fault. Noncatastrophic faults may or may not disable laser operation, depending on the nature and severity of the abnormal condition.

High Voltage Power Supply

To provide the energy necessary to excite the solid-state 2.1 μm holmium:YAG laser rod, a high voltage supply network is required. This network consists of several subcomponents that provide a specific type of pulse energy to the laser head to properly excite the laser rod. This operation is described more thoroughly later.

Cooling System

The sLASE 210 cooling system is comprised of a heat exchanger, water pump, fan, water reservoir, and flow switch. The sole use of the cooling system is to dissipate the excess heat away from the 2.1 μm holmium:YAG laser resonator. A unique feature of the sLASE 210 (twenty watt) system is the option of using the self-contained heat-to-air exchanger, or connecting an external cooling source for maximum efficiency. External cooling may be provided by a stand-alone chiller system that is provided or an external cooling supply such as tap water. Connection of external cooling to the sLASE console is facilitated by two quick disconnect water fittings.

Low Voltage Power Supply

The low voltage power supply provides all of the power necessary for the logic circuits in the system and does not exceed 25 volts. This assembly also performs as the primary interface between the processor unit and all of the various sensors and detectors throughout the system.

Control System

The heart of the sLASE 210 control system is the controller board, which contains the 8085 microprocessor, digital input/output ports, control panel and display interfaces, and circuits for power monitor and interlocks. All of the sLASE 210 system's programming is contained on an EPROM and nonvolatile RAM. The control system also utilizes "watchdog" technology to ensure proper CPU performance (e.g., direct current voltage level, logic timing). If for any reason the watchdog circuit detects an unsuitable condition, the laser is disabled.

External Systems

The external components of the sLASE 210 are those that are required to allow the user to set up, operate, and control the laser. The main features are the control panel and display, emergency off switch, external power detector system, fiberoptic interface system, on/off keyswitch, remote interlock system, footswitch system, circuit breakers, and power cable. All of these features are accessible by the user and must be understood for proper and safe use of the laser system.

Control Panel and Display

The primary user interface is the control panel. Located on the top of the laser console for good visibility, the control panel keypads allows the user to select system status (Standby, Aim, Ready), treatment power level, a fiber calibration routine, pulse repetition rate, exposure time, and Repeat mode. The user can also access stored data pertaining to total pulses delivered, total joules delivered, and total time of exposure. The system continuously accrues all of the values after the laser has been powered up until the reset touchpad is pressed or the system is shut down. A special feature of the sLASE 210 is the ability to operate and continuously monitor the total number of joules delivered for those procedures that require careful monitoring of the total energy transmitted to tissue.

Just above the touchpad controls, a 40-character alphanumeric display provides the user with set parameters, system status, error messages, treatment data, and user instructions. All operational information needed by the user to safely and properly use the laser is provided on this display.

Emergency Off Switch

Based on years of experience and advancement in technology, the modern clinical laser embodies redundant safety circuitry and sophisticated monitor circuits to prevent catastrophic failures from creating a safety hazard for the operating room staff and the patient. The final component in this series of safety controls is the emergency off switch, or panic switch. When this switch is pushed, the laser system is immediately shut down, and laser energy delivery is terminated instantly. This brightly colored switch is mounted on the front panel, toward the surgical team so it can be rapidly identified and accessed.

External Power Detector System

The sLASE 210 is factory-calibrated to display the set power level based on a fixed loss of 15% from the fiberoptic delivery system. However, because it is possible for the fiberoptic efficiency to degrade owing to slight damage or contamination to the fiber system, it is sometimes useful to be able to measure the true output power of that delivery system. The sLASE 210 provides an external power detector that, when Calibration mode is selected, allows the user to measure the actual delivered power from the fiber. The detector head sits on top of a fiber boom (provided for convenient positioning and support of the fiberoptic toward the sterile field) and is at a height that is within acceptable sterile boundaries so calibration can be achieved under sterile conditions. The power detector is connected to the console control system through a BNC connector located on the front panel.

Fiberoptic Interface System

To transfer the holmium energy from the console to the treatment site, the exit beam of the 2.1 μm holmium:YAG laser head is combined internally with the red helium-neon aiming beam and optically focused into the fiberoptic receptacle. When the external fiberoptic delivery system is properly threaded into the interface receptacle, the helium-neon and 2.1 μm holmium:YAG laser beams coincidentally focus into the fiberoptic system.

The fiber interface system also includes two interlock monitors. One monitor is to ensure that a fiber is connected to the interface before enabling the Aim or Ready system operating modes. The second monitor distinguishes whether a high power- or low power (ophthalmic)-type delivery system is installed. If a low power ophthalmic fiber is installed, the control system automatically limits the maximum energy to 200 mJ to protect the small-diameter fiber from thermal damage.

On/Off Keyswitch

The on/off keyswitch is used to power up and shut down the sLASE 210 system. It is operated virtually the same as an automobile ignition switch with Off, On, and Start positions. To start up the sLASE 210, the keyswitch is rotated to the Start position for 1 second and then released. The keyswitch automatically springs back to the On position and the laser starts.

Located just below the keyswitch is an amber indicator lamp that remains illuminated whenever the power cable is connected to a live circuit and both circuit breakers are in the On (untripped) position. This feature is useful when trouble-shooting a system that fails to start up.

Remote Interlock System

All laser systems are required to provide the user with the ability to connect an external interlock switch so the laser is interrupted when an access door to the treatment room fitted with that switch is opened. To meet that requirement, the sLASE 210 has a receptacle that is compatible with a phone plug style connector. Because experience has shown that a laser that shuts off every time someone walks through the door can be more of a problem than a safety benefit, a jumper plug is provided to bypass the need for an external interlock.

Footswitch System

Delivery of laser energy to the treatment site is controlled by a water-resistant footswitch. The footswitch is connected to the rear panel of the sLASE console with a keyed five-pin connector to prevent improper installation. The laser must be in Ready mode for the footswitch to be enabled; and once the pedal is pressed, internal safety shutters are opened to allow passage of the preset energy into the fiberoptic delivery system. The laser energy is then delivered for the preset exposure time and automatically shut off at the prescribed time so long as the footswitch is depressed. If the footswitch is released before the preset exposure time is reached, the safety shutters immediately close, thereby interrupting the exposure cycle and delivery of laser energy. In Continuous mode, the laser energy is delivered indefinitely until the footswitch pedal is released.

Circuit Breakers

There are two circuit breakers located on the rear panel of the console, and they are redundant. However, one of the breakers is a rocker-type switch and doubles as the mainline power switch for the system. When this breaker trips, the rocker switch moves to the Off position and must be reset to On. The second breaker is a plunger-type switch that when tripped must be pushed in to reset it. If either or both of these circuit breakers trip, the amber indicator light on the front panel is not lighted, nor is it possible to start up the system.

Power Cable

Connection to the facility electrical service is done with the system power cable. This cable is hard-wired and strain-relieved to the laser console and, depending on the specific electrical service setup, has the appropriate single-phase electrical plug at its distal end.

Delivery Systems

Of equal or greater importance to the laser console design, the delivery system, like the steel scalpel, is the true surgical tool; and the laser console serves only as a safe, reliable source of energy. Therefore it can be argued that the laser system is only as good as its delivery systems. As with the family of sLASE systems, designed to meet a range of specific economic and clinical requirements, the fiberoptic-based delivery systems are likewise varied for the same reasons.

Fundamentally, the 2.1 μm holmium:YAG laser delivery system utilizes a low-water (or low OH), stepped-index silica quartz fiberoptic. Use of a low-water quartz fiber is essential because lower-cost, standard quartz fibers, which are suitable for 1.06 μm neodymium:YAG and argon lasers, attenuate the 2.1 μm wavelength energy of the holmium:YAG laser to an unacceptable degree. It should be noted that this is a significantly higher fiberoptic cost delivery system over those manufactured with the standard quartz fibers. Furthermore, although the 2.1 μm holmium:YAG laser delivery system emits the transmitted energy as a free beam, it is typically used in a contact or near-contact manner using a hand-held probe (or handpiece) for open procedures, or the jacketed fiber may be inserted through an endoscopic instrument to the treatment site.

Sunrise Technologies has developed single-use, *disposable* fiberoptic delivery systems for those customers whose primary requirement is maximum performance from procedure to procedure or who want to ensure a negligible risk of cross contamination. The company has developed *reusable* fibers to satisfy those customers who are more concerned about cost containment per case and are willing to repair and reprocess used fibers. In addition, these fibers are available in 200, 320, 400, and 550 μm diameters, depending on the surgical application. A series of general purpose, reusable handpieces that support and direct the distal end of the fiberoptic are also available.

At present, sophisticated systems have been designed by Sunrise Technologies for arthroscopy, general surgery, and percutaneous discectomy. They include a variety of suction handpieces, cannulas, stylets, bending tools, and so on to facilitate specific techniques, add versatility, and maximize performance where required.

External Chiller

For the 20 watt sLASE 210 systems, a stand-alone chiller system is provided as a standard accessory; use of external cooling is required for operation of the sLASE 210 above 10 watts. The sLASE 210 laser console was intentionally designed without the more efficient onboard cooling systems because it increases the size and weight of the laser by as much as 75% and adds significant noise immediately adjacent to the surgical field. For example, the chiller may be left in one operating suite for high power applications, and the laser can be easily moved from suite to suite for the more common, low power procedures (the chiller unit is also easily transported from site to site). By separating the chiller unit, the sLASE 210 features a compact, lightweight, quiet 2.1 μm holmium:YAG laser with a high degree of versatility and setup options.

A one-piece, dual-hose assembly interconnects the two consoles (chiller and laser) utilizing keyed quick disconnect fittings for error-free, spill-free installation. Either end of the hose may be used for the laser or the chiller console connection.

sLASE 210 System Operation

Line power is delivered to the laser console through the main power cable. The system is protected from excessive line surges by routing one side of the single-phase electrical energy through two circuit breakers, one of which also acts as the primary line switch for the console. The other side of the electrical service is routed to the console on/off keyswitch, which is used by the operator to start up the laser system for use. This keyswitch operates much like an automobile ignition switch. Once the key is rotated momentarily to the start position, the processor activates the main power relay and the system is powered up.

At this time, the low voltage power supply is activated in addition to the control system. Initialization involves a self-test routine where the microprocessor and a "watchdog" circuit check for improper operation or setup conditions, open interlocks, and other safety violations. Once the self-test is completed any faulty condition is displayed; upon satisfactory completion, the laser defaults to the standby state, in which all laser parameters are automatically set to their minimum value point. The system is now ready for adjustment and use.

In addition, a simmer power supply now continuously maintains a low current plasma in the flash lamp (used to optically pump the solid-state crystal) to eliminate a cold start condition once the command to fire at treatment power levels is applied. This design extends the lifetime of the flashlamp and enhances stability of the laser energy at the onset of firing.

Before the laser can be turned on, it is necessary to connect the remote interlock connector or the remote interlock jumper plug into the remote interlock receptacle. The footswitch must also be connected at this time. Before start-up of the laser, it is recommended to position the laser console as required near the sterile field and install the fiberoptic connector to the fiber interface on the laser console. It is necessary to install the fiber *before* turn-on as the laser automatically enters the low power ophthalmic operating mode if no fiber is installed. If high power delivery is needed and the laser is turned on without the fiber in place, it is impossible to switch out of Ophthalmic mode. Once the high power fiberoptic is connected, the system is now started by use of the on/off keyswitch, as described previously. Once the system goes through its self-test routine, the laser automatically goes to the default Standby mode. It is now necessary to set the laser treatment parameters using the control panel touchpads before the laser is ready for use. It is recommended that the laser be set up in the following order.

1. Set the pulse repetition rate to one of the available values by pressing the appropriate control until the desired value is displayed.
2. Set the exposure time to single-burst operation between 0.1 and 0.5 second if a single burst is desired. The laser will now be delivered to tissue for the set time and then stop until the footswitch is released and pressed once again.
3. If a repetitive burst is desired, set the repeat (off interval) time between 0.2 and 1.0 second. The laser will now be delivered to tissue for the set exposure time, turn off for the set repeat time, and cycle through this on/off sequence until the footswitch is released.
4. If a continuous burst is desired, press the exposure time touchpad until the display indicates Cont. The laser will now be delivered to tissue in continuous bursts of energy so long as the footswitch is depressed (Repeat mode is now deactivated).
5. The final parameter adjustment should be the output power or energy (both watts *and* joules are displayed). Two touchpads allow the laser output to be increased or decreased. Once a level has been set and the touchpad is released, the laser automatically calibrates itself internally for 2 seconds without delivering energy to the tissue and then stops. The laser is now fully adjusted; only the system status must be set to make the laser operational.

At this point, the laser is in its safest operational state, Standby. In this state the footswitch is non-functional, and neither the helium-neon aiming beam nor the 2.1 μm holmium:YAG treatment beam can be transmitted to the fiberoptic delivery system. When the Aim touchpad is pressed, the footswitch is still nonfunctional, but now the helium-neon aiming beam is transmitted through and out from the distal end of the fiberoptic. This condition can be a useful one, as endoscopic location of the fiberoptic tip is readily accomplished without risk of inadvertent firing of the laser (as for procedures requiring triangulation where the tip is not immediately within the field of view in the endoscope). When the Ready touchpad is pressed, the footswitch is now enabled, the aiming beam is continuously transmitted, and the laser is ready to be fired to tissue.

With the laser in Ready mode and the footswitch depressed, a standard firing sequence is initiated. The high voltage power supply provides a specific amount of energy into two main discharge capacitors. The capacitors and a set of inductors comprise a pulse-forming network. To fire the laser, the microprocessor sends its fire signal to a silicon-controlled rectifier (SCR). Once the proper charge is established on the main capacitors and the fire signal is received by the silicon-controlled rectifier, the full discharge of the capacitors is sent to the flashlamp.

The radiant energy of the flashlamp is directed into the solid-state 2.1 μm holmium:YAG rod, thereby exciting the resident atoms within the crystal and establishing the necessary physics for stimulated emission. As with all laser resonators, partial reflector and mirrored optics are positioned at opposite ends of the resonator assembly to oscillate the photon stream (for a complete explanation of laser physics, supplemental literature pertaining to laser theory and design should be read). Laser energy is generated in this manner for the duration of exposure time set by the user. Pulses generated during the first second are not delivered to tissue; they are used as a redundant safety check to ensure that the transmitted energy is the same as the set energy level within a specified degree of accuracy. This safety test is accomplished by placing a light detector at each end of the laser resonator to sample a small percentage of the beam. The detected signal is monitored by the control system and compared with the set value.

A series of safety checks are continuously undertaken at a high frequency while lasing and otherwise, so any faulty condition detected is interrupted within a fraction of second of its occurrence. These safety checks include laser resonator power level, power supply voltage level, remote interlock connection, footswitch connection, excessive exposure duration, safety shutter position, coolant temperature, fiberoptic connection, helium-neon beam operation, and many other internal circuit monitors.

Delivery System Operation

The delivery system is the essential surgical tool to the surgeon, and the laser itself serves as a safe, reliable energy generator. The delivery system is therefore a critical part of the overall system. With 2.1 μm holmium:YAG lasers, the energy is transferred from the laser console to the surgical treatment site through a special type of silica quartz fiberoptic cable. Unlike visible and 1.06 μm neodymium:YAG lasers, which use low-cost, standard quartz fibers, the high water absorption characteristics of the 2.1 μm holmium:YAG wavelength mandates the use of more costly low water (OH) silica quartz fiberoptics. As a result, it may be noted that 2.1 μm holmium:YAG delivery systems often cost substantially more than equivalent delivery systems that use the less expensive fiber material. Sunrise fiber systems are 3 meters long to minimize intrusion of the laser console into the sterile field. In addition, a fiber boom is provided to support the fiberoptic and enhance transition of the fiber from unsterile to sterile conditions while minimizing the risk of contamination.

All Sunrise fiber delivery systems are designed to transmit the 2.1 μm holmium:YAG energy in a free-beam manner. That is, the energy is emitted from the distal end of the fiberoptic and optically transmits through space in a 26- to 27-degree divergent cone angle. The optical energy must be intercepted and absorbed by a target material to produce a thermal effect. Surgically, the fiberoptic may be used in a free-beam, near-contact, or contact manner depending on the surgical application.

For rigid or flexible endoscopic applications, free-beam fibers may be used as is and introduced through existing instrument or biopsy channels of the endoscope. For endoscopic procedures that utilize an endoscope and a second portal for instruments (as for arthroscopy or open procedures), various handpieces are available that support the fiberoptic and enhance control of the emitted energy. These handpieces are available in a range of probe working lengths, diameters, and angled or straight configurations. In all cases, the handpieces are reusable and utilize a mechanical collet to secure the fiberoptic in place after insertion into the handpiece system.

For arthroscopy, a special delivery system kit is available that includes obturators, a rigid handpiece, and a malleable handpiece that can be bent by the surgeon up to 30 degrees (a bending tool is supplied). The handpieces work in conjunction with either 320 or 400 μm presterilized, single-use, sheathed fibers that prevent inadvertent breakage of the fiber tip within the joint.

Because reusable fibers invariably suffer some degradation during use, repair tools are provided to allow the facility to cleave the fiberoptic strand and produce a new distal surface, and thereby restoring performance of the delivery system. After some time the fiber must be replaced because it becomes too short to reach the sterile field (each repair removes 1 inch or so of the fiber end) or from the gradual degradation of the overall fiberoptic transmission that occurs after numerous uses.

The choice of reusable single-use fibers is offered to provide a delivery system option for those facilities concerned about cost per case and that are willing to expend resources to repair and resterilize fibers. Single-use fibers provide peak performance in every procedure and maximum patient safety by minimizing the risk of cross contamination.

Arthroscopic and Soft Tissue Surgery

The sLASE 210 hdolmium:YAG laser is approved by the U.S. Food and Drug Administration (FDA) for marketing for use in arthroscopic procedures: cutting (incision, excision), ablation, and vaporization with hemostasis of soft tissue and firm cartilage. Soft tissues include skin, subcutaneous tissue, striated and smooth muscle, cartilage, mucous membranes, lymph vessels, and organs and glands.

Contraindications

Contraindications for laser arthroscopy are virtually the same as for conventional techniques, with the laser adding no constraints in this regard. It is strongly recommended that the laser system be used only by fully trained, qualified physicians who have undergone training for use of the 2.1 μm holmium:YAG laser, and that the facility comply with recommended practices for safe use as described in the American National Standards Institute (ANSI) document Z136.3.

Suggested Energy Settings

It has been demonstrated clinically that the tissue effect of the 2.1 μm holmium:YAG laser is fairly consistent regardless of the type or vascularization of the target tissue. The depth of tissue absorption and necrosis has been reported to be between 0.4 and 0.6 mm. The depth of incision is largely determined by the amount of energy applied, and the rate is more a function of the pulse repetition rate selected. Therefore incision depth and rate can be optimized by varying both the pulse repetition rates and energy settings on the laser.

Suggested treatment parameters for arthroscopic applications are shown in Table 22-1. The figures assume that the energy is applied in a contact or near-contact mode.

Coagulation is achieved without damaging adjacent tissues and is effected by reducing the power density. The latter is done by reducing the energy and repetition rate settings of the laser or by defocusing the laser beam, which is easily accomplished by moving the distal end of the fiber delivery system away from the target tissue.

Enhanced Delivery System

To enhance delivery of 2.1 μm holmium:YAG laser energy for arthroscopic applications, Sunrise Technologies has developed a delivery system that utilizes reusable stainless steel handpieces and presterilized disposable fibers. The fibers are encased in a small profile stainless jacket to protect the quartz tip from breakage. This system features a set of sharp and blunt obturators to facilitate entry of the delivery system into the joint; one of the handpieces is bendable up to 30 degrees. The company

Table 22-1. Suggested treatment parameters for arthroscopic applications.

Use	Energy (joules)	Pulse repetition rate (Hz)	Power watts
Ablation	0.5–2.5	5–15	2–25
Excision	1.0–2.5	5–15	5–25

also offers delivery systems that utilize repairable fibers but are not sheathed to protect the tip.

Laser Safety Considerations

The most comprehensive and established reference for laser safety guidelines in the medical environment is the ANSI document Z136.3. Although these guidelines are not legally binding, they are based on the experience and wisdom of experts from a variety of medical specialties, and Z136.3 is considered the gold standard for surgical laser safety criteria. It is highly recommended that any medical facility utilizing laser technology obtain a copy of this document and become thoroughly familiar with its contents.

Potential safety hazards from the 2.1 μm holmium:YAG laser can be classified into discrete categories, listed below in a descending order of likely occurrence:

Skin burn
Corneal eye injury
Treatment injury (to patient)
Fire/explosion
Electrocution
Biologic contamination

The following discussion describes the nature of these hazards and offers safety practices that can be employed to minimize their occurrence or risk.

Skin Burn

The surgical laser is absorbed by tissue, resulting in some degree of temperature increase (up to the point of thermal vaporization), and this energy is capable of causing a similar effect when inadvertently aimed and fired at the physician, staff, or patient, resulting in a burn. The closer the 2.1 μm holmium:YAG laser fiber is to the victim and the higher the energy (joules) applied, the more severe the injury is likely to be. The laser is capable of causing a third degree burn at high power levels. To minimize the possibility of a skin burn injury, the following recommendations should be followed:

1. The laser should always be placed in Standby mode when not in use.
2. The laser nurse should always vocalize any change in laser status (Laser Standby, Laser Aim, Laser Ready).
3. The physician should *always* visualize where the laser beam is aimed *before* firing the laser.

Eye Injury

The 2.1 μm holmium:YAG laser wavelength is highly absorbed in water, and therefore its potential hazard to the eye is restricted to injury of the cornea. In addition, the nominal hazard zone (NHZ) of the 2.1 μm holmium:YAG laser is much lower than with high power 10.6 μm CO_2, 1.06 μm neodymium:YAG, or visible wavelength lasers. This fact has caused some degree of controversy concerning the need for safety glasses for personnel who are outside the NHZ. Sunrise Technologies recommends that the ANSI standards be followed, which prescribe that all personnel within the treatment room must wear appropriate eye safety glasses or goggles regardless of the wavelength or power level of the laser in use. These additional steps should be taken to minimize the risk of eye injury:

1. Place a warning sign outside every entrance to the treatment room indicating the type of laser in use, power, wavelength, and so on.
2. Place additional laser safety eyewear at the entrances for personnel entering the room.
3. Safety glasses and goggles worn should be clearly labeled by the manufacturer that they are for the 2.1 μm holmium:YAG wavelength and should specify the optical density (which indicates the degree of protection).
4. Access to the treatment room should be restricted to personnel who need to be there.
5. Laser should be placed in Standby mode when not in use.
6. Windows should be covered with an opaque material.
7. Physicians should see that the laser beam is aimed at the intended target before firing the laser.
8. Laser safety glasses or moistened cottonoids should always be placed over the patient's eyes while the laser is in use.

Treatment Injury

Use of the sLASE 210 system (as with any surgical laser system for that matter) in a manner not in accordance with recommended procedures and training increases the risk of injury, not only to the operating room personnel but to the patient as well. Good communication between physician and laser nurse is essential to ensure that safe operating procedures and parameters are always maintained during the surgical procedure. Adherence to laser training, and the following guidelines are recommended to maximize patient safety during the laser procedure.

1. Laser nurse should always vocalize any change in the system status (Standby, Aim, Ready) and repeat any treatment parameter changes back to the physician before putting laser in Ready.
2. Laser should be in Standby mode when not in use.

3. Physician should always visualize where the laser beam is aimed before firing the laser.
4. Use of reflective instruments should be avoided if possible. Care must be taken not to aim the laser beam toward instruments, as reflected energy can cause thermal injury to adjacent vital tissues.
5. For open procedures, wet drapes are used to surround the treatment area, protecting the patient against inadvertent laser exposure.
6. Laser safety glasses or moistened cottonoids should always be placed over the patient's eyes while the laser is in use.

Fire/Explosion Hazards

The sLASE system should never be used in the presence of flammable gases or chemical agents. The greatest risk of fire is caused by flammable drape materials, so never fire the laser toward the drape material. Several steps can be followed to avoid fire or explosion hazards, and a few precautionary procedures are recommended in case a fire should occur.

1. *Never* use the sLASE in the presence of a flammable anesthetic, chemical agent, or flammable preparatory solution.
2. If possible, use flame-resistant or fire-retardant drapes.
3. Place the laser in Standby any time the delivery system is laid down on the surgical drape.
4. If no aiming beam is visible when the laser is placed in Aim or Ready mode, do not use the laser. Check the integrity of the fiber delivery system.
5. Do not use the laser on patients who have been doused in a flammable material (e.g., automobile accident victims with gasoline residues).
6. Keep a halon-type fire extinguisher in the treatment room during the procedure.
7. Keep a basin of water in the sterile area as a first-line defense should fire break out (such as on the Mayo stand or instrument table).
8. If smoke or arcing sounds are heard within the laser console, discontinue use immediately and unplug the laser from the wall receptacle.

Electrical Hazards

The most significant electrical hazard with any laser is electrocution. This risk may be caused by exposed high voltage wires or components, or interaction of the high voltage with leaking water, which is remotely possible with water-cooled laser systems (even if they are internally cooled). Although it is an extremely unlikely event with modem surgical laser systems, a few words of precaution are appropriate.

1. When plugging the system into the wall receptacle, examine the condition of the power plug for exposed, frayed, or burned wires. Do not use if the power cable is found to be damaged.
2. If water is observed leaking from the laser console, unplug the laser from the wall receptacle immediately and do not use until the leak is repaired (small drips of water may be controlled by placing towels or blankets under the console to catch the water so surgery can proceed as scheduled; however, the laser should be repaired as soon as possible).

Biologic Hazards

There have been several studies on the hazards of the smoke plume that evolves as a by-product of vaporization. Production of smoke plume is the greatest during open procedures with any laser, and the 2.1 μm holmium:YAG laser is capable of creating this plume as well. Although it is not clear whether there is indeed a biologic hazard tc the staff from inhaling the smoke plume, there is evidence that the plume does contain active DNA (at the time of this writing). Consequently, it is recommended that a suitable smoke evacuator always be used during open procedures to remove smoke and steam during vaporization. Appropriate smoke evacuators are commercially available from a variety of manufacturers that specialize in this equipment and claim that their instruments are capable of filtering out the potentially hazardous biologic materials.

Finally, it is important to understand that the 2.1 μm holmium:YAG laser wavelength is nonionizing and is therefore nonmutagenic. There is no risk to pregnant women who are in the vicinity of the sLASE when it is in use, nor are there any other reported chromosomal hazards associated with the spectral emission of the 2.1 μm holmium:YAG laser.

Administrative Safety Responsibilities

To ensure that adequate and proper laser safety procedures are established and complied with, it is important that a laser safety officer or committee be appointed, depending on the size and scope of the laser surgery program. The laser safety administration should be responsible for establishing laser safety policy and procedures, including the following:

Safety policies and procedures established, distributed, and enforced

Laser safety and education programs developed and conducted

Credential requirements for laser physicians and nurses established

Laser access controlled (e.g., access to keys, who uses them)

Laser maintenance policy established and compliance maintained

Follow-up education programs conducted

Annual review of policies and procedures performed
Adverse incidents reported to the FDA

Training Requirements

As described above, it is the responsibility of the laser safety officer or committee to establish the safety requirements at each health care facility, including training. An important educational program is the laser in-service training, usually conducted shortly after installation of the laser system by a qualified representative of the manufacturer. This in-service training is open to physicians, operating room nurses, biomedical staff, and any other personnel the laser safety officer or committee may deem appropriate. Topics recommended include the proper set-up, adjustment, test, and use of the laser, routine maintenance requirements and procedures, and laser safety.

Although this training is good, it is essential that all personnel who operate the laser carefully read and understand the operator manual provided with the laser system. Supplemental in-service sessions are essential to refresh training and to educate new staff. Such training may be done by the manufacturer but is usually performed by experts within the health care facility. The quality of any laser safety program is a direct reflection of the establishment of sound policies and procedures, commitment to education and reeducation, good maintenance practices, and consistent enforcement of established regulations.

Installation Requirements

The sLASE 210 series features a compact, lightweight chassis that is capable of fitting into small treatment rooms. In addition, the sLASE 210 is internally cooled or may be cooled by a separate, self-contained chiller unit provided as standard equipment with the 20-watt laser. Consequently, the sLASE 210 requires no special electrical or water utility services for installation and use.

Electrical Requirements

The sLASE 210 series holmium:YAG laser and chillers can be configured for the electrical services shown in Table 22-2. Laser systems configured for 120 VAC operation have a 20 ampere plug standard and a 15 ampere plug extension cable for lower power operation using conventional 120 volt wall outlets. It is recommended that the 100 and 120 volt sLASE 210 systems be plugged into a dedicated wall circuit to avoid tripping panel circuit breakers, as the current requirement is high. *Never connect anesthesia carts to the same circuit.*

Table 22-2. Electrical parameters for sLASE 210 series holmium:YAG laser and chillers.

VAC	Duty cycle (Hz)	Phase	Amperes
100	50/60	Single	20
120	50/60	Single	20
220	50/60	Single	10
240	50/60	Single	10

Cooling Requirements

The sLASE 210 laser cooling systems are either self-contained or include a stand-alone chiller that requires no connection to external water service. The chiller may be connected to a conventional wall outlet but does not require a dedicated circuit as with the laser console.

Console Dimensions

The sLASE 210 series has a compact console design and can be positioned close to the sterile field with minimal intrusion. The laser console dimensions are 31 inches high by 14 inches wide by 21 inches deep; the chiller units are 19 inches high by 18 inches wide by 30 inches deep.

The design philosophy of the sLASE 210 series intentionally separates the chiller from the main console in order to achieve a quieter, more compact, easily transported system. Because the chiller components are isolated from the laser, unwanted noise and obstruction are minimized immediately adjacent to the surgical table, and the weight is divided between two smaller packages. As a result, the sLASE console is easily moved into position and readied for use when called for by the surgeon; and it takes up little room when stored.

By nature, solid-state lasers tend to exhibit better reliability and durability than do gas lasers, with the mean time between failures often surpassing 24 months or more. Consequently, catastrophic failures are rare, and service calls tend to be made for preventive maintenance rather than for repair of the system. The sLASE 210 uses a flashlamp to optically pump the solid-state YAG rod, and this component has a limited lifetime. The average life expectancy of the sLASE 210 flashlamp is on the order of several million joules before degradation of output power requires a lamp exchange. Other components of the system do not degrade in such a manner and have indefinite lifetimes, depending on the environment in which the system is used, stored, and transported. Use of the external chiller, however, does extend the durability of the system owing to enhanced cooling of the internal optical and electrical components.

System Maintenance

It is recommended that the sLASE 210 undergo an annual preventive maintenance to restore optimum performance and identify any conditions that may lead to degradation or failure of the system. As with the annual automobile tune-up, this preventive measure can add many years of use to the laser system. Sunrise Technologies warrants the sLASE 210 for 1 year, including parts and labor, and offers annual maintenance contracts that provide several service plan options, including no-cost maintenance and system repair during the term of the contract. Because preventive maintenance is the primary requirement, this section describes the various maintenance procedures performed by the service engineer on the sLASE 210 system.

Calibration

The laser power detection system must be calibrated once a year to ensure compliance with regulated accuracy standards. Displayed power must always fall within ±20% of the actual power (or energy). Therefore the calibration is checked against a known power meter (NTSC traceable: verified ±5% accuracy). If necessary, recalibration is performed to bring the system to within specification.

Laser Power

Output power is checked to verify that the laser is delivering specified energy at all settings. If output power is below specification, an inspection is made to determine the cause. Typically, low power is caused by the following three conditions, any of which can be corrected by the service engineer on site:

1. Degraded flashlamp. After several million shots of the laser, it is expected that the flashlamp can no longer efficiently pump the YAG rod. A degraded flashlamp is easy to replace and is inexpensive.
2. Contaminated resonator mirrors. Although rare, it is possible for one or both of the laser resonator mirrors to become damaged by contamination to the extent where laser power is diminished. A contaminated mirror can usually be identified by visual inspection. This condition usually occurs because the laser has been exposed to dusty air environments. Because it is difficult to clean these delicate optical components without special tools and conditions, the contaminated optic is usually replaced. Keeping the laser system covered and dust-free when stored is recommended to avoid contamination of all internal optics.
3. Laser resonator misalignment. If the laser system is subjected to a sharp mechanical shock or repeated rough handling, it is possible for the laser resonator to become misaligned. Potential for this condition is reduced, but only to a certain extent, by using shock-absorbing resonator mounts. Realignment of the mirror mounts restores specified power in this situation.

Fiber Interface Optical System

As with the laser mirrors, dusty air environments, rough handling, or sharp shocks to the system may cause the optics that focus the laser energy into the fiberoptic delivery system to become contaminated or misaligned. These optical components can be removed, cleaned, and realigned on site.

Coolant Fluid

It is recommended that the deionized water in the sLASE 210 internal cooling system and the tap water in the external chiller be drained and replaced annually. Despite the fact that most of the cooling system components do not rust, buildup of particles and rust do occur. Annual replacement prevents these contaminants from becoming excessive and harmful to the laser system.

Delivery System Maintenance

Current sLASE 210 delivery systems combine reusable handpieces with either single-use or reusable fiberoptics. Handpieces are available in a variety of lengths, diameters, and probe shapes but are essentially the same from a maintenance standpoint. Where appropriate, additional ancillary accessories such as obturators and bending tools are also available. All of these delivery systems and accessories are constructed of materials that allow them to be sterilized and cleaned consistent with conventional processing methods.

Reusable Fiberoptics

Available in several fiber diameters, reusable fibers require several reprocessing steps prior to each surgical use. Reusable products are delivered in a nonsterile manner and with a properly cleaved distal tip. Initial use requires only sterilization as prescribed by the package labeling. However, once the fiberoptic has been used, the tip becomes degraded and must be recleaved to restore peak transmission. Fiber repair tools are provided with the laser system to allow protective jacketing to be stripped and the fiber to be cleaved. This process produces a new, mirror-like surface at the distal end.

After surgery, the fiber should be wiped off and cleaned with a disinfectant. Under nonsterile conditions, the fiber is recleaved and evaluated for proper performance before resterilization. After sterilization, the reusable fiberoptic is ready for surgical use. It should be noted that use of higher power 2.1 μm holmium:YAG energy tends to degrade reusable fibers with each subsequent use faster than at lower powers. Typically, these fibers perform well for at least 10 or more procedures before replacement becomes necessary (due to power degradation or shortening of the fiber from multiple repairs).

Disposable Fiberoptics

Single-use, disposable fibers are more expensive on a cost per case basis but have two important benefits. First, single-use products maximize patient safety by minimizing the potential for cross contamination. In addition, single-use fibers always deliver peak power performance during the surgical procedure and require no reprocessing for reuse. Because they are not reprocessed the cost of repairing and resterilizing the fiber is saved, recouping some of the initial expense of the single-use product. Single-use products require no maintenance and should be discarded as biocontaminated waste.

Handpieces/Ancillary Accessories

Currently, all Sunrise handpieces and accessories are reusable. After surgical use, the handpieces and accessories should be terminally cleaned in the conventional manner. In addition, a small-diameter brush may be used to clean the probe lumen on the handpieces to remove any organic debris from within. The handpieces and accessories may then be resterilized as specified in the product manual. If disassembly of the handpiece ever becomes necessary, it is important not to lose the internal Silastic rubber component that is used to secure the fiberoptic to the handpiece system.

All fiber products, handpieces, and accessories should be stored in a clean, safe environment when not in use. Similarly fiberoptics should be maintained in a protective container to avoid the possibility of fiber cable breakage due to kinking or crushing.

Editor's Cautions

1. **Even though many surgeons believe there is no need to wear 2.1 μm wavelength-specific protective eyewear, I do not agree. The 2.1 μm holmium:YAG is a class IV laser, and its wavelength can damage the eye.**
2. **These fibers should be used in a standard liquid arthroscopic environment. Use in a gas environment is not recommended.**
3. **Some fiber products may be fragile and might fracture if not fully protected. Forcing, levering, or using the "probe" as a mechanical probe can result in a fracture and an intraarticular foreign body.**
4. **All fibers have a definitive life-span. Optimal, satisfactory use of this system requires some experience. It is best to start in the laboratory, not with patients. The best techniques, energy settings, and probe selections can be preliminarily determined in this way. The reader is referred to Chapter 4 for a discussion on ablation efficiency.**
5. **Mechanical instruments should be available at all times during arthroscopic laser surgery.**
6. **This chapter is only an introduction to this arthroscopic laser system. The reader is encouraged to study this entire text, follow acceptable training and credentialling procedures, as well as research the subject at hand for additional information and changes before undertaking this arthroscopic laser system's use.**

Suggested Reading

Brillhart AT (1991) Arthroscopic laser surgery, the holmium:YAG laser and its use. Am J Arthrosc 1(3):7–11

Dillingham MF, Fanton GS (1990) The use of the Ho:YAG laser in arthroscopic surgery [abstract]. Coherent, Inc.

JGM Associates (1991) Endoscopic Therapy Applications of Advanced Solid State Lasers. JGM, Burlington, MA, pp 6–72 to 6–83

Lane GJ, Mooar PA (1991) Holmium:YAG laser arthroscopic débridement [abstract]. American Society for Laser Surgery and Medicine, Suppl 3

O'Brien SJ, Miller DV (1991) The contact Nd:YAG laser, a new approach to arthroscopic laser surgery. Clin Orthop 252: 95–100

Owens P, Zacherl A (1991) Holmium laser arthroscopy opens new frontier for orthopedics. Laser Nurs 5(3):97–103

Sherk HH (1990) Lasers in Orthopedics. Lippincott, Philadelphia

Vangsness CT, Huang MS, Smith CF (1991) Light absorption characteristics of the human meniscus: applications for laser ablation [Abstract]. Los Angeles

Whipple TL (ed) (1992) Laser Applications in Orthopaedics. AAOS Course Syllabus, Rosemont, IL

23

Surgical Laser Technologies' Contact ArthroProbe™ and the SLT Contact™ 1.06 μm Neodymium:YAG Laser Systems for Arthroscopic Laser Surgery

Terry A. Fuller

Contact Laser™ technology was developed nearly 10 years ago by Surgical Laser Technologies (SLT; Oaks, PA) as a means of accurately delivering controlled laser energy to tissue for open or endoscopic incision, excision, ablation, or coagulation. The key element of this technology is the family of Contact Laser probes, scalpels, and fibers, whose patented geometric shapes and Wavelength Conversion™ effect surface treatments modulate the thermal characteristics of the 1.06 μm neodymium:YAG laser beam to achieve a variety of therapeutic effects. Contact Laser probes and scalpels are contact tips that are used in conjunction with an assortment of fiberoptic delivery systems and several portable, multispecialty 1.06 μm neodymium:YAG lasers. Some of these contact tips are made of fused silica and others of sapphire.

Contact ArthroProbe Contact Tip

The Contact ArthroProbe for Incision is a specialized adaptation of contact delivery systems for the particular demands of arthroscopic surgery (Fig. 23-1). A single-piece 1000-μm fused silica fiberoptic is mounted in a 2.2 mm external diameter handpiece shaft. A novel application of patented technology incorporates a technical ceramic (zirconia) jacket encasing the distal tip, providing sufficient thermodynamic and mechanical support to withstand the stresses of arthroscopic laser surgery. The Contact Arthroprobe for Ablation is a unitary product comprised of a 600-μm fiber integrally attached to a large fused silica ablation probe tip that is supported by a sleeve of zirconia (Fig. 23-2).

The Contact ArthroProbe for Incision tapers to a 0.4 mm diameter distal surface, where a high, localized power density is created. With the addition of the Wavelength Conversion effect treatment, the probe is effective for tissue cutting with only a moderate degree of accompanying coagulation. A choice of straight and 12, 20, and 40 degree curved shafts facilitates access to all areas of joints.

The substantially larger, blunter, round, fused silica distal tip of the Contact ArthroProbe for Ablation produces its effect over a larger surface area for wide area vaporization or ablation. Shafts are available with 20 and 40 degree curves. It too has been treated to achieve Wavelength Conversion effect.

SLT Contact Laser Systems

The advent of the contact approach to laser surgery made feasible the use of 1.06 μm neodymium:YAG lasers that were more compact and versatile than the massive first generation machines, which required hard-wiring and permanent plumbing connections for cooling. Two SLT systems—the CL MD/110-40W and CL MD/DUAL Contact Lasers—provide the full power range needed for all arthroscopic or open orthopedic procedures. The CL MD/110-40W plugs into any 120 volt alternating current (VAC) outlet and delivers up to 40 watts of power; the CL MD/DUAL delivers 40 watts from a 120 VAC outlet and, interchangeably, up to 60 watts from a 220 VAC line. Each system is self-contained and weighs less than 250 pounds, meaning that both Contact Laser systems can readily be moved to any site where they are needed without wiring or plumbing restrictions. All CLMD/110 series lasers can be field-upgraded to power up to 60 watts, which is accomplished by a cost-effective module added to the customer's existing laser.

All SLT Contact Lasers have an integrated fail-safe fiber calibration port. In addition, for procedures in which coaxial cooling of Contact Laser scalpels and probes is required, a sterile fluid path and filtered path for air or CO_2 gas is provided.

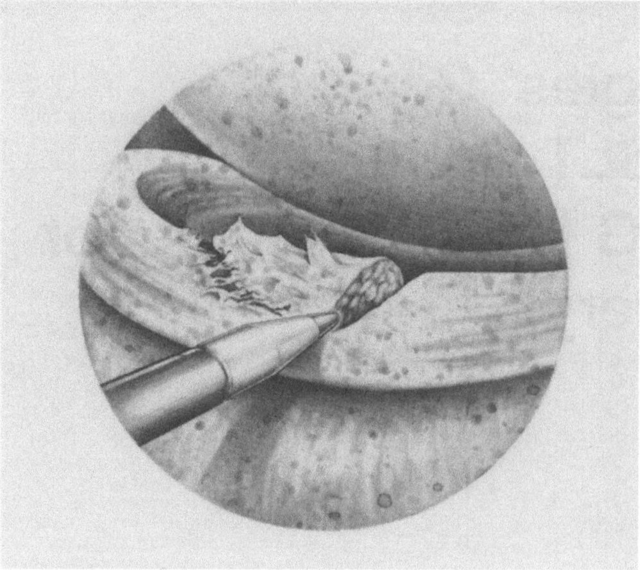

Figure 23-1. Contact ArthroProbe for Incision comprises a one-piece, 1000-μm fiber with a proprietary technical ceramic Contact Probe tip and a handpiece for arthroscopy.

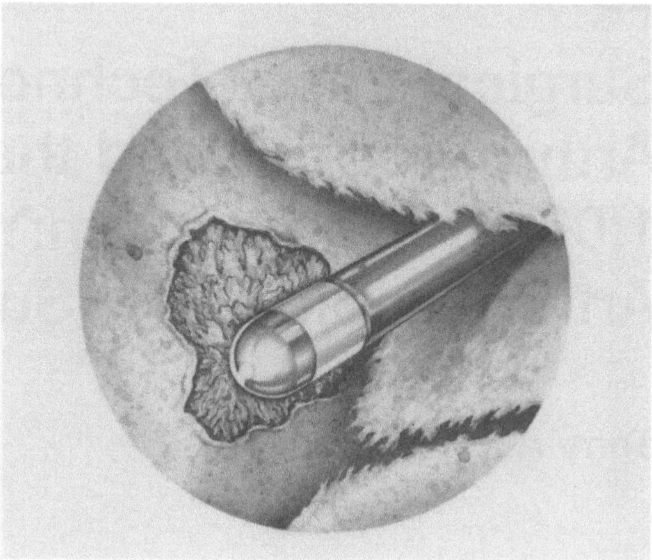

Figure 23-2. Contact ArthroProbe for Ablation.

A microprocessor control unit leads operators through system setup. Power, pulse duration and other parameters are selected and confirmed on the LED panel on the top of the laser. Delivery systems connect to a fiber launch port on the right rear surface of the laser adjacent to the gas/fluid cartridge slot and the fiber management mast, which can, if desired, route the fiberoptic overhead, out of the way.

Physical Principles and Tissue Effects

All thermal lasers create their therapeutic effects through the transformation of light energy into thermal energy at or within the tissue. With the conventional, noncontact mode of delivery, the nature of this transformation is determined entirely by the laser wavelength, power density (which in turn is a combination of the total output power and the spot size), and the optical and thermodynamic properties of the tissue.

Contact Laser technology, in contrast, provides a means of uncoupling the tissue effect from the laser wavelength. It is accomplished by what is referred to as Wavelength Conversion effect treatments. Infrared energy-absorbing surface treatments titrate the relative amounts of light and thermal energy emitted from the Contact Laser scalpel, probe, or fiber to provide the desired thermal profile in the tissue. The native 1.06 μm neodymium:YAG wavelength emitted from a bare, untreated fiber penetrates several millimeters into most soft tissue, which is useful for deep coagulation but unsuitable for more controlled hemostasis, ablation, or cutting. Shaped fibers without surface treatments emit the native wavelength until the tip becomes fouled or deformed, after which they combine light with thermal effects, though in an unpredictable and changing ratio.

An appropriate surface treatment (i.e., an infrared-absorbing substance), on the other hand, can transform predetermined amounts of the 1.06 μm neodymium:YAG light energy into heat at the probe or fiber surface to provide an intense thermal effect at the tissue surface with little radiant energy penetration, comparable to the therapeutic result with the 10.6 μm CO_2 laser (Fig. 23-3). Lesser amounts of surface treatment create other effects, thereby adjusting the thermal profile in a controlled, reliable way to create the desired temperature gradient within tissue. The Wavelength Conversion effect surface treat-

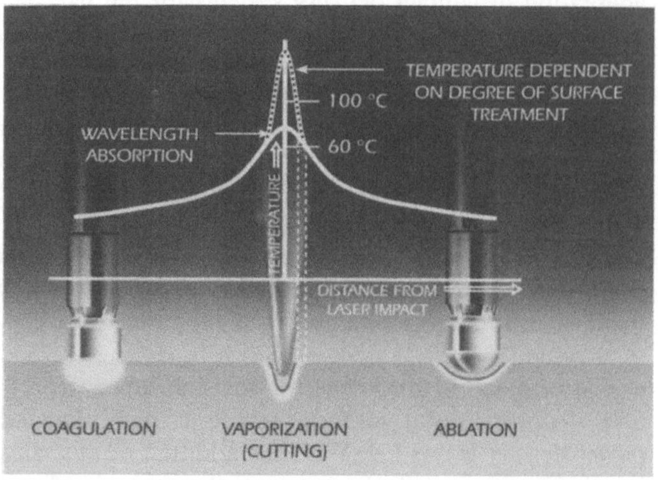

Figure 23-3. Changes in temperature gradient and tissue effect by Wavelength Conversion effect treatments.

ments eliminate the hazards and poor clinical effect of the free-beam 1.06 μm neodymium:YAG laser.

The geometric shapes of Contact Laser devices further determine the spatial distribution of the power density and thermal effect and provide a mechanical advantage not available with noncontact laser modalities. A 2.5 mm diameter flat probe, for example, provides the mechanical ability to tamponade a bleeding vessel as well as a laser power density suitable for coagulation. A 0.2 mm distal diameter conical Contact Laser scalpel, in contrast, provides the high power density localized in a small spot size needed for fine incision with minimal coagulation.

Nevertheless, Contact Laser delivery devices always precisely determine the energy delivered because the spot size is a function of the tip configuration. Moreover, they deliver energy principally when in direct contact with tissue.

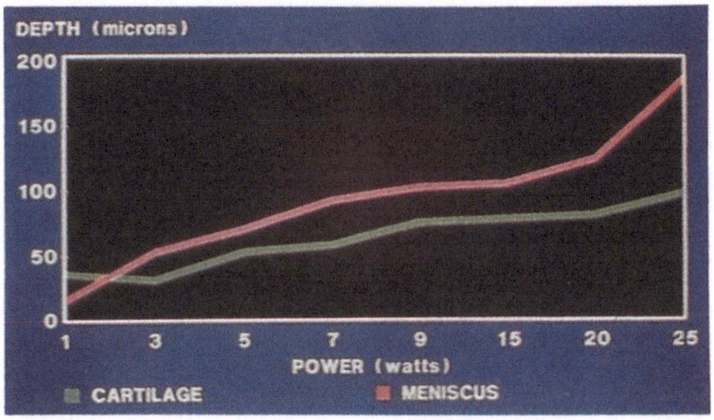

Figure 23-4. Depth of damage chart. At 20 watts, the depth of damage associated with the Contact ArthroProbe is less than 0.5 mm.

Tissue Effects and Applications

Early in vitro studies on bovine and human meniscus (Glick, 1984) and in vivo work with rabbit tissue (Inoue et al., 1983) indicated that the conventional noncontact 1.6 μm neodymium:YAG laser cut poorly while causing an unacceptable amount of thermal damage to adjacent nontargeted tissue. Other studies found that during ablation of fresh human cadaver menisci the zone of lateral damage could be limited to 35 μm, and that for clinical applications the noncontact 1.06 μm neodymium:YAG laser could be employed to smooth degenerated hyaline cartilage, remove the margins of degenerated menisci, and ablate synovial tissue (Sherk and Kollmer, 1990). Relatively low levels of 1.06 μm neodymium:YAG laser energy appear to promote at least short-term proteoglycan, collagen, and noncollagen protein synthesis (Herman and Khosla, 1988; Spivak et al., 1992), a finding supported by in vivo evidence of enhanced regeneration of partial-thickness cartilage defects following 1.06 μm neodymium:YAG laser irradiation (Schultz et al., 1985; Kollmer, 1990).

By limiting and controlling the depth of penetration, Wavelength Conversion effect Contact Laser technology provided the means for circumventing the most troublesome drawback of the 1.06 μm neodymium:YAG laser. This technology made it possible to regulate the nonspecific, deeply penetrating 1.06 μm neodymium:YAG beam.

Fronek and colleagues (1990) used a sapphire Contact Laser scalpel to section 24 macroscopically normal human menisci obtained from patients undergoing total knee arthroplasty for osteoarthritis and found that they were able easily, accurately, and safely to cut the tissue. Microscopic examination revealed necrotic and coagulation layers comparable to those obtained with the 10.6 μm CO_2 laser but without the thick carbon layer (Fig. 23-4).

Bickerstaff et al. (1991), using a chisel-shaped Contact Laser probe, were similarly able to incise 24 human menisci at 25 or 30 watts of power, producing minimal thermal damage to the remaining tissue. The coagulation depth lateral to the cut at both power settings was 105 μm, and the investigators speculated that in a clinical use the constant fluid irrigation from the arthroscope would further dissipate the heat and limit the extent of the lateral coagulation zone.

Miller, O'Brien, and their colleagues have published results of both clinical and experimental work with the Contact Laser. Anatomic specimens from canine knees showed a preferential effect on meniscal tissue over articular cartilage and experimental articular cartilage lesions on the femoral condyle of New Zealand white rabbits demonstrated a significantly enhanced healing response with Wavelength Conversion Contact Laser lesions compared to those created with a steel scalpel or electrocautery (Miller et al., 1989) (Figures 23-5, 23-6, and 23-7). Lesions were bordered by a minimal necrotic margin, and most defects had healed by the end of 12 weeks (O'Brien and Miller, 1990).

In a limited series of clinical studies, these same authors reported successful meniscectomies in 15 patients. Access to difficult areas such as the posterior one-third of the medial meniscus was noticeably easier than with other modalities. Patients returned to full activity within an average of 3 weeks, with no wound-healing problems or postoperative complications at an average of 1 year follow-up (Kelly et al., 1990; O'Brien and Miller, 1990).

Clinical Applications

Contact ArthroProbes are used in light contact with tissue in a fluid medium. For incision, surgeons begin at a power level of 15 watts and increase the power if and as needed to a level of 25 watts. Experienced users typically remain within the 22 to 25 watt range. The Contact ArthroProbe for Ablation is employed at levels between 30 and 40 watts, with 32 to 33 watts about average during normal clinical use.

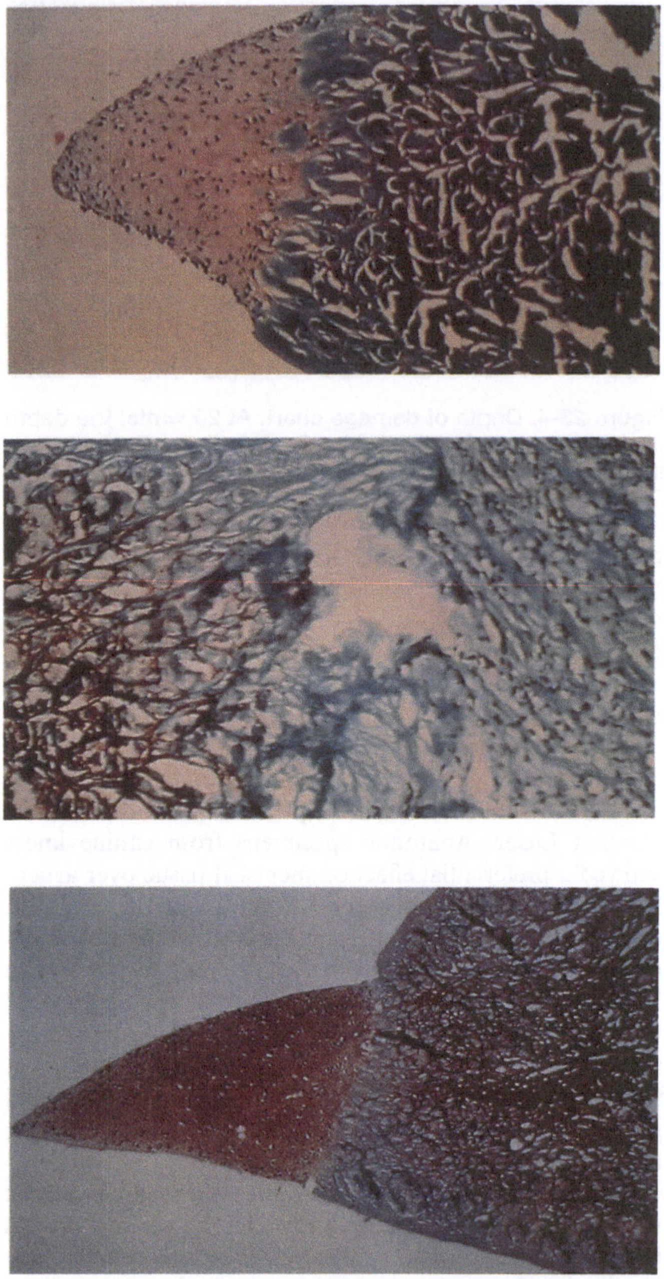

Figure 23-5, 23-6, 23-7. (Top to bottom) Scalpel, electrocautery, and SLT's Contact ArthroProbe menisectomies at 6 weeks. Note the similarity of the scalpel and laser healing responses and the wide band of necrotic meniscus associated with electrocautery.

Contact ArthroProbes fit naturally into the surgical armamentarium of the experienced arthroscopist, requiring little modification of basic surgical technique. The 2.2 mm diameter ArthroProbe shafts are compatible with all normal arthroscopy cannulas and instruments. Because they emit a highly divergent beam, special coated instruments and backstops are not required. Normal electrolytic fluid-distending media such as saline can be used. The tactile feedback of the Contact ArthroProbe provides a more natural experience for the surgeon accustomed to mechanical instruments, in contrast to the free-beam 10.6 μm CO_2 or the 2.1 μm holmium lasers, which add novel constraints and hand–eye coordination factors to already difficult arthroscopic procedures. It is the photothermal energy, rather than the mechanical device itself, that performs the work, so gentle manipulations are sufficient to cut or ablate tissue quickly and easily.

Procedural Advantages of Contact Laser ArthroProbes

Contact ArthroProbes offer a number of significant clinical advantages over conventional mechanical arthroscopy devices.

1. Controlled depth of penetration and reduced damage to surrounding tissue for improved safety
2. No need to change arthroscopic surgical techniques
3. Effective resection in a fluid medium
4. Tactile feedback
5. Reduced mechanical pressure and increased speed of resection
6. Ability to coagulate and reduce blood loss and in some cases eliminate the need for a tourniquet
7. Small size for improved access to joints with less scuffing
8. Ability to accommodate all tissue types found in arthroscopic surgery, decreasing the need to change instruments and the number of instruments needed in many procedures

Because there are no moving parts, the surgeon can cut and remove tissue in close regions of joints with minimal risk of scuffing articular cartilage. Contact Laser incision of meniscal tissue is accurate, does not require the mechanical force needed with a shaver, and leaves a smooth meniscal rim, eliminating the need for secondary trimming. The Contact ArthroProbe for Incision provides enough coagulating thermal energy to cut hemostatically, so knee arthroscopy can routinely be performed without a tourniquet, thereby eliminating ischemic complications. In the absence of bleeding, visualization is better, and the surgeon can check for hemostasis before withdrawing the arthroscope from the joint, which translates into a lower incidence of postoperative complications.

The SLT Contact Laser probes, scalpels, fibers, ArthroProbes, and lasers have received U.S. Food and Drug Administration (FDA) market clearance for the incision and excision of soft tissue during open and arthroscopic orthopedic procedures.

1. Arthroscopic applications in the knee
   a. Arthroscopic meniscectomy
   b. Lateral release
   c. Excision of plica
   d. Excision of scar tissue for arthrofibrosis

   e. Synovectomy
   f. Control of bleeding vessels
   g. Shaving of the patella
2. Arthroscopic applications in the shoulder
   a. Removal of scar tissue in the subacromial space
   b. Labral tears
   c. Synovectomy
   d. Capsular release for adhesive capsulitis
   e. Releasing tissue for shoulder stabilization
   f. Release of coracoacromial ligament during acromionectomy
3. Open arthroplastic and other open applications
   a. Shoulder procedures
   b. Hand and wrist procedures
   c. Knee procedures
   d. Hip procedures

The major uses of the Contact ArthroProbe have been for knee and shoulder arthroscopy, though small joint applications, including temporomandibular joint and wrist procedures, are currently under investigation and should become more feasible with the development of smaller-diameter delivery devices.

Safety Requirements

Any successful laser program must follow appropriate laser safety precautions as established by the American National Standards Institute (ANSI), Occupational Safety and Health Administration (OSHA), FDA, and individual state and hospital guidelines. Such guidelines include the establishment of a laser committee (or in smaller facilities a laser safety officer) and proper training of the clinical laser nurse and other personnel.

Even though the Contact Laser system does not emit a free beam in normal use, there is a small risk of fiber breakage from abuse or misuse. The 1.06 μm neodymium:YAG beam has the ability to pass through transparent ocular media, such as the cornea, lens, and vitreous, causing irreversible retinal damage. Current ANSI standards call for protective goggles or glasses with side guards. Protective eyewear with an optical density of 4.5 is sufficient for surgical use. Patients under light anesthesia may wear eyewear similar to that of the operating room personnel. For patients under general anesthesia, moist saline pads and foil eyeshields are recommended.

Lasers should not be used in the presence of flammable or explosive substances. Ebonized or other special instruments are not required when using the Contact Laser.

Installation, Setup, and Maintenance

The SLT Contact Laser systems were specifically designed for ease and practicality of use. They plug into standard 120 or 220 VAC single-phase outlets and require no external cooling hook-up.

The solid-state design and microprocessor control of these modern 1.06 μm neodymium:YAG lasers makes them reliable and maintenance-free. SLT Contact Laser systems have a modular internal design so if repairs are required it is simple to replace the nonfunctional component.

Each time the Contact Laser system is turned on, the LED display panel leads the operator through the setup procedure, including automatic calibration of selected fibers. In the event of microprocessor failure, all essential basic settings can be manually controlled.

Editor's Cautions

1. **The free-beam mode (in contrast to the contact mode) of tissue application of the 1.06 μm neodymium:YAG laser for arthroscopic surgery has been shown by Raunest to cause severe degenerative changes in articular cartilage in laboratory animals. The free-beam mode has also been shown by Bradrick to cause subchondral fibrosis of bone and noncontact hyaline cartilage burns. (Noncontact, cleaved, bare, or sculptured fibers are not recommended for use on these structures. Noncontact tips should also not be used in the posterior popliteal area or near skin when working from within the joint.)**
2. **Contact tips do emit some free-beam 1.06 μm neodymium:YAG radiation, especially if they have not been in contact with tissue. Use of any probe emitting 1.06 μm neodymium:YAG radiation on articular cartilage may cause problems similar to those mentioned above.**
3. **Probing or levering with any fiber or contact tip will likely result in fracture of the device and an intraarticular foreign body. They are fragile devices and must be handled as such. Forcing the device is not recommended. Contact tips use thermal energy, not mechanical force, to achieve clinical effects.**
4. **Contact tips made of sapphire are not recommended for arthroscopy where the tip may be subjected to thermal shock. Such shock can arise when a heated tip is moved quickly between a liquid environment and an air or gas environment. Such shock can lead to fracture of the tip. The contact ArthroProbe is made from fused silica and thus is suitable for such environments and is recommended for arthroscopy.**
5. **Every fiber or contact tip has a limited life-span. These instruments should not be used without mechanical instruments available.**
6. **This laser should *not* be used without 1.06 μm-specific protective eyewear.**
7. **Satisfactory use of this system for optimal results requires some experience. It is best to start in the laboratory, not with patients. The best techniques, energy settings, and contact tip selections can be preliminarily determined in this way.**
8. **This chapter is only an introduction to this arthroscopic**

laser system. The reader is encouraged to study this entire text, follow acceptable training and credentialling procedures, as well as research the subject at hand for additional information and changes before undertaking this arthroscopic laser system's use.

References

Bickerstaff DR, Wyman A, Laing RW, et al (1991) Partial meniscectomy using the neodymium:YAG laser: an in vitro study. Arthroscopy 7:63–67

Brillhart AT (1991) Arthroscopic laser surgery: the contact neodymium:YAG laser; fourth of four articles. Am J Arthrosc 1(4):7–10

Fronek J (1988) Contact Tip Neodymium:YAG Lasers in Orthopedics. North American Arthroscopy Association, Washington, DC

Fronek J, Krakaver A, Colwall CW Jr (1990) Effects of the neodymium:YAG laser on the meniscus of the knee joint. SPIE Proc 1200:214–220

Glick J (1984) Laser for arthroscopic surgery. In Casocells SW (ed), Arthroscopy: Diagnostic and Surgical Practice. Lea & Febiger, Philadelphia

Herman JH, Khosla RC (1988) In vitro effects of neodymium:YAG laser radiation on cartilage metabolism. J Rheumatol 15:1818–1826

Inoue K, et al (1983) Arthroscopic laser surgery [experimental study]. Department of Orthopedic Surgery, Jichi Medical School, Tochigi, Japan

Kelly AM, O'Brien SJ, Miller DV, et al (1990) Arthroscopic surgery with a contact neodymium:YAG laser. In Shark HH (ed), Lasers in Orthopedics. Lippincott, Philadelphia, 158–168

Kollmer C (1990) Experimental evaluation of stimulatory effects of neodymium:YAG lasers on canine articular cartilage. In Sherk HH (ed), Lasers in Orthopedics. Lippincott, Philadelphia, 140–146

Metcalf RM (1987) Lasers in orthopedic surgery. In Dixon JA (ed), Surgical Applications of Lasers. Year Book Medical Publishers, Chicago, pp 275–286

Metcalf RW, Dixon JA (1984) Lasers for arthroscopic meniscectomy. Lasers Med Surg 3:366

Miller DV, O'Brien SJ, Arnoczky SS, et al (1989) The use of the contact neodymium:YAG laser in arthroscopic surgery: effects on articular cartilage and meniscal tissue. Arthroscopy 5:245–253

O'Brien SJ, Miller DV (1990) The contact neodymium:yttrium aluminum garnet laser. Clin Orthop 252:95–100

Schultz RF, Krishnamurthy S, Thelmo W, et al (1985) Effects of varying intensities of laser energy on articular cartilage: a preliminary study. Lasers Surg Med 5:577–588

Sherk HH, Kollmer C (1990) Arthroscopic surgery with a free-beam neodymium:YAG laser. In Sherk HH (ed), Lasers in Orthopedics. Lippincott, Philadelphia, pp 134–139

Smith CF, Johansen WE, Vangsness CT, et al (1990) Arthroscopic surgery with a free-beam CO_2 laser. In Shark BS (ed), Lasers in Orthopedics. Lippincott, Philadelphia, pp 146–157

Spivak JM, Grande DA, Ben-Yishay A, et al (1992) The effect of low-level neodymium:YAG laser energy on adult articular cartilage in vitro. Arthroscopy 8:36–43

Whipple TL, Caspari RB, Meyers JF (1983) Laser energy in arthroscopic meniscectomy. Orthopedics 6:1165–1169

24

Trimedyne OmniPulse 2.1 μm Holmium:YAG Laser for Arthroscopic Laser Surgery

Vahid Saadatmanesh, Joan L. Hawver, Sanford D. Damasco, and Glenn D. Yeik

The OmniPulse holmium laser operating at a wavelength of 2.1 μm is a versatile orthopaedic surgical tool, combining high ablation efficiency with conventional rugged fiberoptics. The 2.1 μm wavelength is highly absorbed in tissue with a penetration depth of approximately 0.4 mm (Esterowitz et al., 1986). Furthermore, fiberoptic handpieces carrying this wavelength can be utilized in a saline-filled environment, like other conventional tools, which results in tissue ablation with minimal damage to the adjacent tissue. The combination of these advantages along with the OmniPulse 2.1 μm holmium:YAG laser's higher energy pulses allow it to ablate tissue more swiftly and easily than the other previously mentioned lasers.

OmniPulse 2.1 μm Holmium:YAG Laser System Description

The OmniPulse 2.1 μm holmium:YAG laser is a class IV pulsed, solid-state holmium:YAG medical laser system. This laser system is designed to deliver pulsed infrared laser energy at a wavelength of 2.1 μm and a nominal pulse width of 350 μs. Other important factors which have driven the design of the OmniPulse 2.1 μm holmium:YAG laser system are upgradeability, serviceability, reliability, and advanced ergonomic controls. Upgradeability is fundamental in keeping up with the latest technical advances, and serviceability and reliability are requirements of any medical system. Advanced ergonomics, contained in the organization of the control panel and menu driven interface, afford intuitive operation and useful information about selected laser parameters. The selection of pulse repetition rate, output power, and maximum lasing period are performed through the parameter selection menu on the control panel.

Physically, the fiberoptic delivery port, on-board energy/power meter, swiveling control panel, footswitch for initiating laser energy output, and remote interlock system are situated on the front of the system unit. The interior of the OmniPulse laser system consists of a laser energy generation unit, laser power supply with a pulse shaping network, a cooling system, and a fully functional microcomputer for overall system control. These components are integrated into a mobile unit mounted on locking casters. Figure 24-1 shows the OmniPulse 2.1 μm holmium:YAG laser, the OmniPulse-MAX.

Menu Driven Control Console

The menu driven control console has the ability to swivel through 180 degrees, which allows flexible placement of the unit within the operating room and a greater viewing angle. The 0.5 inch character height on the liquid crystal display (LCD) also supports good viewing distances. The control console was designed to support single-handed operation, incorporating tactile and nontactile feedback keys for fast, efficient use. The selection of laser system status and lasing parameters is additionally assisted by a feedback mechanism that illuminates control buttons when selected and correspondingly prompts the user with screen messages that indicate the condition of the system. The menu driven control panel greatly benefits those new to operating a laser by facilitating the learning process. Figure 24-2 shows the OmniPulse 2.1 μm holmium:YAG laser console.

The swiveling control panel contains all of the user-accessible controls except the alternating current (AC) circuit breaker, remote interlock, and footswitch. This panel permits access to the laser status and menu driven laser parameters through touch pad controls. The OmniPulse 2.1 μm holmium:YAG laser system control panel contains a manual emergency shutoff button, 4 × 40 charac-

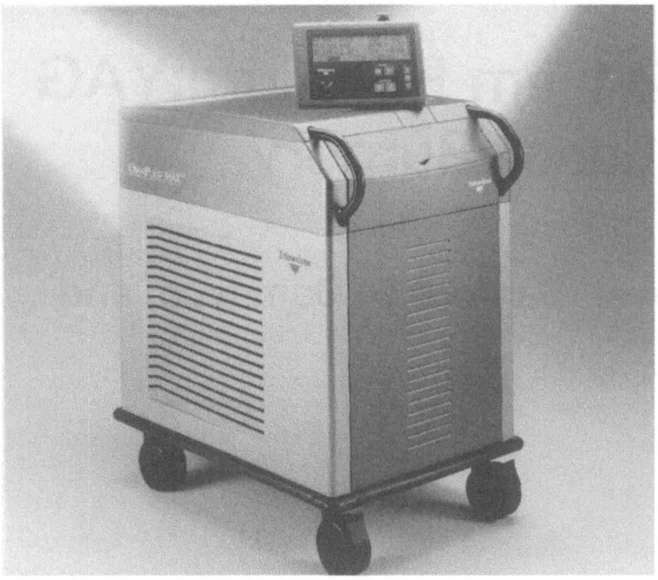

Figure 24-1. OmniPulse-MAX 2.1 μm holmium:YAG laser.

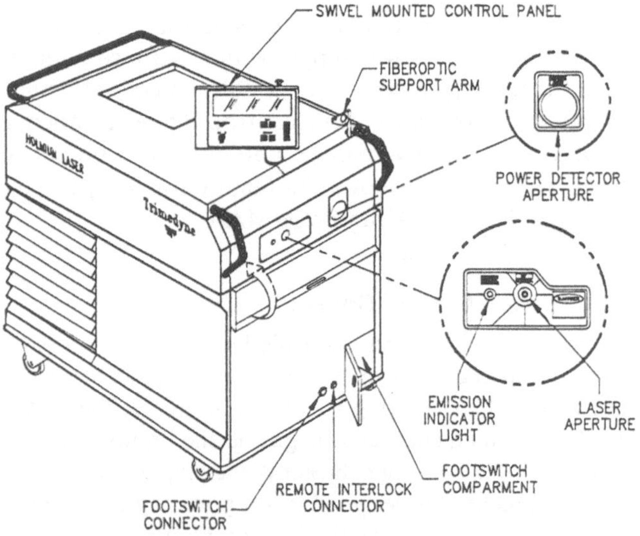

Figure 24-2. OmniPulse 2.1 μm holmium:YAG laser console. The laser aperture cover is open.

ter backlit LCD display, key-actuated power switch, and tactile feedback touch pad controls for the selection of lasing parameters for both the holmium laser and the 0.632 μm helium-neon aiming beam.

Laser System Parameters

The lasing parameters contained in the parameter selection menu are repetition rate (rep rate), power (watts), lasing time (seconds), energy (millijoules), and total energy (joules). All lasing parameters are selectable while the laser is not delivering energy. The relation between repetition rate, energy per pulse, and average power is actively demonstrated on the screen during the selection of the lasing parameters. When a given repetition rate is selected, the corresponding energy per pulse value changes appropriately, with the average power remaining fixed. If the average power is raised or lowered by the user, the corresponding energy per pulse changes accordingly. The user quickly sees the relation of these parameters and can determine that the repetition rate and the power constitutes the energy per pulse: Power = rep rate × energy (40 watts = 12 Hz × 3333 mJ).

Optical System

The OmniPulse optical system consists of the following assemblies: front (output coupler, OC) and rear (maximum reflector, MR) mirror optics, optical pumping module (rod, flashlamp, and laser cavity), optical feedback system, 0.632 μm helium-neon aiming beam, safety shutters, and fiberoptic coupler with connector. All assemblies are mounted on a rigid platform, which minimizes the effects of shock and vibration on the optical system. The combination of the output coupler and maximum reflector optics and the optical pumping module is called the laser resonator. The resonator design in the OmniPulse 2.1 μm holmium:YAG laser is optimized to provide high energies per pulse and high repetition rates. Figure 24-3 shows the OmniPulse 2.1 μm holmium:YAG laser optical system.

Power Supply Unit

The power supply unit consists of a high voltage power supply and a pulse-forming network (PFN). The PFN regulates and shapes the power delivered to the flashlamp, which defines the pulse characteristics of the laser energy emitted from the system. The rate at which the PFN is charged is regulated by a combination of the required lamp driver energy per pulse and the selected pulse repetition rate. The energy emitted is determined by the lasing parameters set by the operator on the control panel. The power required to generate the energies selected is microcomputer-controlled and dynamically regulated on a pulse-to-pulse basis. The power supply contains potentially lethal voltage levels of up to 1500 volts direct current (VDC). Access to these areas of the unit is physically limited by the outer laser cabinet, high voltage power supply cabinet, and PFN unit cabinet; it is electrically limited by cover interlocks.

Cooling System

The OmniPulse uses a self-contained deionized, distilled water cooling system for the removal of waste heat generated by the flashlamp in the pump cavity. The water cooling system also optimizes coolant operating temperatures to achieve maximum lasing system efficiency and is capable of maintaining the coolant temperature within 1°C of the set point. The primary function of the cooling system is to maintain a set coolant temperature accurately at

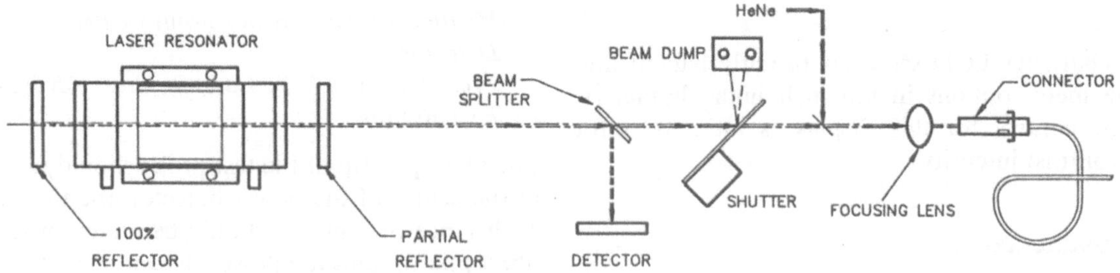

Figure 24-3. OmniPulse 2.1 μm holmium:YAG laser optical system.

any energy level or repetition rate, which enhances the performance of the holmium resonator and is a major factor in determining laser energy reliability and stability. The chiller is intentionally overdesigned so it can accommodate future upgrades of laser energy output from the system.

Microprocessor Control System

The microprocessor control system, as implemented in computer hardware and software, controls all of the subsystems in the OmniPulse 2.1 μm holmium:YAG laser. The primary function of this system is to ensure that the entire system is controlled in a safe manner. The microprocessor control system monitors the control panel for user interaction, controls the output parameters of the laser as selected from the menu driven control console, provides optical feedback control of laser energy and, power and performs periodic checks of the other subsystems to ensure safe system performance. The inputs from the menu driven control console and from various system signals are all organized and prioritized by the microprocessor control system.

OmniPulse Laser System Operation

The OmniPulse emits one pulse of laser radiation each time the flashlamp is fired. An individual laser pulse, which lasts for about 350 μs, consists of a large number of overlapping "spikes" each about 1 μs in duration. The laser pulse, as previously mentioned, refers to the overall pulse waveform. Laser pulses are generated continuously at the pulse repetition rate chosen by the operator while the footswitch is depressed.

Screen and Option Selectors

The menu selection keys allow movement between screens and parameter options and permit the value of selected parameters to be raised and lowered. Movement between screens and parameter options is done by pressing the Next key. The value of the selected parameters can be raised or lowered by pressing the ▲ and ▼ keys, respectively. Figure 24-4 diagrams the swiveling control panel.

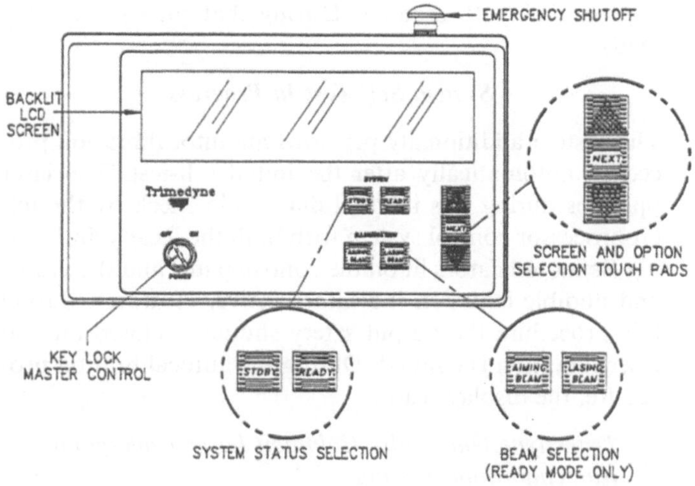

Figure 24-4. Swiveling control panel.

System Status

System status keys illuminate when activated and are not illuminated when deactivated. The system Standby mode, activated by the Stdby key, prevents the laser from being activated by the footswitch. Standby mode is a safe mode in which to place the system when the laser is not be used immediately. The System Ready mode, activated by the Ready key, allows activation of either the 2.1 μm holmium:YAG laser beam or the 0.632 μm helium-neon aiming beam. The Ready mode is the only mode in which lasing is permitted.

Beam Status Selectors

Two beam options are available when the system status is in the Ready mode. The border of the keys or touch pads illuminate when a beam is active and do not illuminate when it is inactive. The 2.1 μm holmium:YAG and the 0.632 μm helium-neon beams may be selected together or separately. In the OmniPulse laser system, Lasing Beam indicates the 2.1 μm holmium:YAG laser, and Aiming Beam indicates the 0.632 μm helium-neon beam. The footswitch must be activated to transmit the 2.1 μm Holmium:YAG beam whereas the helium-neon beam can be transmitted through a fiberoptic by putting the system in the Ready mode and pressing the Aiming Beam key.

LCD Screen

The 4 × 40 character LCD screen is brightly backlit and displays the menu options in 0.5 inch high characters. The contrast control for this display is factory-set for maximum contrast intensity.

Power On Sequence

The power to the system is turned on by turning the master power control key in a clockwise direction to the On position, after which the system performs a self-test for approximately 10 seconds. During that time the display reads:

System Self-Test In Progress

The system additionally performs an autocalibration procedure automatically after the initial self-test. The laser operates during this internal diagnostic check by the microprocessor control system with both the Ready and Lasing Beam indicators lit on the control panel and the visible and audible emission indicators active. However, during this procedure the output safety shutter is closed and no laser radiation is emitted. During the autocalibration procedure, the display reads:

Trimedyne OmniPulse Holmium Laser Undergoing Autocalibration Routine

Once the autocalibration procedure has been completed, the display reads:

Autocalibration Complete

The system remains in the Standby mode (Stdby) upon completion of the autocalibration routine and is now ready for energy verification.

Energy Verification

Although the energy verification process is optional, it is nevertheless recommended to ensure a reasonable level of energy transmission from the laser resonator to the tip of the fiberoptic surgical instrument. Immediately after the autocalibration procedure has been completed, the display reads:

Optional Optical Train Verification Test: Insert Test Probe To Begin Or Press <Next> To Bypass

The optical train verification process is designed to ensure that a proper level of energy is delivered to the target. However, at the discretion of the operator, this step can be bypassed. To bypass energy verification, press the Next key. If Next is chosen, operation of the system continues with the section labeled "Setting Lasing Parameters."

External energy verification is selected when a test probe is inserted into the laser fiberoptic connector port. If external energy verification is selected, the display reads:

Position Probe 3 Inches From Center Of Energy Detector
Press Footswitch To Lase Or Press <Next> To Exit Routine

The fiberoptic tip of the test probe should now be directed at the center of the power detector aperture at this point. A distance of 3 inches should be maintained between the fiberoptic tip and the power detector aperture. This setup prevents unnecessary damage to the energy detector and provides an even distribution of energy on the detector. The energy verification sequence begins when the footswitch is depressed. Hold down the footswitch until the verification sequence is completed, at which time laser energy emission stops automatically. The transmitted energy displayed as follows:

Laser Probe Output Energy At 10 Hz = XXXX mJ

At this point, the display reads one of two possible messages depending on the success of the energy verification process. If the process is successful, the display reads:

Optical Train Test Successful

Alternatively, if the optical train test is not successful, the display reads:

Insufficient Energy Is Measured With
The Current Test Probe
Replace Probe And Retest

A retest can be requested at this point by removing the test fiberoptic probe and replacing it with another test probe. If this step is done, the system repeats the optical train verification test. If the energy verification process was successful, the display advances to read:

Remove Test Probe To Continue

The calibration portion of the system start-up is now complete. Remove the test fiberoptic probe to advance to the next screen.

Setting Lasing Parameters

Upon omission or completion of the optional optical train verification test, the display should read:

Insert Probe
Press <Next> To Select And Enter A Laser Setting

Insert a fiberoptic for use into the laser fiberoptic connection port and select Next to advance to the lasing parameters menu. The system should now be in the standby (Stdby) mode, and the display should read as follows:

Rep Rate = 05 Hz
Power = 3.0 W
Energy = 600 mJ
Lasing Time = 99 Sec
Total Energy = 00,000 J

Standby Mode

Three lasing parameters must be set by the operator to control laser energy delivered to the fiberoptic tip. First, the repetition rate should be set to the desired number of pulses per second to be delivered (ranging from 5 to 55 pulses per second). Second, the power (watts), which represents the number of joules delivered per second, should be set to the desired value. The permissible values for power depend on the selected repetition rate. Third, the desired lasing time should be selected, with values ranging from 1 to 99 seconds, or CL (continuous lasing). The lasing time is the maximum time interval the laser can supply energy to the fiberoptic tip with a single continuous activation of the foot pedal.

Pressing the Next key sequentially moves the flashing cursor through the lasing parameter menu. To choose a parameter, push the Next button, placing the cursor on the equal sign at the parameter of interest. To raise or lower the value of a parameter, press the ▲ or ▼ key to adjust the parameter to the desired setting.

As an example, the operator decides to set the three lasing parameters to the following values:

Power = 10.0 W (The time rate of laser energy delivery is set to 10 watts of power).

Repetition rate = 15 Hz (The repetition rate, or the frequency of the pulses of energy, is set to 15 pulses per second).

Lasing time = 20 seconds (The maximum time interval the system can lase with one continuous activation of the foot pedal is set to 20 seconds).

On the parameter selection menu display both the energy parameter and the total energy parameter are shown for monitoring purposes. The value of the energy parameter adjusts according to set parameters of repetition rate and power. The total energy parameter accumulates the number of joules of energy actually delivered during the time interval in which the system is emitting pulses of laser energy. Consequently, the total energy display keeps a record of the total energy transferred by the laser. To reset this counter, the cursor should be positioned on the equal sign of this parameter by using the Next key and then pressing either the ▲ or ▼ key to reset the total energy to zero (0000).

With the previously mentioned values for the repetition rate, power, and lasing time, the display should read as follows:

Rep Rate = 15 Hz
Power = 10.0 W
Energy = 667 mJ
Lasing Time = 20 Sec
Total Energy = 00,000 J

Standby Mode

Of course, during a surgical operation, these settings vary depending on the basis of the operating requirements that are established for a given procedure. Again, the maximum amount of laser power available varies depending on the chosen repetition rate.

Laser Operation in the Ready Mode

After all parameters have been selected and set, the Ready key should be pressed to place the system into the ready mode and the indicator lights surrounding the Lasing Beam and Aiming Beam keys should be illuminated. The laser system is now in a state of readiness to lase. It is important at this time that the fiberoptic probe or catheter is not pointed into the air or toward anyone in the operating room. Furthermore, all personnel must now be warned that lasing is about to begin, and a visual check should be performed to verify that all personnel are wearing appropriate laser safety goggles. Lasing can now commence by activating the foot pedal.

While the system is lasing, a red emission indicator light is lighted (near the fiberoptic connector port) and an audible alarm sounds for safety reasons.

Before beginning the medical procedure, it is possible to verify the power output of the fiberoptic probe or handpiece if desired. To verify the output power of the probe, the operator must point the test fiberoptic or probe at the on-board detector before depressing the footswitch. This step is the only additional one required to perform this test. The fiber end *must* be held about 3 inches away from the detector. Once the footswitch is depressed, provided the fiber tip is pointed toward the detector, the screen changes and shows the measured pulse energy and power at the bottom of the display. A sample screen is as follows:

Rep Rate = 10 Hz
Power = 10.0 W
Energy = 1000 mJ
Lasing Time = 99 Sec
Measured Power = 10.0 Watts
Measured Energy = 1000 mJ

The measured power and energy represents an average of 1 second of operation.

Safety Interlocks

The cover, flow, remote, emission, optical, and footswitch interlock chains provide operator safety and equipment protection. If any of these interlock chains is interrupted, high-voltage and laser radiation generation are halted immediately. The appropriate fault indicator message is subsequently shown on the control panel display.

Laser Aperture

The OmniPulse 2.1 μm holmium:YAG laser fiberoptic connector is inserted into the laser aperture or fiberoptic probe connector port, as shown in Figure 24-2, and secured by rotating a threaded nut on the connector in a clockwise direction. The connector is designed to be properly aligned at the laser focal point when the nut is fingertight. The use of any other connector not designed specifically for the connector/coupler system is prohibited, as its use may pose a safety hazard and damage the laser system.

Laser Emission Indicators

The laser emission indicators, shown in Figure 24-2, supply a visual and audible indication that the laser resonator is active. The visual indicator is a red light located adjacent to the fiberoptic probe connector port. The visual and audible indicators are activated during autocalibration and while laser energy is being released through a fiberoptic probe.

Adjustable Aiming Beam

The adjustable aiming beam is an adjustable red 0.632 μm helium-neon beam. The adjustability of the aiming beam is important particularly when using the laser for endoscopic procedures. The output power of the 0.632 μm helium-neon aiming beam can be continuously adjusted from 0 up to 5 mW.

Internal Power Meter

An on-board power verification detector, shown in Figure 24-2, is incorporated into the system unit. This meter is utilized during the optional optical train verification procedure and is located on the front panel beside the fiberoptic probe connector port. It can also be used at any time during normal lasing operation to verify output power delivery by simply pointing the fiberoptic probe into the laser aperture and engaging the footswitch. The bottom display shows both the energy and the power exiting the distal end of the fiber, which allows the user to verify the output of any probe at any time during normal usage.

Fiberoptic Support Arm

A retractable fiberoptic support arm is mounted into the cover panel adjacent to the control panel as shown in Figure 24-2. This arm is provided to hold the excess fiberoptic and dispensing reel out of the work area.

Operator Control Panel

The operator control panel, shown in Figure 24-4, is designed to permit convenient access to the laser status and menu driven operating parameters. The panel is mounted onto the top panel of the laser console on a swivel that allows viewing from the front, left side, and rear of the laser.

Master Control Key

The key-actuated power control is used to turn on the power to the laser system, as shown in Figure 24-4. This key can be removed only in the Off position, which condition is intended to prevent unauthorized use. Two keys are provided with each laser system.

Emergency Shutoff

The manual emergency shutoff control is the large red button on the top of the control panel, as shown in Figure 24-4. Firmly pushing down on the shutoff control immediately cuts all power to the laser system. If the shutoff control is engaged, no portion of the laser can be activated by any other control. After activation, the laser system can be reactivated by (1) turning the master control key to the Off position, (2) releasing the emergency shut off control by twisting the button in a clockwise direction, and (3) turning the master control key back to the On position. The laser system begins the full start-up sequence at this point.

Remote Interlock Connector

The remote interlock system, shown in Figure 24-2, is an additional safety feature. It can be connected to a remote interlock switch at the entrance door. Whenever the entrance door is opened, the external switch contact opens, interrupting the laser energy generation.

Footswitch Connector and Mechanism

The footswitch connector, shown in Figure 24-2, accepts a mating locking connector attached to the footswitch mechanism. The footswitch itself is a grounded remote control device that allows direct lasing control by the physician. Lasing parameters cannot be changed while the footswitch is activated. The footswitch is waterproof and is guarded in protective housing to prevent accidental activation. In some configurations, the footswitch and cable can be stored in a compartment located at the bottom of the front (Fig. 24-2).

Power Cord and Circuit Breaker

A built-in, 220 VAC, 30 ampere, single-phase power cord is supplied with the system, as shown in Figure 24-5. Also shown in Figure 24-5, just above the power cord, is the system AC circuit breaker. This circuit breaker must be in the on (1) position to operate the laser. Depressing the lower portion of the rocker switch turns the breaker on, and depressing the upper portion of the switch turns the breaker off.

Protective Housing and Top Cover Panel

The protective housing, detailed in Figures 24-2 and 24-5, is designed to prevent human access to the laser or col-

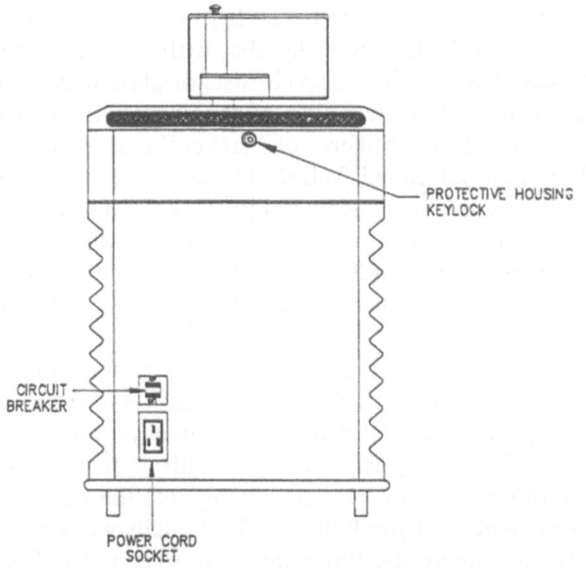

Figure 24-5. OmniPulse laser console (rear view).

lateral radiation. The internal configuration of the unit isolates the laser resonator from the operator control panel, high-voltage power supply, and cooling system. This arrangement eliminates laser exposure to operational or service personnel. All access inside the protective housing through the interlock protected top cover panel is controlled by a key lock different from the master control key. Only qualified service personnel trained by Trimedyne have access to this key.

Hand Grips

Hand grips are positioned at the front and rear of the laser console, as shown in Figure 24-2. These grips are provided for secure handling and control when the laser system is wheeled to a new location. The hand grips are not designed to support the weight of the laser system.

Wheels

The unit is provided with four swivel wheels, shown in Figure 24-2, that can be locked independently. Stepping on the flange located above the wheel locks the wheel, and lifting up on this flange releases the wheel lock.

OmniPulse Laser Delivery Systems

At 2.1 μm, the holmium:YAG laser wavelength is effectively delivered to the target tissue with flexible fiberoptic delivery systems. Access to remote locations in all joints can easily be accomplished with an assortment of tip configurations. Inadvertent joint trauma, surface scuffing, bleeding, and swelling are reduced owing to the small profiles of each delivery system. Unlike sculpted tips used with 1.06 μm neodymium:YAG lasers, the holmium fiber is recessed at the distal end of the probe, eliminating the potential for fiber tip breakage within the joint.

As laser techniques and applications in arthroscopic surgery evolve, delivery systems continue to be refined and developed for increased efficiency, versatility, and cost-effectiveness. Trimedyne manufactures both a disposable and a multiuse line of orthopaedic delivery systems for use with the OmniPulse 2.1 μm holmium:YAG laser.

Tapertip Orthopaedic Handpiece (Single Use)

The Tapertip handpiece is a disposable fiberoptic energy delivery system consisting of a handpiece and laser fiber contained in a metal cannula. The distal end of the fiber is contained in a 12.5 cm long metal cannula assembly that is attached to the handpiece.

Tapertip delivery systems include a lightweight, small-profile handpiece that incorporates longitudinal ridges to facilitate rotation by fingers without slippage. An assortment of distal tip configurations are available, including straight and 20, 30, or 60 degree angles and a 90 degree sidefire probe. Figure 24-6 shows the 30 degree angle and Sidefire Tapertip disposable holmium orthopaedic handpieces. For small joint surgery, the straight and sidefire configurations are available in a "mini" version with a 6.5 cm working length. With the exception of the sidefire probe, each 2.1 μm holmium:YAG delivery system includes two prongs extending lateral to the fiber tip that serve as a tissue manipulation device. A maximum of 10% energy loss can be anticipated with the Tapertip delivery systems due to the mechanical structure of the product.

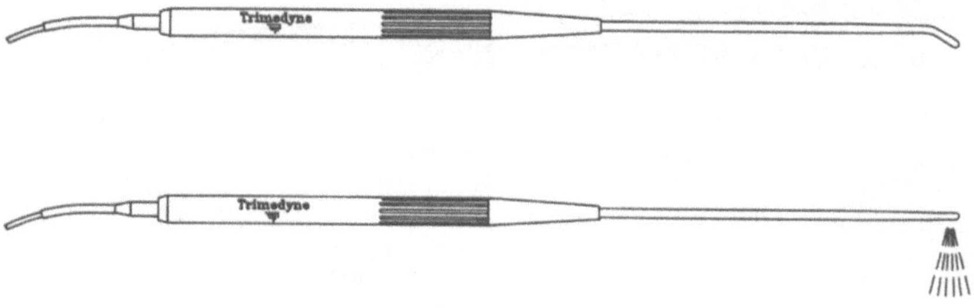

Figure 24-6. Tapertip disposable holmium orthopaedic handpieces (single use).

Omni Switchable System (Multiple Use)

The Omni switchable tip system is a fiberoptic energy delivery system consisting of disposable interchangeable tips (Omnitips) and a limited-use handpiece. The Omnitips contain a near-contact fixed fiber in a protective stainless steel shaft available in the same tip configurations as the Tapertip line. Figure 24-7 shows the Omni multiuse handpiece with an assortment of Omnitips. The proximal end of the interchangeable tip includes a custom fiberoptic connector. Cost-effective and versatile, surgeons can select additional tip configurations within each procedure at a nominal cost.

The Omni multiuse handpiece contains a fixed fiber combined with an indexed connector at the distal end for the attachment of Omnitips. The handpiece is designed with a flattened side that includes an elevated tactile button, which allows surgeons to remain continuously oriented to the angled tip as it approaches the surgical site. A maximum of 15% energy loss can be anticipated with the Omni switchable tip system due to the handpiece–interchangeable tip interface in combination with the mechanical structure of the distal tip.

Fiberoptics

The 2.1 μm holmium:YAG fiberoptic cable is 3 meters in length and consists of three layers. The central region, or "core," is 550 μm in diameter, and is constructed of silica glass (quartz); it transports the holmium energy from the laser fiberoptic output coupler to the surgical site. Containment of the energy within the core is due to the subsequent layer. This next layer, termed the "cladding," serves as a reflective barrier that forces light to remain inside the core through the length of the fiber without significant energy loss. The cladding also consists of glass with a lower index of refraction than that of the core. The outermost layer is called the "buffer," or "jacket," and is made of a Teflon material called Tefzel (Dupont). This layer provides protection and added stability for the internal materials. Figure 24-8 diagrams the fiberoptic design.

Efficient delivery of 2.1 μm holmium:YAG laser energy through an optical fiber requires the use of low-OH quartz fibers. Special measures have been incorporated during the manufacturing process of these fibers to reduce the water content, as the 2.1 μm holmium:YAG wavelength is highly absorbed by water. The outer jacket not only protects the core glass fiber, it shields it from ambient water vapor, which would slowly degrade the fiber.

Trimedyne's 2.1 μm holmium:YAG delivery systems do not require fiberoptic threading. The fiber is fixed in the proper position within the tip for optimum effect. All systems include a proximal end custom connector designed for high energy transmission with an extended damage threshold.

Patented fiber dispensing wheels are attached to all Trimedyne fiberoptic delivery systems. Providing the benefits of fiber containment, protection, maintenance of sterility, and surgeon control, the fiber dispensing wheel is conveniently attached to the sterile field.

Figure 24-9 shows of the multiuse fiber dispensing wheel, which is used exclusively with the Omni multiuse handpiece. The resterilizable wheel is ergonomically designed for ease of fiber removal and allows decontamination and re-reeling of the fiber for sterilization. In addition, the wheel provides a "hole punch" tracking sys-

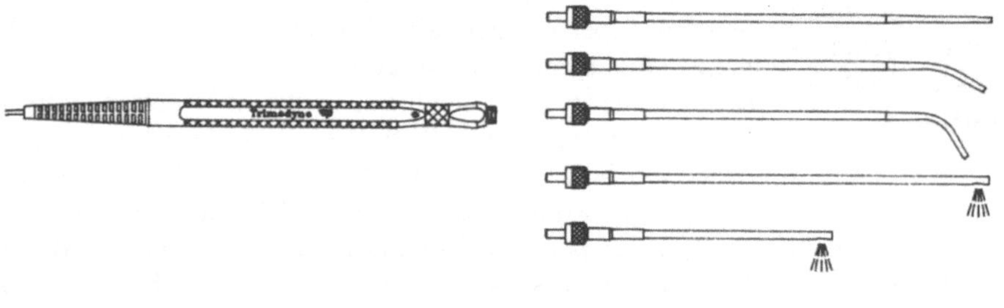

Figure 24-7. Omni switchable tip system.

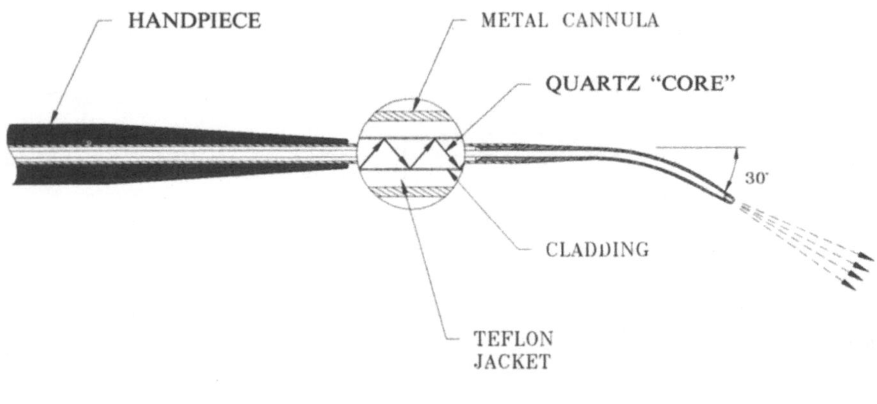

Figure 24-8. Cross section of probe and fiber.

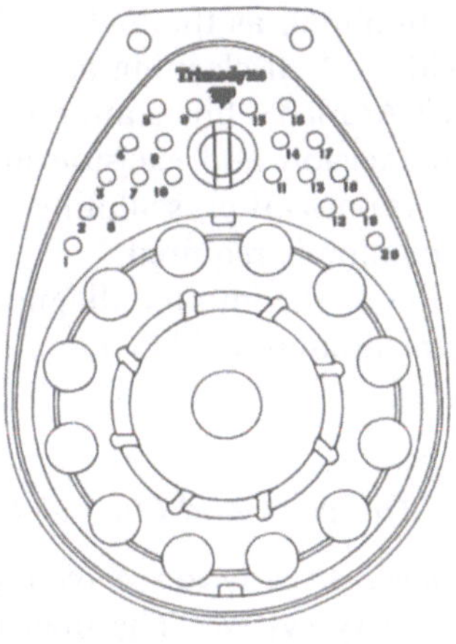

Figure 24-9. Multiuse fiber dispensing wheel.

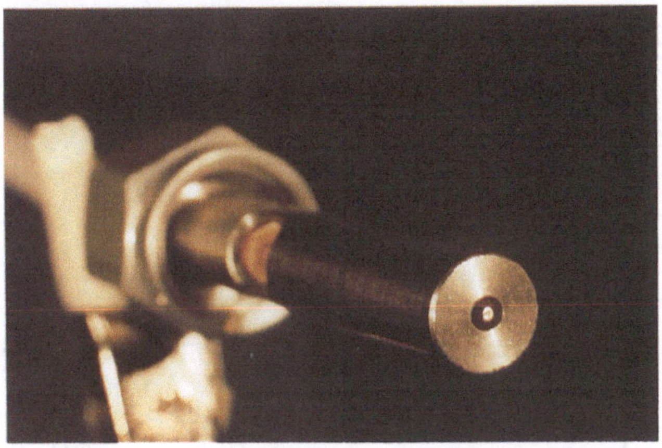

Figure 24-10. Proprietary fiberoptic connector.

tem to accurately count the number of times the product has been sterilized.

Proprietary Fiberoptic Connector

The high repetition rates and pulse energies generated by the OmniPulse 2.1 μm holmium:YAG laser system necessitate use of an extraordinary fiberoptic connector. As pulse repetition rates increase, the divergence of the laser beam exiting the system also increases and makes high energy transmission more difficult. This phenomenon alone would not necessarily require the use of a custom fiberoptic connector.

However, the intense peak pulse energies emitted by this laser system cause unusual problems in effectively coupling laser energy into a fiberoptic probe. As peak powers rise, an increasing amount of laser energy cannot be coupled to the fiberoptic probe. This excess energy in traditional connectors is partially reflected back from the connector and partially absorbed by the metal surrounding the fiberoptic. Excessive peak powers cause even more power to be absorbed by the metal surrounding the fiberoptic, which results in scorching the metal and quickly degrading energy transmission. Furthermore, elevated peak powers can cause pitting in the fiberoptic itself if concentrated in too small an area. Therefore a proprietary connector was designed by Trimedyne for use with the OmniPulse 2.1 μm holmium:YAG laser system. Figure 24-10 shows this proprietary fiberoptic connector.

The proprietary fiberoptic connector was designed to achieve high energy transmission along with an extended damage threshold. High energy transmission is achieved by the extended length of the connector for mechanical support in conjunction with the supplementary glass sleeving surrounding the fiberoptic. This glass sleeving prevents the energy not coupled into the fiberoptic from being absorbed by the enveloping metal connector. The sleeving also allows an extended damage threshold by permitting the laser energy to be coupled into the full area of the fiberoptic to prevent pitting. This approach was used rather than trying to couple all of the laser energy into a smaller portion of the fiber, as is done with other lasers. Thus the proprietary fiberoptic connector on probes intended for use with the OmniPulse system allows a maximum amount of energy to be transferred from the laser system to the delivery device, resulting in maximal energy being available for treatment.

Theory of OmniPulse Operation

The term "laser resonator," sometimes used synonymously with "laser oscillator," denotes the fact that the photons oscillate back and forth between the fully reflective and partially reflective mirrors. The OmniPulse 2.1 μm holmium:YAG laser uses a solid-state crystal, the CTH:YAG, as a lasing medium. The C, T, and H stand for chromium, thulium, and holmium respectively. YAG is an abbreviation for yttrium-aluminum-garnet, which serves as the "host" crystal medium: It does not actively participate in the lasing process but, instead, provides a housing medium for the lasing ions, in this case the Ho^{3+}. The chromium and thulium ions act as sensitizer ions, creating a bridge by which the photon energy from the flashlamp can be transferred to the Ho^{3+} ions in an efficient manner. For simplicity, the CTH:YAG crystal is usually referred to as holmium:YAG.

The energy transfer chain begins with a pulse of electrical current generated by the power supply passing through the flashlamp and thereby causing a burst of photons at various wavelengths to escape into the pumping chamber of the laser. These photons, distributed across a wide optical spectrum, travel through the chilled water and enter the laser crystal. The photon energy is initially absorbed by the chromium ions, which have a wide absorption band. Next, there is transfer of energy from the Cr^{3+} ions to the Tm^{3+} ions. Finally, the energy of these ions is transferred to the Ho^{3+} ions, initiating the lasing process. As the Ho^{3+} ions become excited by the energy transferred

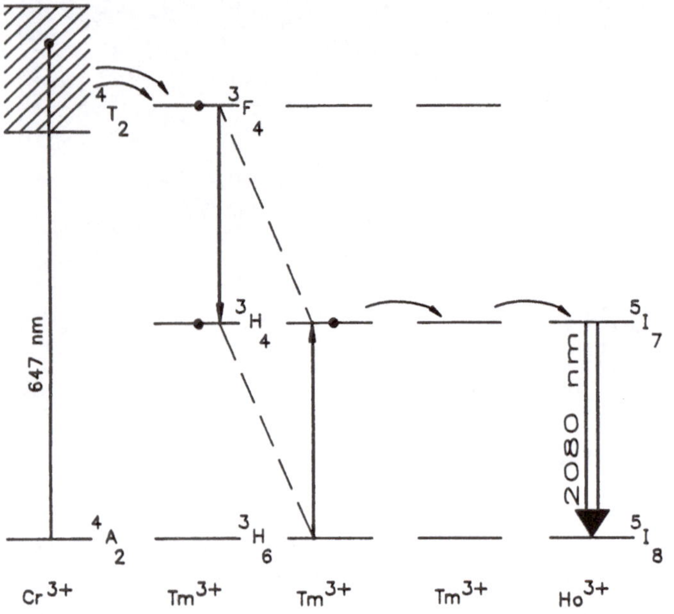

Figure 24-11. Pumping diagram for the CTH:YAG laser.

to them, photons at 2.1 μm wavelength are released and oscillate back and forth between the two mirrors. As these photons collide with the excited ions of the lasing medium, they cause the outer shell electrons of these ions to fall to their unexcited ground level. Through this process these electrons release photons in phase with the original photons and thus emit radiation. This process occurs millions of times in the laser resonator, and during each round trip a portion of the photons circulating in the laser resonator escape through the partial mirror in the form of useful laser energy. The elliptical reflectors form a shell and facilitate transfer of the energy from the lamp into the laser crystal.

It is important to note that the energy is transferred from the flashlamp to the Cr^{3+} through a radiative process mediated by the photons (Fig. 24-11). However, the energy transfer from Cr^{3+} to Tm^{3+} and then from Tm^{3+} to Ho^{3+} is nonradiative.

Operation of the Delivery Systems

Flexible fiberoptic delivery provides freedom of movement as well as the ability to easily access remote areas in arthroscopic surgery. Because 2.1 μm holmium:YAG laser fibers can perform in direct contact with tissue, they can be used in a wet or completely submerged field despite the fact that the 2.1 μm wavelength is absorbed strongly by water. The intervening water layer that might be present is usually too thin to attenuate pulse energy significantly before it reaches the tissue surface or is vaporized out of the way by the initial portion of each laser pulse.

The potential for the fiber tip to overheat or result in debris buildup is minimal, as the high peak power of the laser pulses provide a "self-cleaning action." As a result, 2.1 μm holmium:YAG laser fibers are reliably used in the contact mode for incision and excision and in the near-contact mode for vaporization, sculpting, or coagulation. No coaxial fiber cooling is required.

Upon completion of the internal diagnostic checks, the OmniPulse 2.1 μm holmium:YAG laser displays a message stating:

Insert Probe
Press <Next> To Select And Enter A Laser Setting

At this time, the laser is ready to receive the proximal end of the selected delivery system. The fiberoptic male connector is mounted within the female connector of the output coupler on the laser. This attachment should be secured fingertight. With laser parameters set and the delivery system appropriately positioned, the laser is activated by depressing the footswitch to begin the surgical procedure.

Figure 24-12 represents the 2.1 μm holmium:YAG laser beam profile as it is emitted from a sidefire and 30-degree

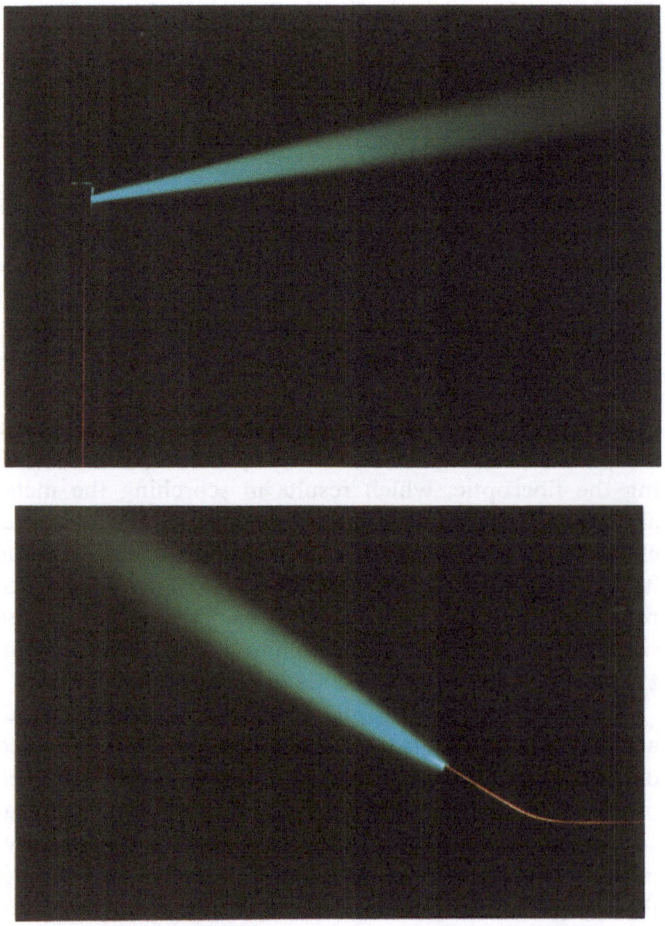

Figure 24-12. Laser energy distribution.

angle delivery system. The energy distribution in the photograph is demonstrated by a 0.488 μm argon laser in an aqueous medium against a black background.

2.1 μm Holmium:YAG Applications in Arthroscopic Surgery

The development of new arthroscopic techniques has revolutionized the treatment of intraarticular pathology. The desire for more powerful, efficient, and accurate cutting instruments has led to continued interest in lasers for arthroscopic use.

Food and Drug Administration Clearances

In March 1991 the U.S. Food and Drug Administration (FDA) cleared the OmniPulse 2.1 μm holmium:YAG laser to be marketed for use in arthroscopic laser procedures for incision, excision, ablation, and coagulation of pathologic soft and cartilaginous tissues in small and large joints. In July 1994, the FDA provided clearance to Trimedyne to market a 80-watt 2.1 μm holmium:YAG laser.

Clinical Applications

The 2.1 μm holmium:YAG laser performs in a standard arthroscopic fluid environment and is powerful enough to cut and ablate orthopaedic tissues while maintaining enough precision to avoid excessive tissue damage. Specially designed delivery systems are maneuverable enough to access the relatively confined areas and curved surfaces of the joints, and the tactile feedback is helpful for tissue manipulation. Lasers are considered useful surgical instruments primarily because they bridge the gap between electrosurgical and mechanical instruments in terms of the surgical precision and hemostasis they provide. Lasers have distinct advantages over electrocautery devices. Electrocautery works best in nonphysiologic fluid, which has been shown to be harmful to chondrocyte metabolism and creates cellular swelling. Additionally, the path of necrosis using electrosurgery is also poorly controlled and may be more extensive than can be visually appreciated.

The 2.1 μm holmium:YAG laser may be used in a contact mode or a near-contact mode of delivery, which allows safe laser application with minimal risk to nontarget tissue. This single instrument, offers the potential to cut, contour, resect, ablate, and coagulate. By varying the pulse rate and energy levels, the 2.1 μm holmium:YAG laser beam can be altered to meet specific needs. A near-contact technique generates a defocused laser beam (larger spot size), which allows more effective cartilage ablation, synovial reduction, and coagulation. This technique is effectively performed simply by varying the distance the laser tip is positioned from the target tissue. Minimal but effective thermal effects ensure excellent hemostatic capability without charring or carbonizing surrounding tissue.

Table 24-1. Laser parameters.

Arthroscopic procedure	Repetition rate (Hz)	Power (watts)
Knee		
Meniscectomy	20–30	40–80
Lateral release	20–30	30–40
Chondromalacia	30–55	20–40
Synovectomy	20–30	40–80
Shoulder		
Acromioplasty	10–16*	60–80
Collagen shrinkage	10–20	10–30
General tissues		
Hard tissue	Low repetition rate (10–26 pulses/s) with maximum power (60–80 watts)	
Semihard tissue (cartilage)	Medium repetition rate (20–30 pulses/s) with maximum power (60–80 watts)	
Soft tissue (synovium)	High repetition rate (30–55 pulses/s) with low to medium power (40–60 watts)	

* Denotes "Double Pulse™" Technology

Surgery with the 2.1 μm holmium:YAG laser can be performed without use of a tourniquet or general anesthesia. Postoperative bleeding, inflammation, and pain may be substantially reduced and so the technique allows faster recovery than does conventional surgery.

Laser Parameters

Table 24-1 is provided as a "guide" by which surgeons may achieve desired tissue effects. Laser parameters should be altered to reflect the tissue type or pathology. When selecting laser parameters, one should consider the tissue density and the desired effect (i.e., cutting versus hemostasis).

Tissue interaction may be modified with any fiberoptic delivery system by adjusting the distance of the fiber tip to the surgical site. A cutting effect may be obtained when in "contact" with the tissue, whereas a contouring effect is better achieved with a near-contact approach, with the probe tip being several millimeters from the tissue surface.

Orthopaedic Procedures Performed with the OmniPulse 2.1 μm Holmium:YAG Laser

Shoulder: labral tear resection; biceps tendon tear débridement; subacromial bursal resection; coracoacromial ligament resection; acromioplasty; Bankhart procedures; rotator cuff débridement; loose body removal; synovectomy; subacromial decompression; removal of scar tissue; release of coracoacromial ligament for acromionectomy; bursectomy; capsular release; chondroplasty

Knee: meniscectomy; abrasion arthroplasty; chondromalacia; chondroplasty; plica removal; synovectomy; resection of the anterior cruciate ligament; excision of meniscal cyst; lateral release; lateral retinacular release

Ankle: removal of osteocytes impinging on the tibia/talus; osteochondral fracture débridement; synovectomy; fracture débridement; partial synovectomy; chondroplasty

Elbow: removal of loose body; débridement of the extensor tendon; synovectomy; chondroplasty

Wrist: débridement of torn triangular fibrocartilage complex; osteochondral fracture débridement; partial synovectomy; chondroplasty

2.1 μm Holmium:YAG Tissue Interaction

The short tissue penetration depth of the 2.1 μm holmium:YAG wavelength (<500 μm) combined with its ease of delivery is the key to its success as an arthroscopy tool. It is transmissible through conventional fiberoptics utilizing fused silica as a core. The advantages of the 2.1 μm holmium:YAG laser as an arthroscopic instrument can be summarized as follows:

1. Short penetration depth in tissue, with high water content (i.e., cartilage)
2. Durable and flexible fiberoptic delivery system
3. High pulse energy
4. High average power
5. Operation in a saline environment
6. Solid-state reliable construction

The short penetration depth of the 2.1 μm wavelength is due to water being the main absorbing molecule for this wavelength.

Safety Requirements

Lasers are not dangerous when properly used and maintained by trained, knowledgeable personnel. As with any piece of medical equipment, there are potential hazards associated with lasers that can cause injury. These hazards can be avoided if measures are taken to prevent their occurrence.

The American National Standards Institute (ANSI) is an organization that sets recommendations and standards for various industries. A system of laser classification has been developed by ANSI categorizing lasers in one of four groups according to their ability to cause biologic damage and their maximum power output capabilities. This classification system has been adopted by the FDA and is recognized as the standard throughout the industry.

Class I includes lasers considered to be incapable of producing damaging radiation levels and therefore are exempt from radiation hazard controls. Class IV includes high powered lasers that require control measures to prevent exposure of direct and reflected laser beam to eyes and skin. Most medical laser systems are class IV and are considered to be the most hazardous and so require specific labeling precautions.

Eye Protection

The eye is the organ most sensitive to damage by laser radiation. Damage can result from an acute incident or a slow degeneration from chronic low power exposures. These slow changes include damage to the lens of the eye, resulting in possible cataract formation, or damage to the retina. Accidental exposure to a 2.1 μm holmium:YAG laser beam may be detected by a burning pain at the site of exposure: the cornea or the sclera. Trimedyne recommends that protective eyewear be worn by all personnel in the laser-use area whenever the laser is activated. The surgeon must not view the procedure by placing his eye next to the scope.

A laser eye protection device can be defined as a filter (lens with absorbers) designed to reduce light of a specific wavelength or a range of wavelengths to a safe level while maintaining adequate light transmission at all other wavelengths. Optical density (OD) is a logarithmic function that explains the degree of attenuation of the specific wavelength as it passes through the lens. For 2.1 μm holmium:YAG lasers, the optical density should be at least 5.0. The optical density and the laser wavelength should appear on all eye protective devices to prevent confusion.

Protective eyewear should be comfortable and prevent exposure to hazardous peripheral radiation. The eyewear should be cleaned and stored upon use and periodically inspected for cracks or breakage, that might decrease its effectiveness.

Skin Exposure

The skin is also subject to damage by class IV laser radiation and is more likely to be damaged simply because of its greater exposed surface area. Accidental exposure is painful but less likely to be as disastrous as eye exposure.

Environment

Where available, warning lights outside the controlled area should be turned on before beginning the laser procedure. Appropriate eyewear for 2.1 μm wavelength should be placed outside each entrance to the controlled area for anyone who may enter the room during the procedure. Access to the controlled area should be limited to necessary personnel and appropriately instructed visitors.

Laser warning signs should be posted on the exterior of each entryway to the controlled area. The design of the sign should be in accordance with the ANSI specifications for accidental exposure prevention signs.

Prepare beforehand with efficient room setup to ensure that equipment can be operated in a safe manner without hindering movement within the operating room. The foot control, fibers, and electrical cord should be positioned for safe and efficient use. The risk of falls, injuries, or equipment damage is minimized when traffic patterns are considered during equipment positioning.

The scope will be damaged if the laser beam is directed into it. A fracture of the lens may occur.

Electrical Fire or Explosion

Cords and electrical wiring should be periodically inspected for integrity. The laser should not be used when electrical cords are loose or frayed, or if any water leakage from the system is noted. So long as the laser console panels are left in place, There is no significant risk of electrical shock to anyone in the room. Only trained service personnel should open the laser system.

A basin of water should be immediately accessible to control fires on nonelectrical items. Personnel should know the location and operation of the nearest fire extinguisher in the event of a fire.

The laser beam should not be used in the presence of flammable materials (e.g., alcohol, certain anesthetic preparation solutions, drying agents, ointments, plastic resins, anesthetics).

Training

Proper training is essential. Both users and operators of surgical lasers should have appropriate training for the particular laser system with which they are involved. Laser credentialing policies vary from one hospital to another. Generally, a surgeon must attend an accredited laser program, which includes both a lecture and a hands-on session with appropriate animate or cadaveric tissues.

Patient training is also important. Although lasers are not new to the medical community, they present a mysterious concept to the lay community. Through brochures, video, or discussions patients can be instructed on what a laser is, how it will be used, and the safety measures that will be followed throughout the procedure. These issues should be discussed especially if the patient will be under local anesthesia.

Delivery Systems

Delivery systems should be inspected upon opening the sterile package. Should a fiberoptic cable fracture during surgery, the outer white jacket glows red under the red aiming beam in the region of breakage. If this situation occurs, the delivery system should be replaced immediately.

Do not clean the fiber tip with alcohol or any other flammable agent.

Caution should be exercised while lasing near an arthroscope to avoid damage to the optical system. Contact with metal objects such as cannulas or introducers should also be avoided.

Laser Operation

During a procedure, the laser should be managed by a dedicated operator. Several commonsense principles must be set forth as a guide for the operator to practice safe and effective use of the laser. A laser safety checklist and a laser log should be maintained for every laser procedure. A safety checklist comprises the practices that should be performed before, during, and after a laser procedure to safeguard against possible hazards. A laser log is a form on which to record pertinent information concerning the procedure, such as type of fiberoptic used, wattage, and total joules.

Clear communication among the surgical team is essential for a safe operating environment. Most accidents resulting from laser use are due to poor communication or poor training. All communication should be two-way. Nothing should ever be assumed.

The laser should always be placed in Standby (Stdby) mode when not actually in use. The standby function allows added control over the laser shutter to prevent inadvertent firing of the laser. The laser key should be stored in a secured area to prevent misuse of the laser by unauthorized personnel.

Laser Installation Requirements

The installation procedure for the OmniPulse 2.1 μm holmium:YAG is neither difficult nor cumbersome. The laser is usually fully operational upon delivery and requires only electricity to begin operation. The setup in the operating room depends only on the desired placement of the laser. Because the OmniPulse has a swiveling control panel, placement of the laser is flexible, and it can be positioned to maximize operating room staff convenience.

Power and Cooling Requirements

The OmniPulse holmium laser requires 220 VAC at 50 or 60 Hz line frequency, single-phase, 30 ampere line service. The wall outlet should provide a ground connection for electrical safety (i.e., three connections consisting of a "hot" line, return line, and a ground). A dedicated outlet would be beneficial and ideal for operating conditions.

The cooling requirements for the laser are self-contained within the system. The operator does not need to provide additional servicing. The laser uses distilled, deionized coolant water, if required.

The system and patient leakage current requirements of UL 544 have been met or exceeded by this system. A built-in isolation transformer provides the required electrical isolation and minimizes leakage current.

Laser Maintenance

Aside from the normal preventive maintenance that is provided, the OmniPulse laser system does not require "postmaintenance" attention. If any problems arise during the initial self-testing or operation, the control console explicitly alerts the staff that a problem has occurred. Problem explanations are clearly identified on the display console.

Laser Safety and Ensurance

The OmniPulse holmium laser has been ETL-tested and approved to meet UL 544 safety standards in reference to medical and dental equipment. Additionally, the system unit has been TÜV-approved per the IEC 601 and 825 international standards of patient safety and system compliance to operational safety.

System Specifications

Laser module: chromium-thulium-holmium: yttrium-aluminum-garnet (CTH:YAG) solid state, pulsed
Lasing ion: Ho^{3+}
Wavelength: 2.1 μms
Approximate pulse duration: 350 μs
Maximum output energy: 3.5 joules/pulse
Output polarization: Random
Pulse repetition range: 5 to 55 pulses/s
Maximum output power: 80 watts to tissue
Energy accuracy: $\pm 10\%$
Aiming beam: 0.633 μm red helium-neon laser; 5 mW, continuously variable
Operational controls: membrane touch keys
External energy meter/probe: pyroelectric detector
Power requirements: 220 VAC, ($\pm 10\%$); 30 amperes, 50/60 Hz, single phase
Product safety approvals: ETL/MET (Domestic); TÜV (International), IEC 601-1

Maintenance of the Laser Delivery System

The Tapertip and Omnitip products are single-use items shipped EtO-sterilized; they are not to be resterilized or reused. The Omni multiuse handpiece is also shipped EtO-sterilized. Products are sterile/nonpyrogenic only if packages are not opened, damaged, or broken.

Resterilization of the Omni Multiuse Handpiece

After completion of the surgical procedure, the Omnitip is detached and discarded. Both the connector and distal end of the handpiece are cleaned with a nonfibrous swab and sterile water. The optical surface is allowed to dry thoroughly before replacing the protective cap of the handpiece. The handpiece should be decontaminated with an appropriate solvent. The product is compatible with EtO sterilization not to exceed 140°F.

The Omni multiuse handpiece has been qualified for up to 20 uses under normal conditions and with proper maintenance. Factors that may shorten the life of the Omni multiuse handpiece include failure to remove contaminants or residues from the fiber surface prior to sterilization, improper sterilization processes, improper handling (i.e., dropping or pinching the fiberoptic, severe bending of the fiber), improper tip attachment (i.e., Omnitip not completely engaged in handpiece when lasing).

Product Durability

The Tapertip and Omni Switchable Tip delivery systems are single-use products. The ability of these delivery systems to efficiently transmit 2.1 μm holmium:YAG laser energy for a relatively long time depends on several factors, such as lasing parameters, total energy transmitted, and lasing against hard surfaces (i.e., bone). Fiber degradation may occur during the procedure; therefore power output should be confirmed if energy loss is suspected.

Precautions

1. The Omni switchable tip system should be handled with care and should not be subjected to severe angle bends, which may result in breaks or fractures.
2. Immediately discontinue the procedure if breaks or fractures appear in the laser fiber or if a sudden drop in power is noted. These breaks or fractures can potentially allow energy to exit at locations other than the tip, rendering the distal tip useless and causing harm to the surrounding environment. *Do not lase in air or attempt to reshape the tip in any way.*
3. If the tip accumulates debris, lasing should be discontinued and the tip carefully wiped with a cotton swab and sterile water.
4. If the handpiece heats up significantly, remove the Omnitip and clean the optical surface of the handpiece with a nonfibrous swab and sterile water.

Editor's Cautions

1. **Even though many surgeons believe there is no need to wear 2.1 μm wavelength-specific protective eyewear, I do not agree. The 2.1 μm holmium:YAG is a class IV laser, and its wavelength can damage the eye.**
2. **These fibers should be used in a standard liquid arthroscopic environment. Use in a gas environment is not recommended.**
3. **Each fiber is fragile and can fracture if not fully protected. Forcing, levering, or using the "probe" as a me-**

chanical probe will likely result in a fracture and an intraarticular foreign body.

4. **All fibers have a definite life-span. Optimal, satisfactory use of this system requires some experience. It is best to start in the laboratory, not with patients. The best techniques, energy settings, and probe selections can be preliminarily determined in this way. The reader is referred to Chapter 4 for a discussion on ablation efficiency.**
5. **Mechanical instruments should be available at all times during arthroscopic laser surgery.**
6. **This chapter is only an introduction to this arthroscopic laser system. The reader is encouraged to study this entire text, follow acceptable training and credentialing procedures, as well as research the subject at hand for additional information and changes before undertaking this arthroscopic laser system's use.**

References

Anonymous (1989) Risk analysis: laser use and safety. ECRI January: 1–7

Anonymous (1990) Eyeglasses, safety, laser. ECRI April: 1–5

Brillhart AT (1991) Arthroscopic laser surgery: the holmium:YAG laser and its use; third of four articles. Am J Arthrosc 1(3):7–11

Esterowitz L, Hoffman CA, Tran DC, et al (1986) Angioplasty with a laser and fiber optics at 2.9 microns. SPIE Proc 605:32–35

Fanton GS, Dillingham MF (1992) The use of the holmium laser in arthroscopic surgery. Semin Orthop 7(2):102–114

Huber G, Duczynski EW, Petermann K (1988) Laser pumping of Ho-, Tm-, Er-doped garnet laser at room temperature. IEEE J Quantum Electronics 24:920–923

JGM Associates (1900) Recent advances in solid-state lasers. JGM, Burlington, MA, pp 5–20 to 5–24

Moore YH (1973) Laser energy in orthopedic surgery. In Proceedings of International Congress of Orthopaedic Surgeons. Excerpta Medica, Amsterdam

Nishioka NS, Domankevitz Y (1989) Reflectance during pulsed holmium laser irradiation of tissue. Lasers Surg Med 9:375–381

Nishioka NS, Domankevitz Y, Flotte TJ, Anderson RR (1989) Ablation of rabbit liver, stomach, and colon with a pulsed holmium laser. Gastroenterology 96:831–837

Nuss RC, Fabian RL, Sarkar R, Puliafito CA (1988) Infrared laser bone ablation. Lasers Surg Med 8:381–391

Stein E, Sedlacek T, Fabian RL, Nishioka NS (1990) Acute and chronic effects of bone ablation with a pulsed holmium laser. Lasers Surg and Med 10:384–388

Stuck BE, Lund DJ, Beatrice ES (1981) Ocular effects of holmium (2.06 microns) and erbium (1.54 microns) laser radiation. Health Phys 40:835–846

Walsh Jr JT, Deutsch TF (1988) Pulsed CO_2 laser tissue ablation: measurement of the ablation rate. Lasers Surg Med 8:264–275

Walsh Jr JT, Flotte TJ, Deutsch TF (1988) Er:YAG laser ablation of tissue: effect of pulse duration and tissue type on thermal damage. Lasers Surg Med 9:314–326

25

Zeiss OPMILAS 144 Surgical Lasers for Arthroscopic Laser Surgery

Dietmar Eisel, C.L. Petersen, and W.L. Nighan

The OPMILAS 144 surgical lasers, which include the OPMILAS 144 and OPMILAS 144 Plus models, are solid-state lasers featuring a pulsed 1.44 μm wavelength (Fig. 25-1). The 1.44 μm wavelength is produced from a neodymium:YAG crystal using a proprietary technology developed by Carl Zeiss. The OPMILAS 144 Plus model offers, in addition to the pulsed 1.44 μm wavelength, a conventional continuous wave 1.06 μm wavelength that is also produced from the neodymium:YAG crystal. The 1.06 μm neodymium:YAG wavelength is *not* recommended for arthroscopic use by the manufacturer. However, the OPMILAS Plus laser provides two wavelengths in one unit for other uses.

Because the 1.44 μm neodymium:YAG and 1.06 μm neodymium:YAG wavelengths are in the infrared region of the electromagnetic spectrum and are invisible to the human eye, the OPMILAS 144 surgical lasers incorporate a 0.670 μm wavelength diode laser to generate a red aiming beam that is particularly useful for noncontact applications.

The OPMILAS 144 surgical lasers have a self-contained cooling system. This system employs recirculating water and a heat exchanger to cool the flash lamps of the laser. In contrast, 2.1 μm holmium:YAG systems require a refrigeration system for operating in the upper range of their average power settings. All circuitry and software of the laser are constantly monitored and controlled by a microprocessor. In particular, the laser power is continuously measured when the instrument is activated with the footswitch, for safety reasons.

The control panel of the OPMILAS 144 surgical lasers features a pressure-sensitive membrane with up/down control keys and LCD displays for easy selection of desired operational parameters. When working with the 1.44 μm neodymium:YAG wavelength, the user adjusts the pulse energy (in joules) and the pulse repetition rate (in hertz). The average power (pulse energy multiplied by the repetition rate), is also displayed (in watts). The intensity level of the aiming beam can be continuously adjusted. A multifunctional LCD display provides prompts and messages to assist the user in system operation. The display also indicates the cumulative laser energy delivered during the procedure. Laser emission is controlled by a footswitch.

Also included in the OPMILAS 144 lasers is a fiber calibration port to enable the user to precalibrate certain types of delivery fibers, if desired. If the user chooses to calibrate the fiber the laser automatically compensates for any loss in transmission, provided this loss is within acceptable limits and does not pose a safety concern.

The OPMILAS 144 surgical lasers employ quartz optical fibers for delivery of energy to the target tissue. Various types of fiber delivery systems are available depending on the particular wavelength selected and the intended application. The proximal end of all the fiberoptic delivery systems are fitted with a standard SMA 905 connector, which threads onto the fiber coupler on the front panel of the laser.

For the 1.44 μm neodymium:YAG wavelength, only low water content fibers may be used owing to the absorption of this wavelength by water. These low water content fibers are available with or without handpieces depending on the application. For arthroscopic procedures, fiber delivery systems have handpieces with the distal portion oriented at various angles to allow access to difficult-to-reach areas of the joints (Fig. 25-2). The fiber or handpiece may be used in contact or noncontact mode depending on the situation and the desired tissue effect. For arthroscopic procedures in a fluid medium, rapid ablation of dense tissue is best accomplished with the delivery fiber in gentle contact with the tissue and using a brush-like technique. Withdrawing the delivery fiber from the

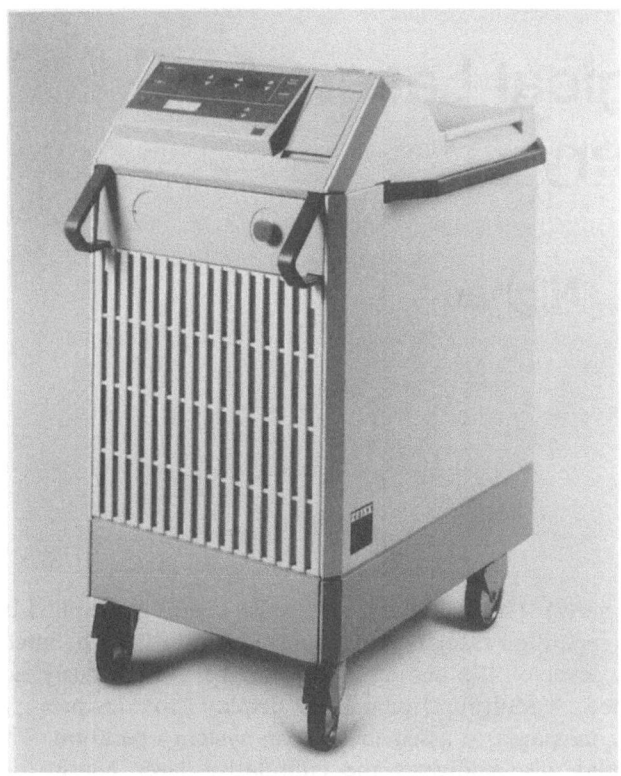

Figure 25-1. Opmilas 144 surgical laser.

tissue results in attenuation of the laser energy and decreased intensity of the tissue effect. Nevertheless, the noncontact technique can be particularly useful for coagulation of bleeders or for ablation of less dense, filamentous tissue.

Laser Hazards and Safety Precautions

As with all surgical lasers, there are various potential hazards associated with use of the OPMILAS 144 laser, including those associated with direct exposure to the laser beam ancillary dangers. Various regulations and standards have been established to minimize the risk of these hazards, most notable of which is the American National Standards Institute (ANSI) document Z136.3, entitled "American National Standard for the Safe Use of Lasers in Health Care Facilities." The user is advised to refer to this and other national and local standards and regulations as applicable.

Eye and Skin Hazards and Precautions

The OPMILAS 144 surgical lasers are high-power surgical lasers capable of causing injury to the eye and skin. Skin injuries may range from mild to severe burns depending on the intensity of energy incident on the skin. Any injury to the eye from the 1.44 μm neodymium:YAG wavelength would occur in the anterior portion of the eye (the cornea and possibly the lens) owing to the relatively high absorption of this wavelength by water. No injury to the retina would be expected to occur with this wavelength. The 1.06 μm wavelength of the OPMILAS Plus, on the other hand, can produce injuries to the retina, as the wavelength readily passes through the nonpigmented ocular media. Retinal injuries are of particular concern, especially if the laser beam is focused on the macula.

The ANSI standards require that eye protection speci-

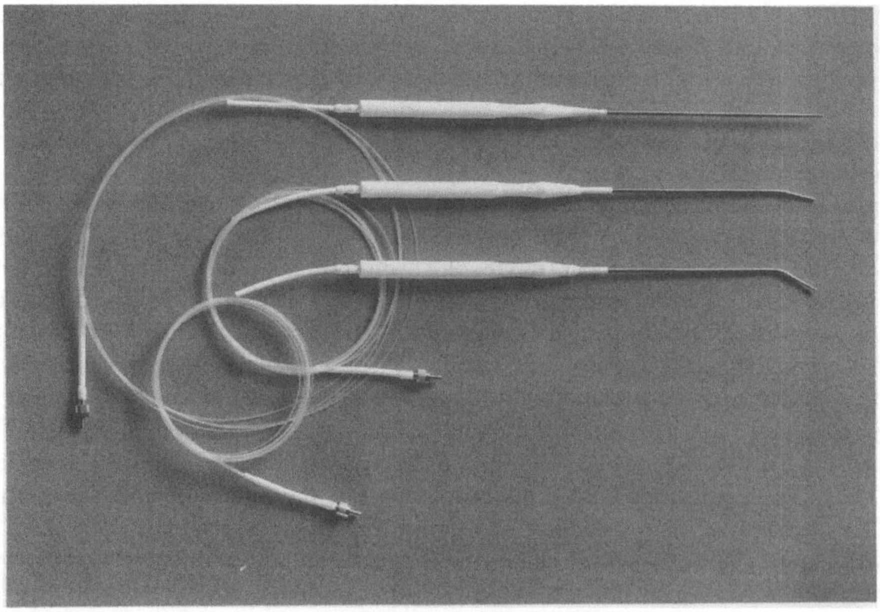

Figure 25-2. Fiber delivery systems with handpieces that allow access to difficult to reach areas of the joints.

fically designed for the wavelength in use be worn by all personnel in the nominal hazard zone (NHZ) when engineering or other procedural controls are inadequate to eliminate potential exposure in excess of the applicable minimum permissible exposure (MPE). The NHZ describes the space within which the level of direct reflected or scattered radiation during normal operation exceeds the applicable MPE. The NHZ can be calculated by the following equation

$$\mathrm{NHZ} = \sqrt{\frac{\mathrm{P}\,\phi \cos \Theta_v}{\pi\,\mathrm{MPE}}}\ \mathrm{cm}$$

where P = the spectral reflectance of a diffuse object at wavelength; ϕ = the average radiant power in watts; and Θ_v = the viewing angle.

Using values that yield a most conservative, worst case scenario (i.e., P = 1.0 and $\Theta_v = 0$ degrees), the NHZ for the 1.44 μm neodymium:YAG wavelength is calculated as 14 cm at an average laser power of 60 watts. Depending on the value used for the viewing angle, the value calculated for the NHZ can vary.

The Nominal Ocular Hazard Distance (NOHD) is defined as the distance along the axis of the unobstructed laser beam from the distal end of the fiber or a broken fiber tip to the human eye, beyond which the irradiation or radiant exposure during operation is not expected to exceed the appropriate MPE. For a fiber with a numerical aperture of NA = 0.22, this distance can be calculated using the following formula (multimode beam):

$$r_{\mathrm{NOHD}} = \frac{1.7}{\mathrm{NA}}\sqrt{\frac{\phi}{\pi \cdot \mathrm{MPE}}}\ \mathrm{cm}$$

For an average output power $\phi = 60$ watts the NOHD is calculated as 1.07 meters.

In accordance with ANSI standards, the protective eyewear should have an optical density (OD) sufficient to reduce the maximum potential eye exposure to below the minimum permissible exposure. The optical density is calculated by the following equation.

$$\mathrm{OD} = \log_{10} \frac{\mathrm{H}}{\mathrm{MPE}}$$

where H = fluence of the radiation based on a 3.5 mm spot size of the beam.

For the 1.44 μm neodymium:YAG wavelength, at an average power of 60 watts the minimum optical density of the eyewear should be 3.8. Protection should also be placed over the patient's eyes. Protective spectacles or goggles or eye shields or patches may be used depending on the particular circumstances of the surgery.

It should be noted that delineation of the NHZ and the requirement for protective eyewear as specified by ANSI is based on the assumption that the laser is being used in an open environment. The ANSI standards do not specifically address the use of a laser in an endoscopic procedure where the laser energy is usually contained within a body cavity. Emission of laser energy outside the body cavity could occur, however, as a result of breakage or damage to the fiber should the fiber be mishandled. Therefore requirements for eye protection during endoscopic laser use should be carefully considered by individuals responsible for laser safety at the time of surgery.

Other measures should be taken to minimize the possibility of accidental eye or skin exposure to laser radiation. Operating room windows should be covered and laser warning signs posted on doors leading into the rooms.

The laser beam should not be directed into the lens. It may damage or fracture it. The surgeon must not view the laser procedure with his eye next to the scope.

Fires and Explosions

The OPMILAS 144 surgical lasers, like most high powered surgical lasers, operate by producing a thermal effect and so create considerable heat at times. Under certain conditions, they are capable of causing a fire or explosion.

Flammable anesthetics and preparatory solutions should never be used in the operating room when the laser is to be used. Flame retardant drapes should be used. If cloth drapes are used, any portion of the drape immediately surrounding the surgical site should be moistened with saline or sterile water. Any sponges, gauze pads, or swabs located near the surgical site should also be moistened. When the laser is not actually being used, the delivery system should be placed on a separate metal or nonflammable surface and not laid on the drape. In addition, the laser system should be placed in the Standby mode when not in use. When the laser is being used for any oral, nasal, laryngotracheal or endobronchial procedures, certain precautions regarding anesthesia must be taken to minimize the risk of fire.

Airborne Contaminants

The plume given off during laser surgery is considered hazardous, and appropriate caution should be taken. The precise nature and extent of the hazard is unclear at this time, but various studies have demonstrated the presence of viable bacteria, virus particles, and mutagenic molecules in tissue aerosols. Generally there is relatively little plume associated with arthroscopic use of the laser. Much of the by-product appears to be trapped by (and carried off with) the fluid medium. The plume generated during use of the laser for open procedures, however, is more prominent and warrants precautions. Such precautions include the use of evacuator suction systems, eye protection to protect from splatter, and masks with effective filtration or other respiratory protectors.

Other Hazards and Precautions

The OPMILAS 144 surgical lasers are high voltage instruments. No one other than a qualified technician should ever attempt to gain access to the internal components. The power supply cord and connections should be inspected prior to each use to ensure their integrity.

Only authorized, thoroughly trained personnel should operate the OPMILAS 144 surgical lasers. Individuals should have in-service training specifically on the use of the OPMILAS 144 in addition to general training on laser science and safety in the operating room.

Installation Requirements

The OPMILAS 144 surgical lasers have a footprint of 33 inches by 22 inches and fit in any moderately sized operating room. There should be adequate space to allow about 24 inches of clearance between the front and rear of the laser and the operating room walls, allowing proper air circulation for system cooling purposes. The OPMILAS 144 surgical lasers operate on a closed-loop water circulating system and require no external water supply.

A dedicated electrical service must be supplied to the laser room to provide three-phase, 208 volt, 50 ampere service for high-powered versions of the laser, and single phase, 208 volt, 50 ampere service for standard versions. The electrical service connection should be located within a radius of 10 feet from where the laser is positioned in the operating room. The laser, in turn, must be positioned within 10 feet of the operating table.

Maintenance

The OPMILAS 144 surgical lasers have been designed to require no maintenance by the user aside from some basic cleaning and visual inspection of the outer components. There are no user-serviceable components inside the laser, and the user is advised against attempting to service the instrument in any way.

The cabinet of the laser may be cleaned periodically using a cloth dampened with a mild antiseptic or mild cleaning solution. This should not be done with the laser plugged into the electrical outlet. Abrasive cleaners or cloths should not be used, and liquid should never be poured over the console. The electrical power cord and footswitch cord should be inspected regularly for any evidence of damage. If damage is indicated, the cord should be replaced or repaired by a qualified technician. The fiberoptic delivery systems for arthroscopy are designed and intended at present to be used as single-use, disposable items. It is expected that a single delivery system will last the length of any typical arthroscopic procedure.

Physics of Laser–Tissue Interactions in the Mid-Infrared Spectrum: Comparison of Pulsed 1.44 μm Neodymium:YAG and 2.1 μm Holmium:YAG Lasers

Mid-infrared lasers have found applications as surgical tools. Lasers in this class are well suited for cutting and ablating biologic tissue because wavelengths longer than approximately 1.4 μms are highly absorbed by water. It is this absorption mechanism that allows effective coupling of the laser energy into the treatment site, as water is the primary constituent of tissue. A constraint on the use of these lasers for many surgical applications is the requirement that their outputs must be delivered through conventionally available low-OH silica fibers. These two considerations create a window between approximately 1.4 and 2.4 μm, which is the wavelength pass band for a fiber-delivered surgical laser operating at a water-absorbed wavelength. At this time, only two mid-infrared lasers operating within this window have been developed into viable surgical products. One is the now familiar holmium-doped YAG laser, and the other represents a new addition to this class of lasers: a specially prepared neodymium:YAG laser operating at 1.44 μm.

The physics of laser–tissue interactions with 1.44 μm neodymium:YAG and 2.1 μm holmium:YAG pulsed mid-infrared lasers are discussed here. The tissue effects can be described in simple physical terms; most of it is not much more complicated than turning water into steam. Minimal thermal damage and a consistent, controllable, safe effect can be achieved with these surgical lasers simply by virtue of their pulsed output and the absorption of the 1.44 μm neodymium:YAG and 2.1 μm holmium:YAG wavelengths in water. The physics of these laser–tissue interactions at the 1.44 μm wavelength of neodymium:YAG lasers and the 2.1 μm wavelength of holmium:YAG lasers are similar, as water and hence tissue absorb both wavelengths equally well. An important difference between the two lasers is the expanded parameter range that is available with 1.44 μm neodymium:YAG lasers (higher average power, higher repetition rates), which is directly attributable to a difference in the properties of the laser crystals themselves.

Absorption Coefficients of Water and Tissue in the Mid-Infrared Spectrum

Mid-infrared wavelength 2.1 μm holmium:YAG lasers have gained U.S. Food and Drug Administration (FDA) clearance for certain surgical procedures. The mechanism for tissue ablation with lasers operating at this wavelength (2.1 μm) is based on absorption by the water in the tissue (Nishioka and Domankevitz, 1989, 1990; Nishioka et al., 1989); this effect is significant, as biologic tissue is typically 80% water. The mid-infrared absorption spectrum of water, after Curcio and Petty (1951), is often cited (Irvine and Pollack, 1968; Hale and Querry, 1973). A table of indices of refraction and absorption coefficients (α in units of centimeters^{-1}) over a larger range is available (Irvine and Pollack, 1968). It is by means of this strong absorption in water that laser energy is converted to heat energy in the tissue. If the energy density in the tissue is high enough, the tissue vaporizes.

The 2.1 μm wavelength of the holmium:YAG laser falls on the long wavelength side of a water absorption peak at approximately 1.94 μm. The 1.44 μm wavelength of a neodymium:YAG laser coincides with a shorter wavelength peak at approximately 1.45 μm. The absorption coefficients for both wavelengths are nearly identical at approximately 26 cm^{-1} and are nearly 200 times greater than that at the 1.06 μm neodymium:YAG wavelength. For comparison, the absorption coefficients at 1.06 and 10.50 μm are approximately 0.13 and 823 cm^{-1}, respectively (Irvine and Pollack, 1968). The characteristic energy absorption depth is $1/\alpha$; thus a large α implies a short penetration depth, which is desirable for efficacious cutting and ablating.

However, a very large and very short penetration depth has a disadvantage in that such wavelengths cannot be used in a fluid environment in near-contact procedures as even a thin film of water between the fiber and tissue will greatly diminish the effective laser power. This is the case with CO_2 lasers, which always require gas insufflation.

The absorption spectrum of the human meniscus (Fig. 25-3) (Vangsness et al., 1991) exhibits the mid-infrared spectral peaks at approximately 1.45 and 1.94 μm, which are characteristic of the water absorption spectrum. The measured absorption coefficient at 1.44 and 2.1 μm is nearly the same in liver as in water ($\alpha \sim 26$ cm^{-1}) (Parsa et al., 1989). It is clear that for either the 1.44 μm neodymium:YAG or the 2.1 μm holmium:YAG wavelength of these lasers, the tissue "looks" like water. Because biologic tissue is typically 80% water, this absorption provides a mechanism for efficient coupling of laser energy into tissue, facilitating removal by ablation (Nishioka and Domankevitz, 1989, 1990; Nishioka et al., 1989; Trauner et al., 1990). This ablation does not rely on the creation of a blackbody radiator ("hot" tip) at the distal end of the delivery system, as is the case with common 1.06 μm contact surgery (Seka, 1990).

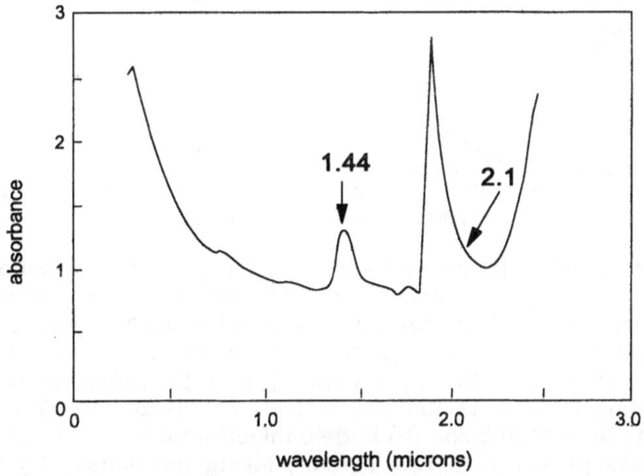

Figure 25-3. Absorption spectrum for human meniscus. Note that the location of the mid-infrared peaks in both spectra are identical to the locations in the water absorption spectrum. (From Vangsness et al., 1991. With permission.)

Energy Density: Spot Size

Most commercially available 2.1 μm holmium:YAG laser delivery systems incorporate 400 μm diameter low-OH silica-clad silica fibers with a numeric aperture (NA) of 0.22, which indicates a maximum full acceptance angle of 25.4 degrees. The delivery systems used with the Zeiss 1.44 μm neodymium:YAG laser incorporate 400 and 600 μm diameter low-OH silica-clad silica fibers of the same numeric aperture. Fiber tips are flat (either cleaved or polished) in the handpieces for both the 1.44 μm neodymium:YAG and 2.1 μm holmium:YAG lasers and are designed to incise and ablate with the fiber tip in contact or in close proximity to tissue. The spot sizes on tissue are therefore approximately equal to the fiber diameter when the handpieces are used as designed for ablation. The beam provided by the combination of laser and multimode fiber delivery system is not pure TEM_{00} but nevertheless exhibits a smooth spatial profile.

If the distal fiber tips are held at some distance from tissue, as is sometimes done for coagulation and some chondroplasty techniques, the spot sizes on the tissue are larger than the fiber diameter, as the beam diverges from the end of the fiber. As with nearly all solid-state surgical lasers, this divergence angle at the fiber output varies with the selected output power; lowest divergences correspond with the lowest average powers due to an effect known as "thermal lensing," which is encountered with all solid-state laser materials. For the Zeiss 1.44 μm neodymium:YAG laser, the divergence angle varies from approximately 11.5 degrees (full angle divergence) at low average power to 17.5 degrees at highest average power. As dictated by the numeric aperture of the fibers used in both the Zeiss and most 2.1 μm holmium:YAG laser handpieces (NA = 0.22), the maximum possible full angle divergence is 25.4 degrees. Again, because the delivery systems for both the 2.1 μm holmium:YAG and Zeiss 1.44 μm neodymium:YAG lasers are designed to put the fiber in contact or close proximity to tissue, the precise divergence angle is not a critical operating parameter. Spot sizes are 400 μm for most 2.1 μm holmium:YAG delivery systems; spot sizes are 400 and 600 μm for the Zeiss delivery systems.

Radiant Exposure: Threshold Radiant Exposure and Above

The "radiant exposure" (also known as energy density or fluence) provided by a single laser pulse is simply the pulse energy divided by the area of irradiated tissue (in units of energy per area, or joules per square centimeter) (Nishioka and Domankevitz, 1989, 1990; Nishioka et al., 1989; Trauner et al., 1990). The "threshold radiant exposure" (F_{th} in joules per square centimeter) is defined as the single pulse threshold for the ablation of biologic tissue (Walsh, 1988; Walsh and Deutsch, 1988; Nishioka and Domankevitz, 1989, 1990; Nishioka et al., 1989; Trauner et al., 1990). For radiant exposures less than this threshold, tissue is not vaporized or ablated but, instead, is heated. For radiant exposures higher than this threshold, tissue is vaporized. Based on the simple physics of the vaporization of water and the absorption of light in water, one can calculate the order of magnitude of F_{th} for biologic tissue. Before going on, we make the approximation that the laser pulse duration is much shorter than the thermal relaxation time of the tissue. We have calculated that it is indeed the case for the Zeiss 1.44 μm neodymium:YAG laser and the 2.1 μm holmium:YAG lasers.

To excise or ablate tissue with a single pulse, the energy carried by the pulse (E_{pulse}, in joules) divided by the area of the irradiated tissue ($A = \pi d^2/4$, in square centimeters, where d is the spot diameter) must be greater than F_{th}:

$$E_{pulse}/A > F_{th} \quad (1)$$

For a given spot size A on tissue, a pulse of energy E_{pulse} ablates the irradiated tissue if the inequality of equation 1 is satisfied. To incise or ablate tissue, the operating parameters of the laser and delivery system should be designed to provide pulse energies and spot sizes that allow radiant exposures of a magnitude consistent with the threshold radiant exposure for ablation. As is shown below, the output characteristics of the typical 2.1 μm holmium:YAG lasers and the Zeiss 1.44 μm neodymium:YAG laser are consistent with these calculated estimates.

The threshold radiant exposure for ablation can be estimated by relating it to the threshold energy per unit volume (in joules per cubic centimeter) for vaporization. For water, the threshold energy per unit volume is a known quantity, approximately 2500 joules/cm³ (Walsh, 1988). This parameter is also called the heat of vaporization, which is the energy per unit volume that is required for the phase change from liquid water to water vapor (including the energy required for raising body temperature water to 100°C (Walsh, 1988). This threshold energy per unit volume is approximately equal to $(F_{th}) \times (\alpha)$ or $(F_{th})/(d)$, as the penetration depth (d) of the laser radiation is approximately $d = 1/\alpha$, where α is the absorption coefficient (α in units of centimeter^{-1}) (Walsh, 1988). At 1.44 or 2.1 μm in water, using α as approximately 25 cm^{-1} and equating $(F_{th}) \times (\alpha)$ with 2500 joules/cm³, we find:

$$(F_{th}) \times (\alpha) \sim 2500 \text{ joules/cm}^3 \quad (2a)$$

$$F_{th}\ (1.44 \text{ or } 2.1\ \mu m) \sim 100 \text{ joules/cm}^2 \quad (2b)$$

This order of magnitude estimate for the threshold radiant exposure for ablation of tissue is based on a calculation for water (Walsh, 1988). It can be used as an approximation for the minimum single-pulse radiant exposure that results in tissue ablation. Some deviation arises when biologic tissue is considered because components other than water are included in tissue. The scattering and additional absorption can result in an effective penetration depth that is somewhat less than $1/\alpha$, although for water the penetration depth still primarily depends on the water absorption coefficient (Parsa et al., 1989). Another factor not considered for equation 2b is the reflection from the tissue, which can result in less effective coupling of energy (Nishioka and Domankevitz, 1989). These effects can contribute to a threshold radiant exposure F_{th} that deviates somewhat from the estimate in equation 2b. However, the estimate in equation 2b can be used to determine the approximate pulse energies and spot sizes that are consistent with ablation, which in turn dictates laser and delivery system design.

Precise experimental determination of absolute values for F_{th} is difficult, as it is derived from an extrapolation of ablation rate versus radiant exposure measurements. These data are obtained from mass loss experiments, as shown in Figure 25-4 (Walsh and Deutsch, 1988; Nishioka and Domankevitz, 1990). The mass of a tissue sample is

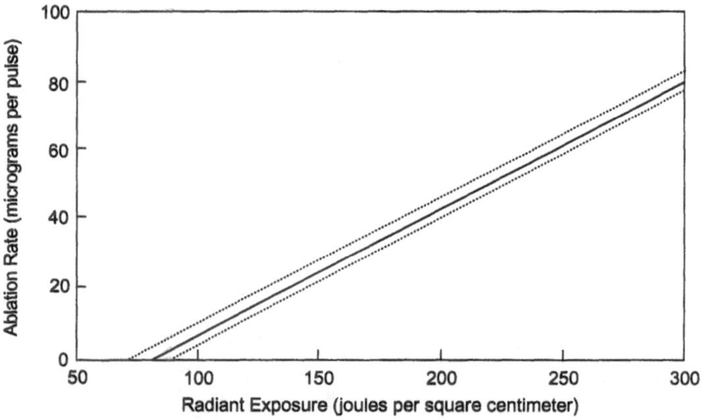

Figure 25-4. Effect of laser radiant exposure on ablation rate. Mass loss experiment: ablation rate versus radiant exposure for fresh chicken liver irradiated by the 1.44 μm neodymium:YAG laser. The threshold radiant exposure F_{th} corresponds to the x-intercept: F_{th} = 79 joules/cm² (corresponding 95% confidence interval of 71–86 joules/cm²). The heat of ablation (H) is determined from the slope: H = ρA/slope which is 12.4 kJ/cm³, taking the density (ρ) of liver as approximately 1.1 g/cm³, the spot size (A) as 4.1 × 10⁻³ cm² the slope as 0.364 μg × cm²/J (corresponding to the 95% confidence interval of 11.6–13.3 kJ/cm³). The values for F_{th} and H are comparable to those that have been reported for the 2.1 μm holmium:YAG lasers in the same tissue. See text. (Courtesy Nishioka, 1989.)

measured as it is exposed to a number of laser pulses at different radiant exposure levels. The ablation rate is determined (in micrograms per pulse) as a function of radiant exposure (in joules per square centimeter) (Walsh, 1988; Walsh and Deutsch, 1988; Nishioka and Domankevitz, 1989, 1990; Nishioka et al., 1989; Trauner et al., 1990). Extrapolation of the data to zero ablation rate yields the threshold radiant exposure. Available values for the biologic tissue at the 2.1 μm holmium:YAG wavelength include approximately 36 and 50 joules/cm^2 for chicken liver (Nishioka et al., 1989; Nishioka and Domankevitz, 1990), approximately 50 joules/cm^2 for bovine articular cartilage, and approximately 11 joules/cm^2 for bovine meniscus fibrocartilage (Trauner et al., 1990). Measurements at 1.44μm indicate that the threshold radiant exposure is approximately 79 joules/cm^2 for chicken liver. All of these values are in the vicinity of the estimate of 100 joules/cm^2 presented in equation 2b. The threshold radiant exposure at 1.44 μm is represented by the x-axis intercept of the data in Figure 25-4. This measurement of ablation rate (micrograms per pulse) as a function of radiant exposure (joules per square centimeter) was performed by Nishioka and coworkers. A description of the behavior of this function (ablation rate versus radiant exposure) for radiant exposures above the threshold radiant exposure follows.

For both the 2.1 μm holmium:YAG and 1.44 μm neodymium:YAG lasers at radiant exposures above the threshold, the ablation rate is observed to increase linearly with increasing radiant exposure (Nishioka and Domankevitz, 1989, 1990; Nishioka et al., 1989; Stein et al., 1990; Trauner et al., 1990). This finding is in agreement with a theoretic model reported by Walsh and coworkers (Walsh, 1988; Walsh and Deutsch, 1988). The theoretic description of this behavior is based on the heating and evaporation of water upon exposure to a laser pulse of a duration shorter than the thermal relaxation time. The ablation rate can be expressed as:

$$R = p \cdot A \cdot (F - F_{th})/H \qquad (3)$$

Here R = ablation rate in mass ablated per pulse (micrograms per pulse); p = density of the target (grams per cubic centimeter); A = area of tissue irradiated by the laser (square centimeters); F = radiant exposure per pulse (joules per square centimeter); F_{th} = single-pulse threshold radiant exposure (joules per square centimeter, estimated by equation 2); and H = heat of ablation in units of energy per unit volume (joules per cubic centimeter). The H term is the efficiency for ablation; for water, this value is 2500 joules/cm^3, or 2.5 kJ/cm^3. As described above, this quantity is the energy per unit volume that is required for the phase change from body-temperature liquid water to water vapor (Walsh, 1988). By measuring the slopes of the plot in Figure 25-4 and using the area (A) of the irradiated spot and the density of the target tissue (p), the heat of ablation (H) can be obtained from the mass loss measurements, where $H = p \cdot A/\text{slope}$. The slope indicates a heat of ablation (H) of 12.4 kJ/cm^3 for fresh chicken liver irradiated by the 1.44 μm neodymium:YAG laser. In 1993, Brillhart reported a similar ablation rate using the 1.44 μm neodymium:YAG laser. The value of 12.4 kJ/cm^3 at 1.44 μm is similar to those previously reported for a 2.1 μm holmium:YAG laser (7 and 10 kJ/cm^3 for fresh chicken liver, 10.49 kJ/cm^3 for bovine articular cartilage, and 11.99 kJ/cm^3 for bovine meniscus fibrocartilage) (Nishioka and Domankkevitz 1989; 1990; Trauner et al., 1990). The rate of ablation for both the 2.1 μm holmium:YAG laser and the 1.44 μm neodymium:YAG laser are therefore in agreement with an accepted theoretic model. Both exhibit a threshold radiant exposure consistent with one that can be calculated for water (as in equation 2), and both exhibit a linear trend above threshold with comparable heats of ablation. Practically, it means that the depth of ablation achieved with a single pulse is linearly proportional to the radiant exposure above threshold, and that the nature of the laser–tissue interaction for both lasers is substantially equivalent.

Pulse Energy

The 400 μm diameter optical fiber delivery systems used in most 2.1 μm holmium:YAG lasers and the d = 400 and 600 μm diameter optical fiber delivery systems used in the Zeiss 1.44 μm neodymium:YAG laser are designed for incision and ablation of tissue when used in contact or close proximity to the tissue. The area (A) of irradiated tissue is simply $\pi d^2/4$, where d is the fiber diameter. F_{th} (from equation 2) multiplied by A provides the single-pulse energy thresholds for ablation for these spot sizes.

$$E_{th} = (F_{th}) \times (A) \qquad (4a)$$

$$E_{th}\ (d = 400\ \mu m) \sim 0.13 \text{ joule} \qquad (4b)$$

$$E_{th}\ (d = 600\ \mu m) \sim 0.3 \text{ joule} \qquad (4c)$$

Both the available 2.1 μm holmium:YAG lasers and the Zeiss 1.44 μm neodymium:YAG laser are designed to provide-single pulse energies between 0.1 and 2.0 joules or more. Thus the single-pulse energies available from either laser are greater than the minimum energies expressed in equations 4b and 4c; and the spot sizes made possible by the 400- and 600-μm delivery systems allow radiant exposures greater than the threshold estimated in equation 2b. The pulse energy from either system can be adjusted with respect to the ablation threshold. From this simple argument, it is expected that the tissue effects obtained with either laser for the same energy and power settings should be comparable.

Although the pulse energies available from these two lasers are nominally the same, an important difference between the two stems from the physics of the laser crystals themselves. A practical implication of this difference is that pulses of a given energy may be delivered at a higher repetition rate from a neodymium:YAG laser at 1.44 μm with little degradation of laser efficiency. This situation is not the case with the 2.1 μm holmium:YAG laser, where an increase in the repetition rate of the laser is accompanied by a decrease in laser efficiency. (This difference is further discussed under Repetition Rate, below.) The behavior can be traced to the energy spacings between the ground-state level and the lower level of the laser transitions in the respective crystals.

Thermal Damage

A common approach to estimating the depth of thermal damage (D) that remains in tissue after ablation is to assume that thermal damage results when a critical temperature is reached (T_c) (Nishioka and Domankevitz, 1990). One can derive the following:

$$D = (1/\alpha) \ln [F_{th} \cdot \alpha/(T_c - T_0) \cdot p \cdot C] \quad (5)$$

where T_0 is the initial temperature of the tissue. By equation 2a, the product $F_{th}\alpha$ is equivalent to the threshold energy per unit volume for the ablation or vaporization of tissue and is therefore depends only on the tissue, not the wavelength or absorption coefficient. By this model, the depth of thermal damage (D) is proportional to the reciprocal of the absorption coefficient. Therefore for the 1.44 μm neodymium:YAG and 2.1 μm holmium:YAG wavelengths, one would expect the thermal damage depths to be comparable because the absorption coefficients at the two wavelengths are nearly identical in water and most biologic tissues (Curcio and Petty, 1951; Parsa et al., 1989). Measurements support with this expectation; for radiant exposures of 250 joules/cm^2 on bovine meniscus, average thermal damage depths were found to be 490 μm for pulses at 1.44 μm, compared to 440 μm for pulses at 2.1 μm. These data are consistent with the model presented in equation 5.

Pulse Duration and Thermal Relaxation Time

The 1.44 μm neodymium:YAG laser and the 2.1 μm holmium:YAG laser are pulsed lasers. Each provides output in the form of high energy pulses that are less than 1 ms in duration. These pulses are delivered at a repetition rate of up to 20 pulses per second for many of the available surgical 2.1 μm holmium:YAG lasers and up to 50 pulses per second for the 1.44 μm neodymium:YAG laser. From the standpoint of laser physics, these lasers must be pulsed in order to achieve a useful output power in a practical, reasonably efficient laser system that is a viable surgical product. From the standpoint of laser–tissue interaction, a pulsed laser output can minimize thermal injury to surrounding tissue and the threshold for ablation.

The argument is simple. First, it is important to realize that the energy at the laser wavelength is converted to heat energy in the irradiated volume of tissue at the end of the fiberoptic delivery system. To ablate that irradiated "target" volume of tissue with a single laser pulse, it is necessary to put enough heat energy into the volume to vaporize it. Second, if there was significant diffusion of this heat energy out of the irradiated volume during the time of exposure (the length of the laser pulse), the amount of thermal injury to surrounding tissue would be increased because heat diffuses out of the irradiated volume the surgeon intends to ablate and into the surrounding tissue, possibly damaging it. Third, any diffusion of heat energy out of the irradiated target volume reduces or drains away the energy density in the target volume of tissue. Heat would leak away from the target tissue while being pumped by the laser pulse. This diffusion effectively diminishes the efficiency with which the laser pulse can vaporize the tissue and therefore acts to increase the ablation threshold (threshold radiant exposure).

The short pulsed output of 1.44 μm neodymium:YAG lasers and 2.1 μm holmium:YAG lasers reduces the potentially detrimental effects of thermal diffusion over the duration of the laser pulse. Diffusion is prevented by the laser pulse durations being much shorter than the characteristic thermal relaxation time of the tissue under treatment (Boulnois, 1985; Walsh et al., 1988; Nishioka and Domankevitz, 1989, 1990; Nishioka et al., 1989). It minimizes the ablation thresholds and the extent of thermal injury to surrounding tissue. By calculating the thermal relaxation time of the tissue, a maximum acceptable laser pulse duration can be determined. The pulse durations of the 1.44 μm neodymium:YAG lasers and the 2.1 μm holmium:YAG lasers are well under this limit, which is part of the reason for their successful application to surgery. It should be noted that these same thermal calculations should be applied to pulsed 10.6 μm CO_2 lasers as well (Boulnois, 1985).

The relevant thermal relaxation time, (τ), is the time required for heat energy to diffuse out of the irradiated target volume of tissue. It is easy to see that this time depends on the diameter of the target and the absorption depth of the laser. Classic heat transfer theory can be used to estimate τ (Carslaw and Jaeger, 1959; Nishioka and Domankevitz, 1990).

$$1/\tau \sim 4\alpha^2 K + 16K/d^2 \quad (6)$$

where α = optical absorption coefficient at the laser wavelength; K = thermal diffusivity of the tissue; and d = diameter of the illuminated spot. This time τ is approximately the length of time required for heat to diffuse one optical absorption depth ($1/\alpha$; it therefore depends on the absorption coefficient at the wavelength of the treatment laser. Because tissue is mostly water, we can use α and K in water as a starting point ($\alpha \sim 25$ cm^{-1} at 1.44 and 2.1 μm, $K \sim 1.4 \times 10^{-3}$ cm^2/s). For spot sizes ranging from 400 μm (fiber in contact or very close proximity to tissue) to infinity (fiber drawn away from tissue), τ is approximately 57 to 286 ms.

For both the typical 2.1 μm holmium:YAG lasers and the Zeiss 1.44 μm neodymium:YAG laser, the output pulse durations (approximately 0.25 and 0.65 ms, respectively) are significantly shorter than the thermal relaxation time. Therefore heat has no time to diffuse on the short time scale of these submillisecond laser pulses. In fact, once the pulse duration has been reduced to a length significantly shorter than τ, tissue effects become independent of the specific pulse duration and primarily depend only on the radiant exposure (fluence) and the optical penetration depth (Walsh et al., 1988). This situation has been reported for 2.1 μm holmium:YAG ablation of soft tissue; no change in the ablation rate was observed for pulse durations that varied from 150 to 500 μms (Vari et al., 1991). Reducing pulse durations to this short pulse regime minimizes the ablation threshold as well as the spatial extent of thermal injury (Walsh et al., 1988). It should also be noted that it is valid to neglect diffusion of heat during the time of a single pulsed exposure only if the pulse duration is significantly less than τ (Boulnois, 1985; Walsh et al., 1988; Nishioka and Domankevitz, 1989, 1990; Nishioka et al., 1989).

Repetition Rate

The average power (P_{av}) of a repetitively pulsed laser is equal to the energy per pulse times the number of pulses per unit time (P_{av} = joules/pulse × pulses/second, in watts). Presently available surgical 2.1 μm holmium:YAG lasers deliver pulses of energy between 0.2 and 2.0 joules at repetition rates of up to 20 Hz. For reasons related to the laser efficiency, not all combinations of pulse energy and repetition rate are possible. The Zeiss 1.44 μm neodymium:YAG laser delivers pulses of energy selectable between 0.1 and 2.0 joules at repetition rates of 5 to 50 Hz. Not all combinations of pulse energy and repetition rate are possible, also for reasons related to laser efficiency. Note that the maximum repetition rate of the 1.44 μm neodymium:YAG laser is much higher than that possible with single head 2.1 μm holmium:YAG lasers.

If a fresh spot is irradiated by each pulse, the single-pulse ablation argument holds. The number of tissue parcels ablated per second is equal to the repetition rate of the laser in pulses per second, or hertz. In this case, increasing the repetition rate to increase the average power delivered to the tissue linearly increases the rate of tissue removal (in micrograms per second).

If a region of tissue is illuminated by more than one pulse, a "buildup" of deposited energy can occur. For example, if the individual pulse energy and spot size provide a fluence below the single pulse threshold radiant exposure (F_{th}), but the interval between pulses at a particular repetition rate is shorter than the characteristic thermal relaxation time (τ), a parcel of tissue may be ablated after a number of pulses has impinged on the tissue. An approximate requirement is:

$$(P_{av}/A) - (F_{th}/\tau) > 0 \qquad (7)$$

where P_{av} = average power (energy per pulse × pulses per second, in watts); τ = thermal relaxation time; A = area of illuminated tissue; and F_{th} = threshold radiant exposure as expressed in equation 2b. [It should be noted that F_{th} may not remain constant in this regime; only the first pulse encounters fully hydrated, native tissue (Walsh, 1988).] Effectively, this criterion indicates that ablation can take place only if energy is supplied faster than it diffuses away. A similar form would apply to a continuous wave (CW) laser. This multiple-pulse ablation regime can be entered at the higher repetition rates with both the available 2.1 μm holmium:YAG lasers and the Zeiss 1.44 μm neodymium:YAG laser; the interval between pulses can be as short as 50 and 20 ms, respectively, which is shorter than the shortest thermal relaxation time that arises from equation 4. Because the thermal relaxation time (τ) is between 57 and 286 ms, a repetition rate greater than 3.5 Hz (1/286 ms) can allow entry into this regime.

As already stated, the maximum repetition rate of the 1.44 μm neodymium:YAG laser is much higher than that possible with the 2.1 μm holmium:YAG lasers. It is because the nature of the 1.44 μm transition in neodymium:YAG allows relatively efficient laser operation at much higher crystal temperatures than is possible with chromium-thulium-holmium (CTH):YAG. The strong temperature dependence exhibited by 2.1 μm holmium:YAG is due to the small energy difference between the ground-state level and the lower level of the laser transitions in the CTH:YAG crystals. These levels are much closer together in CTH:YAG than in 1.44 μm neodymium:YAG. As temperature goes up in a CTH:YAG laser crystal, the population in the lower level of the laser transition increases. Gain decreases, losses increase, and the laser efficiency ultimately decreases. Practically speaking, it is difficult to operate a 2.1 μm holmium:YAG laser at high repetition rates without a significant drop in laser efficiency. For this reason, the maximum repetition rates delivered by presently available single head 2.1 μm holmium:YAG lasers are on the order of 20 Hz, as it is difficult to maintain useful pulse energies at higher rates. On the other hand, with neodymium:YAG operating at 1.44 μm, it is possible to operate a practical laser system at 50 Hz with pulse energies higher than 0.5 joule. Energy and repetition rate settings are provided by the Zeiss 1.44 μm neodymium:YAG laser that are virtually impossible to match with a practical 2.1 μm holmium:YAG laser system.

The higher repetition rate settings that can be provided by the 1.44 μm neodymium:YAG laser result in an output that is nearly quasicontinuous. For certain arthroscopic applications, this level of control provides a useful new tool. High repetition rate, low energy pulses at 1.44 μm have been shown to be useful for chondroplasty, where precise sculpting and shaping is required. The high repetition rate settings of the 1.44 μm neodymium:YAG laser have also been shown to be useful for synovectomy, where effective ablation of soft, "mossy" tissue can be difficult with the more explosive, low repetition rate output of 2.1 μm holmium:YAG lasers.

Conclusion

The physics of laser–tissue interactions at 2.1 and 1.44 μm have been investigated. On the basis of simple physical arguments, the tissue effects achieved with the Zeiss 1.44 μm neodymium:YAG laser and typical 2.1 μm holmium: YAG lasers have been shown to be similar for similar pulse energy and repetition settings. The arguments are based on the following:

1. The similarity of the water and tissue absorption coefficients at 2.1 and 1.44 μm.
2. The similarity of the laser–tissue interaction achieved with the 1.44 μm neodymium:YAG wavelength of the Zeiss laser and that achieved with 2.1 μm holmium:YAG lasers, including the threshold radiant exposure, heat of ablation, and thermal damage.
3. The similar output characteristics for both the 2.1 μm holmium:YAG lasers and the Zeiss 1.44 μm neodymium:YAG laser, including spot size, energy per pulse, and pulse duration.

However, higher average powers and much higher repetition rates are possible with 1.44 μm neodymium:YAG lasers than with single head 2.1 μm holmium:YAG lasers. This difference stems from the energy spacing between the ground-state level and the lower level of the laser transitions in these crystals. The significantly greater spacing in 1.44 μm neodymium:YAG affords an insensitivity to temperature that is readily translated into greater flexibility in the output characteristics of the laser.

The Zeiss 1.44 μm neodymium:YAG system not only matches the high energy, low repetition rates of present single head 2.1 μm holmium:YAG lasers, but it can provide significant average power at much higher repetition rates. This expanded range of operating parameters allows the 1.44 μm neodymium:YAG to be used in a wider range of modalities than was previously possible.

Editor's Caution

1. **At the time of this writing the Zeiss 1.44 μm neodymium:YAG laser was just released for marketing. Limited, though satisfactory, clinical experience exists with this system.**
2. **Probe tips may fracture if they are forced or levered.**
3. **This system should not be used without wavelength-specific protective eyewear.**
4. **The manufacturer does not recommend use of the 1.06 μm neodymium:YAG wavelength for arthroscopy. This warning applies to alternating 1.44 and 1.06 μm wavelengths, but obviously not the 1.44 μm neodymium:YAG wavelength alone.**
5. **I do not recommend that these fibers be used in an air or gas environment.**
6. **All fibers have a definite life-span. Optimal, satisfactory use of this system requires some experience. It is best to start in the laboratory, not with patients. The best techniques, energy settings, and probe selections can be preliminarily determined in this way. The reader is referred to Chapter 4 for a discussion of ablation efficiency.**
7. **Mechanical instruments should be available at all times during arthroscopic laser surgery.**
8. **This chapter is only an introduction to this arthroscopic laser system. The reader is encouraged to study this entire text, follow acceptable training and credentialling procedures, as well as research the subject at hand for additional information and changes before undertaking this arthroscopic laser system's use.**

References

Boulnois JL (1985) Photophysical processes in recent medical laser developments: a review. Lasers Med Sci. 1:47–66

Carslaw HS, Jaeger JC (1959) Conduction of Heat in Solids. Oxford University Press, Oxford

Curcio JA, Petty CC (1951) The near infrared absorption spectrum of liquid water. J Opt Soc Am [A] 41:302–304

Hale G, Querry M (1973) Optical constants of water in the 200-nm to 200-μm wavelength region. Appl Optics 12:555–563

Irvine W, Pollack J (1968) Infrared optical properties of water and ice spheres. Icarus 8:324–360

Nishioka NS, Domankevitz Y (1989) Reflectance during pulsed holmium laser irradiation of tissue. Lasers Surg Med 9:375–381

Nishioka NS, Domankevitz Y (1990) Comparison of tissue ablation with pulsed holmium and thulium lasers. IEEE J Quantum Electron 26:2271–2275

Nishioka NS, Domankevitz Y, Flotte TJ, Anderson RR (1989) Ablation of rabbit liver, stomach, and colon with a pulsed holmium laser. Gastroenterology 96:831–837

Parsa P, Jacques SL, Nishioka NS (1989) Optical properties of rat liver between 350 and 2200 nm. Appl Opt 28:2325–2330

Seka W (1990) Laser energy repartition inside metal, sapphire, and quartz surgical laser tips. SPIE Proc 1398

Stein E, Sedlacek T, Fabian RL, Nishioka N (1990) Acute and chronic effects of bone ablation with a pulsed holmium laser. Lasers Surg Med 10:384–388

Trauner K, Nishioka N, Patel D (1990) Pulsed holmium: yttrium-alminum-garnet (Ho:YAG) laser ablation of fibrocartilage and articular cartilage. Am J Sports Med 18:316–320

Vangsness CT, Huang J, Smith CF (1991) Light absorption characteristics of the human meniscus: applications for laser ablation. SPIE Proc 24:16–19

Vari SG, Shi WQ, Fishbein MC, Grundfest WS (1991) Ablation study of knee structure tissues with a Ho:YAG laser [abstract]. Lasers Surg Med 3:51

Walsh JT (1988) Pulsed laser ablation of tissue: analysis of the removal process and tissue healing. PhD dissertation, Massachusetts Institute of Technology

Walsh JT, Deutsch TF (1988) Pulsed CO_2 laser tissue ablation—measurement of the ablation rate. Lasers Surg Med 8:264–275

Walsh J, Flotte TJ, Anderson R, Deutsch TF (1988) Pulsed CO_2 laser tissue ablation: effect of tissue type and pulse duration on thermal damage. Lasers Surg Med 8:108–118

26

Overview of Arthroscopic Laser Surgery in Europe

Werner E. Siebert

Arthroscopic surgery has become a routine procedure thanks to the availability of excellent video systems and the development of new and efficient instruments (Johnson, 1986). Since early 1980, several groups have undertaken arthroscopic laser surgery because of the advantages of laser instruments for endoscopic techniques. Extremely small but powerful tools with exciting new possibilities inspired the creativity of engineers and surgeons alike (Whipple, 1981; Whipple et al., 1982, 1983, 1984a,b; Smith and Nance, 1983; Glick, 1984; Smith et al., 1984; Frenz et al., 1989).

In Europe, initially, attempts were made to modify the available laser systems, including the 10.6 μm CO_2 laser and the 1.06 μm neodymium:YAG laser, for arthroscopic use. These instruments have been user-unfriendly. Nevertheless, there have been some groups in Europe that use the 10.6 μm CO_2 laser. Philandrianos (1984, 1985) is the surgeon with the most experience with the 10.6 μm CO_2 laser for arthroscopy. As early as 1984 he reported on his clinical experience with this laser for arthroscopic surgery (Fig. 26-1). Many problems arose at that time. The thermal side effects led to ashes in cartilage and synovium, and plume obscured visualization. Nevertheless the 10.6 μm CO_2 laser has proved especially helpful for synovectomy. Most other groups have used 10.6 μm CO_2 systems only experimentally. The technical problems were too many and the advantages too few (Siebert et al., 1990; Rudolph and Herberhold, 1991).

Further investigations by most groups concentrated on neodymium:YAG lasers using 1.06 or 1.32 μm wavelengths. The most experience with neodymium:YAG lasers for arthroscopy in Europe in clinical practice have been demonstrated by Lohnert. He and his coworkers (Lohnert and Raunest, 1988) have shown that partial synovectomy is possible using a free-beam 1.06 μm neodymium:YAG laser in a clinical setting. More than 100 patients were operated on as early as 1988. The modified Lysholm score (modified by W. Klein) was higher with less pain and less swelling in the laser group compared to that experienced after conventional methods. Hefti and Morscher, from Switzerland (1984), reported some interesting possibilities for laser use in hemophiliac patients. The work on articular cartilage and meniscal surgery was not successful, however, using the free-beam 1.06 μm neodymium:YAG laser (Siebert and Kohn, 1988; Raunest and Lohnert 1989, 1990, 1991).

During the late 1980s research for arthroscopic laser systems started systematically (Siebert et al., 1990; Siebert and Thriene, 1991; Siebert and Wirth, 1991). Many groups in Europe showed that tissue damage from free-beam 1.06 and 1.32 μm neodymium:YAG lasers is not acceptable (Fig. 26-2). Many probes and supplies were tested at that time with both wavelengths (1.06 and 1.32 μm), but the results always included severe thermal damage (Siebert and J Wirth, 1991) (Fig. 26-3).

Also during the late 1980s the excimer laser using a 0.308 μm wavelength became popular. It was thought that this system was a "cold laser"and caused no thermal damage. Several groups started experimental and clinical work. In Austria, Kroitzsch and coworkers (1988, 1989) published several case reports, even on cutting the meniscus. In Switzerland, Gerber (1991) investigated the effects of Excimer lasers on porcine knee cartilage. In Vienna, Pelinka (1990) and his coworkers and Buchelt and his colleagues (1991) conducted experimental and clinical studies on "intelligent systems" that could recognize the tissue type (Hohla et al., 1987). Siebert, Klanke, and colleagues (1990) investigated several laser systems, including various Excimer laser systems. Hohlbach and coworkers (1989) investigated the effects on cartilage using Excimer lasers. Clinical reports later concentrated on the use of Excimer lasers for smoothing articular cartilage. The low ablation

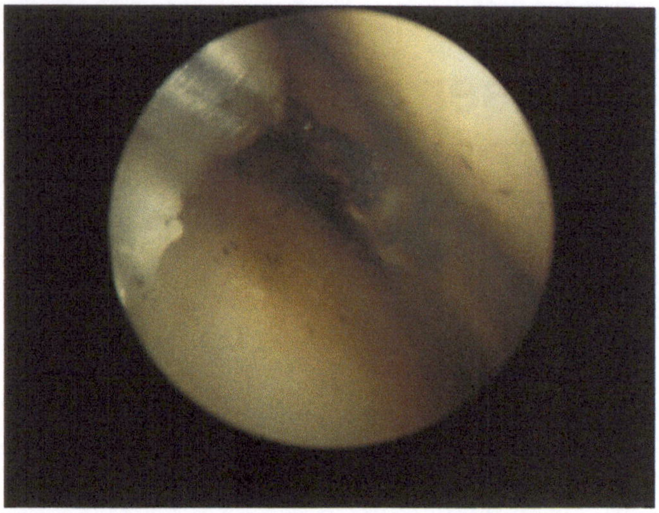

Figure 26-1. One of the first 10.6 μm CO_2 laser partial meniscectomies. (Courtesy G. Philandrianos.)

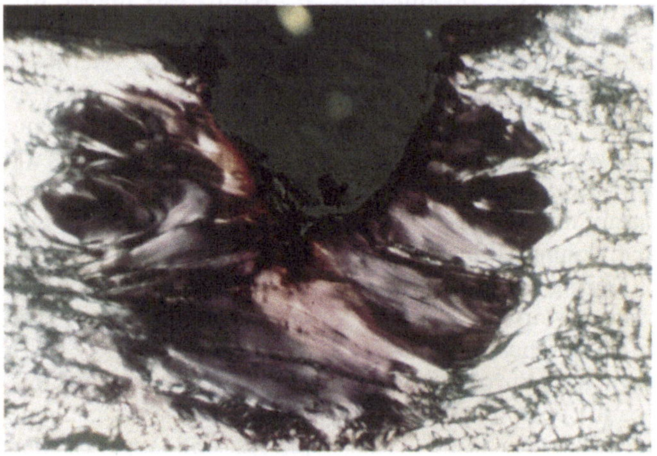

Figure 26-2. Unacceptable tissue damage from free-beam 1.06 μm neodymium:YAG use.

rate made it almost impossible to cut meniscus or tendon tissue.

Imhoff from Switzerland (Imhoff and Leu, 1991) and Raunest and Lohnert (1990, 1991) shared their clinical results with sweeping effects on cartilage. Raunest and Lohnert reported a prospective randomized clinical study on cartilage débridement (1990).

Most results reported at the 1991 International Laser Congress in Hannover, Germany were case reports (Siebert, 1991). Therefore there was a consensus that a multicenter study on the use of lasers in arthroscopy was necessary. These early clinical results were encouraging and raised hope for a better therapy (Kroitzsch et al., 1988, 1989; Imhoff and Leu, 1991; Raunest and Lohnert, 1990, 1991). Work presented by Grifka and Scheier in 1993 based on the work of Raunest again showed excellent clinical results in a prospective randomized study in cartilage damage types IIa–c and IIIa (Fig. 26-4). The low ablation rate was the main fault of the 0.308 μm Excimer laser. A danger for mutagenicity or carcinogenicity did not exist, as Siebert and coworkers had suggested in 1991 (Glick and Harmon, 1991). It is surprising that experimental studies and clinical studies using Excimer lasers had conflicting results. The results of the experimental studies showed low ablation rates and equivocal outcomes in the animal experiments (Siebert and Kohn, 1988; Grothues-Spork et al., 1989; Hohlback et al., 1989; Siebert et al., 1990; Buchelt et al., 1991; Gerber, 1991; Siebert and Wirth 1991).

The search for better laser systems that can also ablate meniscus, bone, and bone cement has been a long tradition in Europe. Horch (1983) was one of the pioneers in this ongoing work, and Clauser (1986), Dittrich and coworkers (especially K. Dinstl) (1988), Grothues-Spork et al. (1989), Schneider (1986) and Siebert (1990; Siebert et al., 1990; Siebert and Wirth, 1991) should be mentioned.

Another interest in lasers in orthopaedics in Europe has been for the treatment of synovitis. Richter et al., (1991) reported on direct techniques, and Siebert invented a photodynamic technique especially for the local treatment of synovitis in rheumatoid patients (Steinmetz and Hofstetter, 1988; Unsold and Jocham, 1988; Siebert and Wirth, 1991). An ongoing goal of a collaborative group in Germany is to devise a laser-enhanced photodynamic treatment for synovitis. Tissue welding had been a dream of laser surgeons in Europe for years (Ulrich et al., 1988), but the solution has become clear only in current experimental studies.

The most promising approach for lasers in arthroscopic surgery is the use of the 2.1 μm holmium:YAG laser. Starting with a Russian prototype and based on theoretic calculations (Siebert and Kohn, 1988; Siebert et al., 1990) I showed that it might be a reasonable system for the future. The first experimental and clinical results were presented in 1991 at the Third International Congress on Lasers in Orthopaedics in Hannover, Germany (Siebert, 1991). The results were promising but also showed the need for prospective randomized clinical studies. Many surgeons in Europe, especially those from Italy, Spain, France, Austria, Switzerland, and Germany, have produced favorable case reports.

Shoulder, knees, elbows, ankles, and especially small joints (wrist) have been treated arthroscopically with lasers. The need for the clinical studies was so obvious that a German and a European study group on lasers in orthopaedics was formed. Multicenter studies for lasers in arthroscopic surgery was started in 1991, and one to study endoscopic and minimally invasive use of lasers for disc and spinal surgery was created as well. The threshold to clinical practice in orthopaedic laser surgery has now been crossed (Limbird, 1990), but lasers must show that their theoretic advantages are matched in practice. This goal not only has been adopted generally in Europe but

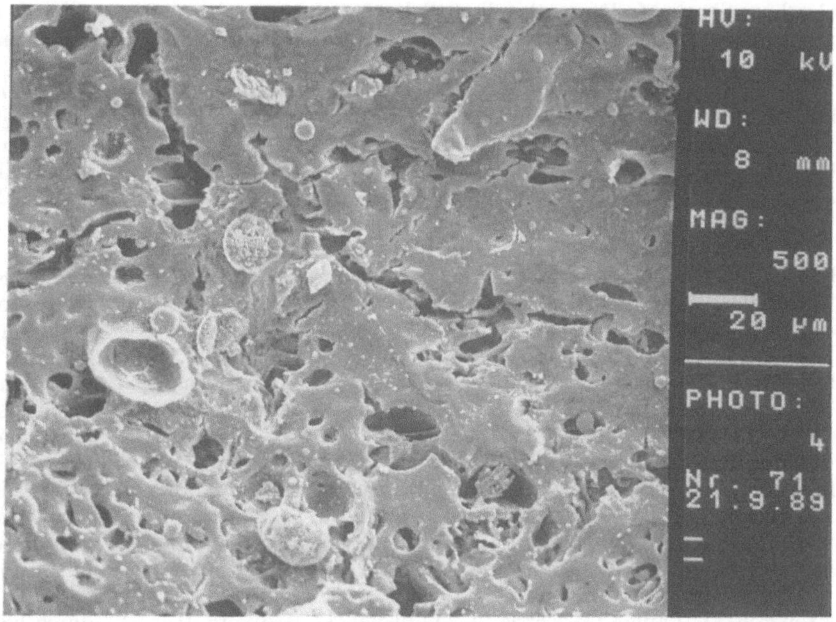

Figure 26-3. Severe thermal damage from free-beam 1.06 μm neodymium:YAG use.

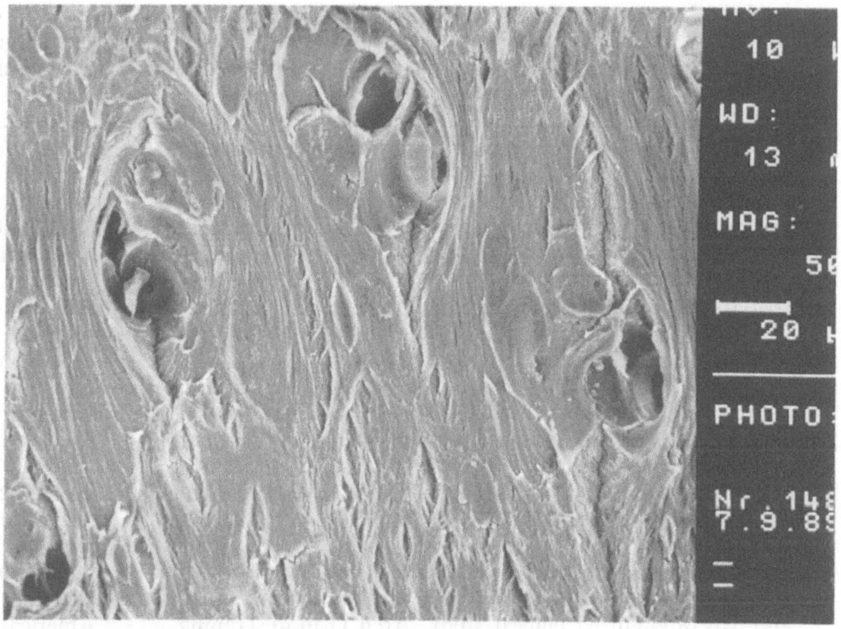

Figure 26-4. Excellent clinical results in cartilage damage types IIa–c and IIIa following 0.308 μm excimer laser chondroplasty.

is also the focus of an international society (International Musculoskeletal Laser Society "IMLAS") founded on April 23, 1993 in Paris. The 1st IMLAS Congress will be held in Neuchâtel, Switzerland in September 1994.

References

Buchelt M, Papaioannou T, Fishbein M, et al. (1991) Excimer laser ablation of fibrocartilage: an in vitro and in vivo study. Lasers Surg Med 11:271

Clauser C (1986) Comparison of depth and profile of osteotomies performed by rapid superpulsed and continuous wave CO_2 laser beams at high power output. J Oral Maxillofac Surg 44:425

Dittrich K, Tuchmann A, Plenk H, et al (1988) Vergleichsstudie Skalpell versus CO_2 laser bei weichteiltumoren im Tierexperiment. Wien, personliche Mitteilung (unveroffentlicht).

Frenz M, Mathelois F, Stoffel MS, et al., (1989) Transport of biologically active material in laser cutting. Lasers Surg Med 8:562

Gerber BE (1991) Ultrastrukturelles bild des Excimer Laser effektes der Knorpelvaporisation. In Siebert WE, Wirth CJ (eds), Lasesr in der Orthopadie. Thieme, Stuttgart, p 62

Glick JM (1984) Use of the laser beam in arthroscopic surgery. In Casscells SW (ed), Arthroscopy: Diagnostic and Surgical Practice, Lea & Febiger, Philadelphia, p 181

Glick JM, Harmon S (1991) The application of carbon dioxide laser and arthroscopy of the knee. Lasers Surg Med Suppl 3:52

Grothues-Spork M, Dinkelaker F, Scholz C, Ramanzadeh R, Muller G (1989) Tierexperimenteller vergleich der heilung nach CO_2, Excimer-Laser und konventioneller Osteotomie am kaninchenmodell. Verhandl Dtsch Ges Lasermed 4:108

Hefti F, Morscher E (1984) Die Anwendung von Laserstrahlen in der Orthopadie. Orthopade 13:119

Hohla K, Henke HW, Pfaff J, Wurth W (1987) Excimer laser for medicine prospects for computer guided surgery. In Proceedings of the 7th Congress International Society for Laser Surgery and Medicine. Springer, Heidelberg, p 15

Hohlbach G, Moller KO, Schramm U, Baretton G (1989) Experimentelle Ergebnisse der Knorpelabrasio mit einem Excimer Laser: histologische und elektronenmikroskopische Untersuchungen. Z Orthop 127:216

Horch HH (1983) Laser-osteotomie und Anwendungsmoglichkeiten des Lasers in der oralen Weichteilchirurgie. In Habilitationsschriften der Zahn-, Mund- und Kieferkeilkunde. Quintessenz-Verlags, Berlin

Imhoff A, Leu HJ (1991) Arthroskopische operationen mit dem excimer laser: erste Erfahrungen. In Siebert WE, Wirth CJ (eds), Laser in der Orthopadie. Thieme, Stuttgart, p 48

Johnson LL (1986) Arthroscopic Surgery (3rd ed). Mosby, St. Louis

Kroitzsch U, Laufer G, Egkher E, Wollenek G, Horvath R (1989) Experimental photoablation of meniscus cartilage by Excimer laser energy: a new aspect in meniscus surgery. Arch Orthop Trauma Surg 108:44

Kroitzsch U, Laufer G, Grimm M, Wollenek G (1988) Photoablation of meniscus tissue by means of a pulsed ultraviolet laser system using a water tissue interface. Presented at the ESKA Congress, Amsterdam

Limbird TJ (1990) Application of laser doppler technology to meniscal injuries. Clin Orthop 252:88–91

Lohnert J, Raunest J (1988) Arthroskopische Synovektomie am kniegelenk unter anwendung des Nd:YAG lasers. Verhandl Dtsch Ges Lasermed 4:294

Pelinka H (1990) Differenzierung verschiedener Kniegelenkstrukturen durch die fluoreszenzspektroskopische Analyse des Laserlichtes. In Siebert WE, Wirth CJ (eds), Laser in der Orthopadie. Thieme, Stuttgart, p 70

Philandrianos G (1984) The CO_2 laser in orthopaedic surgery: 1st results [letter]. Presse Med 13:1151

Philandrianos G (1985) Le laser a gaz carbonique en chirurgie arthroscopique du genou. Presse Med 14:2103

Raunest J, Lohnert J (1989) Arthroskopische Synovektomie unter Anwendung des Neodymium:YAG Laser. Chirurg 60:782

Raunest J, Lohnert J (1990) Arthroscopic cartilage débridement by Excimer laser in chondromalacia of the knee join: a prospective randomized clinical study. Arch Orthop Trauma Surg 109:155

Raunest J, Lohnert J (1991) Arthroskopische behandlung von knorpelschaden mit dem Excimer kaltschnitt laser. In Siebert WE, Wirth CJ (eds), Laser in der Orthopadie. Thieme, Stuttgart, p 57

Richter P, Lange V. Baretton G (1991) Synoviaabtragung am Kaninchenkniegelenk mit dem gepulsten argon Laser. In Siebert WE, Wirth CJ (eds), Einsatzmoglichkeiten des Lasers in der Orthopadie. Thieme, Stuttgart, p 54

Rudolph H, Herberhold HJ (1991) Arthroskopische Operationen im Kniegelenk mit dem CO_2 Laser. In Siebert WE, Wirth CJ (eds), Laser in der Orthopadie. Thieme, Stuttgart. p 74

Schneider D (1986) Comparison of wound healing in thermal knives incisions: contact Nd:YAG laser, superpulse CO_2 laser, saw knife, and electrosurgical knife. Presented to the European Laser Society

Siebert WE (1990) Laserosteotomie mit experimentellen Lasersystemen. Presented at the Habilitationsschrift, Orthopadische Klinik der Medizinischen Hochschule, Hannover

Siebert WE (1991) 3rd International Congress Lasers in Orthopaedics. Hannover, Abstracts. Laseus in orthopaedics in Europe.

Siebert WE, Klanke J, Scholz C, et al., (1990) Rasterelektronenmikroskopische Untersuchungen zur Oberflachenbearbeitung von Knorpelschaden mit Nd:YAG Laser, CO_2 Laser, Excimer Laser, Erbium:YAG Laser und diversen motorgetriebenen Instrumenten. In Proceedings of the 6th Kongress der deutschsprachigen Arbeitsgemeinschaft fur Arthroskopie 13./14. Okt. 1989 Luzern (Schweiz) Buchbeitrag Fortschritte in der Arthroskopie. Enke, Stuttgart, p 82

Siebert WE, Kohn D (1988) Laser as an operative tool in endoscopic operations in orthopaedic surgery. In Waidelich WR (ed), Proceedings of the 7th Congress International Society for Laser Surgery and Medicine. Springer, Berlin, p 192

Siebert WE, Thriene W (1991) Beeinflußung der wundheilung durch helium-neon Laser bestrahlung niedriger Energie. In Siebert WE, Wirth CJ (eds), Laser in der Orthopadie. Thieme, Stuttgart, p 103

Siebert WE, Wirth CJ (1991) Laser in der orthopadie. In Einsatzmoglichkeiten der Lasertechnik bei operativen und diagnostischen Verfahren am Bewegungsapparat. Thieme, Stuttgart

Smith CF, Marshall GJ, Snyder SJ (1984) Comparisons of tissue effects of a surgical scalpel, an electrocautery apparatus and a carbon dioxide laser system when used for making incisions into the menisci of New Zealand rabbits. Lasers Surg Med 3:305

Smith JB, Nance TA (1983) Arthroscopic laser surgery. Presented in part at the Annual Meeting of the Arthroscopy Association of North America, Coronado, CA

Steinmetz M, Hofstetter A (1988) Laserinduzierte verstarkung der wirkung zytotoxischer Substanzen. Lasers Med Surg 2:48

Ulrich F, Durselen R, Schober R (1988) Longterm investigations of laser assisted microvascular anastomoses with the 1318 nm Nd:YAG laser. Lasers Surg Med 8:104

Unsold E, Jocham D (1988) Grundlagen photodynamischer Lasertherapieverfahren. Chirurg 59:76

Whipple TL (1981) Applications of the CO_2 laser to arthroscopic meniscectomy in a gas medium. Presented at the Triannual Meeting of the International Arthroscopy Association; American Arthroscopy Association of North America, Rio de Janeiro

Whipple TL, Caspari RB, Meyers JF (1982) Arthroscopic meniscectomy by carbon dioxide laser vaporization in a gas medium. Orthop Trans 6:136

Whipple TL, Caspari RB, Meyers JF (1983) Laser energy in arthroscopic meniscectomy. Orthopedics 6:1165–1169

Whipple TL, Caspari RB, Meyers JF (1984a) Laser subtotal meniscectomy in rabbits. Lasers Surg Med 3:297–304

Whipple TL, Caspari RB, Meyers JF (1984b) Synovial response to laser induced carbon ash residue. Lasers Surg Med 3:295–295

27

Overview of Current Laser Use in Orthopaedics in the United States

Stephen P. Abelow

10.6 μm CO_2 Laser

The 10.6 μm CO_2 laser is useful in arthroscopy for vaporizing of tissues, cutting, joint débridement, chondroplasty, and meniscectomy. It is an exceptionally useful tool for synovectomy. Whipple (1992) reported that the 10.6 μm CO_2 laser was bactericidal, that superficial wounds could be débrided in the patient's room with only topical anesthesia, and that laser-irradiated wounds healed 4 to 7 days earlier than those treated by conventional methods. In addition to intraarticular use of the 10.6 μm CO_2 laser and wound débridement, the laser has been used for treating skin lesions, excising warts, and treating fungal or infected nails.

The 10.6 μm CO_2 laser has been used for laser-assisted arthroscopic carpal tunnel release and for revision arthroplasty to effect polymethylmethacrylate (PMMA) removal. Utilizing an operating arthroscope, PMMA is almost completely and instantaneously vaporized by the 10.6 μm CO_2 laser. More heat is generated in bone in the setting of the cement than when removing cement with the 10.6 μm CO_2 laser (Sherk, 1990). However, flames of burning methane gas do pose a fire hazard.

2.1 μm Holmium:YAG Laser

The 2.1 μm holmium:YAG laser is useful for vaporizing tissue, cutting, coagulating, and smoothing. It is useful for joint débridement, meniscectomy, chondral ablation, soft tissue release, and synovectomy. With practice, it allows an arthroscopist to smooth and contour a joint surface with elegance.

The 2.1 μm holmium:YAG laser is useful for virtually any joint arthroscopy. With its low profile handpiece, it makes an exceptional tool for small joint arthroscopy. Procedures include the following:

Knee arthroscopy: débridement, meniscectomy, chondroplasty (photochondroplasty), synovectomy, plica excision, lateral release, and cautery of bleeding vessels

Shoulder arthroscopy: coracoacromial ligament release, labral débridement, scar tissue excision and ablation, synovectomy, adhesive capsulitis, frozen shoulder, and SLAP lesion débridement

Ankle arthroscopy: meniscoid lesion, osteochondritis dissecans, synovectomy, spur removal, débridement, and chondroplasty

Wrist arthroscopy: triangular fibrocartilage lesions, chondroplasty, synovectomy, and débridement

Elbow arthroscopy: synovectomy, débridement chondroplasty, and reduction of size of loose bodies

Spine: percutaneous laser nucleotomy and lumbar disc decompression

Oral/maxillofacial surgery: arthroscopic temporomandibular joint surgery

Laser-assisted endoscopic wrist carpal tunnel release

A 1.7 mm diameter flexible 2.1 μm holmium laser/arthroscope is available. It is currently being used for endoscopic disc excision, and with better resolution it may become a useful tool for minimally invasive laser arthroscopic surgery. The 2.1 μm holmium:YAG wavelength is good for laser nucleotomy. Because of its small size, this laser can be used percutaneously or with discoscopy. The 2.1 μm holmium:YAG laser nucleotomy received U.S. Food and Drug Administration (FDA) approval in September 1991.

Ultrasmall combination laser/flexible arthroscopes are being developed. Through a single small portal, laser ablative arthroscopic surgery may become a routine procedure.

1.06 μm Neodymium:YAG Lasers

The 1.06 μm neodymium:YAG laser should be used for arthroscopy only in the contact mode, except for free-beam use for synovectomy. Contact procedures that are done with the 1.06 μm neodymium:YAG laser include the following:

Knee arthroscopy: meniscectomy, lateral release plica excision, excision of arthrofibrotic tissue, synovectomy, cautery of bleeding vessels and chondroplasty

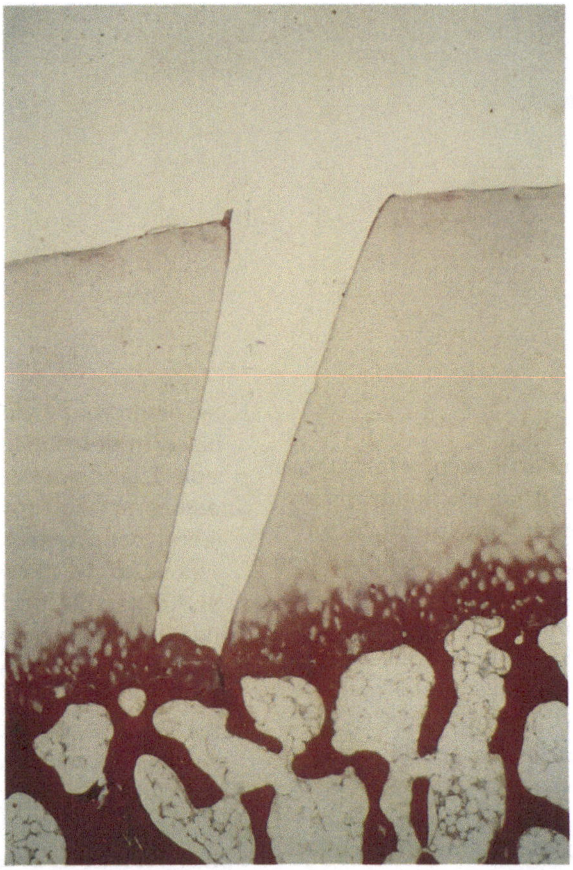

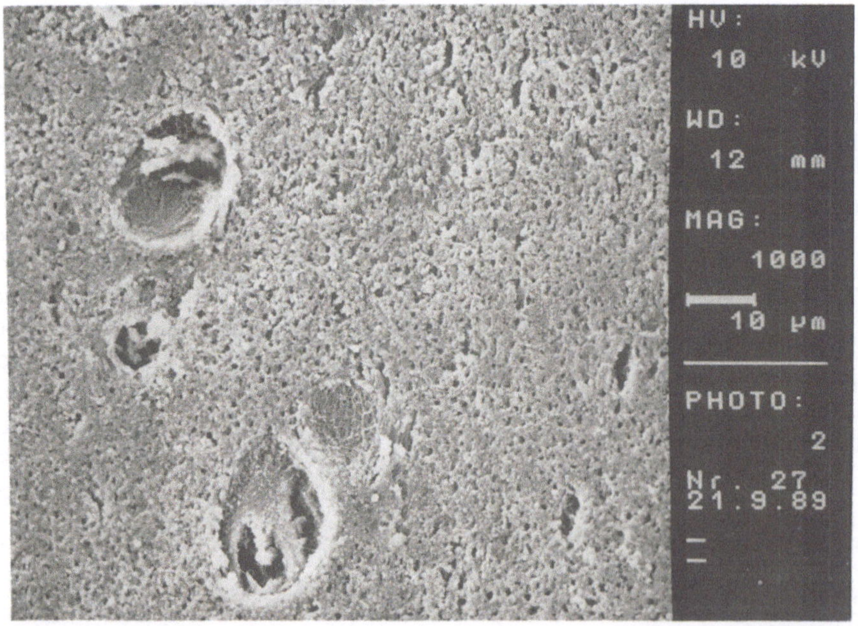

Figure 27-1 and 27-2. Effects of the 2.94 μm erbium:YAG laser on articular cartilage in arthroscopy.

Shoulder arthroscopy: scar tissue removal, débridement of labral tears, coracoacromial ligament release, cautery of bleeding vessels, and synovectomy

The free-beam (noncontact) 1.06 μm neodymium:YAG laser is used in the lumbar spine for percutaneous nucleotomy (with or without discoscopy).

1.44 μm Neodymium:YAG Laser

The 1.44 μm pulsed free-beam neodymium:YAG laser has virtually the same absorption as the 2.1 μm holmium:YAG laser energy. Thus the 1.44 μm neodymium:YAG laser has surgical capabilities similar to those of the 2.1 μm holmium:YAG laser. There is a relatively shallow depth of penetration with the 1.44 μm wavelength, and it can be used to ablate cartilage and other soft tissues. This laser is currently FDA-approved for arthroscopic procedures similar to those approved for the 2.1 μm holmium:YAG laser. It has been approved for percutaneous discectomy.

0.532 μm KTP Laser

The 0.532 μm KTP laser is useful for tissue cutting, coagulation, and disc ablation. An FDA-approved for marketing percutaneous laser discectomy system is available. A side-directed fiber delivery system has been developed to enhance the safety of laser discectomy procedures (a forward-shooting delivery system places the aorta and vena cava in jeopardy of absorbing laser energy). For a simple, uncomplicated disc herniation, percutaneous lumbar laser discectomy may provide a simple outpatient procedure with reasonable outcomes.

With the powers and delivery system currently available, the 0.532 μm KTP laser does not appear to be the most efficient wavelength for arthroscopic surgery. However, the 1.06 μm neodymium:YAG mode of this laser can be used in similar situations as any other 1.06 μm neodymium:YAG laser.

Erbium Laser

Erbium lasers are currently used for experimentation on bone. The 2.94 μm erbium:YAG laser may be market-approved to be used on soft tissues of joints during arthroscopy (Figs. 27-1 and 27-2). No clinical information is available at the time of this writing.

Excimer Laser

The 0.308 μm Excimer laser works well where layers of tissue must be removed; and its use for chondral débridement allows precise sculpting of damaged cartilage surfaces (Glossop et al., 1992). The lased surface seems to "melt." In some cases the 0.308 μm Excimer laser seemed to seal cracks in articular cartilage (Glossop et al., 1992).

The disadvantages of the 0.308 μm Excimer laser are potentially ionizing radiation, low power, cost, and large size. It also tends to be slow for meniscal ablation, and the lasing medium gas is poisonous.

With its ability to cut and ablate tissue precisely, be delivered through flexible fiberoptics in an aqueous medium, produce minimal or no thermal injury, and make a remarkably precise laser cut, it is understandable why the 0.308 μm Excimer laser has incurred so much medical interest. The 0.308 μm Excimer laser is currently experimental in the United States but not in Europe, where it is used arthroscopically for chondroplasty.

Suggested Reading

Abelow S (1993) Use of lasers in orthopedic surgery: current concepts. Orthopedics 16:551–556

Black J, Sherk HH, Meller M, et al., (1992) Wavelength selection in laser arthroscopy. Semin Orthop 7:72–76

Dew D, Supik L, Darrow C. Halpern S (1991) Successful repair of scalpel induced wounds in swine meniscal cartilage using a software controlled 1.3 micron Nd:YAG laser. Presented at the 17th Annual Meeting, American Orthopaedic Society for Sports Medicine, Orlando, FL

Fanton GS (1990) Ho:YAG laser emerges as significant clinical tool for orthopaedic and general surgery cases. Gen Surg News August:8

Fanton GS, Dillingham MF (1992) The use of the holmium laser in arthroscopic surgery. Semin Orthop 7(2):102–116

Garrick J (1992) CO_2 laser arthroscopy using ambient gas pressure. Semin Orthop 7(2):90–94

Glossop N, Jackson R, Randle J, Reed S (1992) The Excimer laser in arthroscopic surgery. Semin Orthop 7(2):125–130

JGM Associates (1991) Orthopaedic surgery applications of advanced solid state laser. JGM, Burlington, MA, pp 5–32

Miller D, O'Brien S, Arnoczky S, et al (1989) The use of the contact Nd:YAG laser in arthroscopic surgery: effects on articular cartilage and meniscal tissue. Arthroscopy 5:245–1253

Sherk HH (ed) (1990) Lasers in Orthopaedics. Lippincott, Philadelphia

Smith CF, Johansen EL, Vangsness CT, et al (1992) "Gas bubble" technique in laser arthroscopic surgery. Semin Orthop 7(2):86–89

Spivak (1991) Metabolic effects of continuous Nd:YAG laser on articular cartilage metabolism. Presented at the Annual Meeting, Arthroscopy Association of North America, San Diego

Whipple T (1992) CO_2 laser surgery. Presented at the Annual Meeting of the American Academy of Orthopaedic Surgeons, Washington, DC

Whipple TL, Caspari RB, Meyer JF (1985) Arthroscopic laser meniscectomy in a gas medium. Arthroscopy 1:2–7

28

1.06 μm Neodymium:YAG Contact Arthroscopic Laser Surgery: 61 Cases

O. Sahap Atik

Because of breakthroughs in 1.06 μm neodymium:YAG contact fiber technology, these lasers have become useful for arthroscopy. They capture the laser energy at the tip of the fiber and convert it to thermal energy. They are capable of producing precise cutting, vaporizing, and coagulating in joint tissues with minimal thermal damage (O'Brien et al., 1991; Sherk, 1991). The purpose of the clinical study reported here was to evaluate the benefits of 1.06 μm neodymium:YAG contact laser for arthroscopy.

Materials and Methods

Sixty-one patients were treated with arthroscopic surgery using the 1.06 μm neodymium:YAG contact laser. Their mean age was 38 years (range 18–66 years). The follow-up period was 4 to 10 months.

The pathology was in knees in 57 patients and in shoulders in 4. In the knee joint, lateral retinacular release was performed in 6 patients, partial synovectomy in 7, chondroplasty in 26, débridement in 24, and partial meniscectomy in 21. Only débridement and partial synovectomy were done in shoulder joints. During these procedures, 15 to 40 watts of laser energy was used. All the surgeries were performed under general, regional, or local anesthesia. Active motion exercises were started, and full weight-bearing was allowed on the first post-operative day.

Results

The 1.06 μm neodymium:YAG laser was used in all cases with no complications. Bleeding and swelling were minimal, and wound healing was normal. There was no complication due to the laser instruments. All of the patients started active joint motions immediately, and all were able to walk with full weight-bearing on the first day after surgery. The recovery and rehabilitation period were short, and their return to work was rapid. There were no infections, severe postoperative swelling, or pain. None of the patients was reoperated. There were no breakages of the probe. The effectiveness of the tips of the probes, however, was not consistent: Some worked well, but some did not.

Discussion

Lasers in arthroscopic surgery have many potential advantages over conventional surgical methods (Trauner et al., 1990; Garcia, 1991; O'Brien et al., 1991; Sherk, 1991; Atik et al., 1992). They include minimal mechanical trauma to cartilage and other tissues, greater accessibility to difficult areas of the joints, and minimal bleeding. The 1.06 μm neodymium:YAG laser operates effectively in a fluid medium, allowing continuous irrigation of the joint with saline (Garcia, 1991; O'Brien et al., 1991; Atik et al., 1992).

In this series, there was no scuffing of the articular tissue, no joint trauma, and no significant bleeding. The results confirm that the recovery time achieved using the 1.06 μm neodymium:YAG contact laser are good.

References

Atik OS, Sener E, Bolukbasi S, Cila E (1992) Laser in arthroscopic surgery. J Arthroplasty 5:1–3

Garcia PG (1991) Arthroscopic laser surgery in treating the knee injuries of leading professional athletes. Am J Arthrosc 9:15

O'Brien SJ, Garrick JG, Jackson RW, et al (1991) Lasers in orthopaedic surgery. Contemp Orthop 1:61–91

Sherk HH (1991) Orthopaedist using lasers in surgery. Am J Arthrosc 9:7–8

Trauner K. Nishioka N, Patel D (1990) Pulsed Ho:YAG laser ablation of fibrocartilage and articular cartilage. Am J Sports Med 3:316–320

29

1.44 μm Neodymium:YAG Arthroscopic Laser Surgery: Initial Impressions

Allen T. Brillhart

The 2.1 μm holmium:YAG laser has been useful for operative arthroscopy of the knee and other joints. It had not been challenged by a "like–kind" alternative until the development of the 1.44 μm neodymium:YAG laser. Both of these systems were developed with the arthroscopist in mind. In October 1992, I performed the first arthroscopic laser surgery with the 1.44 μm neodymium:YAG laser (Fig. 29-1). Since that time, until the time of this writing, fewer than 100 cases have been performed using prototype devices.

Initial Clinical Experience

The techniques of ablation and cutting of meniscal tissue, ablation of synovium, and other joint tissue are the same as for the 2.1 μm holmium:YAG laser. They are described by Fanton, Dillingham, Guhl, Mooar, Thorpe, Larson, and Walker elsewhere in this text. The surgical advantages of this system are similar to those of the 2.1 μm holmium:YAG laser (Fig. 29-2). A detailed description of the device and its delivery system is discussed in chapter 25.

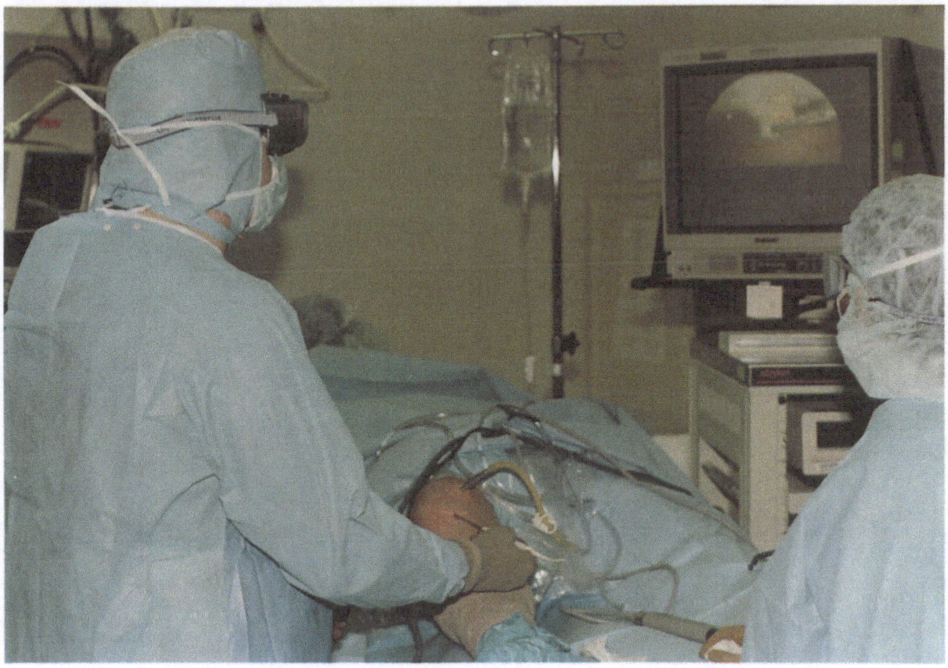

Figure 29-1. Dr. Brillhart performing the first 1.44 μm neodymium:YAG laser arthroscopy.

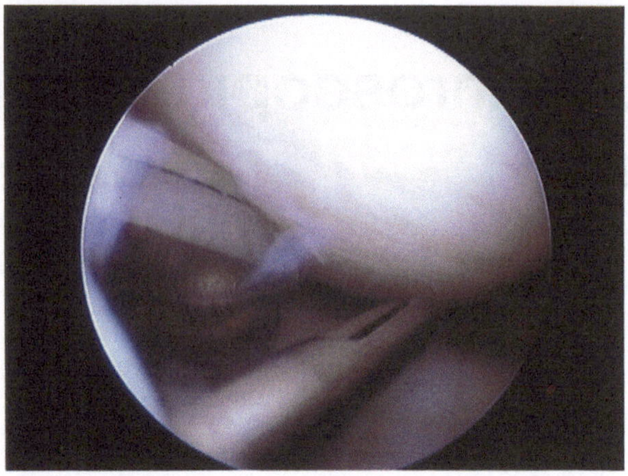

Figure 29-2. Comparison of the size of the 1.44 μm neodymium:YAG laser probe (smaller instrument) and a mechanical shaver (larger instrument).

In my series of fewer than 50 cases, the immediate postoperative results have been similar to those seen with the use of the 2.1 μm holmium:YAG laser. There have been no cases of phlebitis, no infections, no need for reoperation, no need for arthrotomy, no severe postoperative pain, no prolonged recovery, no laser accidents, no patient complication attributable to the laser, and no patient dissatisfaction.

Prototype probes and delivery systems were used. The problems encountered were minor and have been or are being corrected in the commercially available models. They included electrical hookup difficulties, and the prototype rigid probes were actually malleable.

Case illustrations are seen in Figures 29-3 to 29-6. These first procedures included chondroplasty (Fig. 29-3), partial synovectomy (Fig. 29-4), lateral release (Fig. 29-5), and partial meniscectomy (Fig. 29-6).

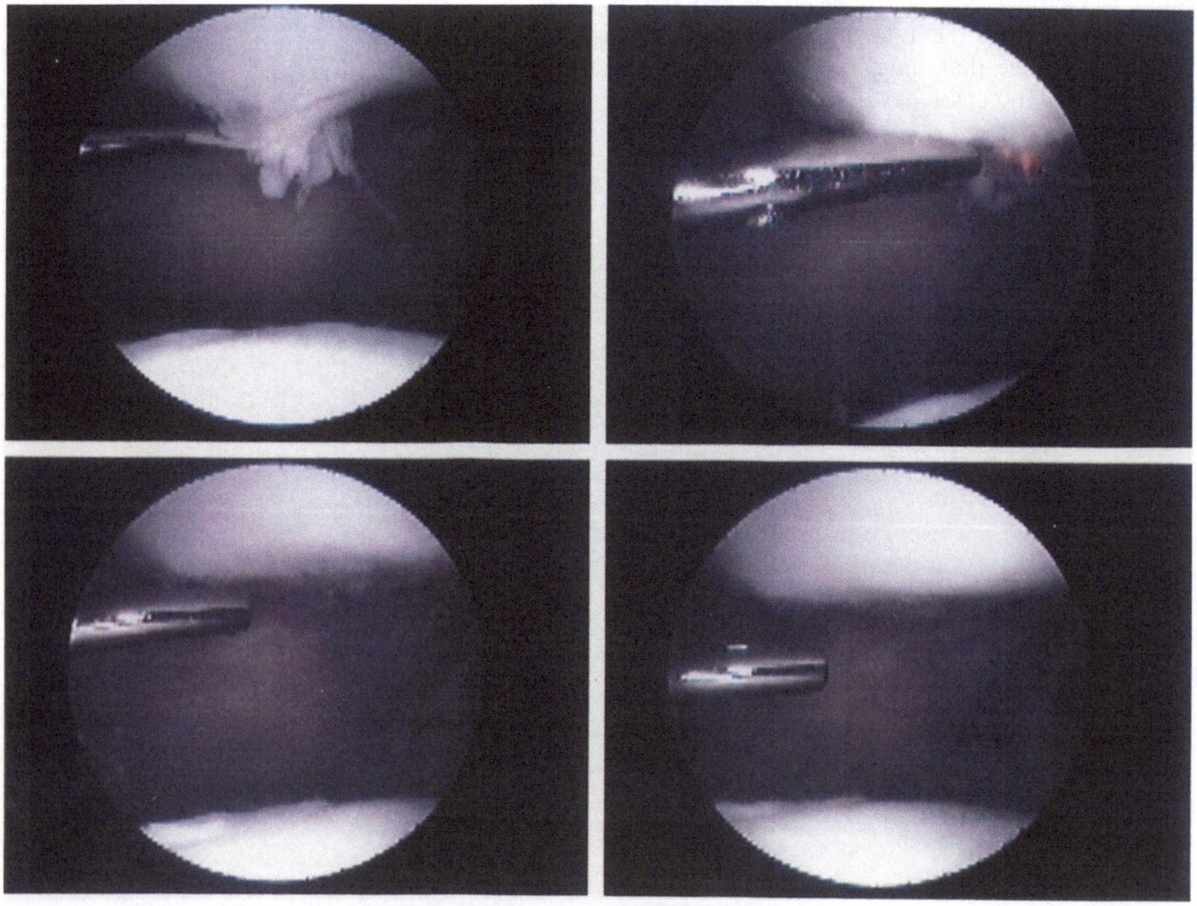

Figure 29-3. Chondroplasty.

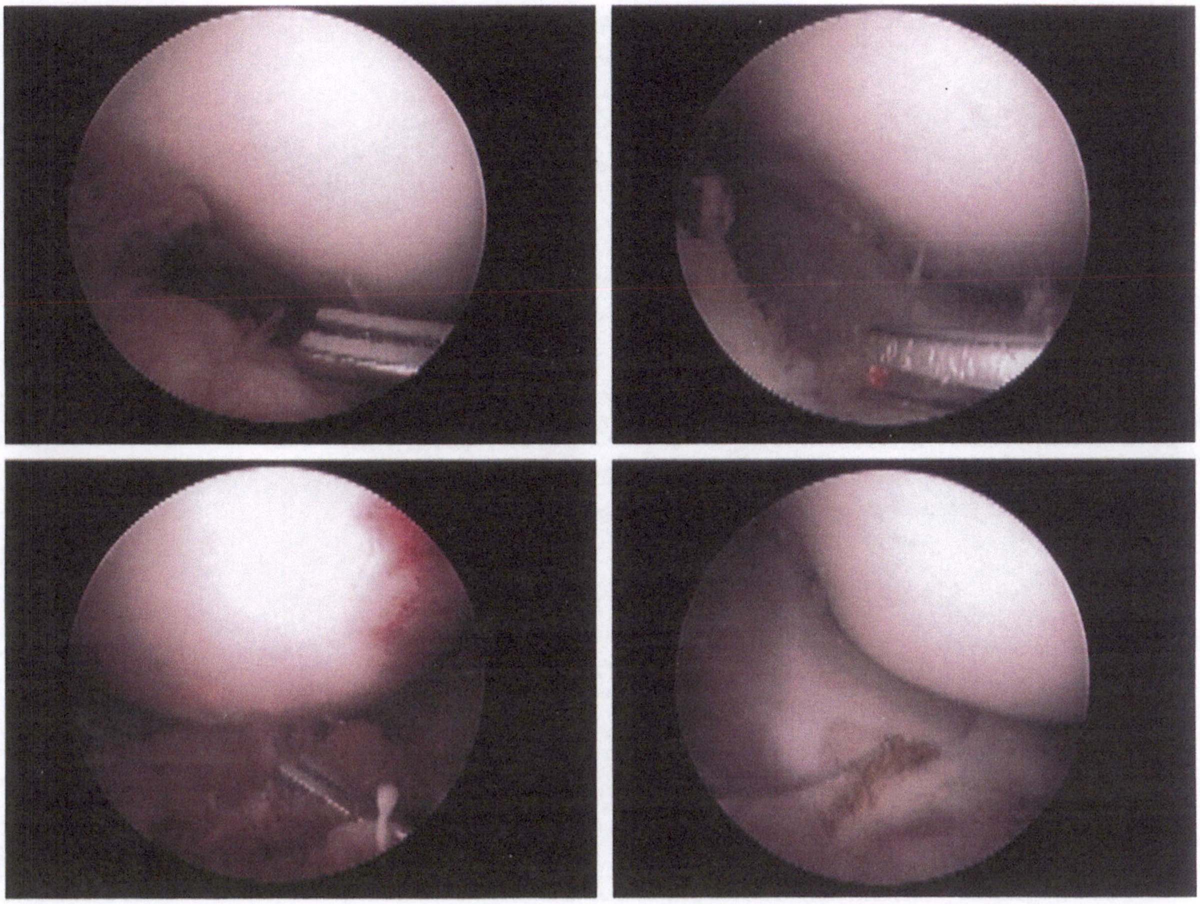

Figure 29-4. Partial synovectomy.

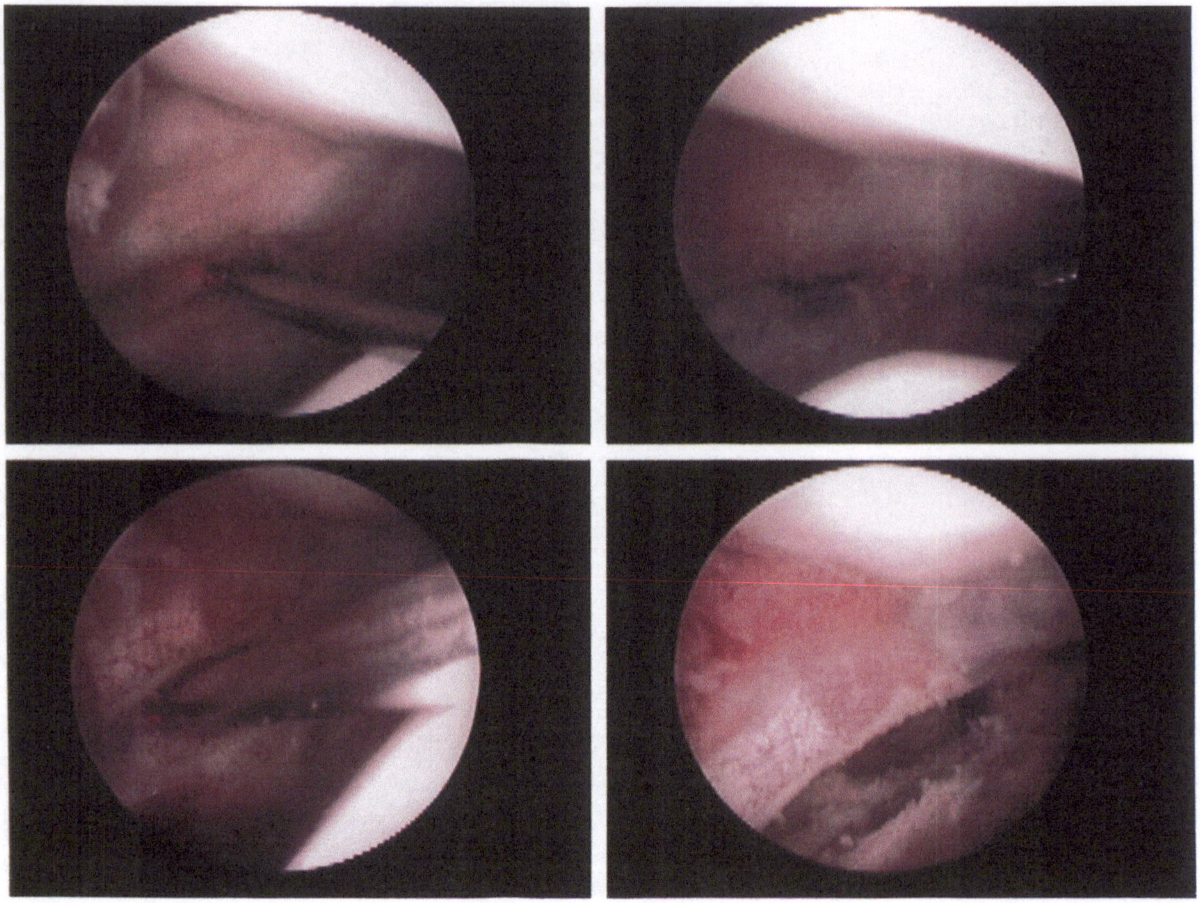

Figure 29-5. Lateral release.

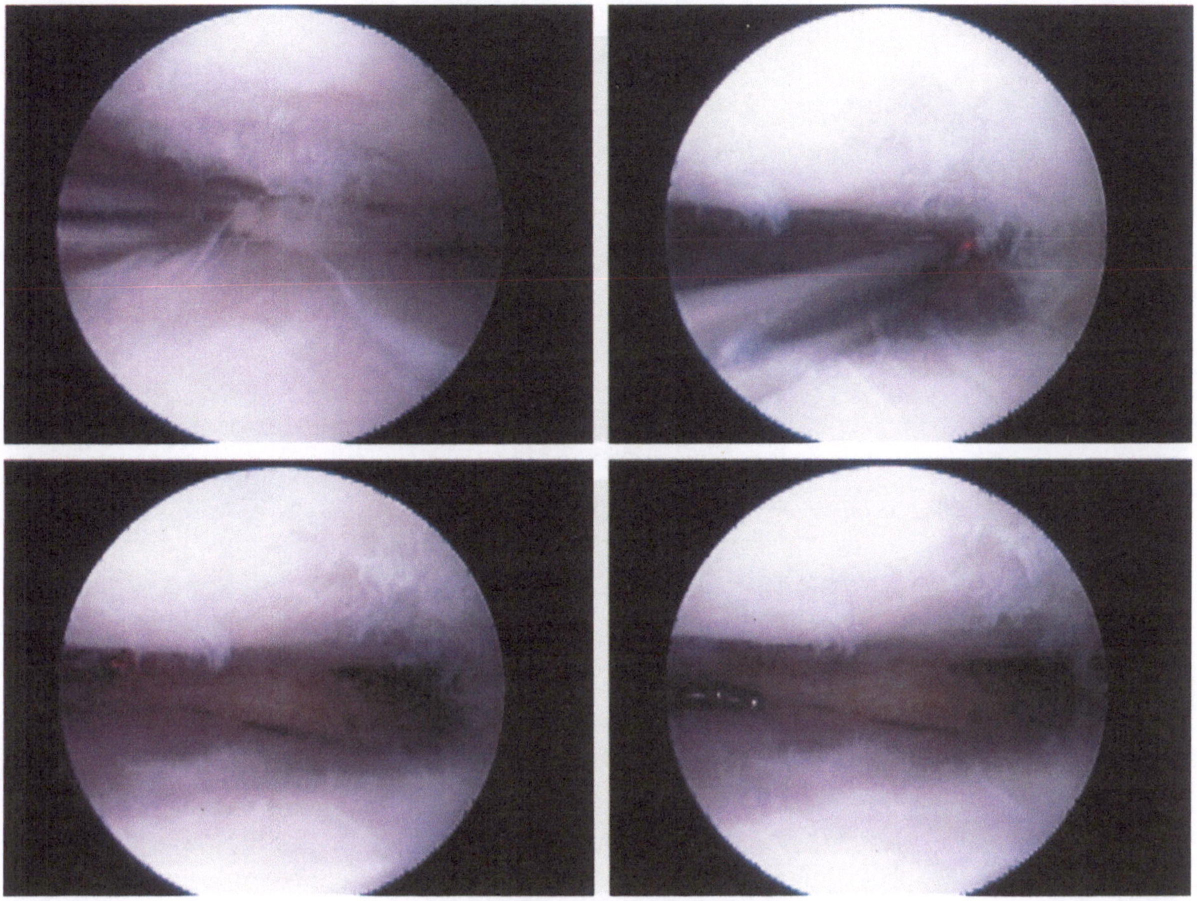

Figure 29-6. Partial meniscectomy.

Conclusion

Based on initial impressions and the excellent immediate postoperative results, I believe that the 1.44 μm neodymium:YAG laser performs initially as well as any other currently available solid-state arthroscopic laser system. Its advantages include less noise, a small size, and a wide choice of energy settings. Long-term results and large clinical series are not available at this time.

Suggested Reading

Brillhart AT (1993a) Ablation efficiency determination using the 1.44 micron neodymium:YAG laser. SPIE Proc 1880:29–30

Brillhart AT (1993b) Arthroscopic laser surgery of the knee using the new 1.44 micron neodymium:YAG laser. Presented at the Second International Symposium on Lasers in Orthopaedics, Boca Raton, FL

Cummings RS, Prodoehl JA, Rhodes A, Black JD, Sherk HH (1993) Nd:YAG 1.44 laser ablation of human cartilage. SPIE Proc. 1880:34–36

30

10.6 μm CO_2 Arthroscopic Laser Surgery of the Knee: Practical and Useful Applications

Raul A. Marquez

Techniques in arthroscopic operative intervention of knee joint pathology have undergone revolutionary changes. The addition of the 10.6 μm CO_2 laser is a complementary adjunct to the instrumentation currently available to the orthopedic surgeon. It has been the most utilized form of laser arthroscopy during the first decade of arthroscopic laser surgery.

Much has been written regarding arthroscopic 10.6 μm CO_2 laser physics, basic surgical principles, possible uses, problems, and complications; but few practical applications, technique suggestions, or clinical results are available. The purpose of this chapter is to share information on proved surgical techniques using the 10.6 μm CO_2 laser for arthroscopic surgery of the knee and to present clinical results to substantiate its efficacy after the use of this technique in 206 cases.

The knee pathology addressed in this study includes chondromalacia, meniscal tears, and pathologic plicas. We suggest that the 10.6 μm CO_2 laser is the instrument of choice for the treatment of chondromalacia. We also believe that there is not an instrument better suited to perform partial meniscectomies of difficult to reach posterior horn tears than the 10.6 μm CO_2 laser.

Technique

The knee is initially distended to 45 to 60 cm^3 with normal saline to facilitate introducing the arthroscope using the distal lateral parapatellar approach. A double-port batwing cannula to control the inflow and outflow proc dures as necessary is preferred. The cannula has a routing ring that allows the surgeon to achieve the greatest visual advantage. A 30 degree arthroscope is inserted via the 5.8 mm cannula to ascertain an adequate field of view (Fig.30-1).

A double-sleeved gas evacuation cannula is introduced via the suprapatellar pouch for fluid outflow. Fluid inflow is achieved by connecting the inflow tubing to a port on the scope cannula. Control of inflow is possible using the bat-wing stopcock (Fig. 30-2).

Normal anatomic structures and pathologic lesions are identified while using the aqueous medium. A third portal is created on the inferomedial parapatellar area for the probe, manual instrument, mechanical débrider, or laser probe insertion. This portal is created under arthroscopic visualization within the joint by inserting a spinal needle prior to creating the stab wound (Fig. 30-3, 30-4, 30-5). This technique allows the surgeon to insert the knife blade under direct vision without damage to the cartilaginous structures.

The final decision to use the laser is made intraoperatively. The saline is evacuated from the knee joint via suprapatellar cannula suction outflow and suction outflow from the port adjacent to the inflow port of the scope cannula. The laser gas/fluid tubing pack allows rapid exchange of fluid with CO_2 gas for laser use (Fig. 30-6).

After saline evacuation is achieved, the laser with a straight or a 30, 60, or 90 degree probe is inserted via the medial parapatellar or lateral suprapatellar portal depending on the location of the lesion to be vaporized. With the laser probe in the appropriate position, CO_2 gas is used to replace the evacuated saline and achieve knee joint distention at a pressure of 1.5 pounds per square inch. The CO_2 gas provides the surgeon with the most precise physiologic view of lesions within the knee, lacking the distortion that is common with saline distention. A tourniquet is used to minimize the chance of a gas emboli. The surgeon directs the aiming beam of the 10.6 μm CO_2 laser at the tissue to be vaporized and controls the power output with a foot pedal. Prior to use, the laser is calibrated to 35 ms of gated energy at 20 watts.

The surgeon must develop the proper sweeping motion

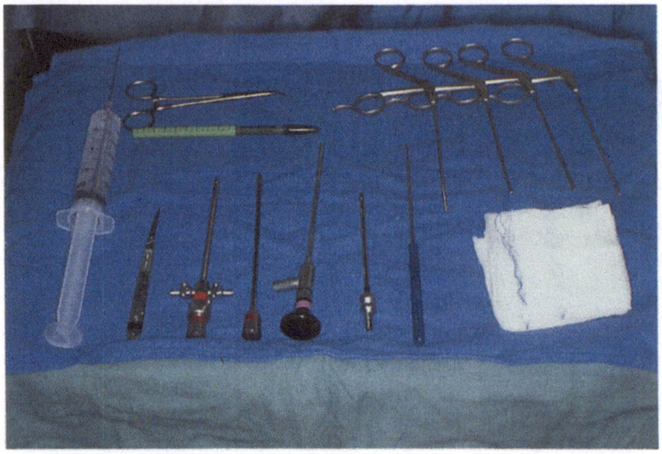

Figure 30-1. Basic arthroscopic instrumentation. (Bottom, left to right) Syringe (60 cc) filled with NS, 18g-3.5; No. 11 knife blade; double-port bat-wing cannula with sharp trocar; blunt trocar; 30 degree arthroscope; gas evacuation cannula; 2 mm probe. (Top, left to right) Hemostat; straight right/left 2.7 mm punch; 2.7 mm grasper.

to enhance the use and efficacy of the 10.6 μm CO_2 laser. Vaporization of pathologic tissue produces carbonization. Once the surface tissue is completely carbonized, the CO_2 gas is replaced by saline lavage, and irrigation of the knee joint is initiated. The carbon must be removed from underlying tissue by irrigation in conjunction with gentle manual débridement using an arthroscopic probe. The above sequence of events may be repeated until pathologic soft tissue is ablated down to healthy tissue. The plume from the 10.6 μm CO_2 laser may be evacuated via the suprapatellar cannula suction or the suction port of the scope cannula.

I prefer a pump lavage system for inflow of fluid due to its ease of use and ability to rapidly exchange fluid within the joint. The presence of two suction outflow ports creates an excellent field of view at all times. The use of the tourniquet is minimized by inflating it only prior to CO_2 gas distention of the knee. Tourniquet use while utilizing CO_2 gas to distend the joint prevents subcutaneous emphysema of the affected extremity from tracking above the level of the tourniquet, and it minimizes the risk of gas emboli. During the postoperative course, the patient is allowed immediate ambulation and full weight-bearing. Occasionally, physical therapy is required to regain full range of motion.

Technique Pearls

Laser technology adds a new dimension to arthroscopic surgery, but like any new technology it has a learning period. The following helpful hints may speed accommodation to this tool:

1. Be skilled at gas arthroscopy before attempting laser arthroscopy in a gas medium.
2. Small "stab wound" incisions allow minimal escape of gas.
3. A double-lumen cannula with the arthroscope is ideal for suctioning fluid where a laser is to be used.
4. Rotate the laser angled probes (38, 60, and 90 degrees) to your advantage.
5. Irrigate and débride (using the probe) the carbonized tissue periodically under saline medium. This proce-

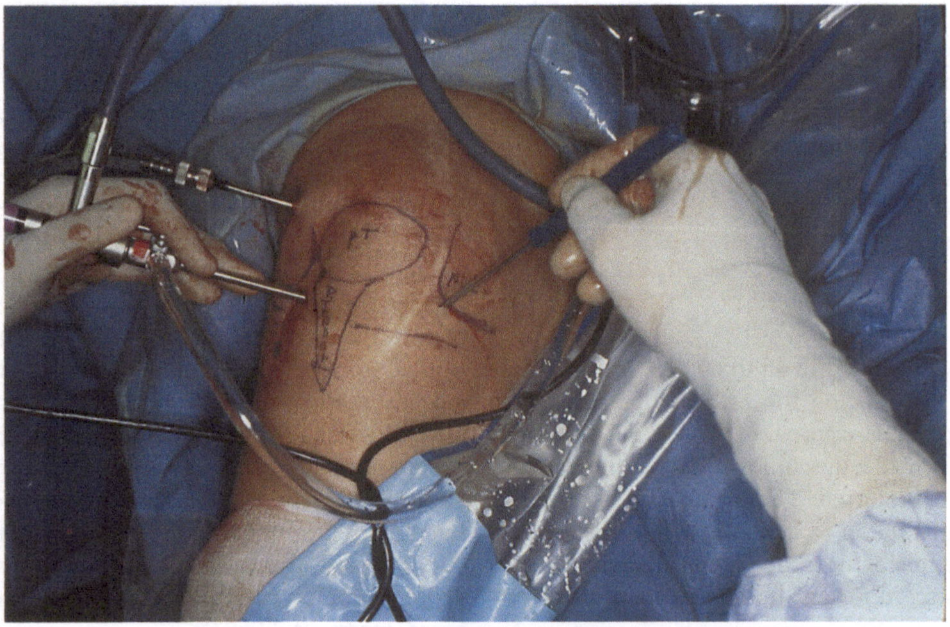

Figure 30-2. Inflow is achieved via a port on the arthroscope cannula. Outflow is achieved via a gas evacuation cannula placed in the suprapatellar pouch.

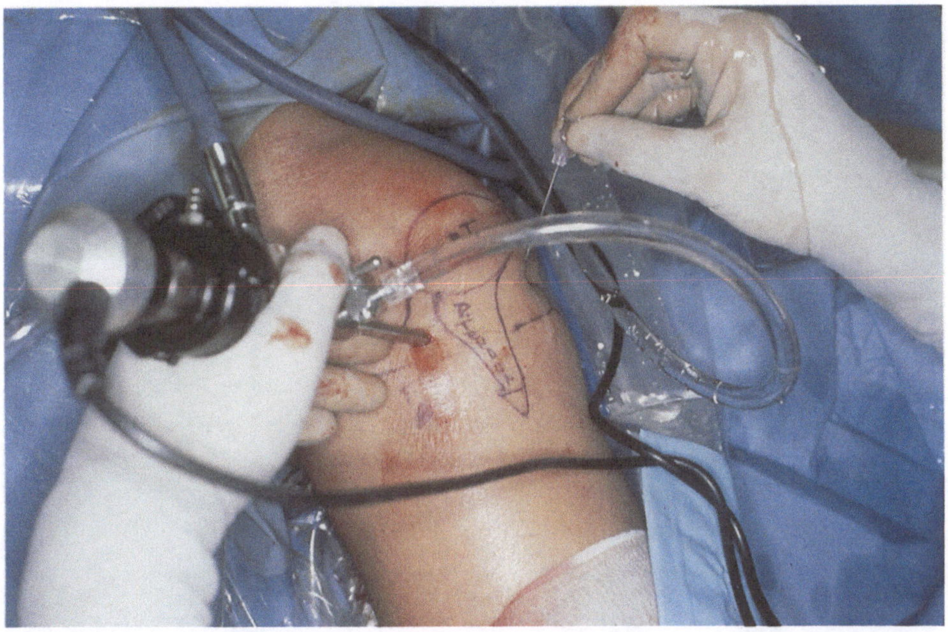

Figure 30-3. Creation of a third portal with the spinal needle under direct visualization.

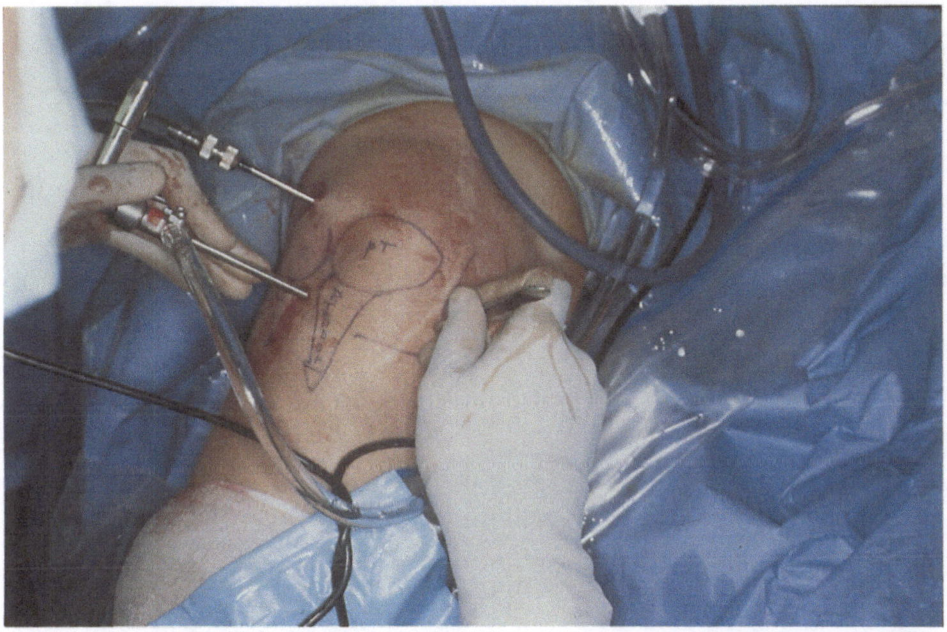

Figure 30-4. Creation of the stab wound for the third portal.

dure (gas–saline–gas) also allows comparison of pathology and review of progress under two visual fields.

6. Should the lens of the arthroscope become clouded by the smoke plume, "clean" it by rubbing it against the synovium.

Laser Safety

1. **Do not use this technique in the shoulder, spine, or temporomandibular joint.**
2. **Do not use gas arthroscopy to repair acute injuries, especially those associated with intraarticular fractures or large open vascular beds.**
3. **Be aware of how to minimize, diagnose, and treat gas emboli intraoperatively and postoperatively. Read the anesthesia literature on this topic.**
4. **Inform the patient before surgery of the rare possibility of gas emboli and permanent neurologic sequelae (including death), even though you may never have personally seen a case.**

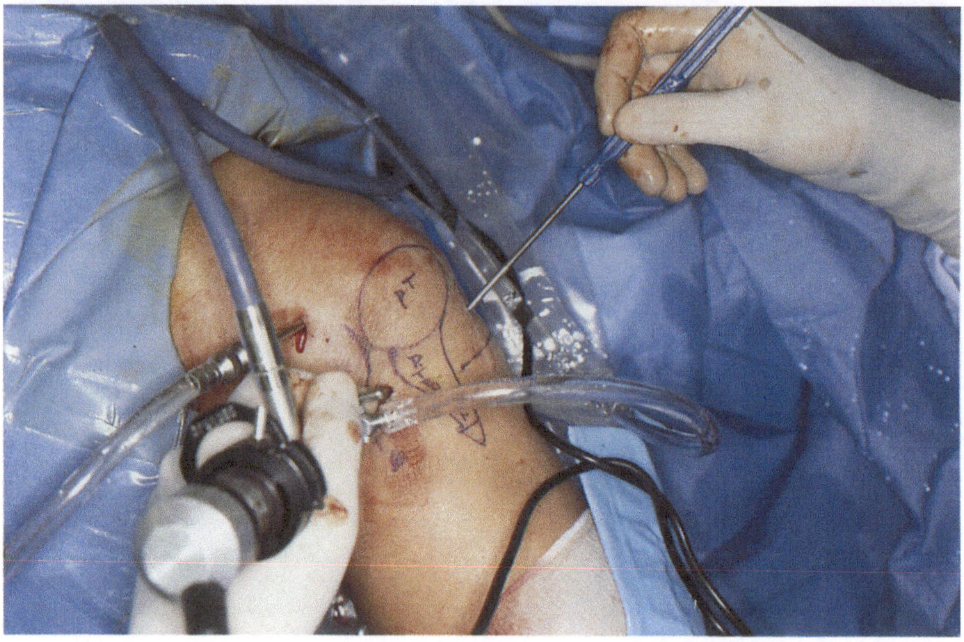

Figure 30-5. Insertion of the arthroscopic probe for manipulation.

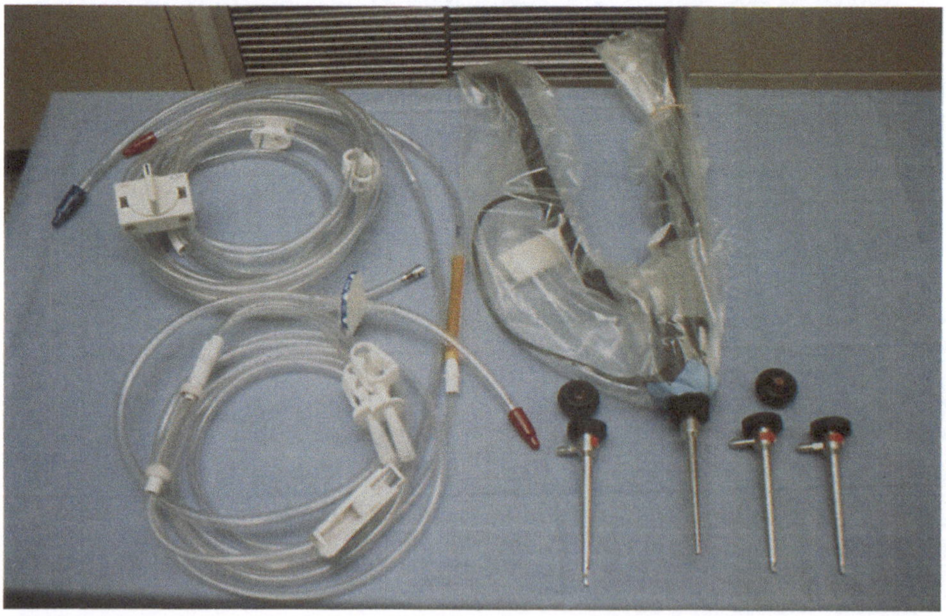

Figure 30-6. (left to right) Laser gas-fluid tubing; laser handpiece with straight, 30, 60, and 90 degree waveguides.

5. Do not deliver pressure over the safe limits (never more than 1.5 pounds per square inch), even if the joint does not distend.
6. Use minimal but adequate CO_2 distention (1.0–1.5 pounds per square inch in the knee).
7. Use a tourniquet when gas distention of the knee is used to minimize proximal dissection of subcutaneous emphysema and the rare possibility of emboli.
8. Use a small amount of continuous intraarticular suction to evacuate the smoke plume and to prevent excessive joint pressure.

Results

The 10.6 μm CO_2 laser was utilized for 206 arthroscopies requiring either a partial meniscectomy, a chondroplasty, or a pathologic plica excision from April 1989 to December 1991. Of the 206 patients, 114 (55%) were male and 92 (45%) female.

Procedures included 116 medial meniscectomies, 50 lateral meniscectomies, 188 chondroplasties, and 29 plica vaporizations. There was a total of 283 of these 10.6 μm CO_2 laser procedures.

Short-term complications included 1 deep vein thrombosis, 1 case of delayed skin healing, 46 episodes of effusions (any degree), 71 cases of mild to moderate pain, 9 patients with decreased range of motion (requiring physical therapist consult), and 19 with subcutaneous emphysema (>3 hours postoperatively). There were no gas emboli, deaths, arthrotomies, or cases of severe pain.

The average surgical time was 35 minutes. The average time for meniscectomy was about 7 minutes. A tourniquet was used in all cases at 200 mm Hg during gaseous joint distention to limit proliferation of subcutaneous emphysema proximally. The average tourniquet time was 15 minutes. Subcutaneous emphysema was absorbed entirely by approximately 90 minutes after operation except in 19 cases, which required no more than 6 hours for full reabsorption.

Our short-term clinical results are encouraging: 93% of patients experienced excellent results, and 7% had good results. The chief complaint in the "good" cases was discomfort over the arthroscopic portals that persisted no longer than 2 to 3 weeks postoperatively.

Discussion

The U.S. Food and Drug Administration's (FDA) market approval of the 10.6 μm CO_2 laser in 1988 has been embraced indifferently by the orthopaedic community. Early frustrating reports labeled carbonized tissue residue and the effects of laser by-products as etiologic agents in postoperative synovitis and tense effusions (Smith and Nance, 1983). We now know that effective débridement and irrigation of charred tissue and the evacuation of the smoke plume make a reactive complication almost unheard of (Garrick and Kadel, 1991). Subcutaneous emphysema lasting longer than a few hours postoperatively has rarely occurred since a CO_2 gas medium replaced the formerly used nitrogen gas medium (Smith and Nance, 1988). There is an unpublished report of permanent neurologic sequelae associated with a gas embolus during CO_2 laser arthroscopy. Abelow (1992) has reported one case of pneumopericardium and pneumoperitoneum. There were no permanent sequelae. At least one case of death has been reported in a nonlaser case using gas distention (Grunwald, 1993). I have never experienced these problems using my technique, but the surgeon must be familiar with how to diagnose and treat gas emboli, and the patient must be informed of this rare possibility preoperatively (Shupak et al., 1984). A surgeon should be skilled in gas and water arthroscopy prior to 10.6 μm CO_2 laser arthroscopy use.

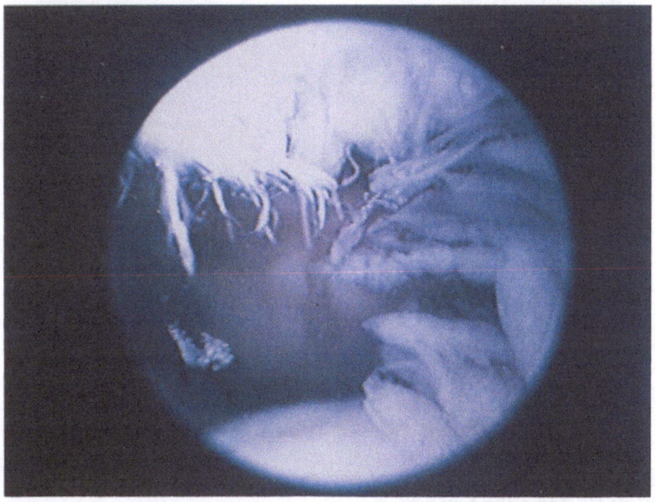

Figure 30-7. Chondromalacia of the patella, grade III; under saline medium.

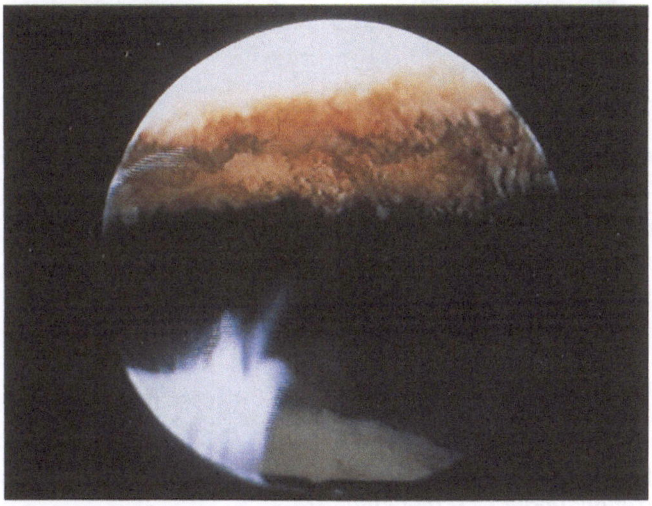

Figure 30-8. Chondromalacia patella after vaporization and cleaning; under saline medium.

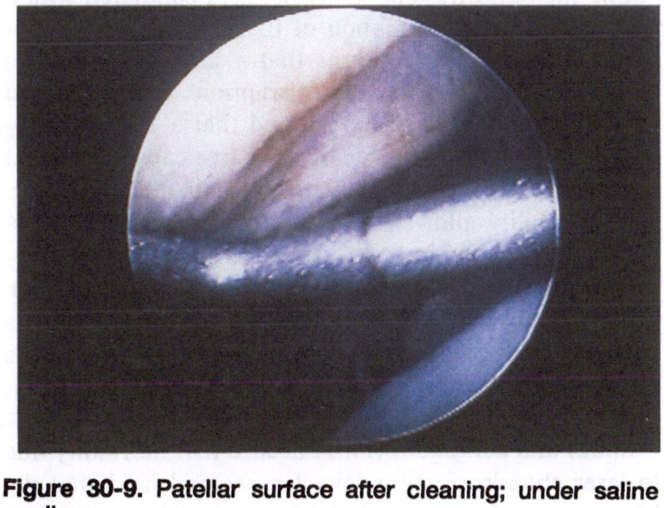

Figure 30-9. Patellar surface after cleaning; under saline medium.

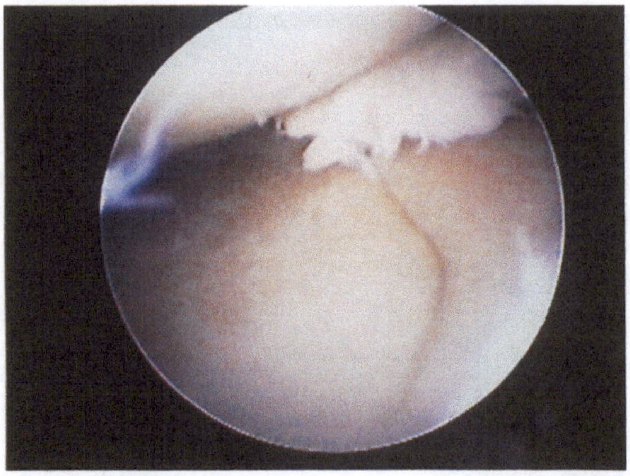

Figure 30-10. Flap tear of the posterior horn medial meniscus; under saline medium.

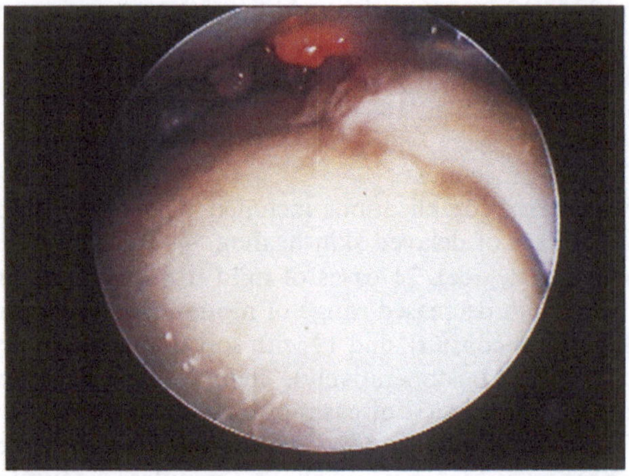

Figure 30-11. Laser beam focused on a flap tear of medial meniscus; under CO_2 medium.

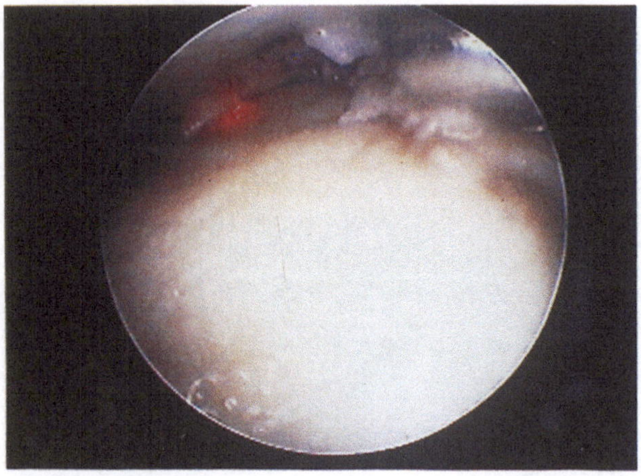

Figure 30-12. Flap tear of the medial meniscus after vaporization; under CO_2 medium.

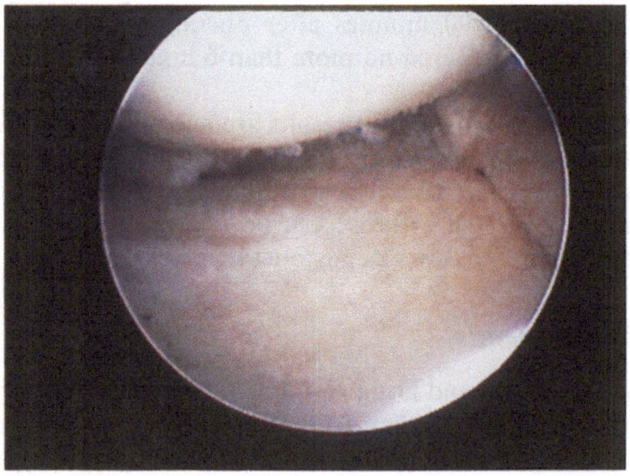

Figure 30-13. Post-operative view of medial meniscus tear; under saline medium.

Riddell (1990) outlined advantages of a CO_2 medium, noting the optically superior visual field compared with a fluid medium and no motion of tissue within the arthroscopic field. Former concerns that a laser may produce insidious wide margin tissue disruption were addressed by Smith et al. (1989), who showed that a 10.6 μm CO_2 laser has specifically directed destructive capabilities that produce a zone of tissue alteration less than 50 μm thick. This capability allows controlled, consistently reproducible depths of incision. By way of comparison, electrocautery produces a zone of tissue alteration 500 μm thick (Miller et al., 1987). In fact, there are some indications that the laser may induce replication of cartilage cells (Norton 1982: Schultz et al., 1985; Herman and Khosla, 1987).

Smith and colleagues (1989) believe that morbidity due to laser chondroplasty is low. I agree and hold that the laser may be the tool of choice for sculpturing the articular surfaces of the femur, tibia, and patella because of its less traumatic effect on healthy articular cartilage (figs. 30-7, 30-8, 30-9).

The 10.6 μm CO_2 laser is useful in areas of limited access, particularly the posterior horn of the medial and lateral menisci. Meniscectomy by vaporization of pathologic tissue using "nontouch" laser techniques can be performed in spaces of about 2 mm (Figs. 30-10 to 30-13).

Other advantages of laser partial meniscectomy over mechanical meniscal débridement include avoidance of damage to nearby articular cartilage and having a smoother, well carved edge on the resected meniscus. The superiority of the laser over mechanical instrumentation regarding treatment of pathologic plicas lies in the fact that pathologic tissue is vaporized rather than débrided; hence there is no loose tissue in the joint requiring removal (Figs. 30-14 to 30-17).

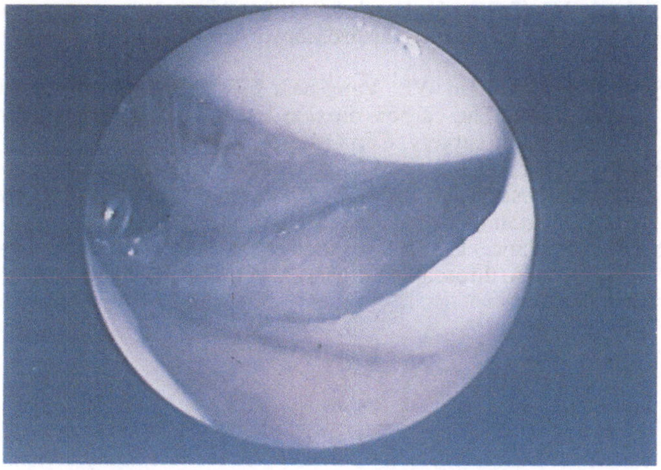

Figure 30-14. Plica; under CO_2 medium.

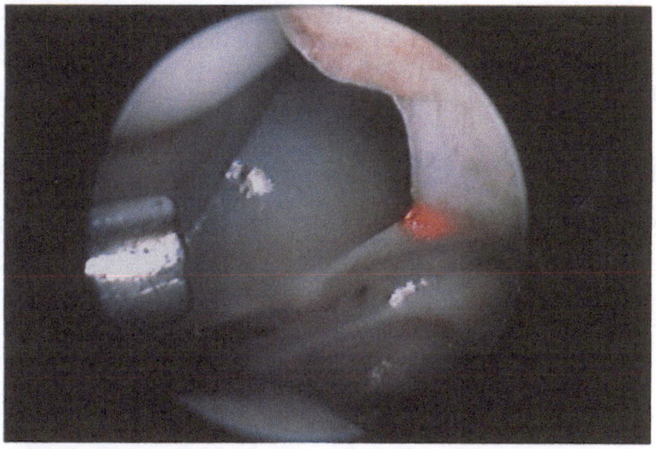

Figure 30-15. Laser beam focused on plica; under CO_2 medium.

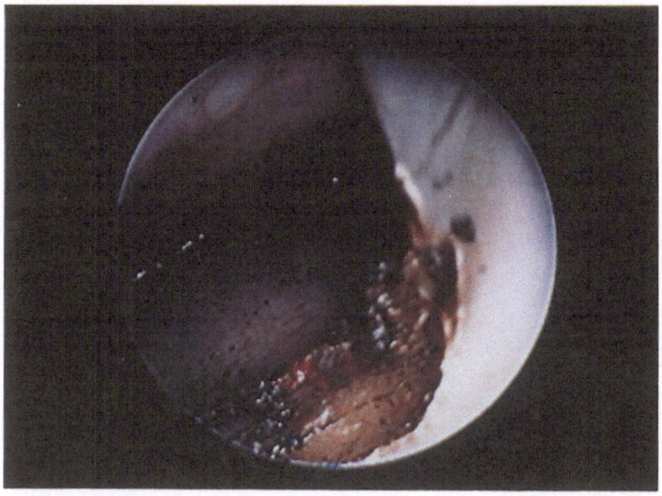

Figure 30-16. Postvaporized plica; under CO_2 medium.

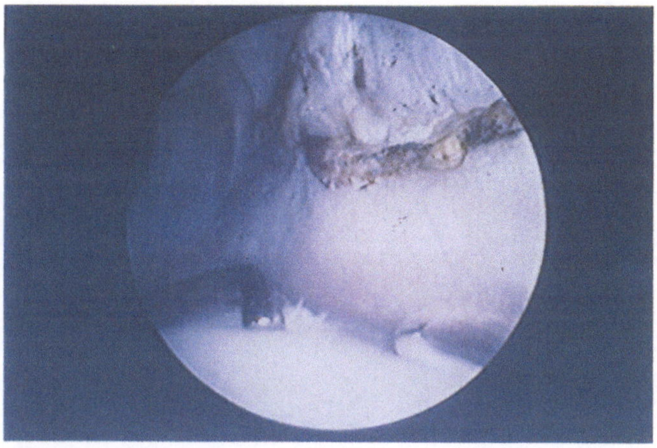

Figure 30-17. Postoperative view of vaporized plica after cleaning; under saline medium.

Conclusion

Arthroscopic knee surgery aided by the 10.6 μm CO_2 laser is a safe, reliable, reproducible procedure in my experience. It is my instrument of choice for sculpting diseased articular cartilage. Not only does the laser leave a smoothly carved surface, it is able to vaporize thin layers of cartilage, thereby leaving as much healthy underlying cartilage as possible. This chapter has described the use of the 10.6 μm CO_2 laser in the knee only. It should not be used in the shoulder, spine, or temporomandibular joint. Use in other joints is not discussed. The most predominant short-term complication, subcutaneous emphysema, has not been clinically significant owing to its rapid reabsorption. We have not seen the rarely reported gas emboli that result in permanent neurologic sequelae or death (Grunwald, 1993). However, surgeons who undertake any form of gas arthroscopy must be familiar with how to minimize recognize and treat these rare complications should they occur (Shupak et al., 1984). The possibility of unforeseen long-term sequelae remains. Nevertheless, the 10.6 μm CO_2 laser is truly a complement to traditional arthroscopic instrumentation, and it is a strong adjunct in the knee arthroscopist's armamentarium when the technique described here is used.

References

Abelow S (1992) Lasers in orthopaedics. Presented at the American Academy of Orthopaedic Surgeons Continuing Medical Education Course, Richmond, VA

Garrick JG, Kadel N (1991) The CO_2 laser in arthroscopy: potential problems and solutions. Arthroscopy 7:129–137

Grunwald JM (1993) Complications during arthroscopy: fatal air embolism. *Complications Orthop* 8:304

Herman JH, Khosla RC (1987) Laser (Nd:YAG)-induced healing of cartilage. Arthritis Rheum 30:s128

Miller GK. Brennan DB, Maylahn DJ (1987) The effect of technique on histology of arthroscopic partial meniscectomy with electrosurgery. Arthroscopy 3:36–44

Norton LA (1982) Effects of a pulsed electromagnetic field on a mixed chondroblastic tissue culture . Clin Orthop 167:280–290

Riddell RR (1990) CO_2 arthroscopy of the knee. Clin Orthop 252:92

Schultz RJ, Krishnamurthy STW, Theimo WRJ, Harvey G (1985) Effects of varying intensities of laser energy on articular cartilage. Lasers Surg Med 5:577–588

Shupak RC, Shuster H, Furch RS (1984) Airway emergency in a patient during CO_2 arthroscopy. Anesthesiology 60:171–172

Smith CF, Johansen WE, Vangsness CT, Sutter LV, Marshall GJ (1989) The carbon dioxide laser: a potential tool for orthopaedic surgery. Clin Orthop 242:43–50

Smith JB, Nance TA (1983) Laser energy in arthroscopic surgery. Presented at the Annual Meeting of the Arthroscopy Association of North America, Coronado, Ca

Smith JB, Nance TA (1988) Laser energy in arthroscopic surgery. In Arthroscopic Surgery. McGraw-Hill, New York

31

10.6 μm CO_2 Laser Endoscopic Carpal Tunnel Release

Charles E. Kollmer

Popularization of the conventional endoscopic technique of carpal tunnel release started with the work of Chow (1989, 1990, 1993) and Okutsu (1989). The benefits of this technique include a rapid return to work, small incisions, little loss of pinch and grip strength, and visualization of the ligament for this limited-incision procedure. New systems are emerging for both single portal and biportal endoscopic carpal tunnel release. The addition of the laser for endoscopic carpal tunnel release (ECTR) provides benefits for hemostasis and decreasing mechanical manipulation during surgery (Strohecker and Piotrowski, 1985).

History

A limited history of carpal tunnel syndrome starts with James Paget, who was the first to describe findings consistent with this syndrome. Carpal tunnel syndrome, however, did not emerge as a commonly treated disease until the 1950s with the work of Phalen (1970).

Popularization of the classic carpal tunnel release and correlation with associated injuries (i.e., repetitive trauma and cumulative trauma) have continued since that time. There are many reports of the conditions associated with this syndrome (e.g., diabetes, pregnancy, thyroid disease, polio, pigmented villonodular synovitis), but discussion of these disorders is beyond the scope of this chapter. Limited-incision techniques started during the early 1970s, but complications soon emerged (Blair, 1988). Talesniak described the most commonly used open incision in 1973 (Franklin et al., 1991) with a curvilinear incision based ulnarly and zigzagging across the wrist. Subsequently, limited open techniques have reemerged with a continued dissatisfaction for these relatively blind procedures.

With the technologic advancement in the fiberoptic fields and increasing surgical experience with arthroscopic/endoscopic procedures, the application of these devices to the carpal tunnel came under investigation. The early experience reported by both Chow and Okutsu began approximately in 1986. Clinical studies relating to carpal canal pressure and relief of carpal tunnel symptoms first appeared in 1989. Some hand surgeons routinely use the endoscopic release unless it is contraindicated.

The criterion for carpal tunnel release for most surgeons is failure of conservative therapy, including resting splints, nonsteroidal antiinflammatory drugs, and occasionally intracanal steroid injection. The presence of abnormal electromyographic findings is also taken into account (Cho, 1989; Richman et al., 1989; Kuschner et al., 1992). However, it should be noted that the most common indication for electromyographic studies is to evaluate the involvement of more proximal levels (Osterman, 1988; Cho, 1989). It should be noted that the protocol for diagnostic testing for carpal tunnel syndrome, particularly the clinical signs, is not yet established. Reports have demonstrated the value of Phalen's test (Kuschner et al., 1992) and the relatively new median nerve compression test (Durkan, 1991), but Tinel's sign appears to be of no clinical significance.

Open Carpal Tunnel Release

Without question, the large open classic incision for carpal tunnel release provides the best visualization of the median nerve and surrounding structures. The possibility of anomalous branches off the median nerve (e.g., Lanz subgroups) clearly is best evaluated with this approach. Richman et al. (1989) demonstrated the changes in the carpal canal morphology after release. The median changes from a relatively flattened appearance to a rounder shape with some intervening soft tissue between the tendons and the nerve are noted postoperatively. Additionally, a change in Guyon's canal is appreciated. This change in shape (i.e., rounding) probably represents a change in the pressure with the carpal region. The relief of associated ulnar nerve symptoms after carpal tunnel release is well documented and may relate to these findings. The other significant advantage to the open release is the extensive history with this procedure. Phalen reported on his own 21 year experience in 1970. With Talesniak's modifications noted above, the open mechanical carpal tunnel release remains the "gold standard."

The problems with the open release relate to the extensive incision. A period of postoperative splinting is required for wound care and to help the bowstringing that is attendant to a properly released ligament. With the significant occurrence of carpal tunnel syndrome in certain occupations, this disease may represent a difficult worker's compensation problem, particularly for those patients who have prolonged pinch and grip strength weakness and those with prolonged pillar pain (Franklin et al., 1991; Hagberg et al., 1991).

Other disadvantages relate to general wound problems (e.g., infection, dehiscence). Skin healing can become a major issue. Blair (1988) discussed keloid formation or thickened scars affecting the result, particularly at the level of the wrist. Hypersensitivity of the scar can cause significant morbidity. Scarring, of course, is also one of the major reasons for recurrence of the carpal tunnel syndrome (Cotton, 1991). A band of scar across the median nerve can lead to significant electrical and clinical deficits (Landloh and Linscheid, 1972).

However, as Blair noted, the most common complication is incomplete release of the transverse carpal ligament. The second most common problem is severance of the palmar cutaneous branch of the median nerve. Lilly and Magnell (1985) reported on this complication, with reexploration and nerve repair required. The nerves at risk during carpal tunnel release include the palmar cutaneous branch, motor branch of the median nerve, radial digital nerve to the ring finger, and communicating branch between the ulnar and median nerve (Lanz, 1977; May and Rosen, 1981; Lilly and Magnell, 1985; Louis and Greene, 1985; Blair, 1988). Reflex sympathetic dystrophy is also seen in approximately 5% of patients after carpal tunnel release.

Laser Open Carpal Tunnel Release

Utilizing the same classic open incision technique with the use of the laser for release of the transverse carpal ligament has been evaluated and reported (Strohecker and Piotrowski, 1985) since the early 1980s. The principal rationale for laser use in this setting is to decrease postoperative hematoma formation and postoperative pain. By decreasing the bleeding at surgery, scar formation also decreases. The thermal effect of the laser seals off small vessels, lymphatics, and nerves, which may also contribute to reducing the incidence and intensity of pillar pain (Kollman, 1985).

Proper protection of the surrounding structures is important and is accomplished with the use of retractors. A small malleable retractor that has been burnished or eburnated placed subligamentously protects the underlying structures from inadvertent exposure to the laser. The work presented and reported in the literature relates to the CO_2 laser (Bergman, 1988). The contact tip neodymium:YAG laser can be used in a similar fashion for carpal tunnel release.

Strohecker studied the ultrastructural histology of the transverse carpal ligament after release with the laser and found a small zone of thermally affected tissue (Strohecker and Piotrowski, 1985), a response seen in any soft tissue exposed to the laser. The CO_2 laser has a high affinity for water and as a result there is a narrow zone of thermal injury (generally in the range of 0.1 mm) at the cut edge. The size of the beam, of course, can be varied by defocusing. However, a well focused beam can be narrowed to 0.2 mm with most of the available CO_2 lasers.

Because this procedure requires release of the overlying skin, palmar cutaneous fascia, and interconnecting support fascia between the thenar and hypothenar aspects of the carpal canal region, there is still difficulty with loss of pinch and grip strength, as is seen with the conventional open release. The lesser pillar pain does not necessarily promote improved strength.

Splinting for postoperative wound protection and good positioning to prevent bowstringing during the early period is still required. Data relating to return to work are not available for the open laser carpal tunnel release procedure.

Proper use of the laser is essential to avoid inadvertent thermal injury to the patient or surrounding personnel. The increased equipment demands also are a disadvantage in comparison to the conventional open release. CO_2 lasers fortunately are present in most hospitals such that obtaining an appropriate laser should not be difficult for most surgeons. Use of the laser does require credentialing and attendance to a training course for each wavelength. The safety and credentialing issues are taken up in other parts of this book.

Limited Open Carpal Tunnel Release

The limited open carpal tunnel release covers a large range of incisions with the common characteristic that they are not as large as the conventional incision. The position of the limited incision is also of importance. An ulnarly based incision in line with the ring finger ray, whether proximally or distally based, is important. With less release of the overlying structures, the loss of pinch and grip strength is reduced. The prevalence of pillar pain remains, and there is still considerable hematoma formation. There is no standard limited open incision, so direct comparison to the classic technique is difficult.

Limited incision means limited visualization, and the "blind" characteristic is the most significant disadvantage to the limited open release. Susceptibility to the anatomic variations with inadvertent nerve injury has been documented (Blair, 1988). With limited visualization, one is also more susceptible to incompletely releasing the transverse ligament. Although patient acceptance of these techniques is higher when everything goes well, the surgeon cannot be as assured of a complete release with adequate protection of surrounding structures as with the conventional incision.

Laser use is not applicable to the limited open incisions, as the surgeon must be able to visualize where the beam is striking at all times. The possibility of damage without tactile feedback is too great in this setting.

Endoscopic Carpal Tunnel Release

The significant advantage of endoscopic release is visualization with a limited incision. There are single portal and biportal techniques. The endoscopic release described by Chow (1989, 1990, 1993) has become the most popular technique with some modifications. Maintenance of the overlying palmar tissue and interfacial tissue probably provides some benefit for retaining pinch and grip strength. The release of the ligament itself without damage to surrounding tissue also appears to contribute to decreasing pillar pain. The reports by Chow (1989, 1990, 1993) described a significantly improved return to work rate with less down time and less postoperative rehabilitation required. The technique involves use of a slotted cannula with subligamentous visualization of the tissue to be incised. The operator may visualize, though incompletely, the carpal canal contents. The incision is made only through appropriately identified ligamentous tissue. In the reports by Chow (1989, 1990, 1993) and Okutsu (1989), no complications were noted (Okutsu and S Nimomiya, 1989).

Increased equipment demands with the endoscopic setup and the obturator/slotted cannula device is required. As previously mentioned, the technique of endoscopy requires a certain amount of operator confidence and knowledge, and this requirement places some surgeons at a disadvantage. The endoscopic technique relies on ulnarly based incisions and identification of landmarks. The possibility of "bowstringing" a tendon or nerve with the obturator makes identification of all structures within the slotted portion of the cannula paramount. Even with the improved visualization, anatomic variations are more susceptible to damage than with the open conventional release. However, the operator has the advantage of appropriately judging the situation prior to releasing the ligament. When the operator is unsure if intervening structures are present, conversion to the open technique is easy. The experience within the surgical community is early, and some presentations have reported morbidity. The most common damage reported is to the flexor digitorum superficialis to the small finger, the radial digital nerve to the ring finger, and ulnar nerve neurapraxia. Moreover, if the palmar arch is proximal to Kaplan's cardinal line, it too is at risk. Overall this technique is gaining acceptance and appears to be a viable option for carpal tunnel release.

Laser Endoscopic Carpal Tunnel Release

Adding use of the laser to endoscopic release provides a less mechanical dissection, decreases hematoma formation, and decreases the incidence of scar formation. The laser also decreases the pillar pain as it seals the small nerves, lymphatics, and blood vessels within the ligament. Endoscopic placement of the cannula and identification of the ligament are unchanged. The laser provides an efficient tool for releasing the ligament. Because the beam can continue for a distance, more complete release (i.e., full thickness) can be expected. Use of the laser combines all the techniques previously described. Few surgeons are currently using the laser for this purpose, however. Active interest from the orthopaedic community and hand society has just begun. Additionally, preliminary investigation into other wavelengths, including the neodymium:YAG and holmium:YAG, continues.

Disadvantages of the laser relate to equipment demands. The surgeon must be endoscopically trained as well as laser trained. The increased equipment in the operating room make this operation a far cry from the simple instrumentation used for the conventional open release. The possibility of thermal damage is always present with laser use, and cost concerns also may have a negative impact. Additionally, experience with the endoscopic laser release is limited. No complications have been reported related to laser endoscopic release.

Laser Endoscopic Carpal Tunnel Release: Kollmer Technique

The approach from proximal to distal allows identification of the ulnar nerve. However the area of the palmar arch is not readily identifiable (Fig. 31-1). The palmar tissue is gently dissected and any intervening structures identified. Patients with palmar arches more proximal than the Kaplan's cardinal line can be identified. The distal leading edge of the transverse carpal ligament is identified; and with the wrist doriflexed, the obturator/cannula is advanced proximally in a subligamentous position. Gentle palpation of the obturator after it emerges from the carpal canal provides placement for the proximal incision. The obturator should not be firmly pushed through the tissue. Rather, a transverse proximal skin incision is made of approximately 1.0 to 1.5 cm. The flexor retinacu-

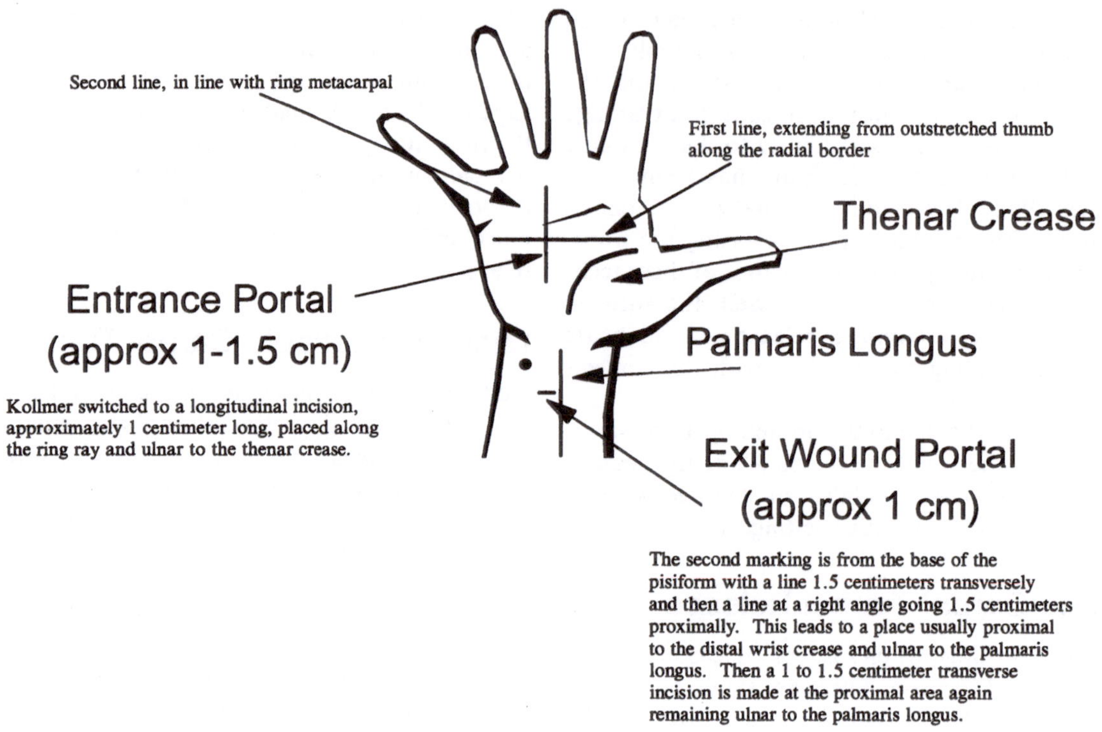
Second line, in line with ring metacarpal
First line, extending from outstretched thumb along the radial border
Thenar Crease
Entrance Portal (approx 1-1.5 cm)
Kollmer switched to a longitudinal incision, approximately 1 centimeter long, placed along the ring ray and ulnar to the thenar crease.
Palmaris Longus
Exit Wound Portal (approx 1 cm)
The second marking is from the base of the pisiform with a line 1.5 centimeters transversely and then a line at a right angle going 1.5 centimeters proximally. This leads to a place usually proximal to the distal wrist crease and ulnar to the palmaris longus. Then a 1 to 1.5 centimeter transverse incision is made at the proximal area again remaining ulnar to the palmaris longus.

Figure 31-1. Distal to proximal portal placement (Kollmer approach).

lum is gently dissected and the tip of the obturator identified. If clear of tissue, it can then be passed through the proximal incision. The reason for the proximal dissection is to ensure that there is no intervening tissue that could lead to hematoma and acute carpal tunnel syndrome (Lourie, 1990).

After the obturator is removed, the identification process for the transverse ligament is as noted above (Fig. 31-2). Following ligament identification, place a groove director along the line of the slot but in a supraligamentous position. It can be done under visualization proximally and distally so the device does not perforate the ligament. The groove director should slide rather easily between the ligament and the palmar cutaneous fascia and provides a ceiling to ensure complete release; it also protects the palmar tissue from the laser beam.

Once the instruments are in place, release of the ligament proceeds (Fig. 31-3 to 31-6). The CO_2 laser with the angled beam and the waveguide at about 15 to 25 watts are used. Smoke evacuation can be performed with wall suction for this type of case. The release proceeds until the groove director can be identified. The ligament can be palpated with probes to ensure complete release. The laser appears to part the ligamentous tissue as it pro-

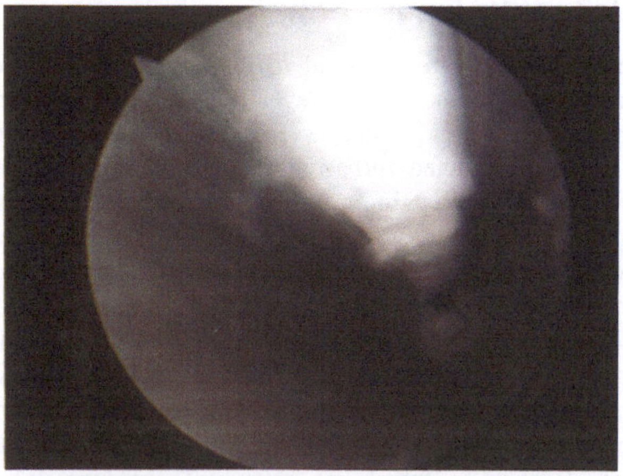

Figure 31-2. Endoscopic cannula in position.

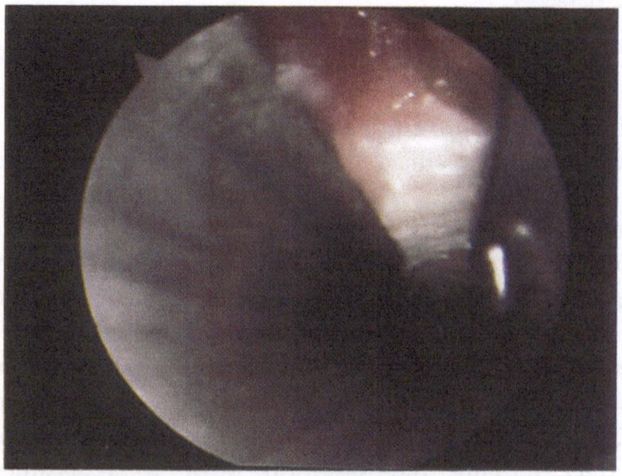

Figure 31-3. Inspecting for longitudinal or oblique structures was also accomplished during this process.

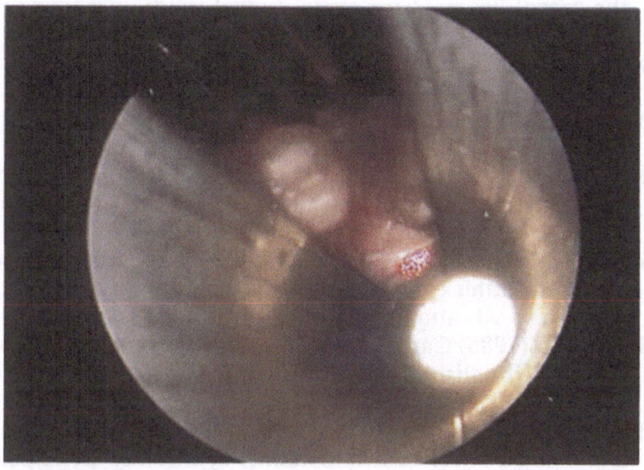

Figure 31-4. Endoscopic view of the laser waveguide with a red helium-neon aiming beam on the TCL.

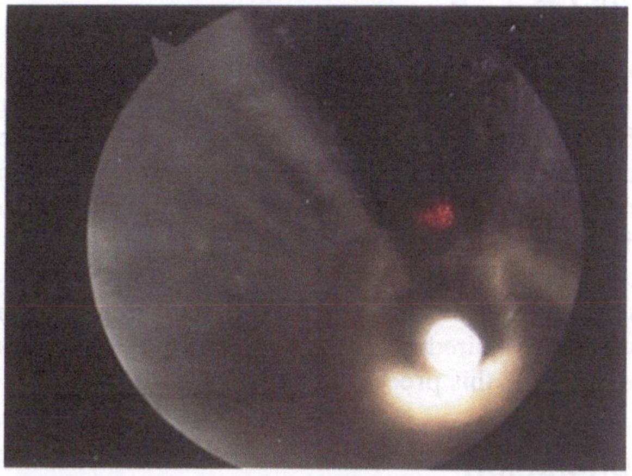

Figure 31-5. During the release, the aiming beam can be visualized as it strikes the backstop after cutting through the underlying ligamentous tissue.

ceeds. Copious irrigation is then undertaken to remove char and debris.

After the release, replace the obturator and remove the groove director and then the slotted cannula/obturator from the wound. With gentle retraction, lifting the wound edges allows limited gross inspection, and the endoscope can be placed to identify and inspect the release and the median nerve. Additionally, photographs can be obtained using the scope. Interrupted sutures are placed in both skin incisions and a gentle, bulky dressing applied.

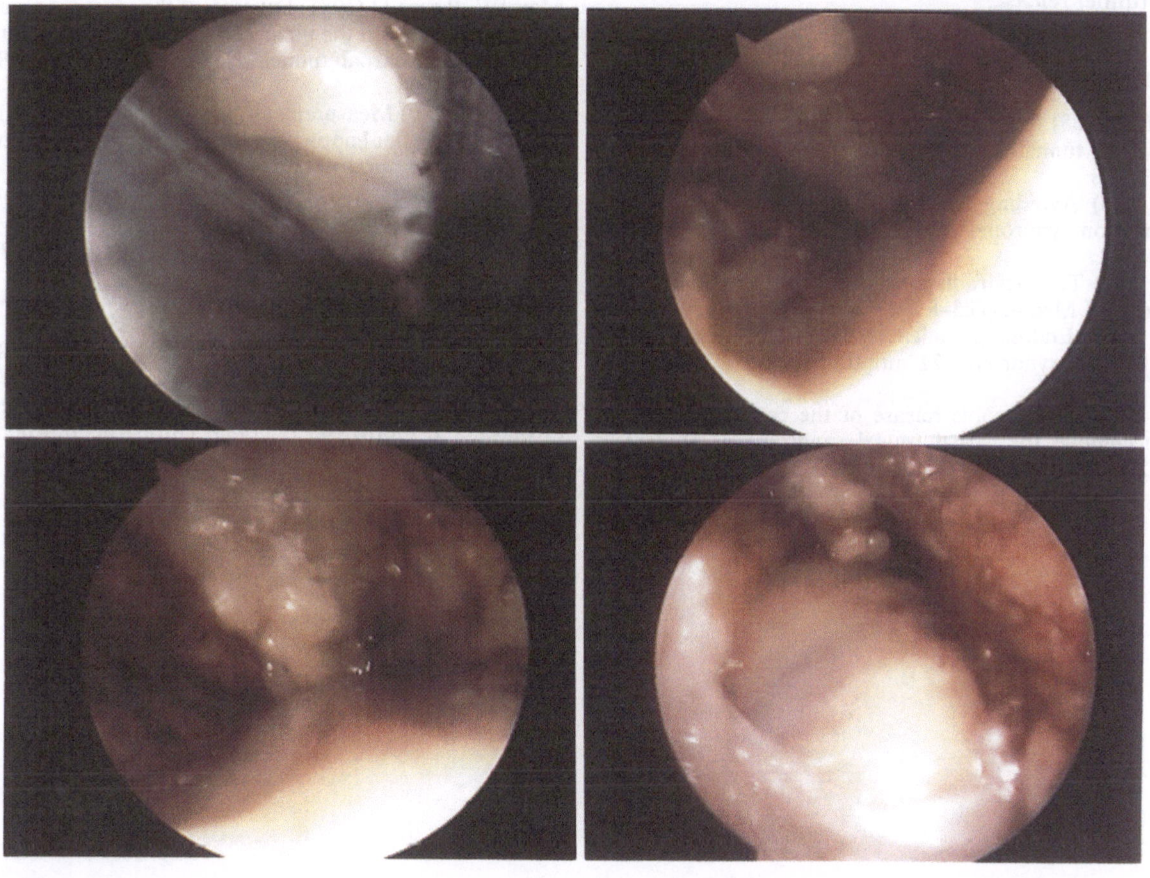

Figure 31-6. (A) Overlying backstop (groove director) is removed, and the palmar cutaneous tissue falls into the slot. (B–D) Endoscopic views after the release and with the slotted cannula removed. The cut edges of the TCL are noted, and the surrounding structures from both the proximal and distal portal can be inspected.

Initial Results

This technique has been used for more than 8 months, involving 33 carpal tunnel releases in 28 patients. The results are comparable to those seen with mechanical endoscopic release, with no complications noted in this limited series. The patients, including those with worker's compensation, return to work within an average of 2 to 3 weeks. Patient satisfaction has been high with this technique. These results are preliminary, and longer term follow-up is required before we can completely understand the place for this procedure.

Conclusion

The use of lasers for carpal tunnel surgery has progressed gradually over the past decade. The new endoscopic techniques provide an alternative for the surgeon where laser use becomes more attractive. Continued study of the role of laser surgery for both endoscopic and open carpal tunnel surgery is required. Also, the role of different wavelengths for this type of surgery is yet to be elucidated. I am now evaluating the 2.1 μm Holmium:YAG laser for use in endoscopic carpal tunnel. The addition of the laser to the endoscopic technique provides yet another method of carpal tunnel release.

References

Bergman RS (1988) Clinical experience with the CO_2 laser during carpal tunnel decompression. Plastic Reconstr Surg 81:933–938

Blair SJ (1988) Avoiding complications of surgery for nerve compression syndromes. Orthop Clin North Am, 19:125–130

Cho DS (1989) The electrodiagnosis of the carpal tunnel syndrome. SDJ Med 42(7):5–8

Chow JC (1990) Endoscopic release of the carpal ligament for carpal tunnel syndrome: 22 month clinical result. Arthroscopy 6:288–296

Chow JC (1989) Endoscopic release of the carpal ligament: a new technique for carpal tunnel syndrome. Arthroscopy 5:19–24

Chow JC (1993) The Chow technique of endoscopic release of the carpal ligament for carpal tunnel syndrome: four years of clinical results. Arthroscopy 9:301–314

Cotton P (1991) Symptoms may return after carpal tunnel surgery [news]. JAMA 265:1922, 1925

Durkan JA (1991) A new diagnostic test for carpal tunnel syndrome. J Bone Joint Surg [Am] 73:535–538

Franklin GM, Haug N, Checkoway H (1991) Occupational carpal tunnel syndrome in Washington State, 1984–1988. Am J Public Health 81:741–746

Hagberg M, Nystrom A, Zetterlund B (1991) Recovery from symptoms after carpal tunnel syndrome surgery in males in relation to vibration exposure. J Hand Surg [Am] 16:66–71

Kollman HB (1985) Carpal tunnel syndrome: causes, symptoms, therapy [English translation]. Wien Med Wochenschr 135:517–521

Kuschner SH, Ebramzedah E, Johnson D (1992) Tinel's sign and Phalen's test in carpal tunnel syndrome. Orthopedics 15:1297–1302

Langloh N, Linscheid R (1972) Recurrent and unrelieved carpal tunnel syndrome. Clin Orthop 83:41–44

Lanz U (1977) Anatomical variations of the median nerve in the carpal tunnel. J Hand Surg [Am] 2:44

Lilly CJ, Magnell T (1985) Severance of the thenar branch of the median nerve as a complication of carpal tunnel release. J Hand Surg [Am] 10:399–402

Louis DS, Greene TL (1985) Complications of carpal tunnel surgery. J Neurosurg 62:352

Lourie GM (1990) Distal rupture of the palmaris longus tendon and fascia as a cause of acute carpal tunnel syndrome. J Hand Surg [Am] 15:367–369

May JW, Rosen H (1981) Division of the sensory ramus communicans between the ulnar and median nerves: a complication following carpal tunnel release. J Bone Joint Surg [Am] 63:836–838

Okutsu I (1989) Measurement of pressure in the carpal canal before and after endoscopic management of carpal tunnel syndrome. J Bone Joint Surg [Am] 71:679–683

Okutsu I, Nimomiya S (1989) Endoscopic management of carpal tunnel syndrome. Arthroscopy 5:11–18

Osterman AL (1988) The double crush syndrome. Orthop Clin North Am 19:147–155

Phalen GS (1970) Reflections on 21 years experience with carpal tunnel syndrome. JAMA 212:1365–1367

Richman JA, Gelberman RH, Rydevik BL, et al (1989) Carpal tunnel syndrome: morphologic changes after release of the transverse carpal ligament. J Hand Surg [Am] 14:852–857

Strohecker J, Piotrowski N (1985) Ultrastructural findings after use of the CO_2 laser in carpal tunnel syndrome. Lasers Surg Med 5:123–128

32

Ambient Air Arthroscopic Laser Surgery Using the 10.6 μm CO_2 Laser

James G. Garrick

Described in this chapter is ambient air arthroscopy using the CO_2 laser. This technique was developed to minimize or overcome the limitations of earlier attempts at CO_2 laser arthroscopy (Smith and Nance, 1983; Smith, 1992), namely subcutaneous emphysema (Smith et al., 1989) and its life-threatening complications (Shupak et al., 1984) and the complexity of the procedure and instrumentation.

The technique utilizes generally two case-specific portals: through one the arthroscope is inserted and through the other an undersized laser waveguide. The first portal is used for the diagnostic part of the procedure. The location of the second portal is chosen based on the location of the tissue to be cut or ablated. To improve the accessibility and visualization, the portals through which the waveguides and arthroscope are inserted may be interchanged.

The advantages of the ambient air technique utilizing the waveguide system include better access to difficult to reach areas with minimal mechanical or thermal trauma (Garrick, 1992). Laser energy can be delivered through small-diameter (1.6 mm) waveguides, allowing access to difficult to reach sites, such as the posterior aspect of the knee. The noncontact property of the CO_2 laser allows the surgeon to treat tissue that can be seen but not physically touched. Mechanical instruments typically have a wider diameter than the small waveguides and may require opening and closing of jaws. Because of their large diameter, mechanical tools sometimes scuff or injure normal tissue (Fig. 32-1). In addition, mechanical tools often require specific angulation for proper effectiveness. The "point and shoot" properties of the laser further augment accessibility compared with mechanical instruments.

The CO_2 laser precisely vaporizes layers of tissue, providing the surgeon with an effective shaping tool for chondral surfaces. Mechanical instruments tear or shave tissue, often sacrificing normal tissue in the process. Other lasers (2.1 μm holmium:YAG, 1.06 and 1.44 μm neodymium:YAG) exhibit deeper penetration than the CO_2 laser.

The CO_2 laser combines cutting, ablating, sculpting, and hemostasis within a single device. Mechanical tools, on the other hand, are typically specialized for cutting, shaving, or tearing and have no ablative or hemostatic effect, which requires the surgeon to exchange several instruments during the procedure, increasing the risk of inadvertent mechanical injury to tissue.

The lessened use of certain disposable equirpment (bags of saline and tubing), the lower cost of other disposables (CO_2 waveguides versus neodymium:YAG and holmium:YAG fibers), the reduced incidence of breakage of certain disposable or expendable equipment (no power instruments, no breakage of fibers), and the smaller capital outlay (existing CO_2 laser or low cost CO_2 laser plus the small waveguides versus a new holmium:YAG laser) makes the ambient air technique probably the most cost-effective means of laser use in arthroscopic surgery. [With just two instruments—the small waveguides for fine tissue removal (particularly effective in tight areas of the knee) and a basket forceps for bulk removal of tissue—more than 100 consecutive arthroscopic surgeries were performed.]

The CO_2 laser is the most widely used for arthroscopy and is also the most frequently used in operating rooms in the United States and Europe. The CO_2 laser cuts and ablates tissue faster and with less adjacent tissue damage than any other laser used today for arthroscopic surgery. In addition, the waveguide probes are smaller and afford better access than either mechanical instrumentation of the fiber delivery systems of the holmium:YAG or neodymium:YAG laser systems.

Despite these advantages, the CO_2 laser has fallen into disfavor with many arthroscopists, both laser and nonlaser users (Whipple et al., 1984, 1985). The reason for

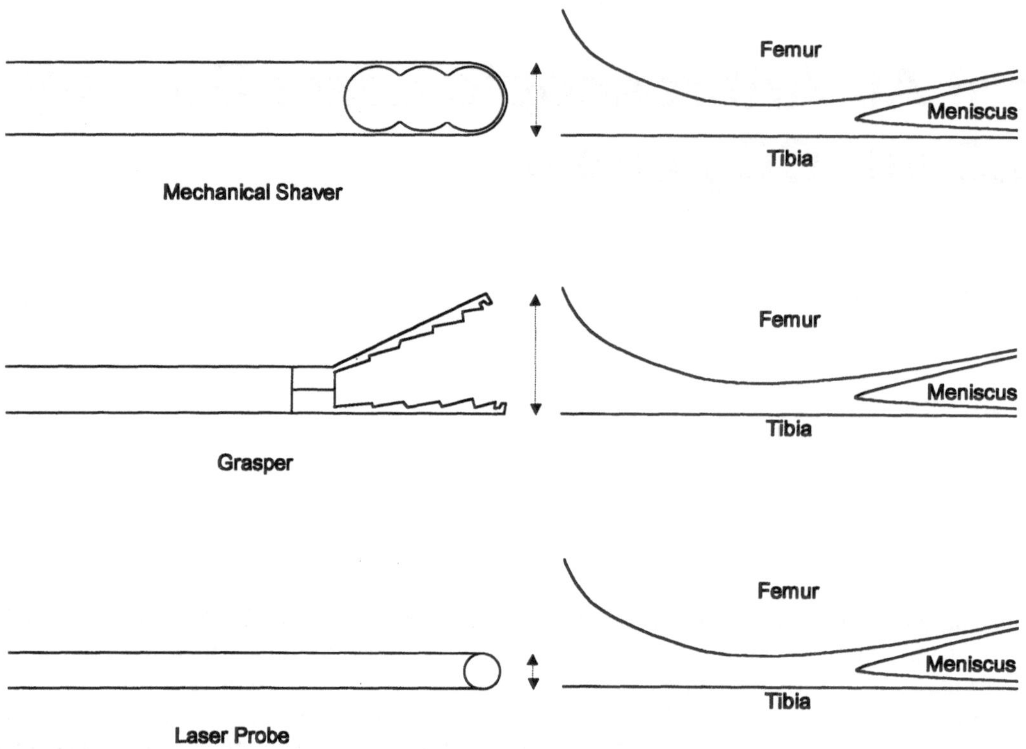

Figure 32-1. Comparison of mechanical shavers, grasper, and laser. Some of the appeal of lasers in orthopaedics is that laser energy can be delivered through narrow fibers in a "point and shoot" mode. This method facilitates access to difficult to reach portions of the knee that are too tight for mechanical instruments.

the CO_2 laser not being embraced centers on the necessity to inflate the joint with gas when CO_2 laser arthroscopy is performed. The high gas pressure used to inflate the knee was reported to cause subcutaneous emphysema after CO_2 laser arthroscopy, which could be life-threatening when the gas escaped the joint.

The presence of CO_2 gas in the joint does not present a clinical problem per se; clinical complications are the result of a pressure gradient large enough to force gas into open vascular beds or violated tissue planes with the subsequent formation of gas emboli. The technique used today permits the gas pressure to equilibrate to ambient air pressure by always providing a gas egress port from the joint to the ambient air. It does not absolutely obviate the potential complications almost universally reported by earlier clinicians but in fact lowers the chance of threatening gas emboli to the point that I know of no cases of gas emboli reported with this technique. Nevertheless, one must still be familiar with methods to recognize and treat gas emboli, and the patient must be informed of this theoretical possibility preoperatively.

Distention is not necessary to view many of the primary structures of the knee, such as the meniscus, tibial plateau, cruciate ligaments, and distal and posterior portions of the femoral condyles. The small outside diameter (1.6 mm) and curved configurations of the CO_2 laser waveguide used for this technique make it easier to access tight spaces within the knee.

Accessing the patellofemoral joint can be achieved by placing the knee in full extension and having an assistant displace the patella laterally or medially. A Stiele probe can be inserted through a separate small stab wound and used to "tent" the synovium.

Although the use of gas as an arthroscopic medium is not popular in the United States, it is popular in many parts of Europe. The advantages of gas as a medium include the following:

1. Bleeding cannot cloud air but can cloud fluid. (In addition, the CO_2 achieves a level of hemostasis not possible with mechanical instruments.)
2. In air, excised particles of cartilage can be easily recovered and removed from the joint by the arthroscopist.
3. Utilizing the ambient air technique, fluid ingress is provided through the arthroscope portal; thereby eliminating one puncture site.
4. The ambient air technique uses gravity flow from a 3-liter bag, thereby eliminating the need for an infusion pump and the additional expenses of disposable tubing and several bags of fluid.

Technique

In addition to the CO_2 laser and small waveguides, the following items are necessary:

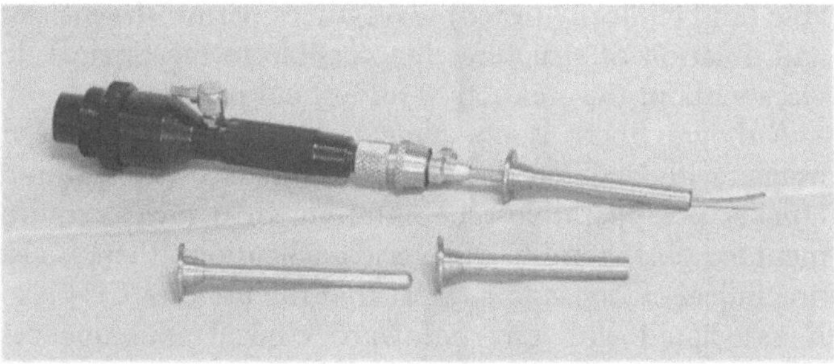

Figure 32-2. Assembled components are placed through the access sleeves to gain access to the knee cavity. An obturator is used to facilitate entry of the access sleeve into the knee. (Courtesy Luxar Corp., 1993.)

1. Dual stopcock arthroscope sheath for fluid ingress and egress.
2. Standard suction and irrigation equipment. A fluid pump is not necessary to perform this technique. Y suction tubing attached to a Frazier tip and an arthroscope is recommended. Typically, no more than three bags of saline are used.
3. Arthroscope.

The procedure requires two access sleeves (Fig. 32-2) that are slightly larger (0.6 mm) than the arthroscope; they are necessary to allow insertion of the waveguides and arthroscope through either portal. The access sleeves are available in varying lengths (20, 40, and 60 mm) to allow for varying thicknesses of subcutaneous fat. The sleeve length should extend into the joint approximately 1 cm beyond the synovial layer.

Establishing Portals

After the diagnostic portion of the procedure is completed and the target tissue selected, the second portal site is chosen while visualizing the target and inserting the tip of the needle, several times if necessary, until the tip touches the target. The portal is established by incising the skin and inserting a mosquito hemostat into the subcutaneous tissue, spreading its jaws and then withdrawing it.

A trocar sleeve is placed into the access sleeve, and a trocar is then placed into the sleeve. The trocar (with assembly) enters the joint under direct vision, allowing the trocar tip to be directed away from the intraarticular structures. The sheath and trocar are then removed, with the access sleeve in place, establishing the portal.

Using Conventional Instrumentation

Where large amounts of tissue are to be removed, the surgeon may prefer to use basket forceps to remove the bulk tissue prior to proceeding with the laser.

Introduction of Gas

By shutting off fluid ingress, opening the suction valve on the arthroscope sheath, and alternately covering and uncovering the opening of the access sleeve, nearly all fluid from the joint can be removed. Leaving the suction on, uncover the second sleeve and then turn the suction off, causing a bubble of room air to be sucked into the joint to allow visualization in a gas medium. If excess fluid is still in the vicinity of the target, a Frazier suction tip (2.5–3.7 mm) may be inserted through the second sleeve to further dry the tissue. The laser waveguide with sleeve may then be inserted through the second portal, and purge gas is turned on.

Using the Laser

The CO_2 laser power should be set initially to 10 watts average power, either continuous wave or superpulsed. Superpulsing yields somewhat less charring at the expense of less hemostasis. The laser power should be adjusted according to the tissue effects observed.

Smoke is probably the most troublesome aspect of laser surgery. It can be removed by opening slightly the suction portal on the arthroscope. Too much suction, however, causes soft tissue to be pulled over the lens of the arthroscope, obscuring vision. **Never fire the laser if you cannot see your target.** Sometimes smoke and other debris collect on the lens, blocking visualization. By wiping the lens on adjacent synovium, the lens may be cleared. If even better visualization or accessibility is desired, improvement can sometimes be achieved by interchanging the portals of the arthroscope and waveguide.

Keep the laser in the standby mode when the laser is not in use.

Cleansing the Target

The by-product of lased tissue, in addition to vapor, is carbonized particles (char). Char should never be lased over as it cannot be vaporized and leads to additional (unintended) thermal damage of surrounding tissue. Char also interferes with visualization of the target and should be removed as it develops. Char can be easily removed by turning off the suction, opening the fluid portal, and using the CO_2 gas bubbles emanating from the waveguide to scrub the target. Care should be taken here, as elsewhere in the procedure, to not block gas flow from the waveguide. **Fluid in the waveguide can hinder transmission and may even cause the waveguide to overheat.**

Meniscectomy

The CO_2 laser with small diameter waveguides is particularly useful for treating degenerative or torn menisci in the difficult to reach posterior aspect of the knee. The laser combines multiple functions, allowing the surgeon to cut (i.e., bucket-handle tears) and smooth meniscal tissue.

Chondromalacia

The affinity of the CO_2 laser for water-laden cartilaginous tissue makes it an efficient tool for ablation of patellar and femoral chondromalacia. The fixed curve on the distal end of the curved guide matches the curve of the femoral condyle, allowing the arthroscopist to sweep back and forth within the joint to remove the diseased tissue.

Chondroplasty

The CO_2 laser offers a fast and precise smoothing tool for grades 2 and 3 degenerative cartilage in conjunction with the mechanical abrasion of grade 4 surfaces. The vaporization effect of the laser allows the surgeon to sculpt chondral tissues. This effect is difficult to achieve with traditional mechanical tools.

No published clinical research has documented quicker healing or tissue regeneration. Indeed, most studies (not necessarily involving arthroscopy) show somewhat slower healing of lased tissue. From the patient's point of view, the slight delay seems inconsequential. On the other hand, most of the clinical difficulties associated with arthroscopy using the CO_2 laser can be traced to high gas pressure. The ambient air technique should significantly decrease this source of problems.

Summary

Used arthroscopically, the CO_2 laser rapidly and precisely incises and ablates tissue, adding a measure of hemostasis not possible with mechanical instruments. Currently available (and clinically tested) waveguides permit the incision and ablation of structures inaccessible to mechanical devices without the creation of additional portals.

Although there is no clinical documentation of laser usage with enhanced healing or tissue regeneration, quicker postoperative rehabilitation. or a lower requirement for postoperative analgesic medications, there is also no clinical evidence to suggest that the use of a CO_2 laser is associated with any untoward clinical consequences. The problems associated with CO_2 laser use are exclusively those associated with the use of a gas medium, and by using gas at ambient (room) pressures even these problems can be avoided.

References

Garrick JG (1992) CO_2 laser arthroscopy using ambient gas pressure. Semin Orthop 7(2):90–94

Shupak RC, Shuster H, Funch RS (1984) Airway emergency in a patient during CO_2 arthroscopy. Anesthesiology 60:171–172

Smith CF, Johansen EL, Vangsness CT, et al (1992) "Gas bubble" technique in laser arthroscopic surgery. Semin Orthop 7:86–89

Smith CF, Johansen WE, Vangsness CT, et al (1989) The carbon dioxide laser: a potential tool for orthopaedic surgery. Clin Orthop 242:43–50

Smith JB, Nance TA (1983) Laser energy in arthroscopic surgery. Presented at the Annual Meeting of the Arthroscopy Association of North America, Coronado, CA

Whipple TL, Caspari RB, Meyers JF (1984) Synovial response to laser induced carbon ash residue. Lasers Surg Med 3:291–295

Whipple TL, Caspari RB, Meyers JF (1985) Arthroscopic laser meniscectomy in a gas medium. Arthroscopy 1:2–7

33

10.6 μm CO_2 Arthroscopic Laser Surgery: 1222 Cases

Chadwick F. Smith and C. Thomas Vangsness Jr.

Between February 1, 1984 and January 1, 1990 a total of 1222 laser arthroscopic surgical procedures were undertaken by us at the shoulder, knee, elbow, and hip (Smith et al., 1987). The procedures reviewed encompass all patients treated surgically during this period with the exclusion of those with ligamentous instability, a primary synovitic problem, a primary arthritic problem, or a primary instability problem. All patients with neoplasms, pigmented villonodular tenosynovitis, rheumatoid arthritis, and hemophilia were also excluded. The procedures were undertaken as shown:

Knee (meniscal and chondromalacic)	1185
Shoulder (impingement and rotator cuff)	28
Elbow	6
Hip	3

During the initial period of this study, 100 of the patients were evaluated under an investigational device exemption for a U.S. Food and Drug Administration (FDA) protocol. After completion of the FDA protocol, all patients have since been treated without the need for FDA or Investigational Review Board (IRB) control. In 1985 the CO_2 hand-held laser device was determined to be safe and effective at all joints with the exception of the shoulder (Cofield, 1983; Andrews et al., 1985; Smith et al., 1987).

Although a randomized double-blind study was not undertaken, it was not thought by the treating therapist or surgeon that any of the patients experienced more rapid rehabilitation in terms of return to full activities when compared to mechanical technique. It was, however, frequently noted by the treating therapist and by the surgery center personnel that the laser patients demonstrated lower morbidity and more rapid progression sometimes with exercises better than did the standard arthroscopy patients.

There were no known lasting complications in any of the patients. The complications from these procedures can be related to the use of gas arthroscopy and in only one instance to the nature of the laser (transient 2 cm skin ulceration at the knee). In each instance in this series a CO_2 laser tool was utilized (either the hand-held Directed Energy, Pfizer device at 20 watts or a Heraeus Cooper Lasersonics tool at 50 watts, both with the use of gated energy) (Andrews et al., 1985). The complications are divided here into nonshoulder joint and shoulder joint problems. The following reflects the complications at the shoulder utilizing gas arthroscopy:

Subcutaneous emphysema	100%
Extensive subcutaneous emphysema	21%
Pneumothorax	7%
Arthrotomy	0%

None of the nonshoulder joint patients had morbidity that affected their clinical course adversely. In 100% of the patients undergoing gas arthroscopy, however, careful palpation identified gas subcutaneously (subcutaneous emphysema). Frequently, the patient was not aware of this extension from the joint to the subcutaneous tissue, but the gas present during gas arthroscopy appears in soft tissues 100% of the time (as does fluid adjacent to the joint during aqueous arthroscopy). The only other complications at nonshoulder joints were one case of a 2-cm knee skin ulceration (which healed within 2 weeks) and one case of phlebitis (which healed with anticoagulation therapy). The shoulder laser surgery complication that caused significant morbidity and caused us to change the technique was extensive subcutaneous emphysema in six cases and pneumothorax on two occasions. Although none of these eight complications was lasting, the dramatic and extensive subcutaneous emphysema in the six cases and the two pneumothoraces dictated a change in technique.

The complications and their incidence with this technique are as follows:

Subcutaneous emphysema	100%
Metastasizing emphysema	0%
Phlebitis	0.0008%
Skin ulceration	0.0008%
Arthrotomy	0%

It should be emphasized that no patient in this series and no patient to our knowledge in the world has been noted to have metastatic gas problems with a properly functioning tourniquet and a properly functioning insufflation device in use at the knee. There are, however, four cases in which gas spread from the knee to the abdomen in elderly individuals with a loosely fitting tourniquet.

It can be concluded from this series of patients undergoing arthroscopic surgery at the shoulder, elbow, knee, and hip that CO_2 arthroscopic laser surgery is safe and effective in all joints except the shoulder. The tool is small and precise, and anecdotally the procedure allows a decrease in early morbidity and shorter operating time. The small size and the efficiency of the tool decreases the chance for damage to adjacent normal tissues (Smith et al., 1987, 1989). No patient in this series required arthrotomy and the results compare favorably to the use of standard tools.

At the present time, CO_2 laser therapy should not be undertaken at the shoulder unless the "gas bubble" technique or the "ambient air" technique is utilized (Whipple et al., 1982; Smith et al., 1984, 1992). All CO_2 laser arthroscopic surgery at the shoulder is considered experimental at this time and must be conducted under the supervision of the FDA and an IRB.

References

Andrews JR, Broussard TS, Carson WG (1985) Arthroscopy of the shoulder in the management of partial tears of the rotator cuff: a preliminary report. Arthroscopy 1:117–122

Cofield RH (1983) Arthroscopy of the shoulder. Mayo Clin Proc 58:501–508

Smith CF, Johansen WE, Sutter LV, Marshall GJ (1987) Meniscal repair utilizing a handheld carbon dioxide laser. Poster presented at the 54th Annual Meeting of the American Academy of Orthopaedic Surgeons, San Francisco

Smith CF, Johansen WE, Vangsness CT, Marshall GJ, Sutter LV (1989) The carbon dioxide laser: a potential tool for orthopaedics. Clin Orthop 242:43–50

Smith CF, Johansen EL, Vangsness CT, et al (1992) "Gas bubble" technique in laser arthroscopic surgery. Semin Orthop 7:86–89

Smith CF, Marshall GJ, Snyder SJ, et al (1984) Comparisons of tissue effects of a surgical scalpel, and electrocautery apparatus and a carbon dioxide laser system when used for making incisions into the menisci of New Zealand rabbits. Lasers Surg Med 3:305

Whipple TL, Caspari RB, Meyers JF (1982) Arthroscopic meniscectomy by CO_2 laser vaporization in a gas medium. Orthop Trans 6:136

34

0.308 μm Excimer Laser for Arthroscopic Laser Surgery

Neil D. Glossop and Robert W. Jackson

Excimer lasers have found applications in many diverse fields over the years. Their use in the medical profession includes angioplasty, photorefractive surgery, and orthopaedics. Some nonmedical uses include photolithography, atmospheric sensing, pumping dye lasers, micromachining, and stimulating various photochemical reactions. However, they are not U.S. Food and Drug Administration (FDA) market approved for arthroscopy even though they are used for this purpose in Europe.

Excimers are complex devices. They are more complicated than most of the other lasers, both optically and physically, which makes them more expensive and more fragile. The attraction of excimers stems from some of their unusual properties. They offer several unique advantages over other laser systems that have made them particularly attractive to the medical, industrial, and scientific communities. Scientific users appreciate the high energy and short wavelengths these lasers provide. This situation is otherwise possible only when using complex nonlinear optical systems or special dye lasers. The short pulse length can be used advantageously to deliver large amounts of energy in a short time.

Industrial applications make use of the precision of the excimer. The short wavelength is less limited by diffraction than visible lasers and results in a beam that can be accurately focused and masked to etch precise patterns. Major industrial users of excimers include manufacturers of small parts and the electronics industry. Here, excimer laser photolithography is used to set down the patterns for electronic chips and circuits.

Excimer Laser System: Description

The excimer lasers bear more than a passing resemblance to the 10.6 μm CO_2 laser. Like the 10.6 μm CO_2 laser, the excimers are gas lasers and produce invisible light. The mechanism of excitation (i.e., "optically pumping" the gas) is similar, usually being carried out using a transverse electrode.

Several excimers exist. Although the construction is almost identical, they produce different wavelength radiation and use different laser media. Optics, power supplies, and cavity sizes also sometimes differ among the various types, although some "multipurpose" excimers have been built that require only a gas change and some small adjustments, in order to be used at a different wavelength.

All versions of excimers use a gas medium consisting of a rare gas such as xenon, krypton, or argon and a halogen such as chlorine or fluorine. Different combinations of gases produce different wavelength excimers. KrF (0.248 μm), ArF (0.193 μm), and XeCl (0.308 μm) are among the best known. XeF (0.351 μm and 0.353 μm) and XeBr (0.282 μm) are also available. Efficient optical fibers are available for the longer wavelength devices, including the XeCl and XeF.

Laser Action

Lasing with excimers results from the radiative decay of an excited dimer. Dimers result when two ions (e.g., Xe^+ and Cl^-) that do not normally bond do so under special conditions. These ions combine only when they are in a highly energetic state, brought about by exciting or "pumping" the gas with an intense electrical discharge.

At least two forms of dimer exist. The excited dimer (XeCl*) is metastable and spontaneously decays to a nonexcited dimer (XeCl). When it does so, it emits a photon of light, which can stimulate emission of more photons from other excited dimers. The nonexcited dimer is the other form. It is also in a higher energy state than the ions and monatomic molecules. It decays quickly—on the order of 10^{-12} second—in a nonradiative manner.

No light energy is released, and the energy is dissipated thermally. This thermal energy goes into heating the excimer gas and is completely separate from any thermal effects of the light beam. Enough heat is produced from this and the electrical discharge that excimers typically contain a gas circulation system within the cavity to ensure good heat transfer.

When the nonexcited dimer decays, it decomposes into the constituent ions such as Xe^+ and Cl^-. These ions may then go on to form Xe and Cl_2 or complexes with other materials in the laser gas or chamber walls.

The nature of the excitation leads to the excimer lasers being pulsed lasers. Excimers are always pulsed lasers, although it is sometimes possible to pulse them rapidly. The length of the pulse is generally 10 to 80 nanoseconds (ns) long, depending on the construction of the laser. Elaborate measures are often used with excimers to prolong the pulse length and thus to enable more energy to be delivered to the tissue. Longer pulse lengths are also kinder to optics and optical fibers.

Gas and Gas Handling

Excimer gases contain components in addition to the halogen and rare gas. They usually contain a buffer gas (e.g., hydrogen) to increase the pressure. Unfortunately, buffers react with the halogen during the discharge, depleting it in time. These complexes also tend to absorb the precise wavelength that is being generated, diminishing the intensity of the laser light. As a result, it is necessary to inject halogen into the gas mixture and remove some of the complexes. There are several ways to do this, but the course generally followed for commercial medical excimers is to replace the gas in the chamber periodically, which requires an elaborate gas handling system to evacuate the old gas and replace it with fresh gas. Storage of both the exhausted gas and the new gas is a problem, as both tend to be toxic and corrosive. Fortunately, it is possible to filter the reactive components from the exhausted gas.

Two approaches have been taken for handling the gas in excimers. The integrated gas handling system is preferred because it is possible to renew the gas in just a few minutes. With this system, a gas canister and an appropriate vacuum system are built into the laser. Gas in the system is evacuated and filtered, and an electronically controlled valve is actuated to release the new gas into the system. The entire process can be controlled by the push of a button.

The other approach requires a separate gas recharge apparatus that is wheeled up to the laser on a cart. This apparatus contains a vacuum pump and gas cylinders. Hoses are fitted between the laser and the gas system, and the used laser gas is evacuated. Fresh laser gas is then introduced into the system.

These systems enable the size of the laser to be reduced but are usually cumbersome to use. Also they require a skilled technician and make it difficult or impossible to change the gas during surgery. The more convenient integrated gas handling systems are more hazardous. It is necessary to contain the gas supply within an airtight housing (in case of leaks) and periodically ensure that all filters are still active.

Optics and Fibers

Excimer laser optics must be more rugged than conventional laser optics. The beam quickly erodes most lenses and mirrors, particularly for high peak energy pulsed (i.e., short pulse length) lasers. Transmissive optics, such as lenses, are generally made from excimer-grade fused silica, and expensive high energy coatings must be applied to mirrors and filters. The efficiency of these optical components is still below that of conventional optics, and light is lost for every component that must be used. Even the high efficiency optics must be periodically replaced because of beam-induced damage.

Optical fibers suffer from the same problems as conventional optics (Pini et al., 1987). Only the 0.308 μm XeCl and the 0.351 and 0.353 μm XeF Excimer lasers can be efficiently delivered with optical fibers so far. It is important to realize that the current state of excimer fibers has been achieved only after much effort.

The large diameter fibers that can best conduct the laser energy are inflexible and ill suited to arthroscopy. Thinner fibers are liable to be damaged by the incident laser beam and cannot conduct as much energy. Several ingenious solutions have been developed to solve these problems: tapered fibers (Jahn et al., 1990), bundles of small fibers (Koort, 1991), and various types of single fibers. The fiber technology has advanced to a state where delivery system problems are not as severe as they once were with these lasers. In addition, the development of longer pulsed excimers has reduced the demands on the fibers by lowering the peak energy that must be transmitted. Losses in coupling to fibers and absorption within the fiber are still high. It is common to deliver less than 40% of the energy issued from the laser head to the tissue.

Beam Characteristics/Special Properties

Optical cavity constraints cause the beam produced by most excimers to have a large, square profile. It is often fairly uniform and roughly a few centimeters in dimension. The beam is focused and conditioned for injection into an optical fiber. Beam conditioning and the precise method of injecting the light into the fiber is vital, as incorrectly focusing the beam on a fiber surface can destroy the fiber after just a few shots.

Beam delivery through an optical fiber is totally different from delivery with a free beam. Whereas free beams can be focused and conditioned precisely, fiberoptics normally completely alter the energy profile. All fibers in use with all lasers cause the transmitted beam to diverge as it exits from the fiber, even if the divergence of the laser itself is small. The numeric aperture of the fiber is a measure of this divergence, which can easily be 20 degrees or more (total divergence angle) for a 600 μm fiber.

Because of the beam divergence, the energy density (also known as radiant exposure) drops off substantially with increasing distance from the fiber tip. It is impossible to ablate material more than a few millimeters away from the tip. Keep in mind that although the total energy (measured in joules) delivered through a fiber may be constant, the energy density (measured in joules per square centimeter) changes if this energy is delivered over a larger area. Therefore large fibers that can deliver more total energy than small ones may not cut as well because the energy is delivered at a lower energy density owing to the increased diameter. This problem may render them ineffective for ablation.

Modal interference also affects the energy pattern emerging from the fiber. This effect is related to the "speckle pattern" that is observed when looking at the spot produced when visible laser beam hits a wall or screen. The actual distribution of light at the end of the fiber consists of several bright and dark spots instead of a square or uniform gaussian-type curve. Again, this occurs with all fibers and lasers, though the effect can be diminished by ensuring "mode mixing" and using larger diameter fibers.

Excimers interact with tissue through the mechanism of photoablation. This effect relies on rapid delivery of a large amount of energy to a substance. Photoablation is accomplished by depositing energy in the tissue faster than it can be thermally dissipated into adjacent cells. It is characterized by disruption of atomic and molecular bonds and a "microexplosion" in which cells, cell fragments, and a variety of atomic, molecular, and ionic species are ejected from the tissue surface at high speed. Although not limited to excimers, this effect is more pronounced with them because of their intrinsically short pulse length and high peak energy. It is possible to cause thermal effects with the excimer at high repetition rates (Kaufmann and Hibst 1989) or at low energies such as those found near the peripheries of the beam. For the most part however, photoablation is a "cold" process.

Medical Applications of the Excimer Laser

The greatest medical advantages of excimers are their ability to remove thin layers of tissue without a significant rise in temperature. Excimers do not typically "cut", instead, they etch (Table 34-1) or ablate a relatively large area, usually a few square millimeters at a time. The depth of the ablation can be controlled precisely and may range from a few micrometers to a millimeter or more with every pulse.

Table 34-1. Etch rates for different tissues for 0.308 μm XeCl Excimer laser.

Tissue	Medium	Etch rate (μm/pulse)	Zone of thermal change (μm)
Bone	Saline	2[a]	2–3[b]; 25–40[a]
	Air	5[c]	15[c]
Intervertebral disc	Air	12[d]	5–40[d]
Meniscus	Saline	32[e]	<50[a]; 4[e]; 96[f]
	Air	27[g]	267[h]
Articular cartilage	Saline	49[e]	16[e]

[a] Twenty hertz; 6 joules/cm^2; 300 ns pulse; 1000 μm tapered fiber (Dressel et al., 1991).
[b] Forty hertz; 20 to 60 joules/cm^2; 120 ns pulse; 1000 μm fiber (Yow et al., 1989).
[c] Ten hertz; 3.9 joules/cm^2; 20 ns pulse; free beam (Sankar et al., 1989).
[d] Twenty hertz; 5.5 joules/cm^2; 85 ns pulse; 400 μm fiber (Wolgin et al., 1989).
[e] Five hertz; 5 joules/cm^2; 135 ns pulse; 600 μm fiber (Vari et al., 1991).
[f] Twenty hertz; 2.8 joules/cm^2; 130 ns pulse; 600 μm fiber (Vangsness et al., 1992).
[g] Twenty hertz; 6 joules/cm^2; 130 ns pulse; 600 μm fiber (Buchelt et al., 1991b).
[h] Twenty hertz; 2.8 joules/cm^2; 130 ns pulse; 600 μm fiber (Vangsness et al., 1992).

The 0.193 μm ArF Excimer laser is used for ophthalmology (Marshall et al., 1985). Several ophthalmologic excimers are currently under investigation primarily in the area of corneal sculpting. A huge market exists for photorefractive surgery. These lasers are currently undergoing clinical trials as investigational devices in the United States. Excimers offer the most promising technique for this surgery. Other ophthalmologic studies have investigated the use of the 308 nm wavelength for cataract surgery (Bath et al., 1988).

Ophthalmologic lasers differ from orthopaedic excimers. The laser light is precisely conditioned, masked, and focused using complex conventional (nonfiber) optics. Beam uniformity is of primary concern, in contrast to orthopaedic excimers where the main concern is the total amount of energy delivered.

Excimers designed specifically for angioplasty have also been produced. There are definite advantages to using excimers for unblocking obstructed arteries, but it is still unclear whether excimers—or even lasers—represent the best technology for this task. Fluorescence guiding and precise cutting are two principal advantages of excimer angioplasty (Clarke et al., 1988; Hohla et al., 1988). In addition, laser fibers can be combined with angioscopes, fluorescence monitoring, irrigation, and guidewires to produce an elegant, compact, functional instrument.

Some work has been performed using excimers in dermatology (Kaufmann and Hibst, 1989). It is still unclear if the known mutagenic properties of 308 nm in skin make it a good candidate for this work (Francis et al., 1988) (Table 34-2).

Table 34-2. 0.308 μm XeCl Excimer laser and x-ray-induced mutagenic changes in the BALB/3T3 cell line

Parameter	Control (no radiation)	X-ray (2 Gy)	308 nm Excimer: 2 mJ, 10 Hz[a]
Total no. specimens checked	96	96	288
Foci/5000 cells	4	127	7

Data are from Hendrich et al. (1991).
[a]Two millijoules is a sublethal dose; 5 to 10 mJ produced cytolysis; more than 10 mJ caused ablation.

Orthopaedic Laser System

The system we use is the Arthrex Arthrolase Max-10 (Arthrex, Naples, FL), pictured in Fig. 34-1. This device has been approved for human use in Europe and Canada for several years but is not available in the United States pending FDA clearance. It is a large instrument and is representative of the first generation of medical excimers.

The laser contains an integrated gas handling system and a secondary containment system for confining any gas leakage. The unit is capable of a 200 pulse/s repetition rate, and the beam can be delivered with either an optical fiber or an articulated arm assembly. Energy at the laser head can reach 120 mJ and about 40 to 60 mJ at the fiber tip. The actual energy available at the tip depends on the pulse repetition rate, fiber alignment, fiber end condition and type of fiber in use. The pulse length is 60 ns at 0.308 μm.

Energy can be delivered either using a fiber bundle system (MedLas GmbH, Bonn) or single fibers of diameter 600 or 1000 μm (Arthrex). The fiber bundles are much more flexible and deliver only slightly less energy. The tips of fiber bundles can also be molded to different shapes for different applications (Koort, 1991). Solid fibers are inserted into the handpiece as shown in Fig. 34-2, and bundles are contained in an integrated handpiece.

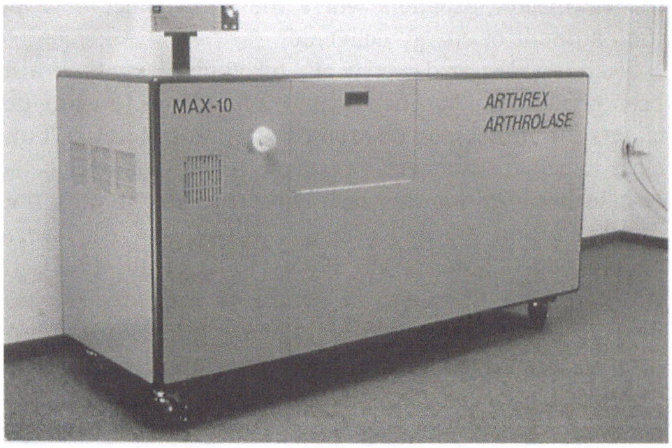

Figure 34-1. Arthrex Arthrolase (MAX-10) 0.308 μm XeCl Excimer laser. The optical fiber is inserted into the swivel arm at the top of the laser.

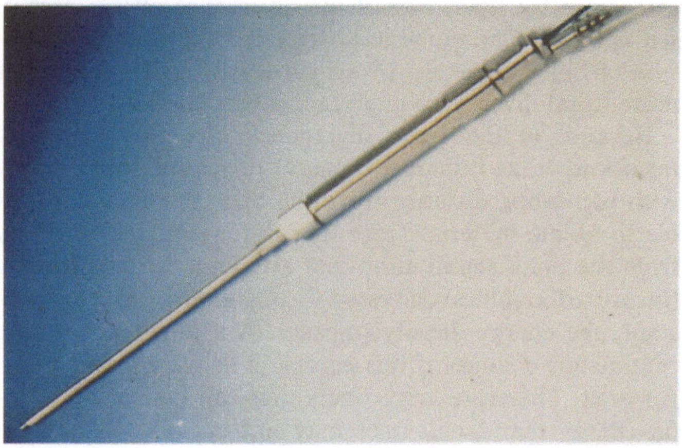

Figure 34-2. Fiberoptic handpiece. Fibers can be inserted into this reusable handpiece, which has a built-in irrigation port that provides concentric fluid flow around the fiber when attached to an arthroscopy pump.

Clinical Applications

The most successful clinical applications of the 0.308 μm XeCl Excimer so far have made use of the unique properties of the excimer laser. Many operations can be carried out, but those that do not make use of these properties may not offer significant advantages over conventional or other laser methods. As with other lasers, many effects of 0.308 μm XeCl Excimer laser radiation are not clearly understood, particularly when dealing with cells that are irradiated but not destroyed.

It has been mentioned that the 0.308 μm XeCl Excimer is a precise laser: It can remove thin layers of tissue—a few micrometers at a time if necessary. In conventional orthopaedics such detailed control might seem radical, but circumstances do arise, especially with arthroscopy, when precision is required.

The 0.308 μm Excimer wavelength is completely compatible with arthroscopy. It can be delivered by fiberoptics in a near-contact mode and can be used effectively in arthroscopic fluids and gases.

It is also possible to make use of the fluorescent signature of many tissue types to differentiate between them. This procedure is more useful in angioplasty, where it is important to discriminate between plaque and lumen, but may have application in some areas of orthopaedics, especially disc surgery.

Because so little heat is produced by the excimer, this laser is not hemostatic. Ancillary thermal effects such as bubbling, carbonization, and risk of fire are also absent.

The excimer can be used for all cutting operations to which other lasers have been applied. Etch rates (Table 34-1) and damage zone sizes for different tissues are summarized. The numbers listed are extracted from a multitude of sources and sometimes conflict with one another.

It is important to keep the laser and fiber parameters in mind when making any comparisons.

Disadvantages and Complications

Orthopaedic applications of current excimers are limited, although this situation promises to change as technological improvements are made. Presently, the lasers have limited power and are large and expensive. Although they excel at certain operations, it may be difficult to justify the cost if the power is insufficient to perform more diverse surgical tasks.

The lack of detailed knowledge of the full effects of the excimer is certainly a problem. There are possible mutagenic effects (Kochevar, 1989), although early studies have shown that this threat is small. No evidence of mutagenic change has been discovered in Europe after a combined experience of several thousand cases.

There are also no details of the nature of the chemical and particulate debris created by the 0.308 μm XeCl Excimer when ablating substances. It is known (Kokosa and Doyle, 1988; Sherk and Lane, 1989) that lasers can produce highly toxic debris when ablating tissue and bone cement.

Surgery time is generally increased with the use of the laser. Raunest and Lohnert (1990) found that laser cases took an average of 48.1 minutes compared to a nonlaser average of 37.1 minutes ($p < 0.01$). Although the time increase is large, much of it can be attributed to the technical requirements and low ablation rate of the particular laser employed.

A complication that was experienced with some early studies was fiber tip fracture. The shock wave extending back from the tissue occasionally shattered the tip of glass fiber, and it became necessary to retrieve the broken fragments. Power at the tip also fell off dramatically as the light was scattered randomly. This problem has been eliminated with the design of special shock-absorbing fiber holders.

Chondroplasty

The initial appearance of excimer laser-débrided cartilage is superior to anything that can be obtained with electrocautery or mechanical instruments (Fig. 34-3). Fibrillated cartilage can be smoothed with only minor damage to the underlying matrix. It apparently seals the surface. Hyaline cartilage is also more aggressively ablated than other tissues, a finding that concurs with our clinical experience and animal studies.

Because of the apparent advantages of excimer laser chondroplasty, the authors have conducted experiments to discover the nature of the laser effect. They are discussed below.

Disc Decompression

Little in vivo work has been done with the excimer for disc nucleotomy. It is known that 308 nm can ablate the disc nucleus (Wolgin et al., 1989). Wolgin et al. found low ablation rates compared to other tissues however, they used a small fiber with a short pulse width. It is possible that the removal speed is higher with modern apparatus.

In an in vitro study, Buchelt et al., (1991a) found that fluorescence spectroscopy can be used to distinguish nucleus pulposus from annulus fibrosis. This distinction can assist the surgeon in preventing inadvertent penetration of the annulus, which might lead to nerve damage.

Meniscectomy and Degenerative Meniscus

Experience with meniscectomy has led us to conclude that the excimer is useful primarily for smoothing degenerating fibrocartilage. It is possible to resect menisci with the excimer, but there currently are no clear advantages to doing so. A micrograph of lased meniscus is shown in Fig. 34-4.

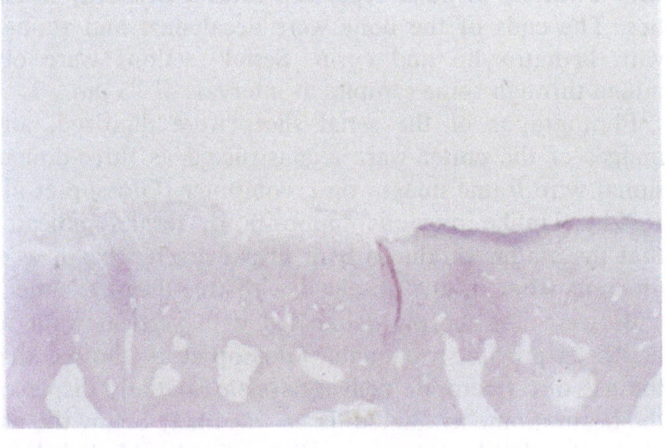

Figure 34-3. Light micrograph of fibrillated rabbit articular cartilage under hematoxylin eosin stain. The laser was used only on the right side of the photograph, causing smoothing without significant reduction in cartilage thickness.

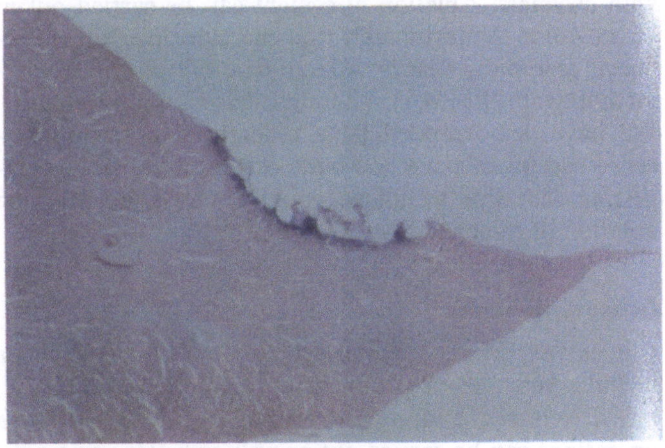

Figure 34-4. Sample of rabbit meniscus that has been exposed to the 0.308 μm XeCl Excimer laser.

The beam emerging from an optical fiber is divergent, usually a few square millimeters in area. Cutting with a divergent beam is not productive, as it requires ablation of a large volume of material. A wide channel must be excavated in the tissue before it can be separated. Notwithstanding the occasional situation where the geometry of the joint and defect substantially hinders the use of a blade or basket forceps, the laser is usually less efficient than these devices.

The rate of ablating the meniscus is lower than that for articular cartilage, but it is still much higher than that for bone. It generally takes about twice as long to ablate a given volume of fibrocartilage than hyaline cartilage.

Bone

As with the other lasers in use, the ability of the 0.308 μm XeCl Excimer laser to cut bone is limited. Although excimers have shown potential for microsurgery in hard tissues, it is still impractical to consider them bone lasers.

Ablation of bone using excimers has been investigated (Sankar et al., 1989; Yow et al., 1989; Jahn et al., 1991) with and without optical fiber delivery. Although it is possible to ablate bone, the etch rate is low. Typical etch rates are about 2 μm/pulse (0.308 μm, 15 joules/cm^2, 250 ns pulse, 20 Hz) (Jahn et al., 1991) or less. At this rate it would take approximately 25 seconds to drill a 1 mm deep, 1 mm diameter hole. This speed is generally too slow for orthopaedics, with the exception of precision bone sculpting.

Free beam (in contrast to fiber delivered) excimers transfer more energy, but they are still not able to ablate a significant volume of bone. Again, improvements in the technology will expand the excimers' role in bone surgery but probably not to the extent of replacing current techniques.

Bone Cement

Yow et al. (1989) studied the ablation of bone cement with excimers. Ablation of cement can be carried out in air or saline. Unfortunately, the energy delivered is insufficient to rapidly destroy a large quantity of polymethylmethacrylate (PMMA), although it is efficiently ablated. We have demonstrated large differences in the fluorescence spectra of bone and bone cement (see below), suggesting that this technique could be used for selective ablation of cement.

Other Operations

Clinical experience with the 0.308 μm XeCl Excimer includes removal of pedunculated bodies, synovectomy, lateral releases, and resection of plicae. Most of these operations can be carried out as well or better using conventional manual and power instruments. Although more powerful lasers enable these surgeries to be carried out without resorting to other instrumentation, there are few other advantages. The tendency to use the excimer (and other lasers) as a general purpose tool in these situations seems to be one of its chief attractions.

Clinical Experience

Clinical experience in Canada with the excimer includes 70 patients. Fifteen of them were admitted to a study (Cinats and Jackson, 1989) that evaluated débridement using mechanical and excimer laser techniques. Differences in physical examination scores were not statistically significant, but there were significant differences in the Lysholm knee scores. Both groups were improved 6 months postoperatively, but the laser group showed an average Lysholm score of 81 postoperatively (SD 7.2) compared to a score of 60 (SD 4.5) for the mechanical group. Statistically, the laser group was significantly superior to the mechanical group ($p < 0.01$). These results are similar to those obtained by Raunest and Lohnert (1990) in a more rigorous prospective study.

These investigators also found a significantly lower ($p < 0.05$) postoperative incidence of pain in the laser-treated group. At follow-up, 33% of their patients reported total absence of pain compared to 17% in the control group, and there was less joint effusion during the follow-up period. Forty-five percent of the laser cases had effusion compared to 65% in the control group ($p < 0.01$).

Laser–Tissue Interaction: In Vitro Effects

Studies investigating in vitro effects on cartilage (Glossop et al., 1992b) were conducted using cartilage and meniscus collected from freshly killed New Zealand White (NZW) rabbits. Cartilage was immediately placed in sterile saline and lased with a fiber delivery system. Several holes were drilled in the cartilage and the meniscus using the laser with a variety of pulse repetition rates and energy densities. The ends of the bone were decalcified and stained with hematoxylin and eosin. Serial sections were obtained through some samples at intervals of 15 μm.

Photographs of the serial slices were digitized, and images of the crater were reconstructed as three-dimensional wire frame images on a computer (Glossop et al., 1992b). Unlike previous suppositions, results indicated that the craters produced by a fiber-delivered beam were different from results obtained with free-beam excimers. Cuts were not sharply delineated with vertical walls as had been previously thought. Glossop et al. showed that the use of a fiberoptic delivery system spatially dispersed the beam. Some irradiated tissue was likely below the ablation threshold, and many cells received sublethal doses of 308 nm radiation.

An in vitro study was carried out to determine the fluorescent signature of various tissue types under

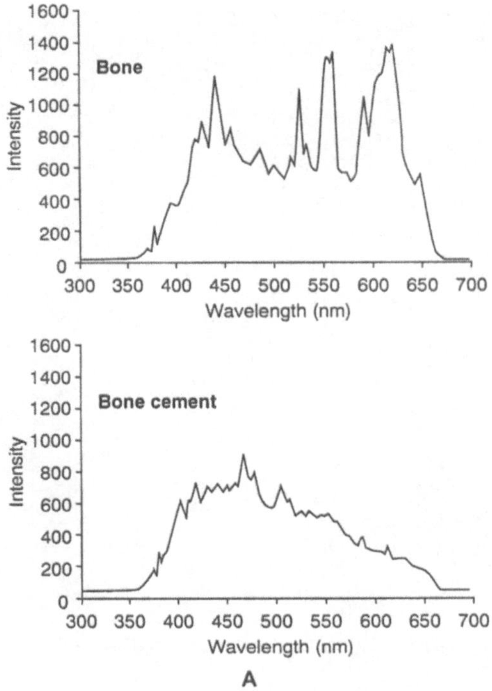

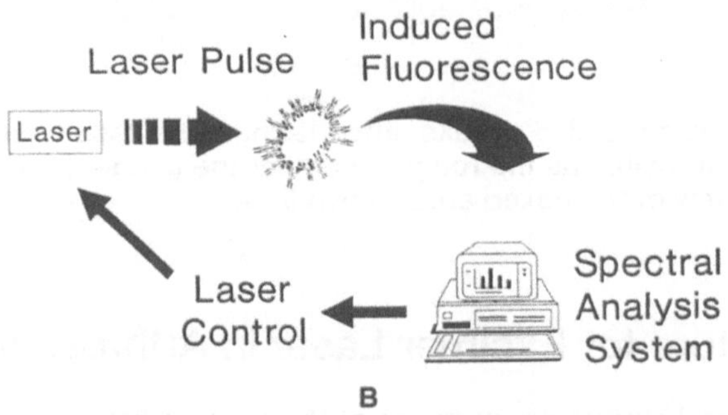

Figure 34-5. (A) Fluorescent spectral profile of bone and bone cement ablated with the excimer laser. High intensity fluorescent emissions occur in bone at 626, 552, and 442 nm when compared to PMMA. Ratios of the intensities at these wavelengths can be used to identify the materials without having to analyze the complete spectra. (B) Computer-guided surgery. The ablated tissue emits a characteristic fluorescent signature that may be used to determine the tissue type and control the laser. Tissues may be ablated selectively using this technique.

0.308 μm XeCl Excimer illumination (Glossop et al., 1992a). This experiment demonstrated the differences in the laser-induced fluorescent signal between bone and bone cement (Fig. 34-5A). The spectral variations were large enough to differentiate one substance from the other based on the intensity ratios at three wavelengths. This result potentially eliminates the need for an expensive multichannel analyzer (as required for angioplasty) in computer-guided surgery in favor of three inexpensive optical band-pass filters.

Metabolic Effects

Experimental studies on in vivo metabolic effects of the 0.308 μm XeCl Excimer laser are far from conclusive. We have conducted some short-term studies into the effects of the laser on rabbit articular cartilage. For the first of these in vivo experiments (Reed et al., 1994), an arthritis model was created in 18 NZW rabbits by performing an arthrotomy, cutting the anterior and posterior cruciate ligaments and removing the medial meniscus. The wounds were closed and rabbits returned to cage activity. Fibrillation was allowed to develop over several weeks.

Two of the rabbits were killed after 6 weeks to evaluate the arthritis model, which was found sufficiently developed to treat. The fibrillated cartilage in half the remaining 16 rabbits was débrided with the XeCl Excimer laser while being flushed with saline. Although the rabbit knees were too small to arthroscope, this technique simulated the operation. Eight of the rabbit knees were used as controls and lavaged. Rabbits were killed at 1, 2, 6 and 12 weeks to evaluate the surgery. Samples of the lased and control articular cartilage were sectioned and stained for light microscopy, and other samples were prepared for scanning electron microscopy.

The studies showed that initial smoothing of fibrillated cartilage occurred with minimal loss in cartilage thickness, but this surface disappeared after several weeks. Although the fibrillation did return, it is possible that the laser débridement temporarily sealed the surface, extending the life of the cartilage. In essence, the treatment was "buying time" for the joint.

A second experiment (article in preparation) examined the propensity of the laser to induce regeneration in partial-thickness cuts made in the articular cartilage. Some researchers (Schultz et al., 1985; Miller et al., 1989; Buchelt et al., 1991b) have found that laser wavelengths stimulate chondrocyte regeneration. This experiment was designed to test the excimer for these properties. In the absence of external stimulation or continuous passive movement, cartilage regeneration in partial-thickness cuts is sluggish or nonexistent.

Scalpel cuts were made in the femoral condyles of 18 rabbits, half of which were subsequently lased. The rabbits were returned to their cages and killed at intervals ranging from 1 to 12 weeks after surgery. The lased portions of the articular cartilage were collected and examined with the scanning electron and light microscopes. Scanning electron micrographs of the lased cuts are shown in Figure 34-6.

No evidence of regeneration or stimulation of the partial-thickness cuts was observed despite contrary observations in a study of fibrocartilage by a German research team (Buchelt et al., 1991b). In autoradiographic studies, no metabolic changes in lased cartilage were detected when comparing the results with unlased cartilage (Fig.

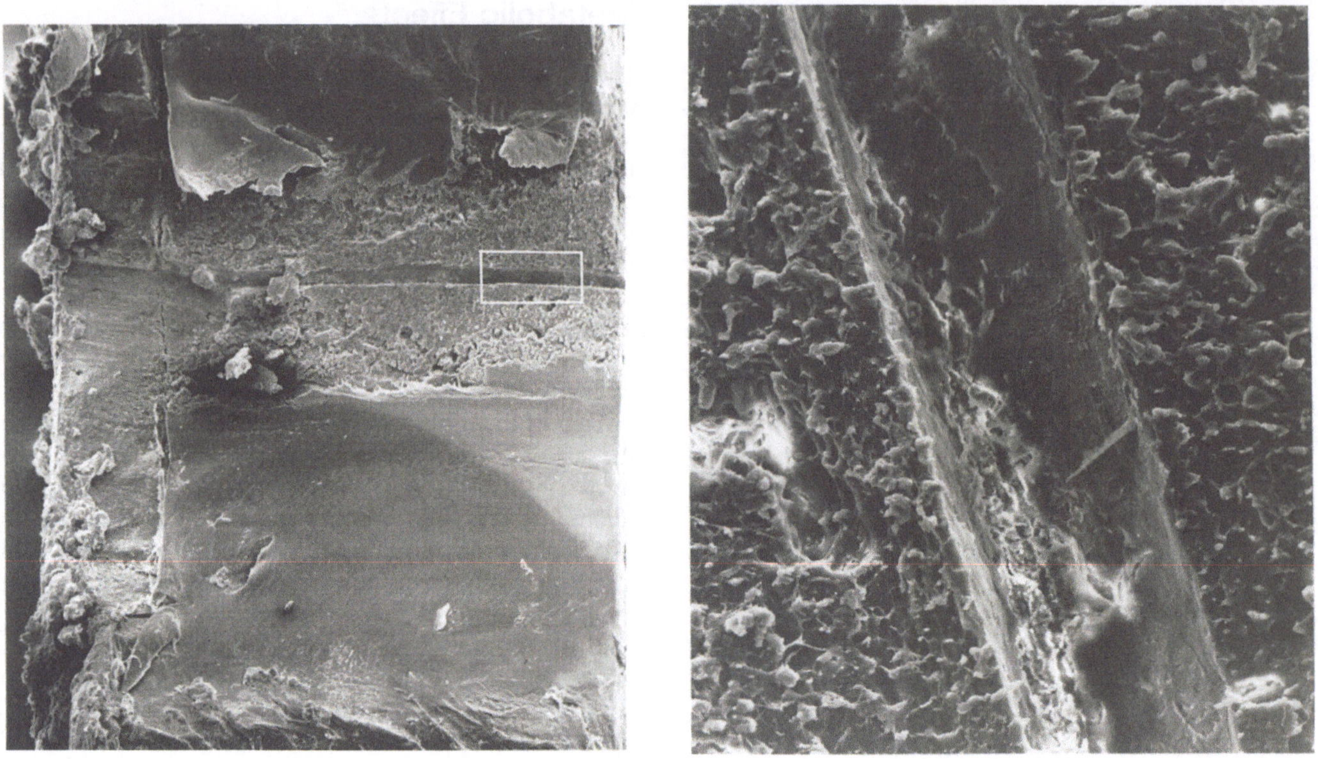

A B

Figure 34-6. (A) Scanning electron micrograph of a scalpel cut in rabbit articular cartilage that has been lased with the excimer laser. The specimen was taken from a rabbit that was sacrificed 6 weeks after lasing. The lased area is clearly visible as the rough area near the gouge. (B) Close-up view of the boxed area shown in (A).

34-7). These studies were, however, carried out at a single energy density setting. It is known that different results occur for different power and energy settings (Schultz et al., 1985), so stimulatory effects are still possible with the excimer set at different radiant exposures.

Future for Excimer Laser in Arthroscopy

Several studies are required of the excimer before its entry into commercial applications. As with the other lasers, it is imperative that detailed animal experiments be carried out

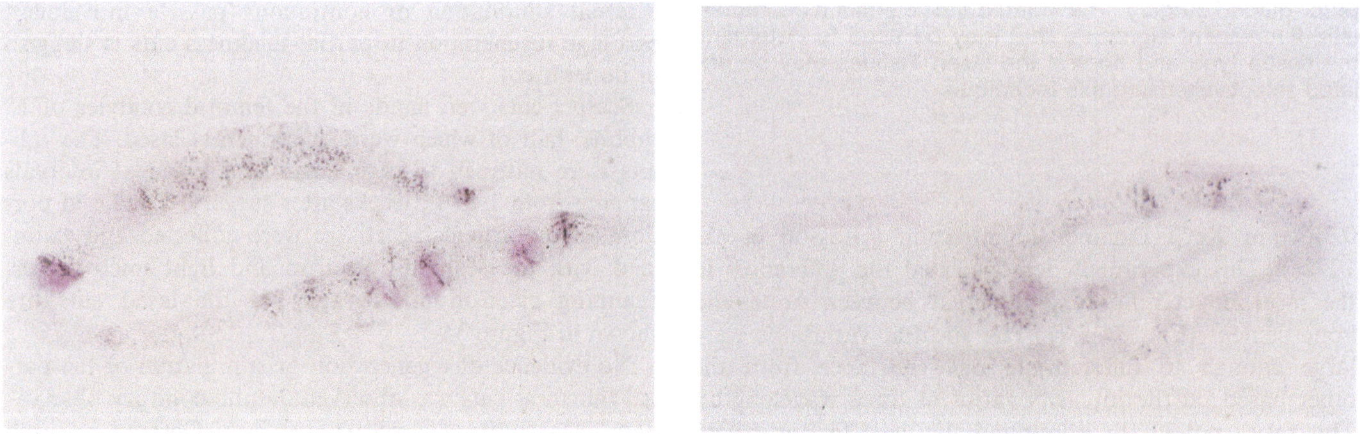

A B

Figure 34-7. (A) Autoradiogram of rabbit articular cartilage that was subjected to laser ablation. This section is from a rabbit that was sacrificed 6 weeks after laser treatment. (B) Autoradiogram of normal rabbit articular cartilage.

to evaluate its in vivo effects on cartilage and other tissues of interest. It is also important to describe the chemical debris produced by the excimers and their various effects.

There are many promising indications for the use of the excimer in arthroscopy. It is unquestionably the "cleanest" laser in our experience. Unlike other mechanical devices and lasers, it is able to ablate material with exacting precision. It does not replace conventional instrumentation, nor should it. Developments in technology are key to the success of this device, and it is certain to supplant many other lasers currently in use once some of these technological barriers are surmounted. Koort (1991) has tabulated the progress made in one excimer laser system in recent years. If this trend continues, it is likely that formidable laser systems will be available during the next few years.

References

Bath P, Mueller G, Apple D, Stolzenburg N (1988) Excimer laser application for cataract surgery. SPIE Proc 908:72–74

Buchelt M, Katterschafka T, Horvat R, et al (1991a) Fluorescence guided excimer laser ablation of intervertebral disks in vitro. Lasers Surg Med 11:280

Buchelt M, Papaioannou T, Fishbein M, et al (1991b) Excimer ablation of fibrocartilage: an in vitro and in vivo study. Lasers Surg Med 11:271–279

Cinats J, Jackson R (1989) Arthroscopic laser surgery in a fluid medium. Poster Presentation, Canadian Orthopaedic Association Annual Meeting, Toronto

Clarke R, Isner J, Gauthier T, et al (1988) Spectral characterization of cardiovascular tissue. Lasers Surg Med 8:45

Dressel M, Jahn R, Neu W, Jungbluth K (1991) Studies in fiber guided excimer laser surgery for cutting and drilling bone and meniscus. Lasers Surg Med 11:569–579

Francis A, Carrier W, Regan J (1988) The effect of temperature and wavelength on production and photolysis of a UV-induced photosensitive DNA lesion which is not repaired in xeroderma pigmentosum variant cells. Photochem Photobiol 48:67–71

Glossop N, Jackson R, Randle J, Reed S (1992a) The excimer laser in arthroscopic surgery. Semin Orthop 7:125–130

Glossop N, Jackson R, Randle J, Reed S (1992b) The excimer laser in orthopaedics. Clin Orthop (in press)

Hendrich C, Mommsen J, Stürmer M, Hagemann G, Siebert W (1991) Mutagenität durch laserstrahlung? I. Untersuchungen für Excimer-Lasersysteme. In Öffentliche Sitzung des Arbeitskreises 29: Lasertechnik in der Orthopädie, Deutscher Orthopädenkongreß 1991, Hamburg

Hohla K, Laufer G, Wollenek G, et al (1988) Simultaneous tissue identification and ablation with excimer laser. SPIE Proc 908:128–136

Reed S, Jackson R, Glossop N, Randle J (1994) An in vivo study of the effect of excimer laser irradiation on degenerate rabbit articular cartilage. Arthroscopy 10:78–84

Jahn R, Dressel M, Fabian H (1990) Excimerlaser und taperfaser—ein effizientes Instrument für die Ablation von Knorpel und Knochengewebe. Lasers Med Surg 6:77

Jahn R, Dressel M, Neu W, Jungbluth K (1991) Elaboration of excimer lasers dosimetry for bone and meniscus cutting and drilling using optical fibers. SPIE Proc 1424:23

Kaufmann R, Hibst R (1989) Pulsed Er:YAG and 308 nm Uv-excimer laser: an in vitro and in vivo study of skin-ablative effects. Lasers Surg Med 9:132–140

Kochevar I (1989) Cytotoxicity and mutagenicity of excimer laser radiation. Lasers Surg Med 9:440–445

Kokosa J, Doyle D (1988) Chemical by-products produced by CO_2 and Nd:YAG laser interaction with tissue. SPIE Proc 908:51–53

Koort HJ (1991) Excimer laser in the arthroscopic surgery. SPIE Proc 1424:53

Marshall J, Trokel S, Rothery S, Schubert H (1985) An ultrastructural study of corneal incisions by an excimer laser at 193 nm. Ophthalmology 92:749–758

Miller D, O'Brien S, Arnosczky S, et al (1989) The use of the contact Nd:YAG laser in arthroscopic surgery: effects on articular cartilage and meniscal tissue. J Arthrosc 5:245–253

Pini R, Salimbenei R, Vannini M (1987) Optical fiber transmission of high power excimer laser radiation. Appl Opt 26:4185–4189

Raunest J, Lohnert J (1990) Arthroscopic cartilage débridement by excimer laser in chondromalacia of the knee joint: a prospective randomized clinical study. Arch Orthop Trauma Surg 109:155–159

Sankar R, Fabian R, Nuss R, Puliafito C (1989) Plasma-mediated excimer ablation of bone: a potential microsurgical tool. Am J Otolaryngol 10:76–84

Schultz R, Krishhnamurthy S, Thelmo W, Rodriguez J, Harvey G (1985) Effects of varying intensities of laser energy on articular cartilage: a preliminary study. Lasers Med Surg 5:577–588

Sherk H, Lane G (1989) Clinical uses of lasers in orthopaedics. Medical College of Pennsylvania, course notes

Vangsness C, Akl Y, Nelson S, et al (1992) An in vitro analysis of partial human meniscectomy by five different laser systems. Semin Orthop 7:77–80

Vari S, Shi W, van der Veen M, et al (1991) Comparative study of excimer and Erbium:YAG lasers for ablation of structural components of the knee. SPIE Proc 1424:33

Wolgin M, Finkenburg J, Papaioannou T, et al (1989) Excimer ablation of human intervertebral disc at 308 nanometers. Lasers Surg Med 9:124–131

Yow L, Nelson J, Berns M (1989) Ablation of bone and polymethylmethacrylate by an XeCl (308 nm) excimer laser. Lasers Surg Med 9:141

35

2.1 μm Holmium:YAG Laser for Arthroscopic Laser Surgery of the Knee

Michael F. Dillingham and Gary S. Fanton

The first human clinical trial with a free-beam fiber-transmitted laser in fluid medium was carried out by us beginning in 1987 using the 2.1 μm holmium laser. This study compared laser-assisted meniscectomy with a conventional arthroscopic technique. The application of holmium technology to the knee was seen to have obvious advantages even then, and its use has expanded greatly since our original study. To fully utilize the 2.1 μm holmium laser's potential in the knee, a specific array of equipment and a specific fund of knowledge are necessary.

Equipment

In addition to the laser itself and routine arthroscopic instruments, the following instrumentation is necessary.

Heavy-duty nerve hook
Reciprocating power shaver
Operating room setup allowing good fluid flow, especially in posteromedial and posterolateral compartments
Leg holder

Knowledge

Although it is best to thoroughly understand the relevant laser physics, minimally one needs a "feel" for tissue effects, depth of penetration, power density, spot size, focusing and defocusing the laser beam, power settings (joules), repetition rate settings (hertz), and the effect of contact and near-contact technique. One needs to know the tissue effect of a given setting in terms of ablation, tissue reduction, coagulation, and carmelization in order to fully utilize the wonderfully variable tissue effects of the laser during various procedures. These effects are achieved by varying the power, repetition rate, and spot size (power density). One must be aware of the angle of incidence to the target surface to safely achieve the goal. For instance, the laser is commonly used perpendicular to meniscal tissue for ablation but is used tangential to the articular surface for chondroplasty to avoid damage to underlying articular material.

With a basic scientific background, the "feel" of the laser comes, as with any surgical procedure, with experience. This chapter presents techniques developed by us during more than 1000 laser-assisted cases with the valuable input of other colleagues with rich laser surgical experience.

Arthroscopic Setup

The patient is prepared and draped in a leg holder as for conventional arthroscopy. The laser is generally to the left or right of the surgeon, according to personal preference. The laser handpiece cable is placed through a loop or clamped to the drapes. If we are not certain the laser will be utilized, we delay opening the handpiece until the initial diagnostic portion of the arthroscopy validates the desirability of laser use. The foot pedal controls are conveniently placed at the surgeon's feet.

Depending on the laser, a several-minute cooling period may be necessary. Thus it is best to precool the laser if its use is likely. With the 2.1 μm holmium laser, local custom and regulation determine the need for protective eyewear.

The full array of handpieces should be in the operating room so as not to delay the case. A conventional arthroscopic shaver should be available. We generally set up the shaver but delay opening the disposable blade until we are sure of its necessity. A 30 degree, 4 mm arthroscope is used routinely.

A sign indicating laser utilization is placed on the door of the operating room. Our experience indicates that when properly set up and equipped, laser-assisted arthroscopic surgery is achieved with in a time period comparable to that of conventional arthroscopic surgery, with the frequent added benefit to the patient of reduced postsurgical morbidity and reduced time of rehabilitation.

Handpieces

Various handpieces are available.

1. Thirty degree curved handpiece. The 30 degree, angled, 400 μm handpiece is the standard equipment utilized in most of our cases. It offers good access to all parts of the knee because of its ability to maneuver around curved surfaces. Other handpieces are used as well.
2. Straight handpiece. Although not as versatile as a 30 degree handpiece, the straight handpiece is valuable for occasional applications.
3. Fifteen degree curved handpiece.
4. Forty-five degree curved handpiece. The curve here is a bit too extreme for routine use, although it could be useful for certain unusual applications, particularly in the front of the knee where its increased angle of incidence allows increased ease of laser utilization.
5. Seventy degree side-firing handpiece. Next to the 30 degree handpiece, the 70 degree device is the most useful. It is exceptionally helpful in small joints such as the wrist and ankle. In the knee it offers some real advantage when working in the notch and especially when working in the anterior portions of the knee and the anterior portions of the menisci (Fig. 35-1).

Some handpieces have been designed that aid in gathering tissue and presenting it to the laser tip. These devices have the look of a Smiley knife and tend to be hooked and help guide the laser.

Fiber diameter differences also exist. Variation of fiber diameter from 200 to 1000 μm is being studied. As increased pulse powers become available, larger-diameter fibers can be utilized without loss of power density. This change offers even shorter surgical times with more efficient tissue coverage per pulse. Alternatively, truly large spot sizes may be utilized at lower power densities to expedite procedures that do not require high power density.

Interchangeable fiber tips are also available. The availability of low-cost interchangeable tips for the free-beam laser is a critical step in expanded flexibility of use, as the surgeon can "afford" more than one type of fiber tip per case, offering greater efficiency and precision during surgery.

Anodized arthroscopic instruments are available. We

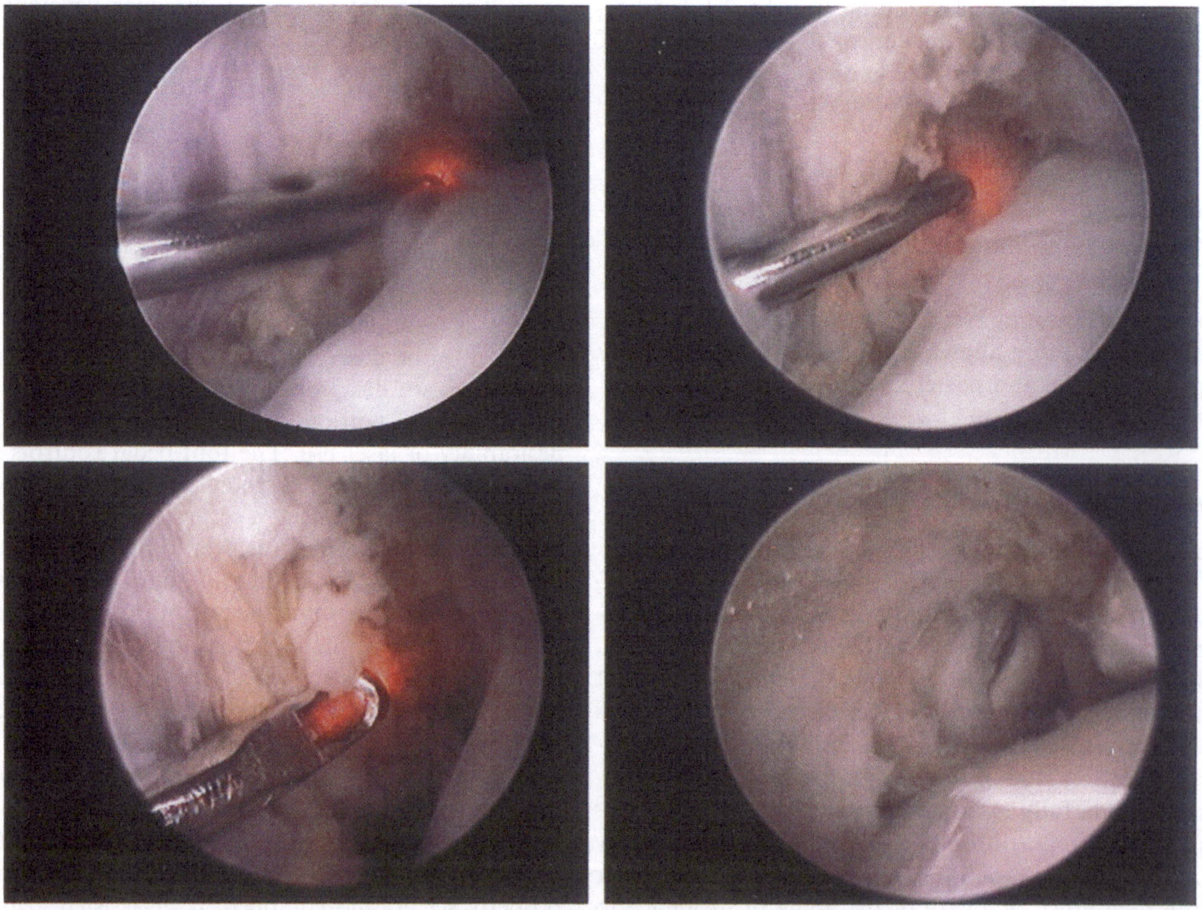

Figure 35-1. Use of the 70° side-firing handpiece in the anterior knee.

have not found it necessary, however, to use anodized instruments for 2.1 μm holmium laser-assisted surgery of the knee.

Techniques

Degenerative Meniscus

The degenerative meniscus has multiple cleavage planes. Our technique takes advantage of this situation. Initially the laser is used to create a radial cut posteriorly toward the notch, weakening or ablating the posterior attachment of the degenerative material. A heavy duty nerve hook is then used to tear the material free, creating a flap tear. This flap is then reduced or totally ablated with a laser. If excess material remains, it can be removed with a power shaver (Fig. 35-2).

Alternatively, the meniscus may be cut at the anterior extent of the lesion and the flap displaced toward the notch for removal. The laser handpiece can easily reach under and around the posterior femoral condyles. After the abnormal tissue has been removed, the rim of the meniscus can be contoured and, if necessary, coagulated with the laser. Simple direct ablation of the abnormal meniscal tissue is also possible and efficient if adequate pulse power (>2 joules per pulse, preferably up to 3 joules per pulse) is available (Fig. 35-3) with adequate repetition rates.

Note: When working in the back of the knee especially, debris from high power or high frequency laser use can obscure vision unless adequate fluid flow is established

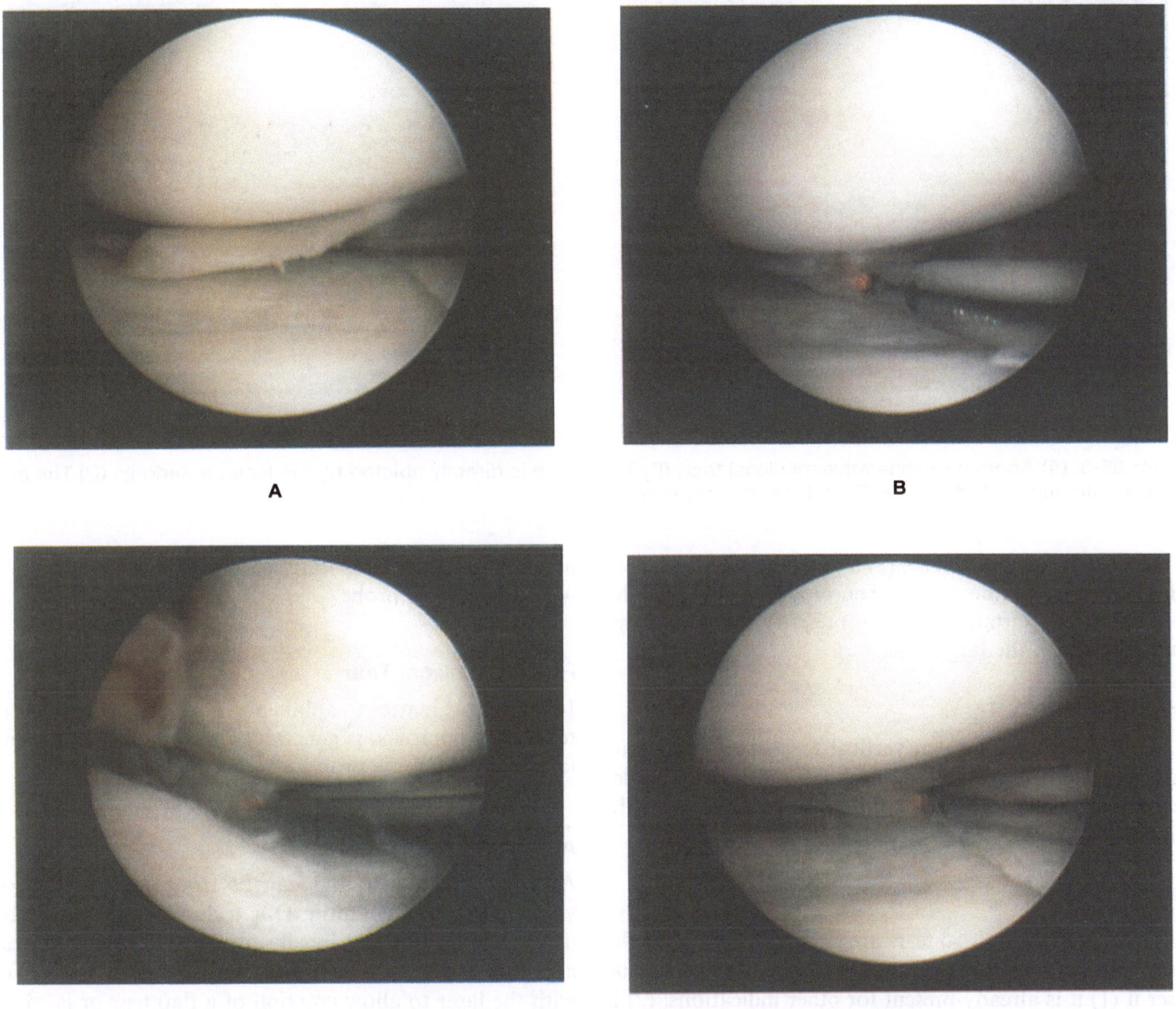

Figure 35-2. (A) Degenerative meniscal tear. (B) The laser is used to create a radial cut toward the notch. (C) A heavy duty nerve hook may then be used to tear the material free. (D) This material is then ablated with the laser or removed mechanically.

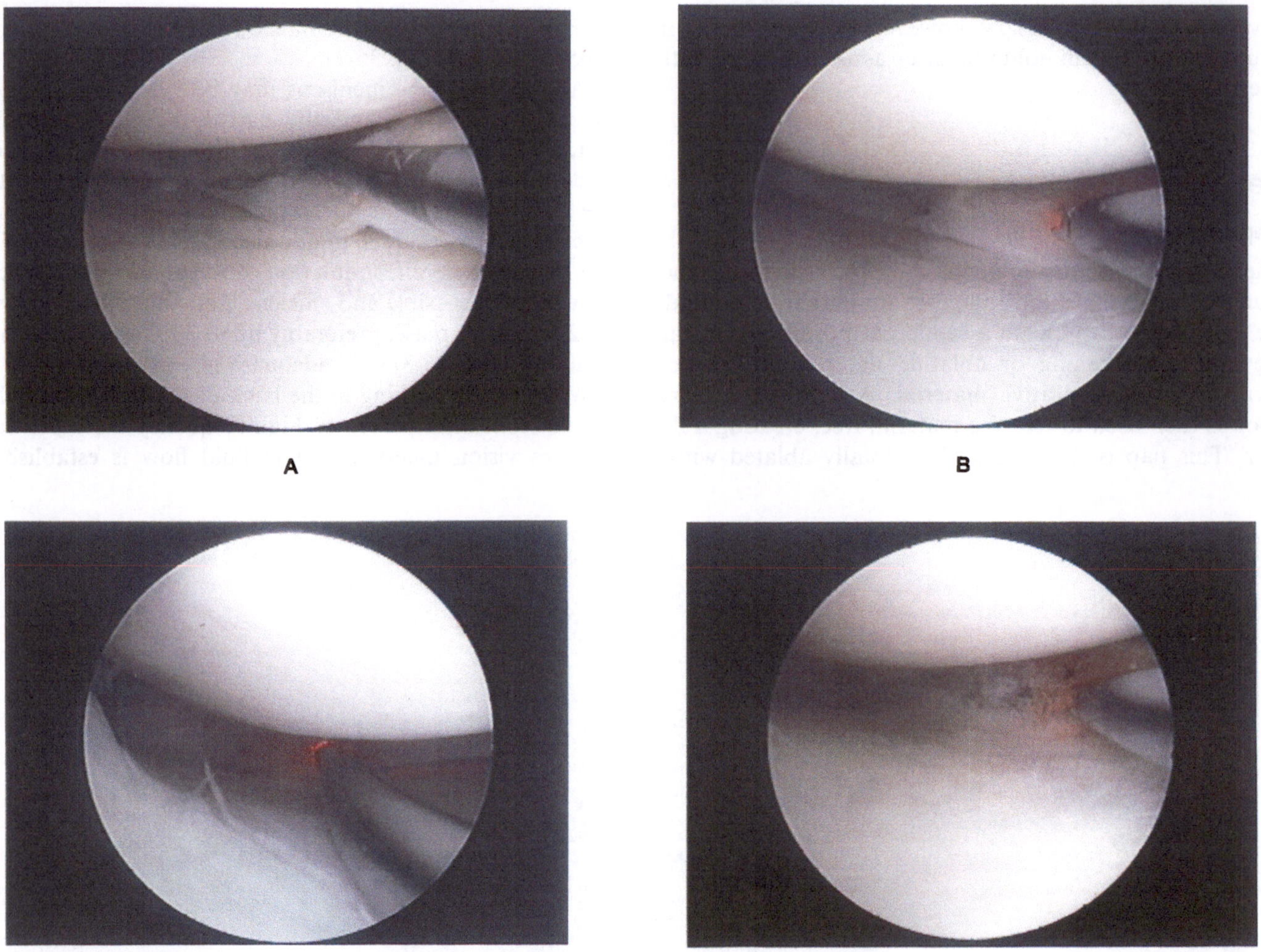

A B C D

Figure 35-3. (A) Another degenerative meniscal tear. (B) The tissue is directly ablated by the laser, anteriorly. (C) The ablation is continued posteriorly. (D) The edges are further trimmed.

by: (1) intermittent drainage; (2) a posterior drainage portal; (3) suctioning the area (a neurologic tip laser in the laser working portal); or (4) a pressure pump forcing fluid away from the target site.

Vertical Meniscal Tears

If for some reason a clean vertical tear of the meniscus cannot be repaired, excision is carried out as for the degenerative meniscus; that is, a flap tear is created and subsequently removed.

Flap Meniscal Tear

Although many meniscal tears are so simple to remove the laser may not offer an advantage, one may elect to use the laser if (1) it is already present for other indications; (2) it would be possible to ablate the fragment in a reasonable amount of time utilizing high pulse powers and avoiding any other instrument damage in the knee; or (3) the fragment would be difficult to reach using conventional instruments. The laser is generally used via the isolateral portal with a 30 degree probe.

Radial Meniscal Tear

It is a simple matter to ablate and contour radial meniscal tears. The approach is generally via the contralateral portal with a 30 degree probe.

Anterior Meniscal Lesions

Anterior meniscal lesions can be troublesome with conventional instrumentation. Our techniques involve débridement of the fat pad locally to allow exposure utilizing a power shaver. The anterior horn segment is then cut with the laser to allow creation of a flap tear or is wholly or partially ablated utilizing the laser. Both 30 and 70 degree probes are useful when utilizing isolateral and contralateral portals. A 70 degree arthroscope is also useful at times.

Bucket-Handle Tear

The laser is used in lieu of cutting instruments to detach the bucket handle consistent with the surgeon's preferred technique, that is, beginning anteriorly or posteriorly. After removing the flap, the rim is contoured with the laser. A 30 degree probe is therefore used via contralateral and isolateral portals.

Plica Technique

The medial plica is easily ablated with the surgical 2.1 μm holmium laser. Two techniques are commonly used. With the first technique, a small stab wound is made just through the skin proximal to the superolateral pole of the patella, and then the laser is used to cut into the knee through the lateral portion of the suprapatellar pouch, creating only a tiny deep portal. The superolateral suprapatellar pouch is visualized during this time with a 30 degree arthroscope that has been placed in the inferolateral portal. Once the laser is in the knee it is brought across the suprapatellar space, and the medial shelf is ablated in an orderly fashion beginning at the superomedial origin and taken down to its insertion in the fat pad. Any remnants or debris may be removed with a rongeur or a shaver (Fig. 35-4). Alternatively, the arthroscope may be placed in the superolateral parapatellar portal and the laser used via the inferolateral portal with a similar approach and resection of the shelf (Fig. 35-5).

We have used a pulse power of up to 3 joules per pulse for plicectomy. However, it is possible to resect the plica using power of 1 to 2 joules.

Lateral Retinacular Release

The release of soft tissue highlights one of the great advantages of the 2.1 μm holmium laser: its ability to coagulate. In our study of lateral release, laser lateral release reduced pain, effusion, and rehabilitation time compared

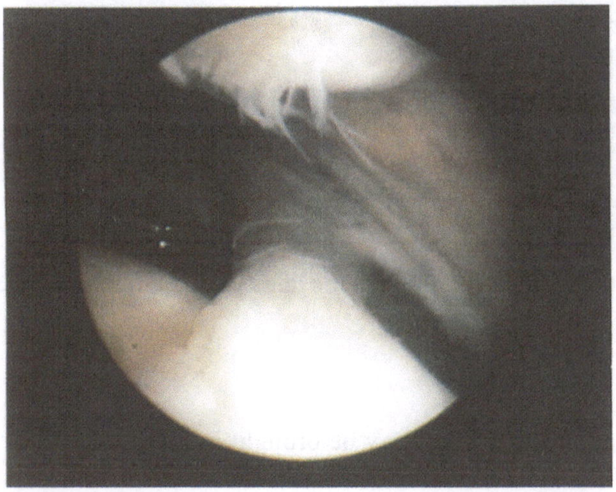

A

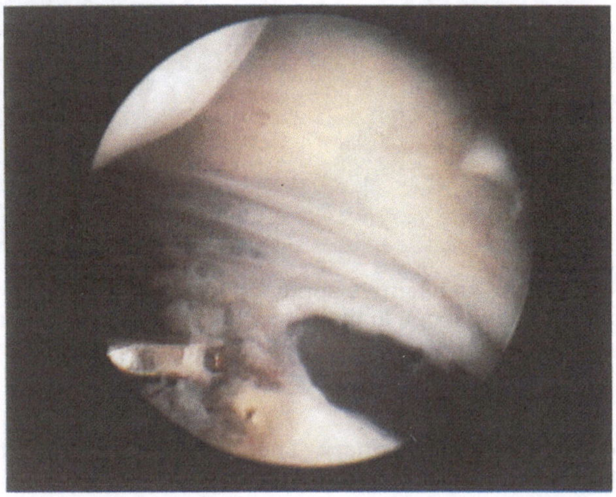

B

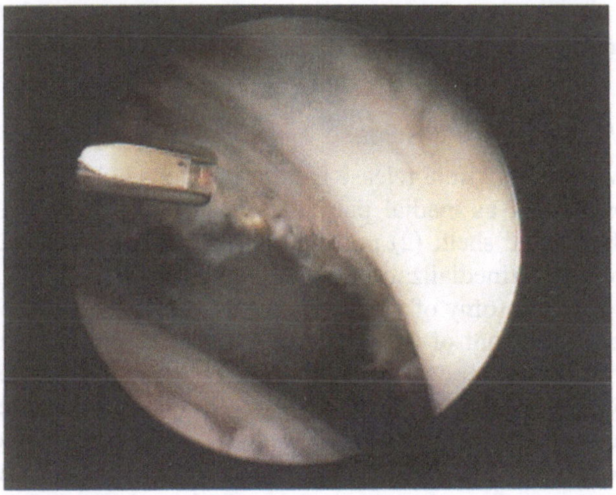

C

Figure 35-4. (A) A medial pliça is easily ablated with the 2.1 μm holmium:YAG laser. (B) The laser probe is brought across the knee from the lateral suprapatellar pouch. (C) The plica is ablated in an orderly fashion beginning at the superomedial origin and taken down to the fat pad.

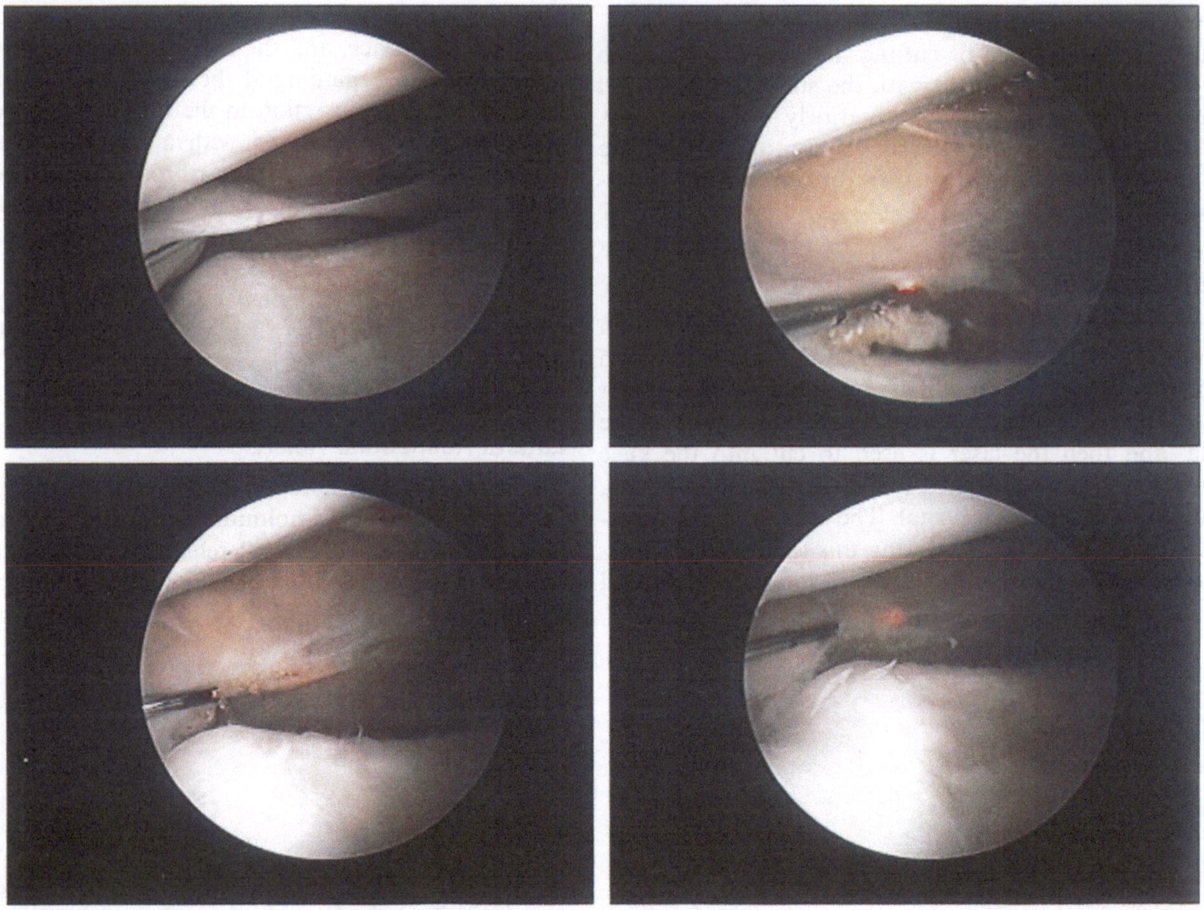

Figure 35-5. An alternate approach to ablate a medial shelf is to place the laser probe in the knee via the inferolateral portal and the arthroscope in the superolateral parapatella approach.

to cold cutting or cautery. The actual time spent cutting the retinaculum is 2 to 5 minutes.

In most patients, local anesthesia is utilized without tourniquet. All other procedures necessary are completed prior to the lateral release. Patellar tracking is evaluated passively, with active extension and active resisted extension. This method allows final determination of the need for and the degree of release as a function of true dynamic analysis of patellar tracking. Once it has been determined that the patella tracks laterally, it has an excessive tilt, or it presents with a clear lateral pressure lesion on the patellar or trochlear surface, a release is carried out.

The first step is to excise the inferolateral fat pad and fat in the lateral parapatellar area using the power shaver. Although the laser ablates this fat, it is inefficient because of the volume of tissue involved and obstruction of vision as fat is exploded and placed in emulsion. Once the fat is excised, local coagulation is achieved with the laser. The laser is then used to cut, coagulate, and ablate the desired amount of lateral retinacular tissue via the inferolateral portal. We prefer this technique (Fig. 35-6). Alternatively, the laser may be brought into the knee from the superomedial portal in the retinacular release.

Postoperatively, a gentle compression dressing is applied, and weight-bearing begins as tolerated. Physical therapy begins the next day.

Generally, a 30 degree angled laser is used. A hook-type endpiece may also be used.

Medial Capsule Release

A medial capsule release is indicated for (1) local fibrosis presenting as medial parpatellar pain mimicking that of the medial shelf; (2) postoperative fibrosis; and (3) iatrogenic overmedialization of the patella.

The anatomy of the medial fat pad and retinaculum differs from that of the lateral fat pad. The approach, however, is similar. At times it is simpler on either the medial or lateral side to incise a short distance of the inferior retinaculum using a No. 15 blade, a Smiley knife, or some equivalent instrument and then coagulate the area with the laser. Once this step is done, the laser is used to finish the release.

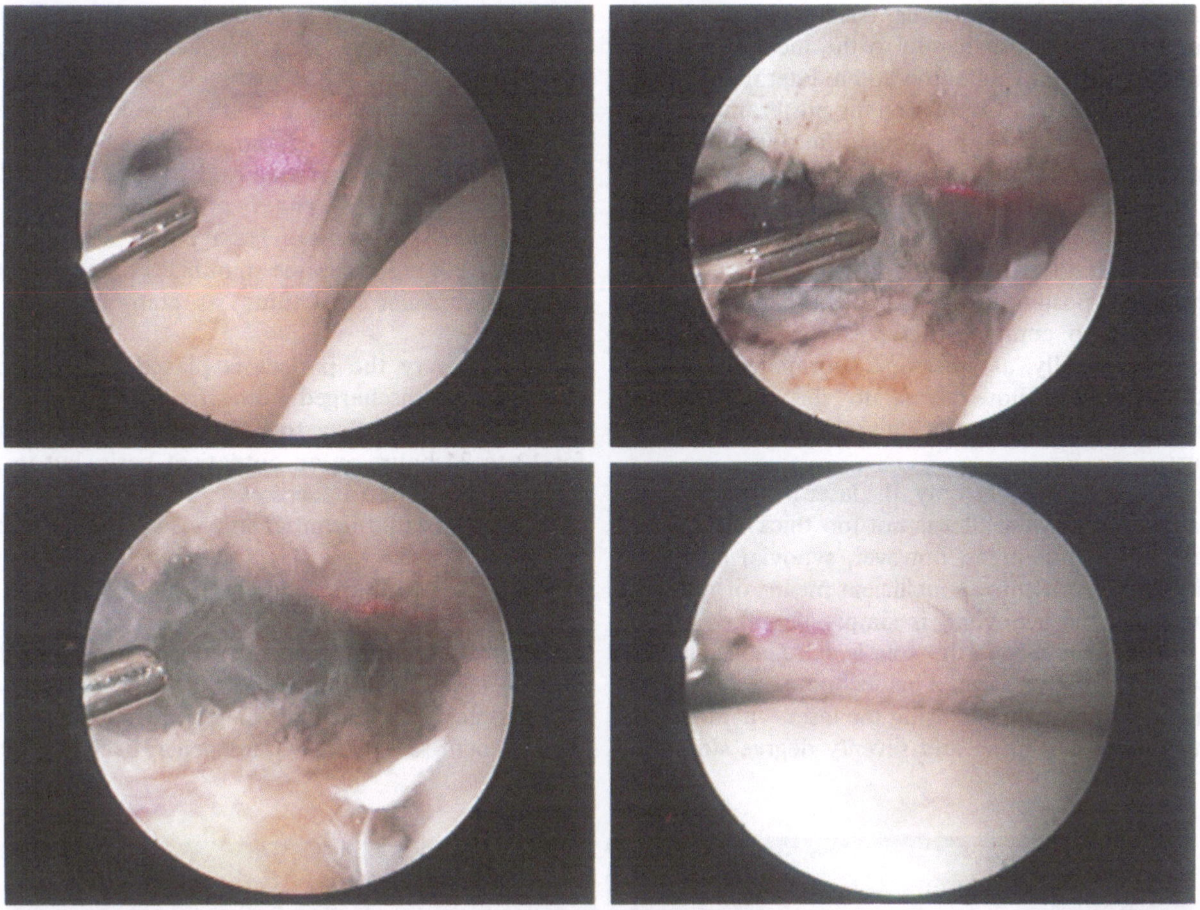

Figure 35-6. For a lateral retinacula release the laser probe is inserted inferolaterally after the lateral fat pad is excised with a power shaver. The laser is then used to cut, coagulate, and ablate the lessened amount of tissue from distal to proximal.

Most soft tissue releases performed medially are limited to the inferior one-half of the retinaculum or less, as the goal is usually the release of painful scar and soft tissue, not lateralization of the patella. The degree of release in an iatrogenically medialized patella must be individualized to the patient. This judgment is best made with the patient under local anesthesia so active tracking can be evaluated.

Synovectomy

Arthroscopic synovectomy for chronic inflammatory synovitis has been shown to offer a dramatic reduction in morbidity compared to open synovectomy. The arthroscope offers access to virtually all areas of the knee with preservation of the menisci. Performed with conventional instrumentation, arthroscopic synovectomy substantially reduces the need for a hospital stay and reduces postoperative morbidity, particularly fibrosis. The addition of laser allows easy, safe access to the notch under the menisci, into the popliteal recess, and so forth. Most importantly, perhaps, it offers efficient coagulation, reducing the degree of postoperative hemarthrosis, which in turn allows early effective physical therapy and reduction of the tendency to fibrosis and loss of range of motion.

The patient is set up as for routine arthroscopy. Remember that in a rheumatoid patient or a patient with another form of inflammatory synovitis, the suprapatellar pouch may extend much further above the patella than usual, so generally the leg holder is placed high on the thigh. Additionally, it must be emphasized that many patients with inflammatory synovitis have significant osteoporosis, so the limb must be manipulated with care. It is important that the surgeon be at ease with multiple portal arthroscopy, including posteromedial and posterolateral portals, as these portals are essential when carrying out adequate synovectomy. These cases are relatively tedious, sometimes lasting 2 hours. Several laser handpieces may be utilized as may several mechanical shavers, as these instruments sometimes wear out during the case. An assistant surgeon should be present to help manipulate the leg and, in extreme cases, even to operate simultaneously.

A tourniquet should be placed on the leg in case it is necessary. Thirty and seventy degree arthroscopes should be available.

A defined approach is established. It is our habit to begin with routine anterior portals, starting in the medial gutter and moving subsequently to the medial compartment, anterior compartment, the notch, lateral gutter and lateral compartments; we approach the posteromedial and posterolateral compartments through the notch and then carry out as much work as possible in the suprapatellar pouch. By doing all possible work via the anterior, medial, and lateral portals prior to establishing other portals, soft tissue fluid extravasation is limited.

At this time, posteromedial and posterolateral portals are established to complete the posterior compartment synovectomy. Finally, as necessary, suprapatellar portals are established to allow access to the often greatly enlarged suprapatellar pouch. Several portals may be necessary.

When doing the synovectomy, the laser is used to ablate and coagulate synovium that is not too thick for efficient tissue effect. In some areas, however, synovial bulk is so great the laser represents an inefficient means of removal. In these areas the synovium is simply debulked with a power shaver: The base of the area is debulked, and then it is coagulated with a laser. This technique achieves one of the main objectives when using the laser—hemostasis.

Thirty degree end-firing and seventy degree side-firing laser handpieces should be available. Large diameter fibers giving a large spot size help speed the process. Ablation of the thinner areas of synovium and effective coagulation of the base of debulked areas can be achieved with an angle of beam incidence well off the perpendicular, and in some areas (e.g., the gutters and suprapatellar space) this angle of incidence is virtually tangential to the surface. High power settings assist in this regard. This technique minimizes damage to the underlying capsular structures so common with power shavers.

After surgery the patient is placed in a compressive dressing and discharged home from the recovery area. The surgeon may elect to use portable suction drainage for 12 to 24 hours on an outpatient basis, but in general we have not found it necessary. Physical therapy begins the next day, with the initial emphasis on range of motion.

Chondroplasty

It was implied during early advertising for the application of CO_2 lasers in orthopaedics that utilizing the laser for chondroplasty to "melt down" the articular surface provided benefit to patients with degenerative arthritic condi-

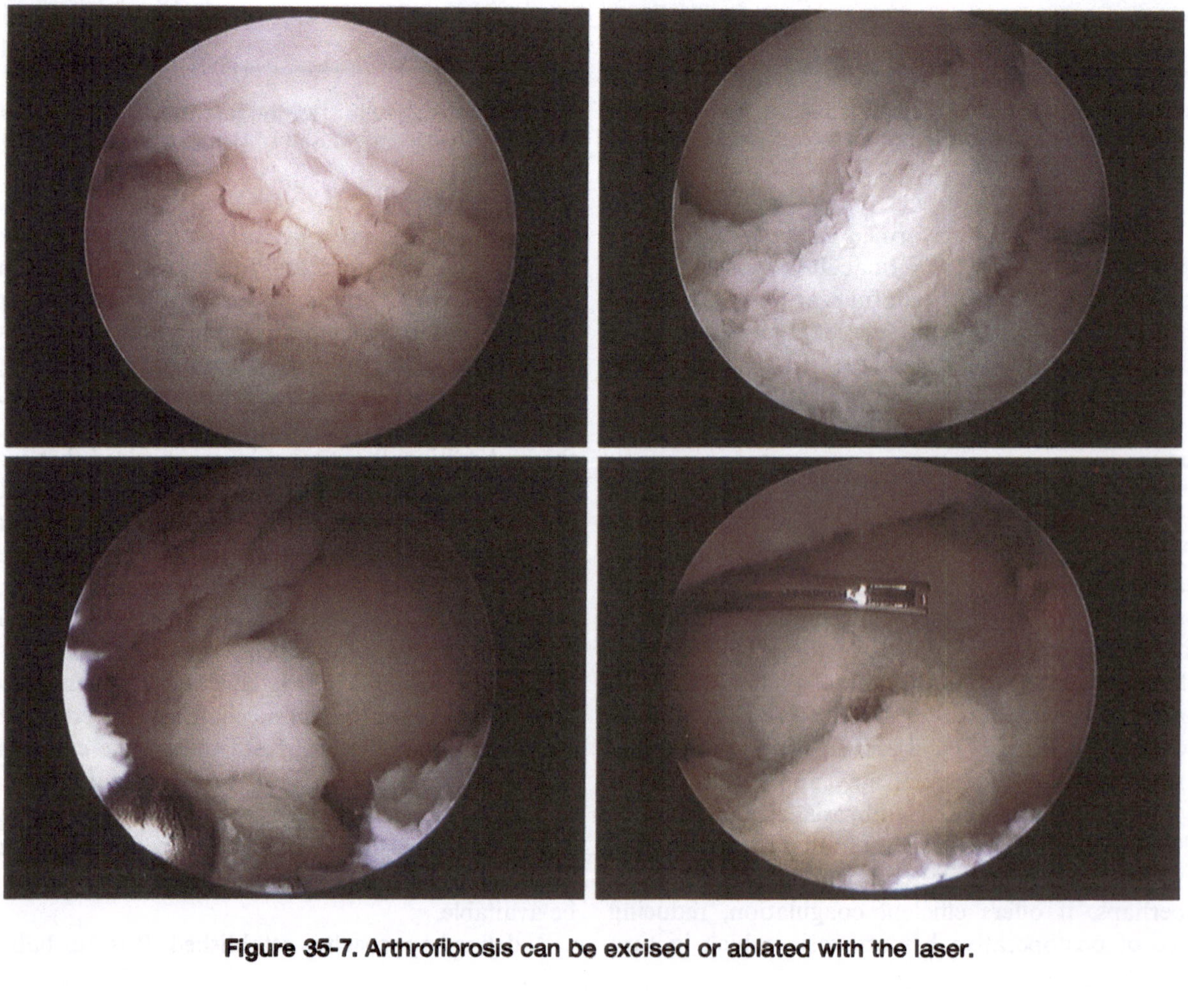

Figure 35-7. Arthrofibrosis can be excised or ablated with the laser.

tions. No evidence was presented to substantiate this claim, however, and it was highly irrational to think that relatively unlimited thermal energy applied to an articular surface could lead to improvement in symptoms once the surface was smooth and tidy. It is equally evident that débridement of an arthritic articular surface does not "cure" arthritis, as it does nothing to improve the load-distributing or load-bearing potential of the articular surface. It is accepted, however, that débridement (chondroplasty) is useful in cases of osteoarthritis or traumatic arthritis to (1) reduce pseudolocking and catching; (2) reduce or eliminate annoying crepitus in selective severe cases; or (3) remove debris that almost certainly will cause synovitis and the associated symptoms of effusion and inflammation.

The laser is ideally suited for these tasks. Relatively low power (e.g., 0.6 joule/pulse) may be used to ablate fronded articular material and to "melt back" articular flaps. The angle of incidence for simple ablation of articular fronds should be 30 degrees or less so no significant thermal damage is done to underlying or surrounding viable articular cartilage. When reducing flaps, more direct beam application may be necessary. The laser is able to do a more precise job in flap reduction than can conventional instrumentation.

To date, no convincing evidence exists that photothermal stimulation of cartilage leads to repair, though this possibility is being researched. What seems to have been established at this time is that at low levels of laser energy débridement can be achieved without worrisome significant collateral damage. Work done by us and our associates has provided preliminary evidence of DNA stimulation by low levels of 2.1 μm holmium laser energy delivered to human chondrocytes in tissue, cultures indicating possible repair potential. This study is preliminary, and further work is needed.

The most commonly used handpiece for chondroplasty is the 30 degree device used via alternating portals to allow easy, safe access to the various articular surfaces. It also allows an advantageous angle of incidence to be utilized. Laser energies from 0.6 to 2.0 joules and more have been used. If higher energies are elected, it is important that the surgeon be familiar with focusing and defocusing the laser beam (that is, moving it closer to or farther from the tissue in order to change the power density delivered to the surface).

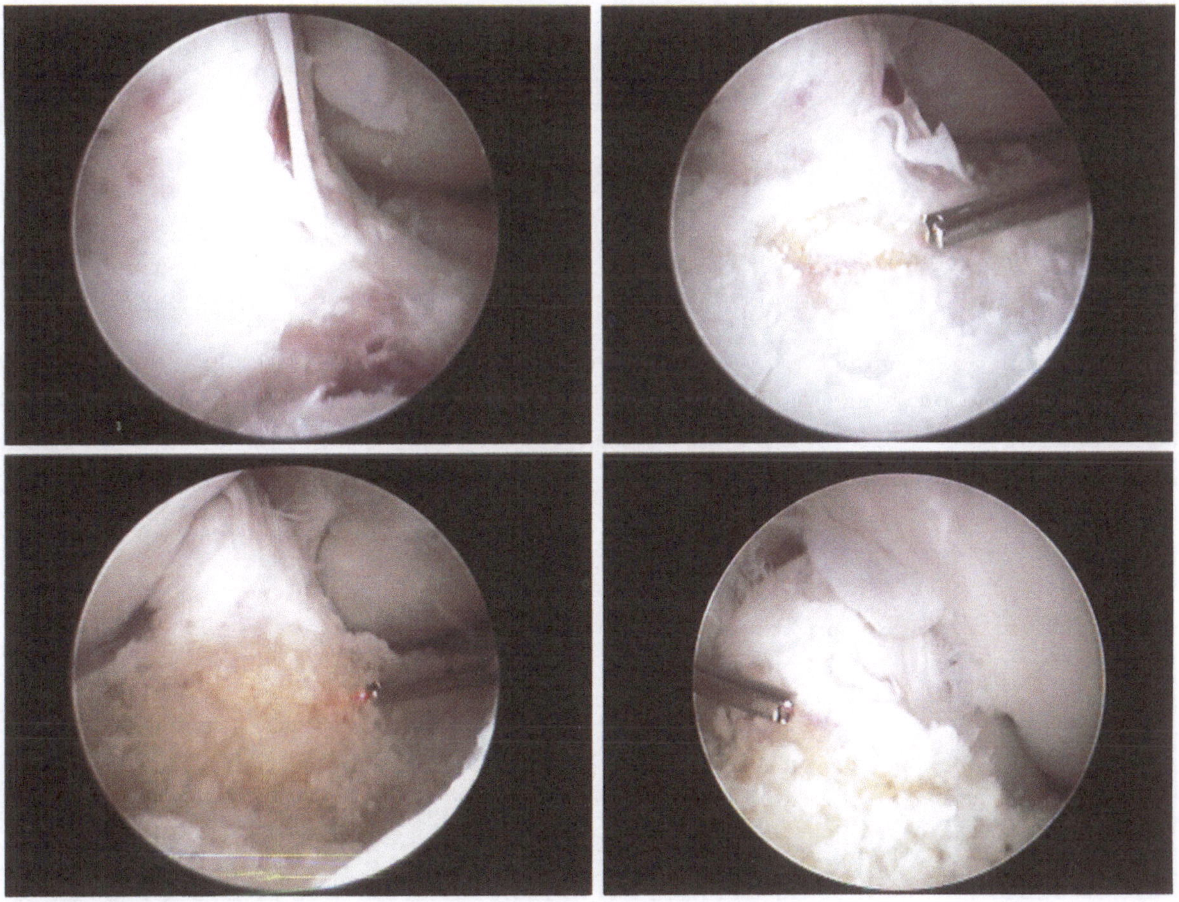

Figure 35-8. Laser débridement of a "cyclops" lesion.

Notchplasty

Débridement and enlargement of the lateral and superolateral intercondylar notch is commonly practiced in a variety of anterior cruciate ligament reconstructive techniques. The laser can facilitate this portion of the procedure, with ablation of tissue and reduction of bleeding often allowing a tourniquet-free technique.

Our technique begins by using the laser to ablate the desired amount of articular cartilage along the lateral and superior notch, followed by ablation and coagulation of soft tissue with the laser. Pituitary rongeurs or power shavers may facilitate removal of large volumes of tissue. A rasp is then used to "clean" the bone to be ablated. Alternatively, a power burr may be used. Placing a small neuro suction tip on the notch to provide simple gravity drainage helps keep the area clear of debris.

Arthrofibrosis

Arthrofibrosis represents a poorly understood genetic variant or extreme of the posttraumatic inflammatory process that leads to debilitating posttraumatic or postoperative fibrosis. Soft tissues fibrose, contract, and thicken. Traditional approaches involve prolonged physical therapy, manipulation under anesthesia, or arthroscopy with cold cutting or electrocautery. Postoperative bleeding is a significant problem when trying to achieve early postoperative range of motion. Additionally, blood is a stimulant to further inflammation and fibrosis (Fig. 35-7).

The laser has proved to be a powerful aid in this setting. Soft tissues can be cut and a large volume of fibrotic tissue ablated with good hemostasis. This method has been our preferred approach when appropriate trials of physical therapy and when manipulation under anesthesia itself either have not proved fruitful or are thought to be insufficient to achieve the results we desire.

Alternatively, a large mass of scar can be cut and resected with traditional instrumentation and the laser used to coagulate the remnant more successfully than can be achieved with cautery. We have adopted this technique if forced to because of the volume of tissue present, particularly in the presence of massive thickening of the parapatellar retinacular tissue. Additionally, ablation of anterior impinging fibrotic lesions (so-called cyclops lesions) after anterior cruciate reconstruction along with further notchplasty or roof plasty, as necessary, is easy to achieve without significant postoperative hemarthrosis (Fig. 35-8).

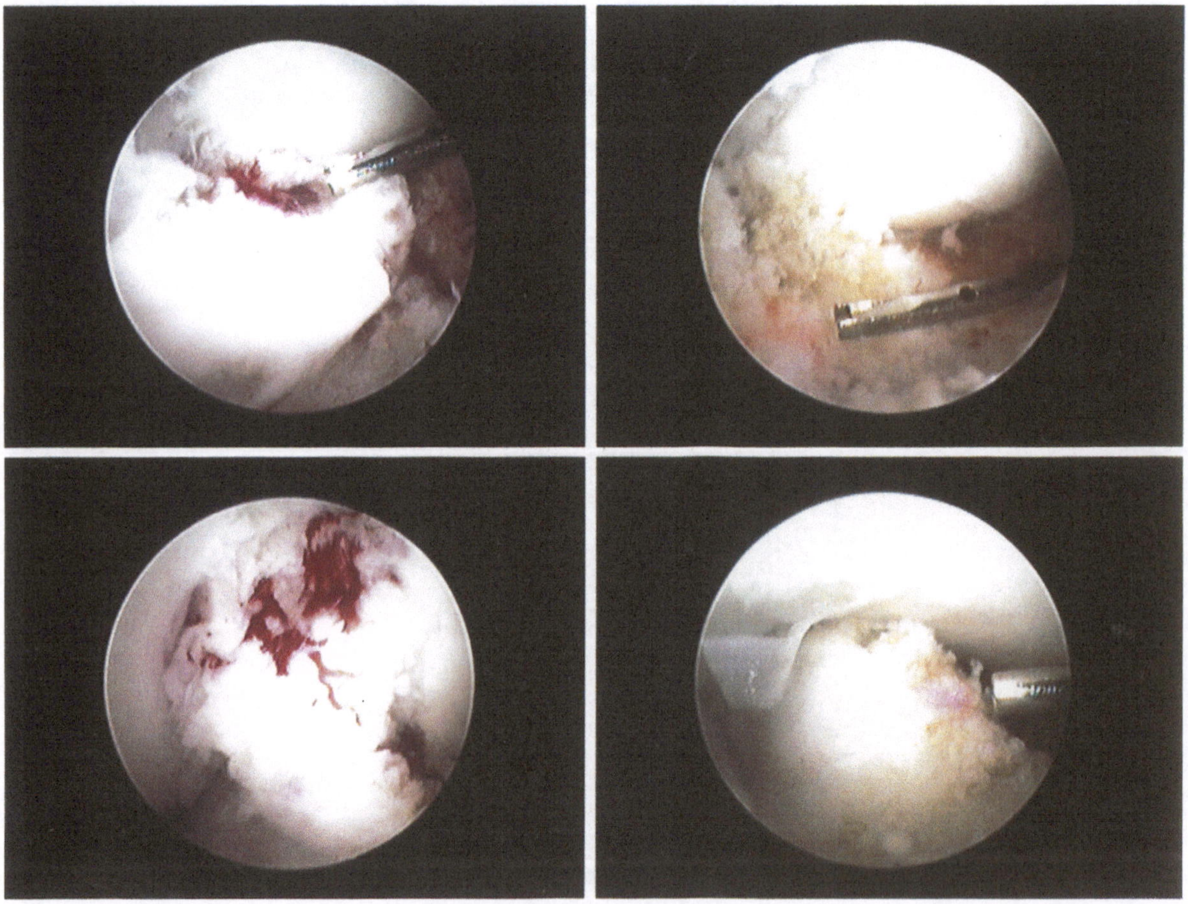

Figure 35-9. Laser ablation of a recurrent hemangioma.

Vascular Anomalies and Cysts

We have successfully resected, coagulated, and ablated areas of recurrent invasive hemangioma and a variety of small vascularized soft tissue masses and intraarticular ganglion type cysts with the 2.1 μm holmium laser with no postoperative hemarthrosis (Fig. 35-9).

Bleeding Disorders

The 2.1 μm holmium laser has been used in cases of von Willebrand's disease to remove soft tissue lesions successfully without associated hemarthrosis. These cases had previously been complicated by postsurgical hemarthrosis. Appropriate platelet activators were used perioperatively.

Clinical Experience

In 1990 we conducted a short-term study of partial meniscectomy and showed that these patients had a faster postoperative recovery than did those with mechanically treated lesions. There was also a faster resolution of effusion and diminished postoperative pain. As of this time, more than 800 laser-assisted arthroscopies of the knee have been performed. The longest follow-up is 4 years and the shortest 1 day. The average follow-up is 18 months.

No significant complications involving the patient, surgeon, or other personnel were attributed to laser use. There were no infections, but there were two large effusions. No patient required reoperation because of laser-related problems. No arthrotomies were performed because of failure of laser use. There were three cases of thrombophlebitis. Probe tips were noted to fail after exceeding tolerance limits, but no adverse sequelae involving the patient has been noted. There was one delivery system failure and no laser device failure. There were no prolonged recovery times attributable to laser use. Most importantly, there were no unhappy patients because of laser use. These results also support our initial favorable impressions of the use of the 2.1 μm holmium:YAG laser for arthroscopic surgery of the knee.

Suggested Reading

Berns MW (1991) Laser surgery. Sci Am 264:85–90

Brillhart AT (1991a) Arthroscopic laser surgery. Am J Arthrosc 1:5–12

Brillhart AT (1991b) Arthroscopic laser surgery: the CO_2 laser and its use. Am J Arthrosc 2:7–12

Brillhart AT (1991c) Arthroscopic laser surgery: the Holmium:YAG laser and its use. Am J Arthrosc 3:7–11

Decklebaum LI, Isner JM, Donaldson RF, et al (1985) Reduction of laser-induced pathologic tissue injury using pulsed energy delivery. Am J Cardiol 56:662–667

Fanton GS (1991) Uses of the holmium laser in arthroscopy: multiple joint applications. Presented at the Coherent Symposium on Advances in Laser Arthroscopy: New Techniques in Orthopaedic Surgery, Anaheim, CA

Fanton GS, Dillingham MF (1990) Arthroscopic meniscectomy using the holmium:YAG laser: a double-blind study. Presented at the Arthroscopy Association of North America Annual Meeting, Orlando, FL

Fanton GS, Dillingham MF (1992) The use of the holmium laser in arthroscopic surgery. Semin Orthop 7(2):102–116

Goldberg VM (1987) Arthritis. In Orthopaedic Knowledge Update II. American Academy of Orthopaedic Surgeons, Chicago, pp 35–47

Goldman JA, Chiapella J, Casey H, et al (1980) Laser therapy of rheumatoid arthritis. Lasers Surg Med 1:93–101

Gross AE, Farine IM (1984) Arthritis. In Orthopaedic Knowledge Update I. American Academy of Orthopaedic Surgeons, Chicago, pp 29–40

Hobbs ER, Bailin PL, Wheeland RG, et al (1987) Super-pulsed lasers: minimizing thermal damage with short duration, high irradiance pulses. J Dermatol Surg Oncol 13:955–964

Jackson RW (1991) Symposium: lasers in orthopaedic surgery. Contemp Orthop 22:77

Lane GJ, Mooar PA (1991) Holmium:YAG laser arthroscopic débridement [abstract]. Am Soc Laser Med Surg (suppl 3)

Lane GJ, Sherk HH, Mooar PA, et al (1991) CO_2 vs holmium:YAG laser arthroscopic débridement [abstract]. Am Soc Laser Med Surg (suppl 3) 52–53

Lord MJ, Maltry JA, Shall LM (1991) Thermal injury resulting from arthroscopic lateral retinacular release by electrocautery: report of three cases and review of the literature. Arthroscopy 7:33–37

Mankin HJ (1982) The response of articular cartilage to mechanical injury: a current concepts review. J Bone Joint Surg [Am] 64:460–465

Meller M, Black H, Sherk H (1991) Wavelength selection in laser arthroscopy. Presented at the American Society for Laser Medicine and Surgery, San Diego

Miller GK, Drennan DB, Maylahn DJ (1987) The effects of technique on histology arthroscopic partial meniscectomy with electrosurgery. Arthroscopy 3:36–44

Moller KO, Lind B, Shurman U, et al (1991) Holmium-laser synovectomy of immune synovitis in rabbits [abstract]. Am Soc Laser Med Surg (suppl 3) 51

Nishioka NS, Domankevitz Y (1989) Reflectance during pulsed holmium laser irradiation of tissue. Lasers Surg Med 9:375–381

Nishioka NS, Domankevitz Y, Flotte TJ, et al (1989) Ablation of rabbit liver, stomach and colon with a pulsed holmium laser. Gastroenterology 96:831–837

Norton LA (1982) Effects of a pulsed electromagnetic field on a mixed chondroblastic tissue culture. Clin Orthop 167:280

Rand JA, Gaffey TA (1985) Effect of electrocautery on fresh human articular cartilage. Arthroscopy 1:242–246

Reagan BF, McInerny VK, Treadwell BV, et al (1983) Irrigating solutions for arthroscopy. J Bone Joint Surg [Am] 65:624–631

Schultz RJ, Krishnamurthy S, Thelmo W, et al (1985) Effects of varying intensities of laser energy on articular cartilage: a preliminary study. Lasers Surg Med 5:577–588

Schurman DJ (1990) Arthritis. In Orthopaedic Knowledge Update. American Academy of Orthopaedic Surgeons, Chicago, pp 57–66

Sherk HH (1990) Lasers in Orthopaedics. Lippincott, Philadelphia

Smith CF, Marshall GJ, Synder SJ, et al (1984) Comparisons of tissue effects of a surgical scalpel, an electrocautery apparatus and a carbon dioxide laser system when used for making incisions into the menisci of New Zealand rabbits. Laser Surg Med 2:305

Stein E, Sedlacek T, Fabian RL, et al (1990) Acute and chronic effects of bone ablation with a pulsed holmium laser. Lasers Surg Med 10:384–388

Trauner K, Nishioka N, Patel D (1990) Pulsed holmium: yttrium-aluminum-garnet (Ho:YAG) laser ablation of fibrocartilage and articular cartilage. Am J Sports Med 18:316–321

Van Leeuwen TG, van der Veen MJ, Verdasdonk RM, et al (1991) Noncontact tissue ablation by holmium:YSG laser pulses in blood. Lasers Surg Med 11:26–34

Vari SG, Shi WQ, Fishbein MC, et al (1991) Ablation study of the knee structure tissues with a Ho:YAG laser [abstract]. Am Soc Laser Med Surg (suppl 3)

Walsh TJ Jr, Flotte TJ, Anderson RR, et al (1988) Pulsed CO_2 laser tissue ablation: effect of tissue type and pulse duration on thermal damage. Lasers Surg Med 8:108–118

36

2.1 μm Holmium:YAG Arthroscopic Laser Surgery of the Ankle

James W. Stone, James F. Guhl, Naomi N. Shields, and Shari Gabriel

The development of arthroscopic surgical techniques for the ankle joint has lagged behind that of other joints such as the knee and the shoulder. The combination of tight ligamentous restraints, highly congruous joint surfaces, and complex curved surfaces makes arthroscopic instrumentation of the ankle joint more difficult than that of the relatively capacious knee joint or the relatively lax shoulder joint. Two major innovations during the 1980s contributed to the more widespread application of arthroscopic surgical techniques to the ankle joint. First, Guhl popularized the use of joint distraction techniques, which facilitated the passage of instruments in the joint. Since the original description of his technique utilizing threaded pins placed in the tibia and calcaneus, the use of distraction has evolved to utilize either a noninvasive or an invasive form. We have found that noninvasive means of joint distraction are sufficient in approximately 90% of arthroscopic surgical cases. The second major advance has been the development of high resolution, small diameter, wide angle arthroscopes. These instruments provide excellent visualization while decreasing the incidence of iatrogenic articular cartilage injury and facilitating passage of the arthroscope across this tight joint.

The application of laser techniques to arthroscopic ankle surgery was initially investigated by Guhl in 1990, with clinical application by Stone and Guhl starting in 1991 using the 2.1 μm holmium:YAG laser. We were interested in determining whether the use of the laser could facilitate procedures on soft tissues, articular cartilage, and bone while potentially decreasing the incidence of complications associated with arthroscopic ankle surgery. The last consideration is not a trivial one. Studies by Ferkel, Guhl, and others have documented an incidence of complications of up to 15% (Martin et al., 1989). The complications frequently involve use of the invasive distraction apparatus or placement of arthroscopic portals. Neurovascular complications may result in areas of hypesthesia or the formation of neuromas. In addition, sinus formation and superficial infection are more common in the ankle than other joints, possibly related to the minimal soft tissue envelope and the dependent nature of the joint. The use of laser might decrease such complications by decreasing the need for multiple instrument passes through the soft tissues, by the hemostatic nature of laser surgery, and by the lessened incidence of articular cartilage injury due to the low profile delivery handpiece.

Laser Alternatives for Arthroscopic Ankle Surgery

Three types of laser can be considered for use in arthroscopic ankle surgery. The 10.6 μm CO_2 laser has excellent soft tissue, bone, and cartilage effects, but its use in the ankle joint is limited (Philandrianos, 1985; Whipple et al., 1985; Smith et al., 1989; Vangsness et al., 1991). The 10.6 μm CO_2 laser requires an articulated arm for delivery of the laser beam as it cannot be passed via a fiberoptic cable. The laser must also be used in a gas environment, to which most arthroscopic surgeons are unaccustomed. A gas bubble technique that allows use of the 10.6 μm CO_2 laser in a fluid with a localized gas environment at the laser tip has been used in the knee joint but to our knowledge has not been applied to the ankle joint. We have not used the 10.6 μm CO_2 laser in the ankle because of these limitations.

The 1.06 μm neodymium:YAG laser has found wide application in laparoscopic surgery, and some orthopaedic surgeons have used it extensively for knee and shoulder arthroscopic surgery (Miller et al., 1989; O'Brien and Miller, 1990). The 1.06 μm neodymium:YAG laser requires use of a contact tip for arthroscopic applications. In essence, the laser energy is converted to heat energy at the tip. This laser has deeper tissue penetration than the 10.6 μm CO_2 laser, and the hot tip cannot be used in a noncontact or a near-contact mode. This laser has limited potential for tissue ablation, contouring of articular cartilage, or synovectomy in our experience.

We believe that the 2.1 μm holmium:YAG laser provides several advantages over the 10.6 μm CO_2 and the 1.06 μm neodymium:YAG lasers. The 2.1 μm holmium:YAG laser operates well in a fluid environment and uses a small-diameter fiberoptic cable enclosed in a durable metal sheath for laser beam delivery (Stein et al., 1990; Trauner et al., 1991; Dillingham and Fanton, 1991; Lane et al., 1991; Moller et al., 1991). The durability of the delivery system allows the handpiece to be used as an arthroscopic probe and a laser delivery tool. The probes are available in 0, 15, 30, and 70 degree beam angles. The 15 and 30 degree probes are useful for passing over the curved surfaces of the ankle. The 70 degree probe is a "side-firing" straight probe. The 2.1 μm holmium:YAG laser is a pulsed delivery system that minimizes heat conduction by allowing the fluid environment to be cooled between pulses. The laser is used in a free-beam mode, either near contact or contact. The amount of energy delivered to the tissues depends on the distance at which the laser energy is applied. This quality of the 2.1 μm holmium:YAG laser makes it a forgiving instrument with precise energy application. Soft tissues can be ablated with ease while simultaneously achieving hemostasis. Articular cartilage can be débrided and contoured using this laser. With higher power devices, bony lesions can be resected.

Technique for Arthroscopic Ankle Surgery

The patient is placed supine on the operating table, and either spinal or general anesthesia is administered. The hip is flexed, and the knee is supported in a well padded genitourinary leg holder so the foot and ankle are in a plantigrade position and the entire leg can be draped in a sterile fashion. We recommend placement of the noninvasive ankle distractor in most cases of ankle arthroscopy. The straps are applied to the hindfoot and midfoot and then secured to the sterile post attached to the operating table. Distraction force sufficient to achieve joint opening is then applied.

The positions of the anteromedial and anterolateral portals are located at the medial border of the tibialis anterior tendon and the lateral border of the peroneus tertius tendon, respectively. An 18 gauge needle is introduced at each location, and the appropriate angle of introduction is determined by the ease with which the needle can be placed across the joint. Each portal is then created by first incising the skin only and then gently spreading the subcutaneous tissues with a small curved clamp to avoid injury to superficial nerves. The portal is completed by inserting a small joint cannula with a dull obturator. Sharp obturators are not necessary in the ankle because there is little soft tissue between skin and joint, and the capsule is thin. Use of the dull obturators makes iatrogenic articular cartilage injury less likely.

A posterolateral portal is then placed under direct visualization. An 18 gauge needle is introduced adjacent to the lateral border of the Achilles tendon. The point of entry is usually approximately 1 cm distal to the location of the anterior portals. A cannula is then placed in the method described above.

A complete, systematic examination of the joint is performed, starting with the arthroscope in the anteromedial portal, then in the anterolateral portal, and finally in the posterolateral portal. The use of an interchangeable cannula system facilitates portal switching and minimizes the chance of neurovascular injury secondary to multiple passes of instruments through the soft tissues. A careful examination of the entire joint for pathology should be performed before concluding that a particular abnormality is responsible for the patient's symptoms.

We use the 2.1 μm holmium:YAG laser for soft tissue débridement, synovectomy, ossicle removal, débridement of degenerative joint disease, débridement of osteochondritis dissecans with contouring of the articular cartilage, and occasionally excision of osteophytes. These applications are detailed below. The laser probe is introduced through the routine arthroscopic portals. If multiple passes are required, we recommend using a plastic cannula with a fluid dam to minimize fluid extravasation and soft tissue injury. The laser is used in conjunction with mechanical instruments such as basket forceps, scissors, loose body forceps, rongeurs, arthroscopic knives, and motorized instruments such as shavers and abraders.

Synovitis

Anterior joint synovitis can exist as an entity by itself, frequently occurring after trauma, and at times it becomes a chronic process. It may also accompany other pathologic ankle conditions, such as loose bodies, osteochondritis dissecans, anterior osteophytes, and synovial impingement lesions. Anterior synovitis may make initial visualization of the ankle joint difficult. Débridement must initially be carried out to achieve adequate visualization. In the past, motorized shavers were most useful for carrying out the débridement. However, significant bleeding frequently accompanied their use. In addition, care must be exercised not to débride too aggressively and cause injury to the anterior neurovascular structures. Some patients, such as those with rheumatoid arthritis, may have particularly fragile anterior capsular structures and are more prone to this complication.

In contrast to the nonspecific or posttraumatic synovitis discussed above, forms of specific synovitis such as rheumatoid arthritis, pigmented villonodular synovitis, crystal-

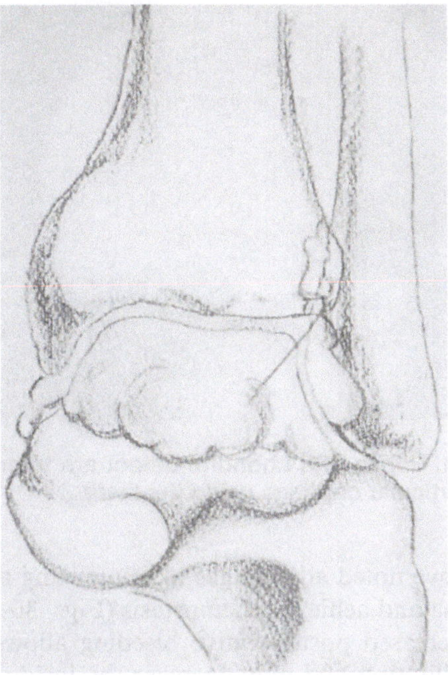

Figure 36-1. Origin of the lateral soft tissue lesion from the superior synovial recess of the lateral talomalleolar joint. This lesion often occurs after a minor ankle sprain or fracture and is the source of continued disabling pain. It is also present to various degrees in most ankles with posttraumatic pathology. Excision of the lesion usually results in dramatic symptomatic relief.

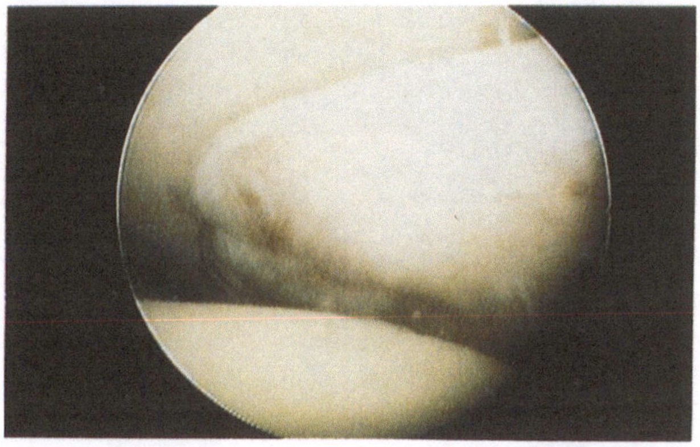

Figure 36-2. Arthroscopic view of the 2.1 μm holmium:YAG laser at 15 watts removing a lesion impinging on soft tissue laterally.

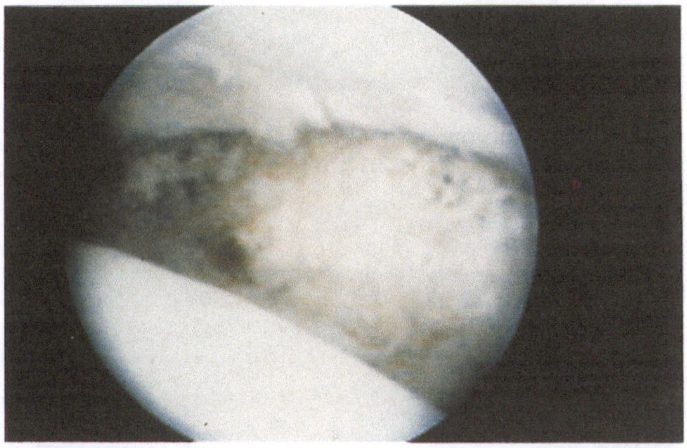

Figure 36-3. Arthroscopic view of lateral soft tissue impingement after lesion was removed.

line synovitis, and synovial chondromatosis may require synovectomy. Such a synovectomy generally requires joint distraction and multiple portals for access to the anterior and posterior reaches of the joint.

The laser is helpful for débriding the soft tissue synovitis because it achieves hemostasis while ablating the tissue. Even when initial débridement is performed with mechanical instruments, the laser is particularly useful for performing precise synovectomy and achieving hemostasis. With more complete synovectomy and less postoperative bleeding and effusion, more rapid rehabilitation can be pursued with less chance of recurrence.

Adhesions

Intraarticular adhesions form after trauma and are most frequently seen after ankle sprain or ankle fracture. The adhesions can be in the form of a single band of tissue or multiple bands forming a dense network of fibrous connective tissue throughout the joint. The single bands can be responsible for symptoms of internal derangement of the joint, including recurrent catching, swelling, and giving way. In their most dense form adhesions may result in arthrofibrosis, which causes significant restriction of motion that may simulate ankylosis.

Arthroscopic techniques have been useful for débriding such adhesions, and mechanical instruments such as basket forceps and the synovial resector are useful as well. However, the laser appears to provide significant advantages over mechanical instrumentation because it allows precise tissue ablation while achieving simultaneous hemostasis. The small profile laser probe allows this instrument to be used even in the posterior reaches of the ankle joint where larger mechanical instruments may be difficult to reach. The precision of the instrument is important because injury to normal joint structures is minimized, and the hemostatic properties allow an earlier, more rapid rehabilitation program to be pursued.

Soft Tissue Impingement Lesions

The history of soft tissue impingement lesions in the ankle joint dates back to the 1950s when Wolin described the meniscoid lesion. Since that time, soft tissue impingement lesions have been cited in the literature. The advent of arthroscopy of the ankle has allowed more precise definition of these lesions. In addition, arthroscopists have found that the formation of soft tissue impingement lesions is

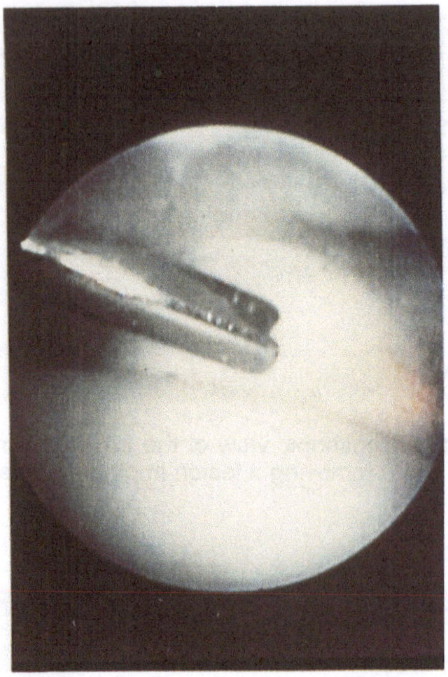

Figure 36-4. Arthroscopic view of an entrapped loose body being removed using the 2.1 μm holmium:YAG laser at 18 to 20 watts.

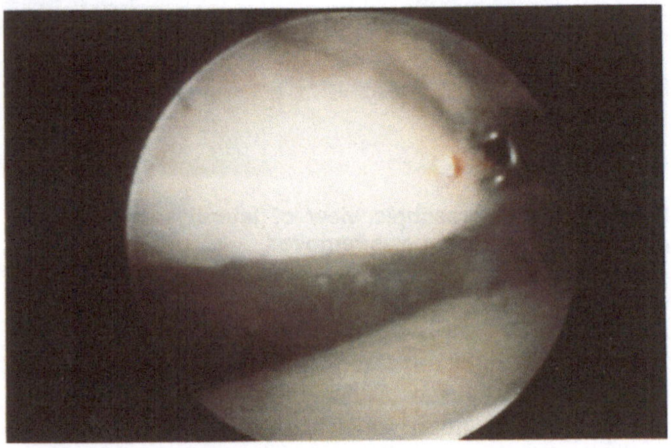

Figure 36-5. Arthroscopic view of the 2.1 μm holmium:YAG laser removing an anterior tibial osteophyte.

not uncommon after relatively minor trauma, including sprains and fractures. The most common site for synovial impingement lesions is in the lateral gutter, most frequently arising from the distal tibiofibular joint (Fig. 36-1). They are noted to be firm masses of tissue that protrude into the joint, causing mechanical symptoms with anterolateral joint pain, catching, and giving way.

A symptomatic lesion that has not responded to conservative treatment, including activity modification, nonsteroidal antiinflammatory medications, rehabilitation modalities, and corticosteroid injections, can be resected arthroscopically. Laser resection is easily performed and has the above noted advantages of minimizing associated joint trauma and achieving hemostasis (Figs. 36-2 and 36-3). The decreased postoperative bleeding allows accelerated rehabilitation and may decrease the incidence of recurrence of the lesion.

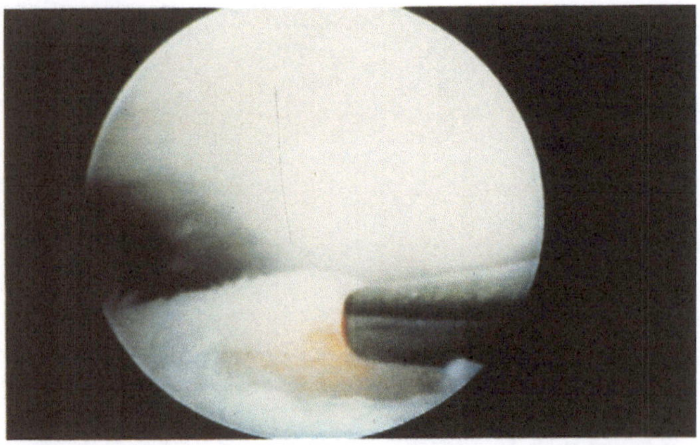

Figure 36-6. Edges of a chondral defect are trimmed back to normal articular cartilage using the laser.

Fixed Osteochondral Impingement

Fixed osteochondral impingements include ossicles, entrapped osteochondral loose bodies, and avulsed fragments of bone. Their removal can be facilitated with the laser (Fig. 36-4). They frequently occur in the medial and lateral gutters, where it may be difficult to place mechanical arthroscopic instruments. The small profile laser probe can be more easily inserted into the gutters, and the laser can be used to shell out the bony lesion.

Anterior Tibial Osteophytes

Anterior tibial osteophytes can be removed with the laser alone or in combination with mechanical instrumentation. The laser probe is smaller than mechanical instruments, and the decreased crowding of instruments in the anterior joint is an advantage. The anterior osteophyte may be well visualized with the arthroscope in the posterolateral portal and the instrumentation positioned anteriorly (Fig. 36-5). An accurate resection with hemostasis is achieved.

Degenerative Joint Disease

The role of arthroscopic débridement of degenerative joint disease has not been resolved, but patients with mild to moderate degenerative changes may benefit for some time by removing osteophytes and loose bodies, and débriding loose and damaged articular cartilage. We do not recommend arthroscopic débridement when a clear bone-on-bone radiographic appearance is present. The laser provides easy access to the entire surface of the talus and tibial plafond, and it facilitates débridement and contouring of the articular cartilage. If a small area of cartilage is

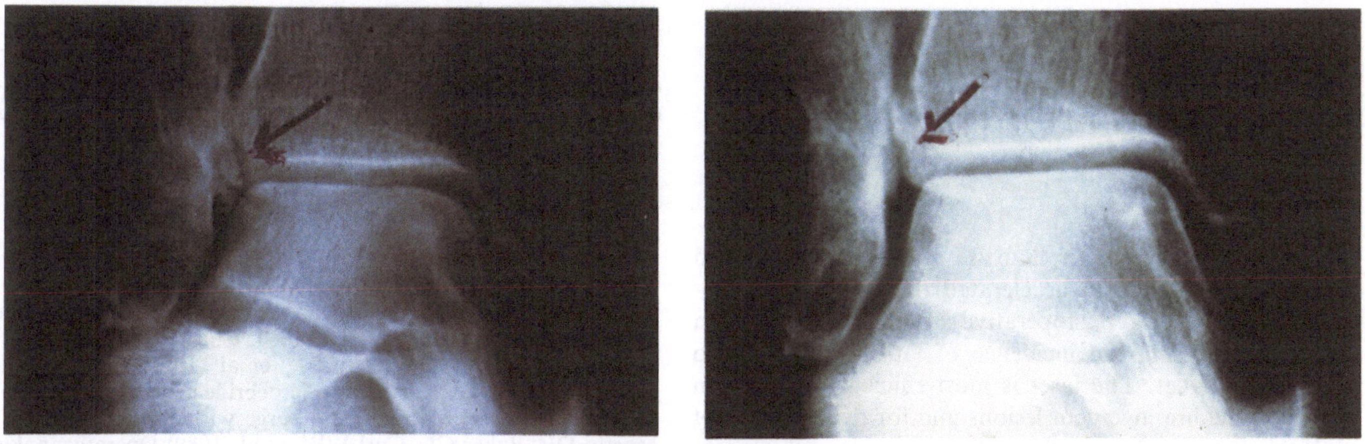

Figure 36-7. Preoperative and postoperative anteroposterior radiographs illustrating removal of a fracture osteophyte arising from the distal fibula in a woman with malunion of a distal fibular fracture.

denuded down to bone, the laser can be used to contour the edges and the base can be abraded or drilled to encourage the ingrowth of fibrocartilage (Fig. 36-6).

Arthrodesis of the tibiotalar joint may be the only alternative for a patient with advanced degenerative changes in the ankle. Advances have allowed the procedure to be performed arthroscopically in patients who do not have significant deformity, producing less morbidity than is experienced with open procedures. In cases where islands of articular cartilage remain, the laser can be used effectively for the initial débridement, especially using the 70 degree side-firing probe. This method may be particularly useful in the posterior aspect of the talus where mechanical instruments are more difficult to place. After laser débridement, the area must be abraded slightly using a burr to ensure the presence of a viable bone bed.

Chronic Fracture

For treatment of chronic fracture and fracture defects, laser débridement creates a working space with less bleeding and fewer recurrences and with better maintenance of motion. Areas of pseudarthrosis can be débrided better and scuffing reduced. Better sculpting and contouring of articular cartilage is possible. Interchanging with mechanical instruments is often necessary. Fracture malunion can result in bony prominences that can enlarge and act as impinging osteophytes. Arthroscopic resection of such bony prominences can provide significant symptomatic relief in cases where nonoperative treatment has failed (Figs. 36-7 and 36-8).

Subtalar Joint Pathology

The subtalar joint is especially well suited to treatment with laser because of the space limitations with mechanical instruments. The larger shavers and basket forceps pose a significant risk for articular cartilage damage. We have used the laser to débride synovitis and arthrofibrosis

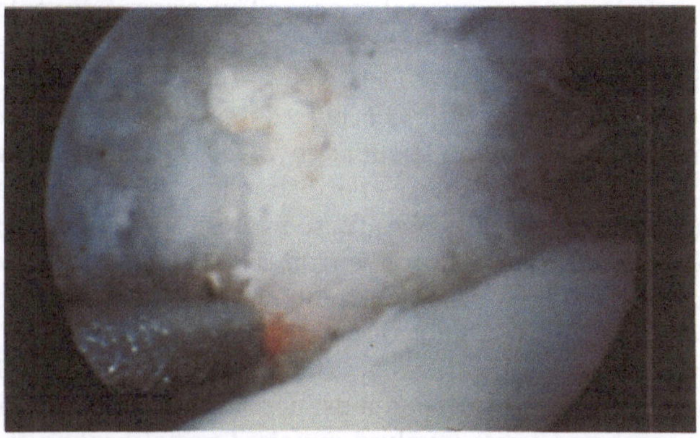

Figure 36-8. Arthroscopic view showing the laser dissecting the fracture osteophyte in the patient whose roentgenograms are shown in Figure 35-7.

of the subtalar joint with good results in a small number of patients. Others have described arthroscopic débridement of the sinus tarsi anterior to the talocalcaneal interosseus ligament using the shaver and mechanical instruments. The laser may provide a significant advantage here because postoperative bleeding would be minimized after efficient soft tissue ablation. We also see a potential role for the laser in arthroscopic subtalar arthrodesis.

Results

The 2.1 μm holmium:YAG laser was introduced into our practice of ankle arthroscopy in January 1991. During the 2-year period from that date until January 1993, the laser was used for ankle and subtalar joint arthroscopy in 56 of 85 arthroscopic cases. The types of surgical procedures performed are detailed below:

Lateral soft tissue impingements	9
Adhesions/synovitis	1
Pigmented villonodular synovitis	1

Chondromalacia	1
Osteochondral defect	18
Osteophyte	7
Loose body	4
Ossicle	3
Arthritis	2
Chronic fracture	10

The clinical impression is that use of the laser decreased postoperative pain and accelerated rehabilitation, probably by decreasing postoperative bleeding and effusion and by decreasing the incidence of iatrogenic injury to the joint surfaces. The laser is most efficient for excision of soft tissue impingement lesions and for débridement of articular cartilage lesions. In addition, ossicles, which represent fixed osteocartilaginous bodies, are easily identified and shelled out using the laser. Use of the laser increases the precision of the surgery and minimizes collateral damage to normal tissues. The elapsed time for surgical cases is approximately the same using laser as using mechanical instruments.

Only two complications occurred during the 2-year period cited. Both complications involved cutaneous nerve damage secondary to skeletal distraction, and none was due to the use of the laser. These figures represent a 3.6% complication rate, a decrease from 11.2% when both mechanical and laser cases are combined (350 cases between 1975 and 1992). Cutaneous nerve injury resulting in a small area of paresthesia accounted for 22 of these 39 complications. The second most common complication in the combined series involved impaired portal healing secondary to superficial infection or drainage leading to a sinus tract. These complications were all minor in nature. No laser cases demonstrated this complication. The major change over the 2 years that contributed to the lower incidence of complications is the use of noninvasive means of mechanical distraction, which significantly decreases the likelihood of cutaneous nerve injury. This decrease is not attributed to laser use. It is possible however, that use of the laser decreases the incidence of the complications secondary to damage that occurs after portal trauma or postoperative effusion and drainage. Nevertheless, complications are less when the 2.1 μm holmium:YAG laser is used for ankle arthroscopy.

References

Dillingham MF, Fanton GS (1991) The holmium laser in arthroscopy. Presented at the Arthroscopic Surgery of the Shoulder and Ankle: Update 1991, Chicago

Lane GJ, Sherk HH, Mooar PA, et al (1991) CO_2 vs holmium:YAG laser arthroscopic débridement. American Society for Laser Medicine and Surgery (Suppl) 3:52–53

Martin DF, Baker CL, Curl WW, et al (1989) Operative ankle arthroscopy: long-term follow-up. Am J Sports Med 17:16–23

Miller DV, O'Brien SJ, Arnoczky SS, et al (1989) The use of contact Nd:YAG laser in arthroscopic surgery: effects on articular cartilage and meniscal tissue. Arthroscopy 5:245–253

Moller KO, Lind B, Schramm U, et al (1991) Holmium laser synovectomy of immune synovitis in rabbits. American Society for Laser Medicine and Surgery (Suppl) 3:51

O'Brien SJ, Miller DV (1990) The contact neodymium yttrium-aluminum-garnet laser: a new approach to arthroscopic laser surgery. Clin Orthop 252:95–100

Philandrianos G (1985) Carbon dioxide laser in arthroscopic surgery of the knee. Presse Med 14:2103–2104

Smith CF, Johansen WE, Vangsness CT, et al (1989) The carbon dioxide laser: a potential tool for orthopaedic surgery. Clin Orthop 242:43–50

Stein E, Sedlacek T, Fabian RL, et al (1990) Acute and chronic effects of bone ablation with a pulsed holmium laser. Lasers Surg Med 10:384–388

Trauner K, Nishioka A, Patel D (1990) Pulsed holmium yttrium-aluminum-garnet (Ho:YAG) laser ablation of fibrocartilage and articular cartilage. Am J Sports Med 19:316–320

Vangsness CT, Smith CF, Marshall GJ, et al (1991) The biologic effects of CO_2 laser surgery on rabbit articular cartilage. American Society for Laser Medicine and Surgery (Suppl) 3:52

Whipple TL, Caspari RB, Meyers JF (1985) Arthroscopic laser meniscectomy in a gas medium. Arthroscopy 1:2–7

37

2.1 μm Holmium:YAG Arthroscopic Laser Surgery of the Shoulder

Gary S. Fanton and Michael F. Dillingham

Arthroscopy has long been recognized as a useful diagnostic and therapeutic technique for many shoulder disorders. Arthroscopic surgery is now considered the standard of care for many specific shoulder conditions, including cartilage tears, instability, loose bodies, arthritis, rotator cuff disease, impingement syndromes, and arthritis of the acromioclavicular joint. With a growing number of applications and surgical procedures there has been a parallel growth of interest in instrumentation that can help expedite these procedures while ensuring safe and reproducible results.

With the advent of laser surgery and new arthroscopic delivery devices, the application of this modality to shoulder surgery seemed obvious. There are several special considerations of shoulder surgery that make the use of lasers especially appealing. Shoulder joint surfaces are more curved than most other joints, and straight-line instrumentation can require repetitive instrument swapping, aggressive joint distraction, or cumbersome instrument manipulation to reach the areas of pathology. Bleeding can significantly impair visualization; and without the available use of a tourniquet for hemostasis, constant control of even small bleeders is mandatory. Likewise, soft tissue swelling can be dramatic. Large portals, excessive bleeding, poor visualization, repetitive instrumentation, and the use of fluid pumps to enhance flow can contribute to soft tissue edema.

The 2.1 μm holmium:yttrium aluminum garnet (Ho:YAG) laser is ideally suited for shoulder arthroscopy. Being fiberoptically transmitted, the free-beam 2.1 μm holmium:YAG laser is easily delivered through a variety of straight, curved, and angled handpieces to reach nearly every aspect of the joint or subacromial space without the need for accessory portals or camera-instrument swapping. In contrast to the CO_2 laser, which requires straight-line delivery in a gas medium, the 2.1 μm holmium:YAG laser is utilized in the standard arthroscopic fluid medium and requires no special fluid pumps or vasoconstrictive agents. The 2 mm wide handpieces can easily reach all areas of the glenohumeral and subacromial space. Operating at a wavelength of 2.1 μm, the holmium:YAG laser is an excellent hemostatic instrument that allows cutting, ablating, and contouring of tissues or bone while maintaining clear, blood-free visualization. The shortened operating time minimizes soft tissue swelling, and the decreased bleeding controls postoperative pain and inflammation. Free-beam application optimizes tissue ablation without contact and can be "defocused" to enlarge the area of effect, in contrast to the neodymium:YAG systems, which are delivered through a hot-tipped cutting device. Because of the significant limitations presented by the neodymium:YAG and CO_2 laser systems for shoulder arthroscopy, we have exclusively utilized the fiberoptically delivered 2.1 μm holmium:YAG laser for shoulder arthroscopy since 1989 and have found it to be effective and expeditious for a wide variety of surgical techniques.

Surgical Setup

Arthroscopy of the shoulder is typically performed utilizing a general anesthetic, which allows a complete shoulder examination to evaluate range of motion and stability prior to positioning. The patient can then be positioned either in the lateral decubitus position or the beach chair position, depending on the surgeon's experience or desire. We prefer the lateral decubitus position with longitudinal traction in a shoulder suspension device. No more than 5 to 7 pounds of traction is required to counterbalance the weight of the arm, although occasionally 10 pounds is used in heavy or muscular individuals. Minimizing the amount of suspension weight lessens the risk of postoperative nerve traction complaints, especially in patients with previously known cervical spine or nerve root pathology. All nerve areas and the axilla are carefully padded, and the neck is cushioned in a neutral position. Approximately 30 degrees of abduction and 10 to 15 degrees of forward flexion allows complete visualization of both glenohumeral joint and the subacromial space.

The joint is inflated with 30 to 40 cc of Ringer's lactate solution through a posterior approach using a 17 gauge Tuohy spinal needle. Because the laser delivery probe is as easy, if not easier, to manipulate than a nerve hook, the standard arthroscopy portals are utilized. A 30 degree arthroscope through a large-bore sheath is introduced posteriorly and a disposable utility cannula is established through the anterior superior portal just below the biceps tendon. This anterior cannula allows introduction of a nerve hook, débriding instruments, or the 2.1 μm holmium:YAG fiberoptic handpiece interchangeably while minimizing soft tissue fluid extravasation. Adequate outflow is also achieved. In fact, nearly every aspect of the joint can be reached with the 30 degree laser handpiece through this anterior portal, including the six o'clock position on the lowest aspect of the glenoid labrum and the undersurface of the rotator cuff. The handpiece and arthroscope positions can easily be reversed if needed in tight joints. If desired, a superior portal behind the acromioclavicular joint can be created but is rarely necessary. The versatility of the narrow laser fiberoptic probe leaves no area of the joint inaccessible. In the subacromial space, the standard portals are also used. With the arthroscope introduced posteriorly into the subacromial bursa, an accessory lateral portal is made approximately 1 inch below the lateral edge of the acromion process at its midpoint. This portal is kept low to allow the 30 degree probe easy access to the coracoacromial arch. Again, the disposable cannula is useful initially, but after several minutes the portal is "self-established" and instrument swapping di-

1-3

4-6

7-9

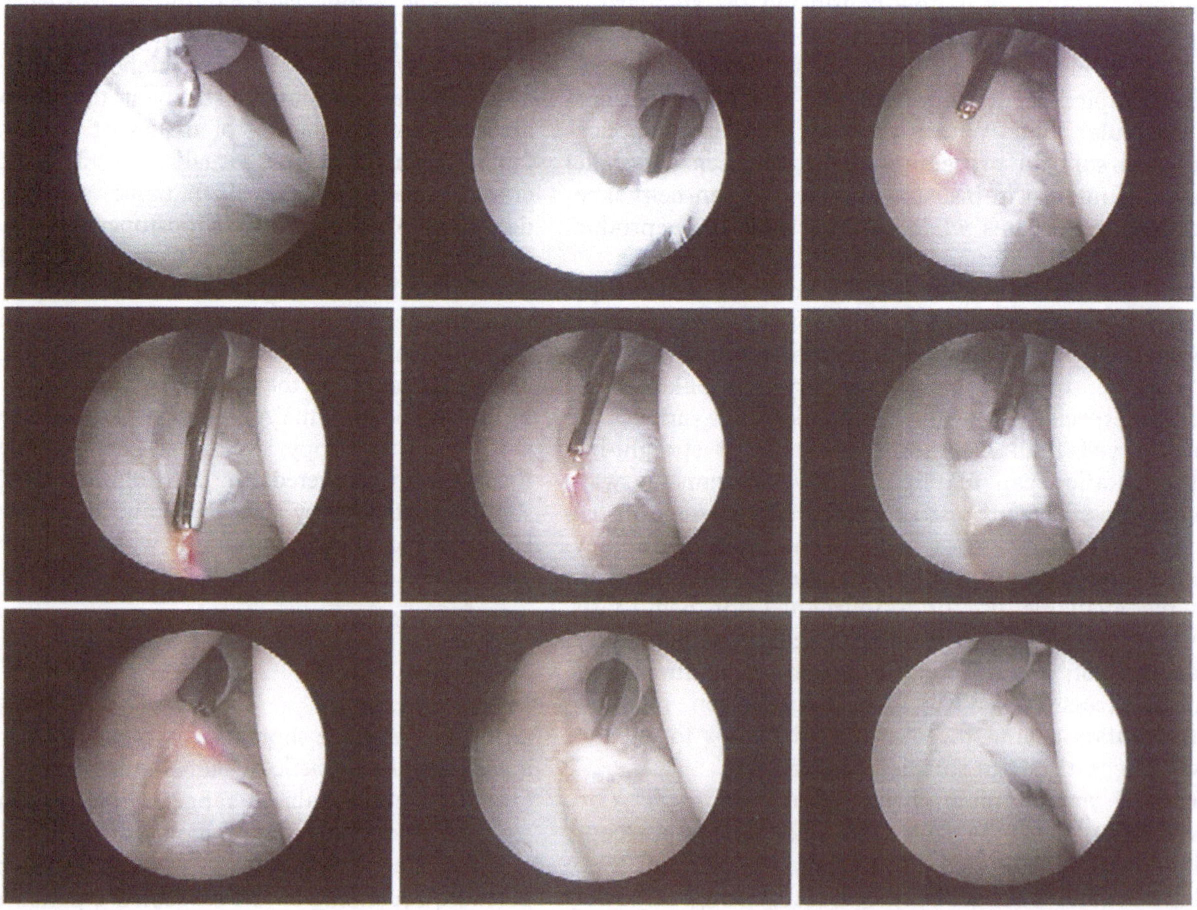

Figure 37-1. Sequential resection of a bucket-handle tear in the glenoid labrum, right shoulder. (Plates 1 and 2) Identification of a large bucket-handle tear in the glenoid labrum of the right shoulder extending from the anterior inferior aspect to the posterior superior aspect. The humeral head is on the right and the glenoid labrum on the left. (Plates 3–6) Incision and detachment of the posterior portion of the glenoid labrum. (Plates 7 and 8) Resection of the anterior portion of the glenoid labrum tear. (Plate 9) Final appearance of the glenoid labrum rim with an intact capsule and biceps attachment.

rectly through the skin puncture is easy. The 17 gauge needle is sometimes inserted to provide a low rate outflow and clear visualization.

Typically, the 2.1 μm holmium:YAG laser is set up at the foot of the table, allowing the handpiece to be brought anteriorly, posteriorly, or laterally as needed throughout the case. The fiberoptic cable has a tendency to "whip" during manipulation or rotation of the handpiece, so it is usually clamped to the drapes below the arm. The laser refrigerant needs to "cool down," and the machine is turned on a few minutes prior to its anticipated use. A dedicated line of 220 volts is the preferred power source. The circulating nurse unpackages the sterile, disposable handpiece while the laser machine self-calibrates and test-fires. The fiberoptic cable is simply screwed into the front machine panel and is set to the desired energy level (joules per pulse) and pulse repetition rate (hertz). As a free-beam pulsed laser, the 2.1 μm holmium:YAG laser provides precise application of heat energy with minimal thermal spread. The energy level and pulse rate can be easily adjusted up or down using the touch pad on the control panel depending on the proximity or laser "sensitivity" of the target tissue. A red helium-neon aiming beam is provided at three intensity levels if desired. The "ready" or "standby" modes on the control panel are controlled by the circulating nurse, but laser activation is performed via a footswitch positioned for easy access by the surgeon. Typically, power settings of 28 to 40 watts (1.4–2.4 joules/pulse) are used for most soft tissue procedures. Defocusing the laser by withdrawing the probe away from the target tissue is the simplest way for the operating surgeon to contour and ablate more photosensitive tissues or to achieve a larger area of effect. Advancing the probe to near contact increases the power

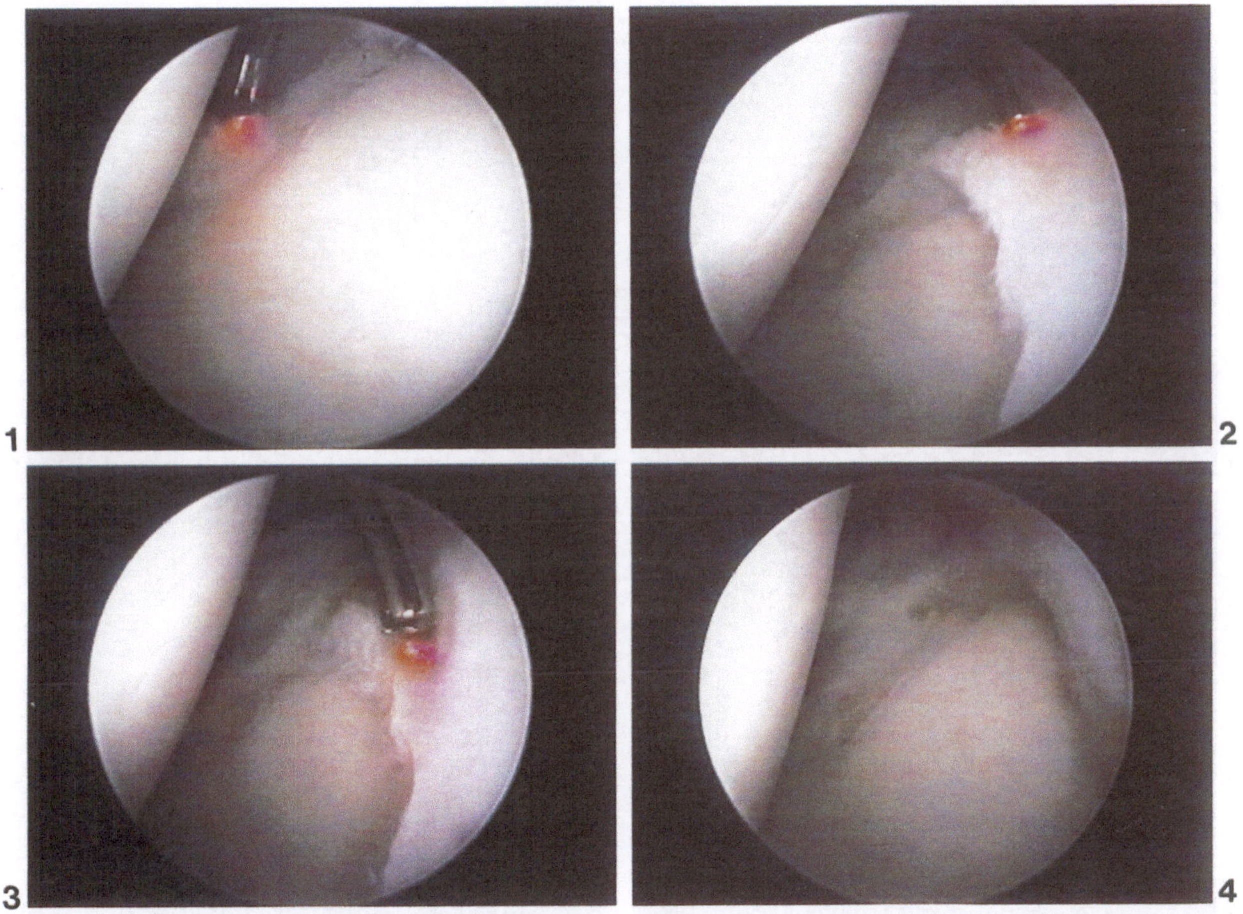

Figure 37-2. Photoablation of a degenerative type I SLAP lesion of the left shoulder, with an intact biceps tendon anchor. The tear extends from the anterior inferior aspect to the posterior superior aspect of the glenoid rim. Posterior visualization with the laser handpiece directed below the biceps tendon. (Plate 1) Photoablation and contouring of the anterior inferior labrum. The capsular attachment to the glenoid is not disturbed. Precise contouring is achieved. (Plate 2) Photoincision and dissection of the superior labrum is done below the biceps tendon anchor. (Plate 3) Extension of the labral resection to the posterior superior aspect. A degenerated piece of labrum is detached from the labral rim and biceps anchor. (Plate 4) Final appearance of the remaining labral rim. There is no damage to the biceps anchor or the underlying articular cartilage.

density, providing an intense thermal effect for cutting or coagulation. Bubbles or haze from tissue ablation are readily evacuated by the assistant or nurse through outflow tubing or a previously placed outflow needle. Upon completion of the procedure, total energy utilized is recorded and the handpiece disposed. "Caramelized" edges of soft tissue that have been laser treated may be further smoothed with small motorized débriding instruments.

Intraarticular Procedures

A complete diagnostic arthroscopy is performed first through the posterior portal with a nerve hook placed anteriorly for tissue manipulation. The biceps tendon, bicipital-labral complex, anterior and inferior labrum, subscapularis tendon, anterior glenohumeral ligament complex, axillary recess, posterior and superior labrum, glenohumeral articular surfaces, and undersurface of the rotator cuff are systematically inspected. If necessary, the arthroscope is then brought anteriorly to view any previously unseen joint surfaces, the posterior capsular labral complex, the posterior rotator cuff, and the anterior inferior glenoid rim.

Glenoid Labrum Tears

Glenoid labrum tears are a common source of pain, popping and catching in the shoulder instability. There are several patterns of injury to the anterior, posterior, and superior labrum and biceps anchor (SLAP lesions) that can be significantly symptomatic. Most of them are successfully treated with 2.1 μm holmium:YAG laser débridement or resection (Fig. 37-1). Because the labrum is less fibrous and more photosensitive than the meniscus of the knee, lower power settings are usually used. We begin with 1.4 joules/pulse at 16 Hz and increase the joules as needed. With the laser probe positioned approximately 2 mm from the target tissue, the labrum is easily and gently

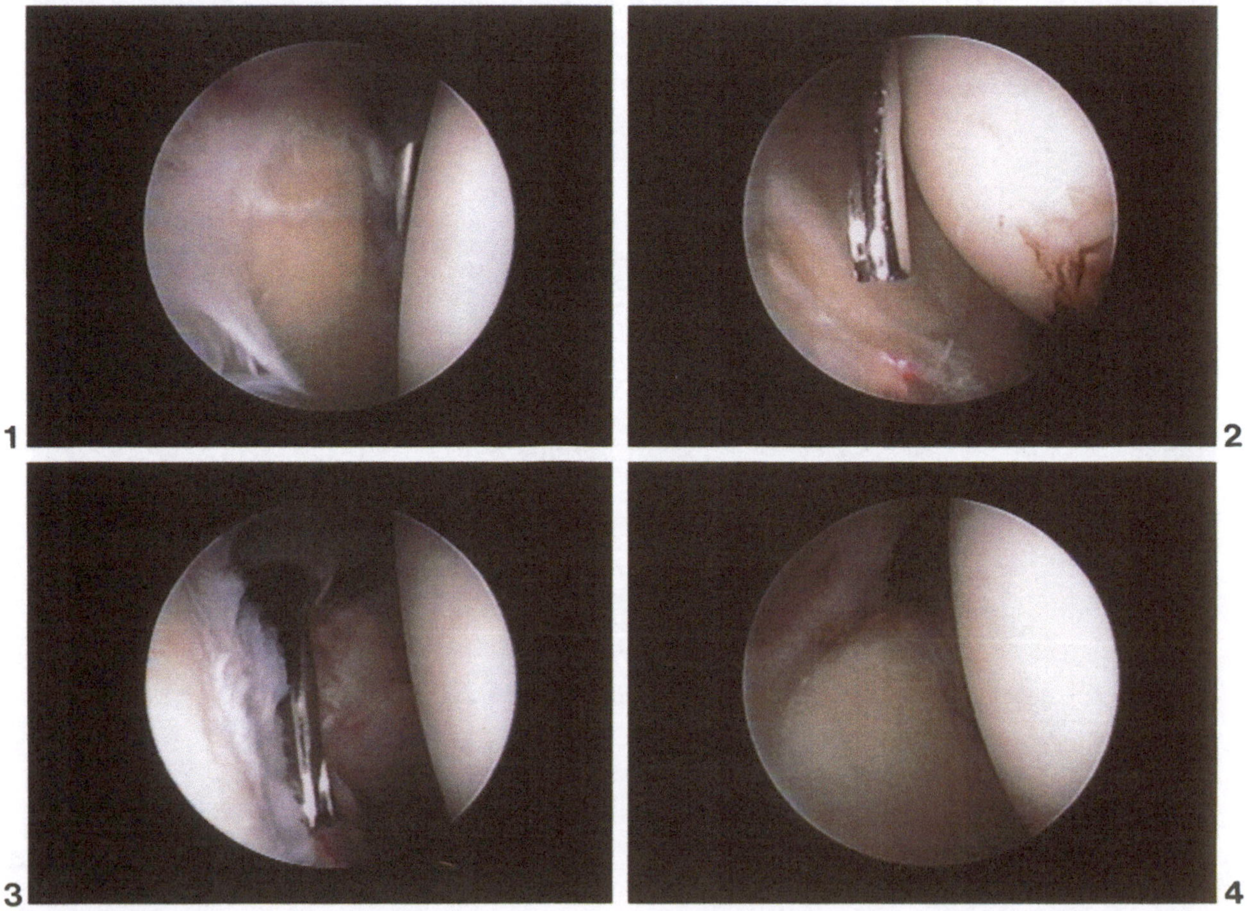

Figure 37-3. Extensive degenerative tear of the glenoid labrum from the anterior inferior to the posterior inferior aspect in the right shoulder. The humeral head is on the right and the glenoid socket on left. A disposable cannula and 30 degree laser handpiece are introduced through the standard anterior portal. (Plate 1) There is an extensive degenerative tear of the anterior superior and posterior glenoid labrum extending to the inferior portions. (Plate 2) Holmium laser ablation of the posterior inferior labral tear. (Plate 3) Photoablation and contouring of the anterior inferior labrum. (Plate 4) Final appearance of the now smoothly contoured labral rim. The biceps tendon anchor was débrided with the laser.

ablated back to a good solid rim or to the capsule without risk of further detaching the capsule from the glenoid margin.

Type I lesions present with frayed and degenerated labral tissue that is vaporized back to the intact substance of the lesion. A 30 degree probe is introduced through the plastic anterior cannula and then rotated anteriorly for anterior tears and superiorly for superior and posterior tears (Fig. 37-2). Precise ablation preserves the remaining capsulolabral attachment and the base of the biceps tendon.

Type II lesions are common and are similar to type I but include detachment of the biceps anchor. These lesions are resected back, as for type I lesions, but in addition degenerative tissue underneath the biceps tendon anchor is also ablated (Fig. 37-3). Many times the degenerative portions appear to congeal into a much smoother rim that creates less synovial irritation. If desired, this procedure can be combined with mechanical abrasion of the superior glenoid rim and the tissue transfixed arthroscopically to promote healing of the biceps anchor.

Type III and IV lesions involve bucket handle tears of the superior labrum. For these tears, increased power density may be required to cleanly transect anterior or posterior portions of the tear. It is usually performed by advancing the 2.1 μm holmium:YAG laser delivery probe to direct or nearly direct contact with the labrum at the point of transection or by increasing the energy to 1.8 joules/pulse, which allows the laser to act as an interarticular "knife." The posterior portion is transected first to prevent the fragment from flipping posteriorly in front of the lens (Fig. 37-4). The anterior portion is then cut with the laser and the fragment removed with a grasping instrument. The remaining labrum can be smoothed and

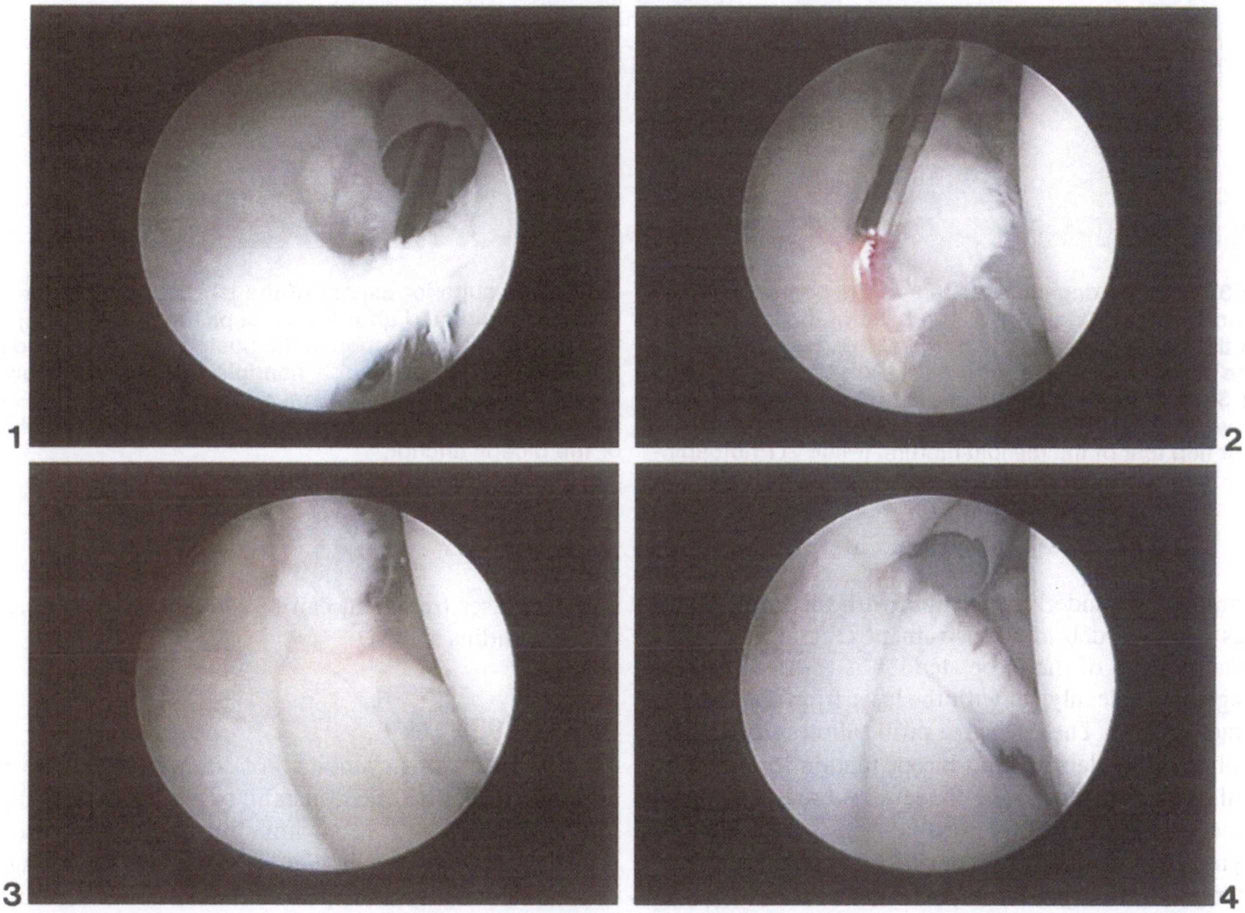

Figure 37-4. Type III SLAP lesion of the right shoulder with a bucket-handle tear from the anterior inferior to the posterior superior labral rim. The biceps anchor is intact. (Plate 1) Demonstration of the bucket-handle tear, with intraarticular displacement. The humeral head is on the right and the glenoid socket and labrum on the left. (Plate 2) Laser incision of the posterior superior attachment of the torn labrum. The laser handpiece is directed anteriorly to posteriorly through a disposable cannula below the biceps tendon. (Plate 3) Laser detachment of the anterior portion of the torn labrum. Note the smooth remaining rim of the posterior superior labrum after detachment. (Plate 4) Final smooth appearance of the labral rim after excision of the bucket-handle tear.

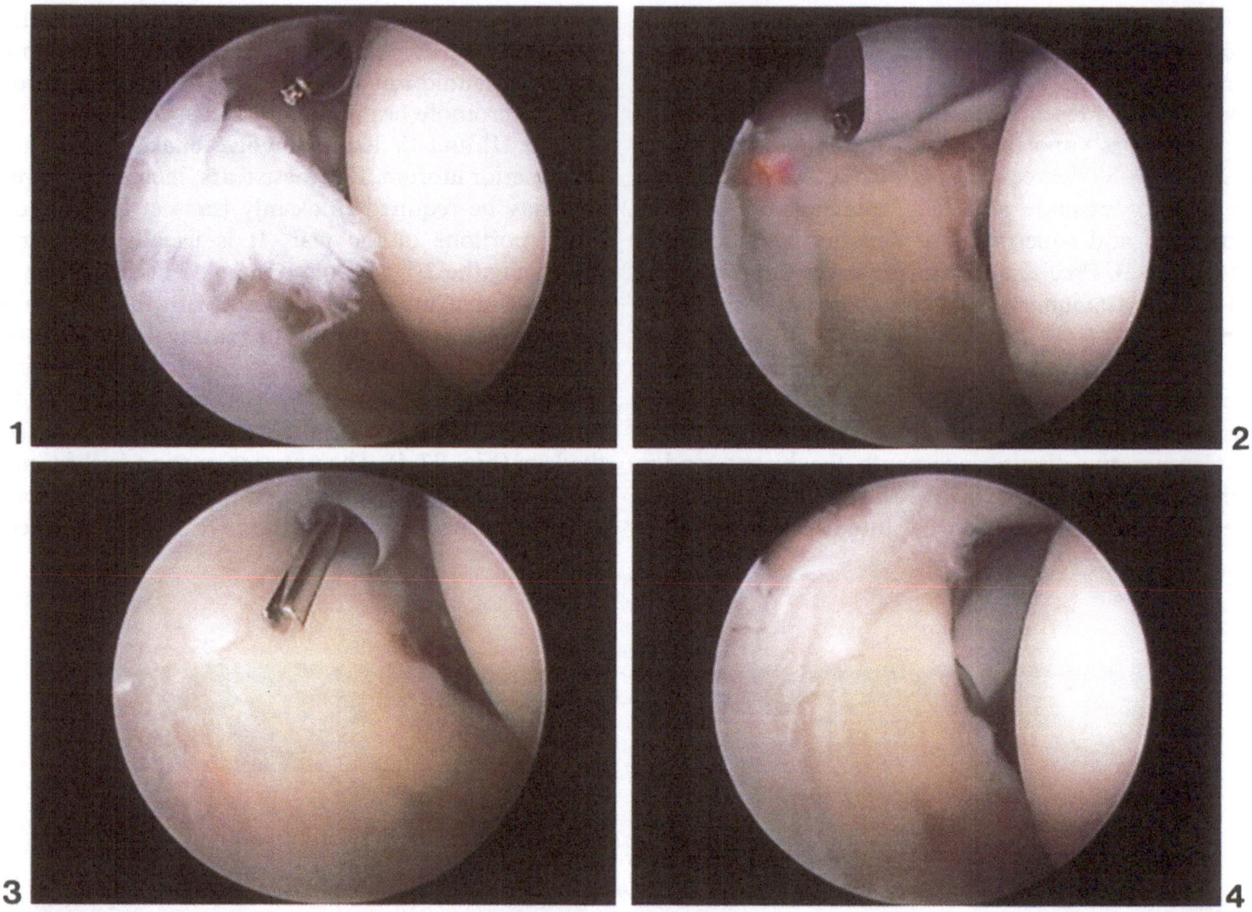

Figure 37-5. Large degenerative tear of the posterior superior glenoid labrum extending to the base of the biceps tendon in the right shoulder. The humeral head is on the right and the glenoid socket on the left. A disposable cannula with a 30 degree laser handpiece and a standard anterior portal were used. (Plate 1) Large degenerative posterior superior flap tear of the glenoid labrum. (Plate 2) Photoablation of the superior aspect of the labral tear, with the laser handpiece directed above the biceps tendon. (Plate 3) Continuation of labral ablation to the posterior superior and mid-posterior labrum, with the handpiece directed below the biceps tendon. (Plate 4) Final appearance of the posterior superior labrum without disturbing the capsular attachment or the biceps anchor.

contoured to the underlying glenoid with the lower power settings or small débriding instrument (Fig. 37-5). If the proximal portion of the biceps tendon is torn as well, the torn segment is cleanly cut with the laser from the remaining intact portion. The 30 degree probe allows the surgeon to manipulate the labrum and biceps tendon to obtain an optimal angle of approach as the laser is fired. Any synovial reaction adjacent to the torn labrum is photoablated (see Synovectomy, below).

Anterior inferior, posterior inferior, and direct inferior degenerative tears (Fig. 37-6) or flap tears (Fig. 37-7) are also photoresected or vaporized as for type I SLAP lesions. The small probe size usually allows direct access to all of these tears through the anterior portal cannula, and the 30 degree curve bends nicely around the posterior curvature of the humeral head to the most inferior aspects. If desired, any caramelized portions of the labrum remaining after laser treatment can be removed with a small 3.5 mm full radius shaver.

Synovectomy

Localized areas of synovitis are commonly seen in association with labral tears, instability, chondromalacia, and loose bodies. The 2.1 μm holmium:YAG laser provides the best method of synovial reduction by shrinking and devascularizing hypertrophic and inflamed tissue without creating troublesome bleeding (Fig. 37-8). Usually located above or anterior to the biceps tendon, the anterior portal provides the greatest ease of access. A defocused technique works the best with the 2.1 μm holmium:YAG laser fiberoptic tip positioned 3 to 4 mm from the target tissue. At this distance, at least 1.6 joules/pulse is utilized with the maximum repetition rate. The inflamed synovial

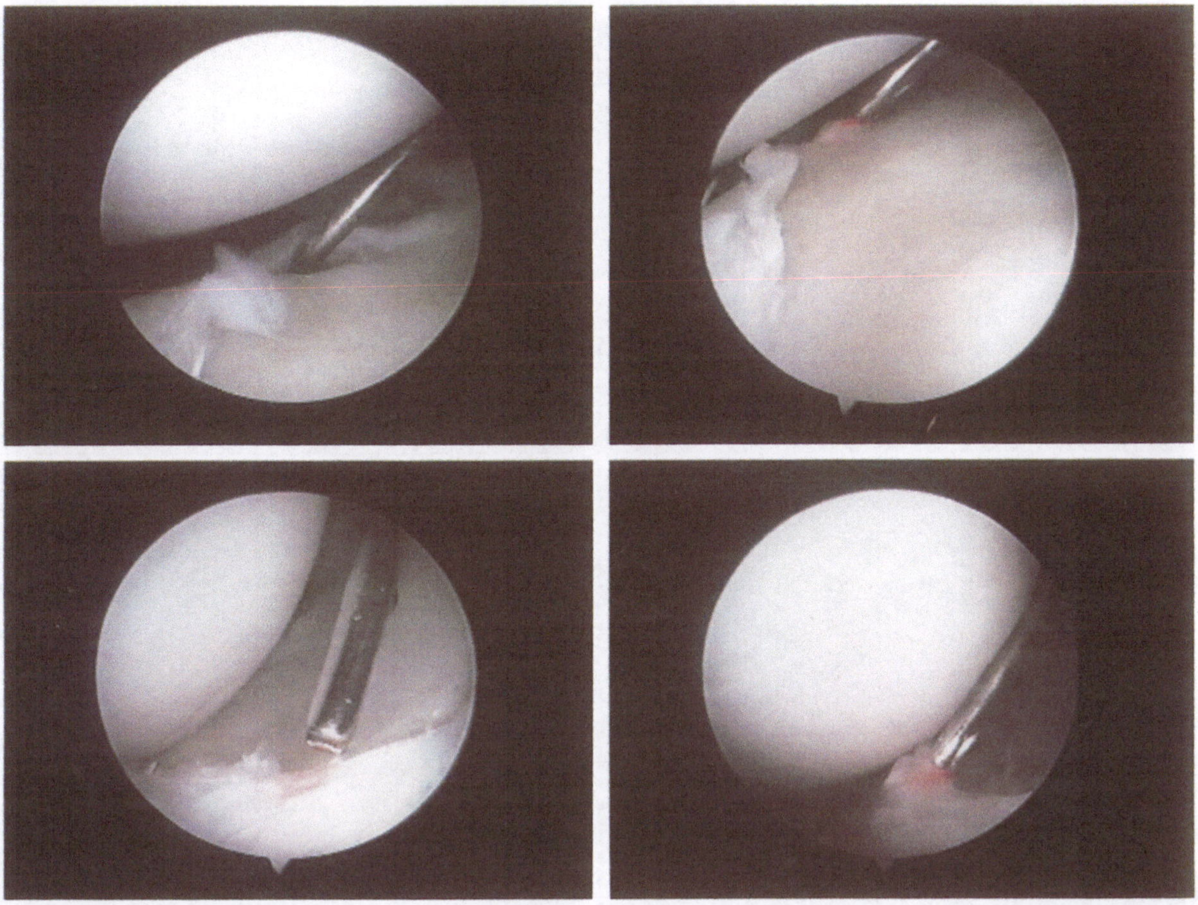

Figure 37-6. Degenerative inferior tear of the glenoid labral rim from the anterior inferior aspect to the posterior inferior aspect, with associated instability of the glenohumeral joint. The humeral head is on the upper left and the glenoid socket on the lower right. (Plate 1) Anterior inferior glenoid labrum tear, with detachment and extension of the tear to the lowest portion of the glenoid. (Plate 2) Laser ablation of the anterior inferior tear, with the laser handpiece directed through standard anterior portal below the biceps tendon. (Plate 3) Photoablation of the posterior inferior labrum. (Plate 4) Photoablation of the inferior labrum at the six o'clock position. Note the relatively easy access to the lowest portion of the labrum through the standard anterior portal using a 30 degree curved handpiece.

tissue is "sprayed" with the laser beam until it shrinks to a nearly flat, avascular layer. No troublesome bleeding or loss of visualization is encountered.

Chondral Débridement

Although little is known about the short- and long-term effects of débriding areas of cartilage fibrillation and degeneration, there is clinical evidence that joint pain, swelling, and synovitis can be lessened by removing diseased cartilage tissue. Whether these symptoms are chemically mediated, the result of mechanical synovial irritation, or both is still under study. Laser photochondroplasty offers the best technique to smooth and contour articular cartilage defects, taper sharp cartilage step-offs on the joint surface, and "congeal" areas of grade III fibrillation. Visually, a smooth surface is created that almost appears to seal the surface, perhaps decreasing the release of cartilage breakdown products and enzymes. Although encouraging histologic and animal studies have been performed to investigate chondrocyte regeneration and biostimulation, much more work is needed before we can extrapolate such effects to the long-term treatment of cartilage disease and arthritis in humans.

Soft Tissue Release

Because of its excellent cutting and coagulation potential, the 2.1 μm holmium:YAG laser makes a versatile and easily manipulated intraarticular "knife." Adhesions, fibrotic bands in the capsule, and tendon contractures can be easily cut using power settings in the 1.6 to 2 joules range. The 0.5 mm depth of penetration allows for a precise cut that can easily be controlled and redirected during surgery. The small delivery device also permits manipula-

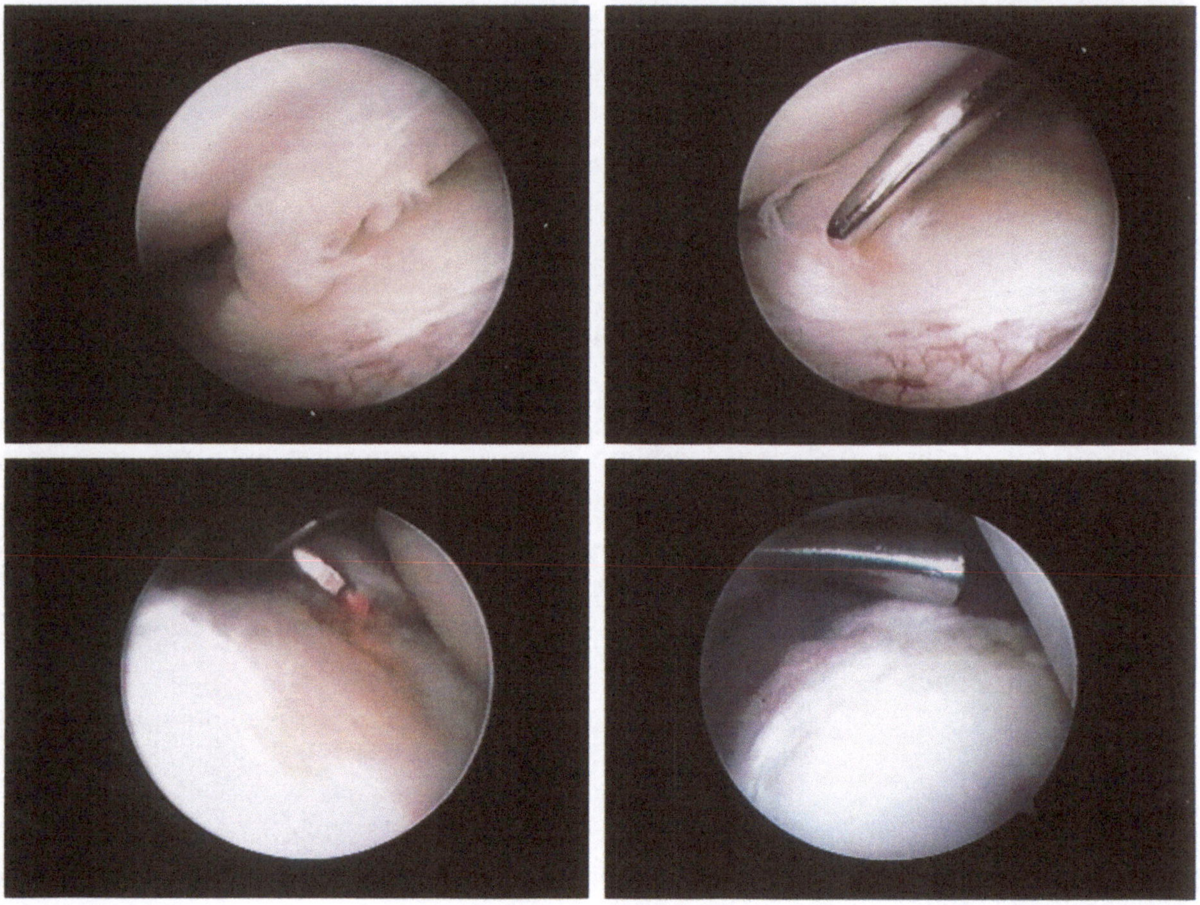

Figure 37-7. Posterior inferior flap tear of the glenoid labrum. (Plate 1) Large posterior inferior flap tear of the glenoid labrum, with intraarticular entrapment. The humeral head is on the upper left and the glenoid socket on the lower right. Visualization is through the posterior portal. (Plate 2) Laser resection of the base of the labral flap tear. The 30 degree handpiece is introduced through the standard anterior portal below the biceps tendon. (Plate 3) Visualization is through the anterior portal with final transection of the posterior inferior tear. The handpiece is introduced through the posterior cannula. The humeral head is on the right and the glenoid socket on the left. (Plate 4) Final appearance of the posterior inferior labrum visualized through the anterior portal. The torn flap has been entirely removed without damage to the articular surface of the humeral head or the glenoid socket.

tion of the joint as the release is being performed, if desired.

Subacromial Space

One of the greatest advantages of 2.1 μm holmium:YAG laser surgery in the shoulder lies in its utilization in the subacromial space. Arthroscopic coracoacromial arch decompression has become the standard of care for rotator cuff disease, impingement, and chronic bursitis. The use of the fiberoptic laser technique allows for excellent control of bleeding, optimal fluid flow and visualization, and precise dissection that significantly shortens surgical time and expedites recovery.

Setup for arthroscopic arch decompression is no different from mechanical instrumentation methods. An accessory lateral portal is created about 1 inch below the lateral border of the acromion process. A 30 degree curved handpiece is preferred and easily reaches every recess of the subacromial and subdeltoid space as well as the acromioclavicular joint capsule. A 70 degree handpiece is also available, but it is usually easier to work more tangentially with the 30 degree handpiece on the underside of the acromion and coracoacromial (CA) ligament. Most patients have a thick, fibrotic subacromial bursa that is débrided first with a 4 mm full radius shaver to create space and afford visualization. A 17 gauge Tuohy needle is sometimes placed anteriorly for gentle fluid or bubble outflow. The 2.1 μm holmium:YAG laser is set at maximal power, 1.8 to 2.0 joules/pulse, and beginning laterally the CA ligament is peeled off the underside of the acromion while firing in a medial direction (Fig. 37-9). A contact technique is used. The laser effectively peels portions of the CA ligament and bursa off the undersurface

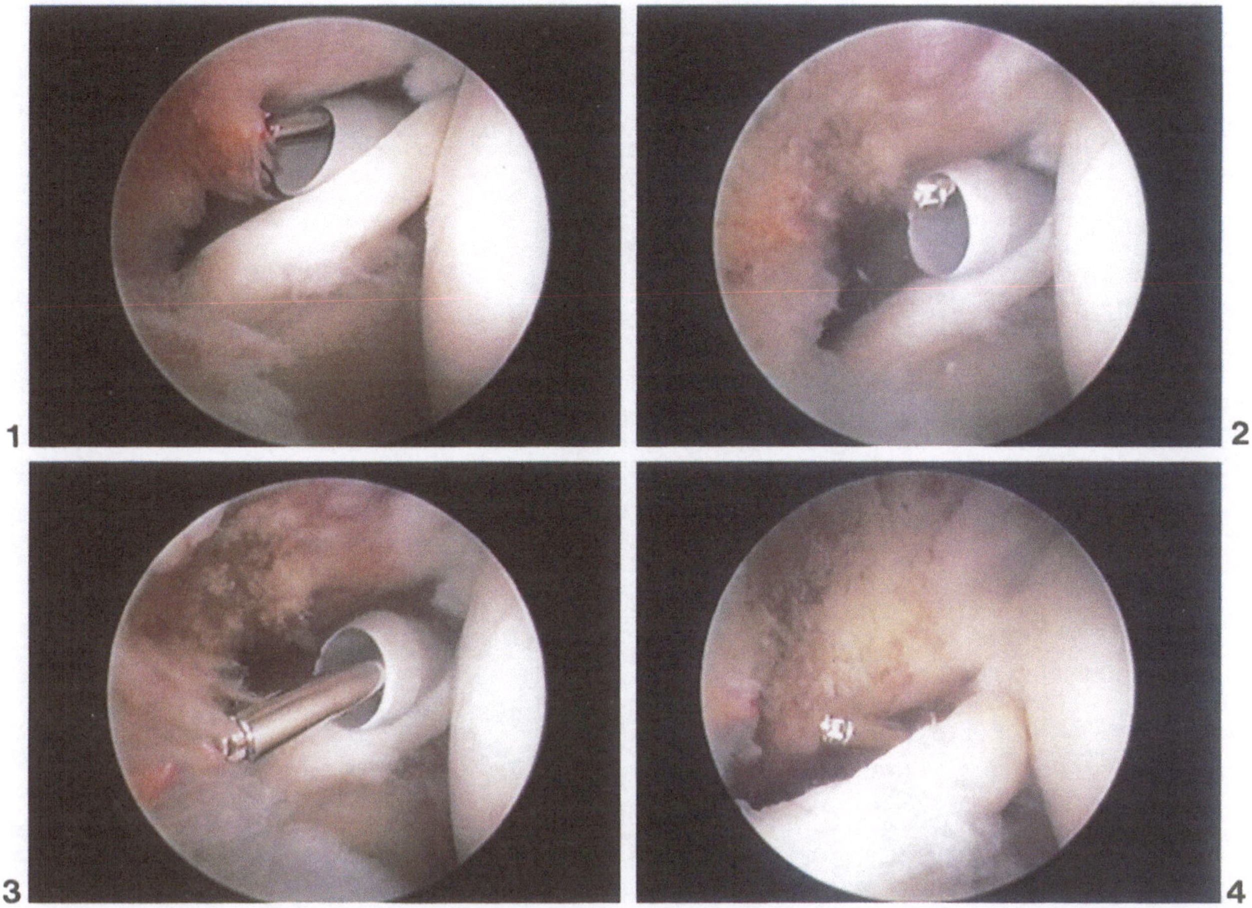

Figure 37-8. Photosynovectomy for glenohumeral synovitis with a posterior superior labrum tear. Visualization is through the posterior portal. Note the synovitis in the posterior superior capsule and the inferior aspect rotator cuff. (Plate 1) Holmium laser handpiece directed posteriorly through a disposable cannula above the biceps tendon. (Plate 2) Laser ablation of superior synovitis underneath the rotator cuff. Note the shrinkage and blanching of the synovium without bleeding. (Plate 3) Laser ablation of posterior synovitis and degeneration in the posterior superior labrum. Clear visualization is maintained. (Plate 4) Final laser ablation and contouring of the synovium. Note the pale, smooth areas of synovium, decreased vascularity, and shrinkage of synovial layer.

of the acromion and deltoid muscle anteriorly without disturbing troublesome muscle bleeders that are often sucked into mechanical shavers. If bleeding does occur, it is quickly stopped with near-contact photocoagulation. The entire bursa–CA ligament flap is continually peeled in a medial direction over to the acromioclavicular joint capsule. The final avascular piece is then simply pulled free from the space with a pituitary rongeur or grasping instrument. This maneuver leaves a blanched, dry acromial surface that can be inspected for bone spurs, acromial overhand, or os acromiale. A mechanical high speed pear-shaped burr is used for acromioplasty or spur resection. If spurs are noted preoperatively at the AC joint, the capsule must be lifted off the undersurface of the joint to expose them. The laser débridement is continued further medially, bleeding is controlled, and soft tissue is removed. These spurs can then be smoothed down with mechanical abraders or an arthroscopic rasp. With power outputs of 60 watts available at over 2 joules per pulse, we have been able to perform the actual bony acromioplasty and spur resection entirely with the 2.1 μm holmium:YAG laser removing a layer of bone that can be resected in one piece (Fig. 37-10). This technique minimizes postoperative bleeding and inflammation.

Partial-thickness rotator cuff tears have been described on both the articular and bursal sides of the tendon. Débridement of these tears has been described as being palliative in some athletes. Although we do not believe that simple débridement alone has much clinical or mechanical effect on tendon function, it can be a useful technique as an adjunct to other procedures or to a biomechanically sound rehabilitation program. Débridement of fibrillated tissue does help keep tendon debris from creating synovial irritation and affords better visualization of the extent and depth of the tear (Fig. 37-11).

Likewise, calcific deposits that are extruded from the

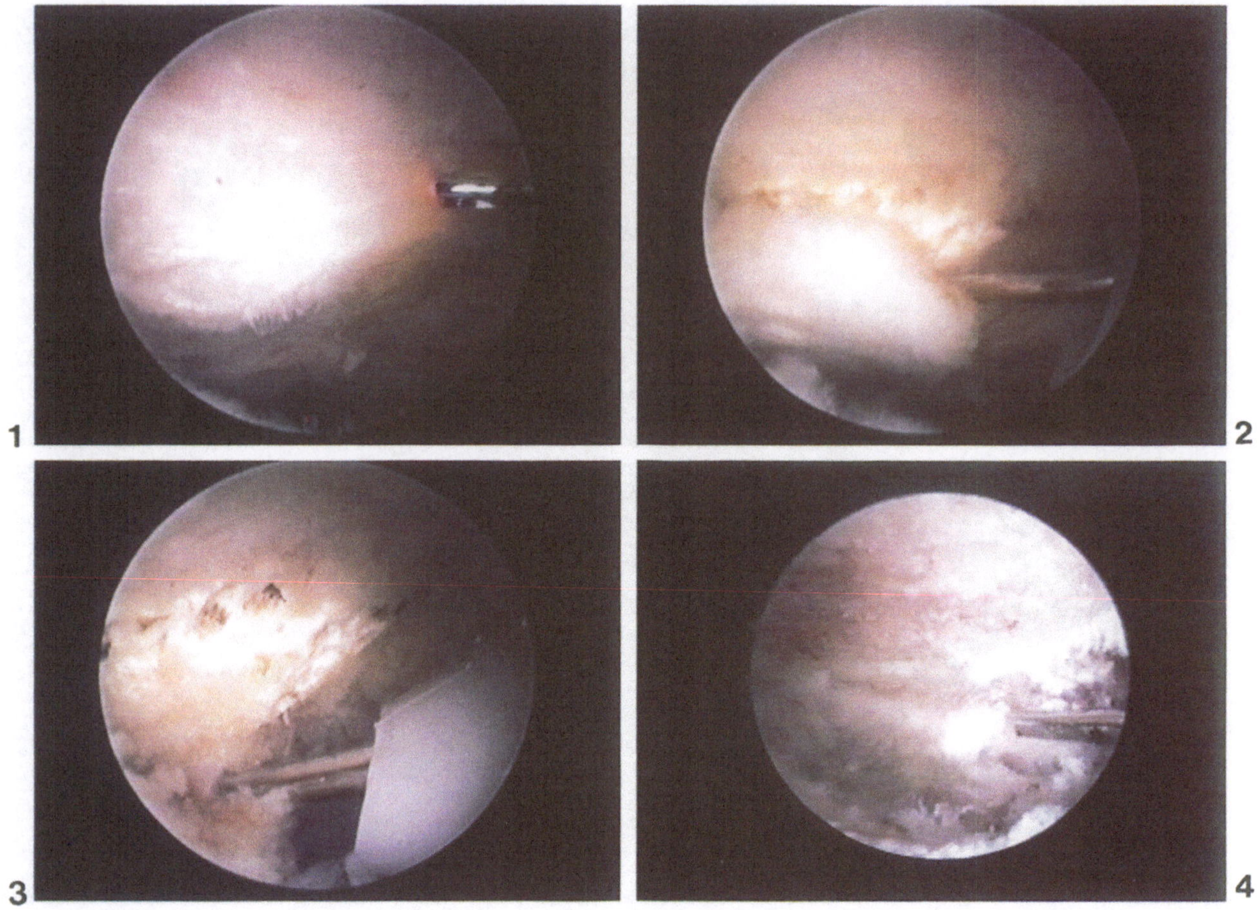

Figure 37-9. Laser resection of the coracoacromial (CA) ligament and bursa in the right shoulder, with posterior visualization. A 30 degree handpiece is introduced through a disposable cannula using the midlateral portal. The subacromial bursa has already been débrided. The CA ligament is above and the rotator cuff below. (Plate 1) Initial incision, lateral aspect, the CA ligament. (Plate 2) Development of a CA ligament flap directly off the undersurface of the acromion. (Plate 3) Complete detachment of the CA ligament from the undersurface of the acromion and dissection of the ligament from the undersurface of the deltoid. (Plate 4) Status after acromioplasty with final photoablation of the anterior CA ligament and bursa. Note the clear visualization maintained throughout the procedure. Minimal bleeding was encountered.

rotator cuff tendon leave a degenerative defect. Because calcium reflects and poorly absorbs laser energy, it must be mechanically removed. The surrounding degenerative tendon can be effectively smoothed with the 2.1 μm holmium:YAG laser in a near-contact fashion (1.6 joules). Currently, studies are being designed to evaluate the possibility of tendon fibroblast stimulation and healing with low power laser induction.

Clinical Experience

More than 200 arthroscopic shoulder procedures have been performed by us using the 2.1 μm holmium:YAG laser. The average follow-up is at least 24 months. Overall, 95% of the patients expressed satisfaction with the procedures. Unsatisfactory results were similar to those cases of the authors' during which only mechanical instruments were used.

Three patients required operation for failure to adequately decompress the subacromial space. Five patients had symptoms consistent with shoulder instability and went on to open capsular stabilization. Three patients had persistent symptoms from intrinsic rotator cuff pathology that required open repair. One patient required superficial débridement of a painful portal site.

Complications related to the use of the laser device were infrequent. In two cases, the handpiece failed intra-operatively and the procedure was continued with a new handpiece. There was one portal site infection that responded to local débridement. No deep infections were encountered and there were no laser safety failures or accidents. There were no unusual or unanticipated side effects or complications related to the use of the laser.

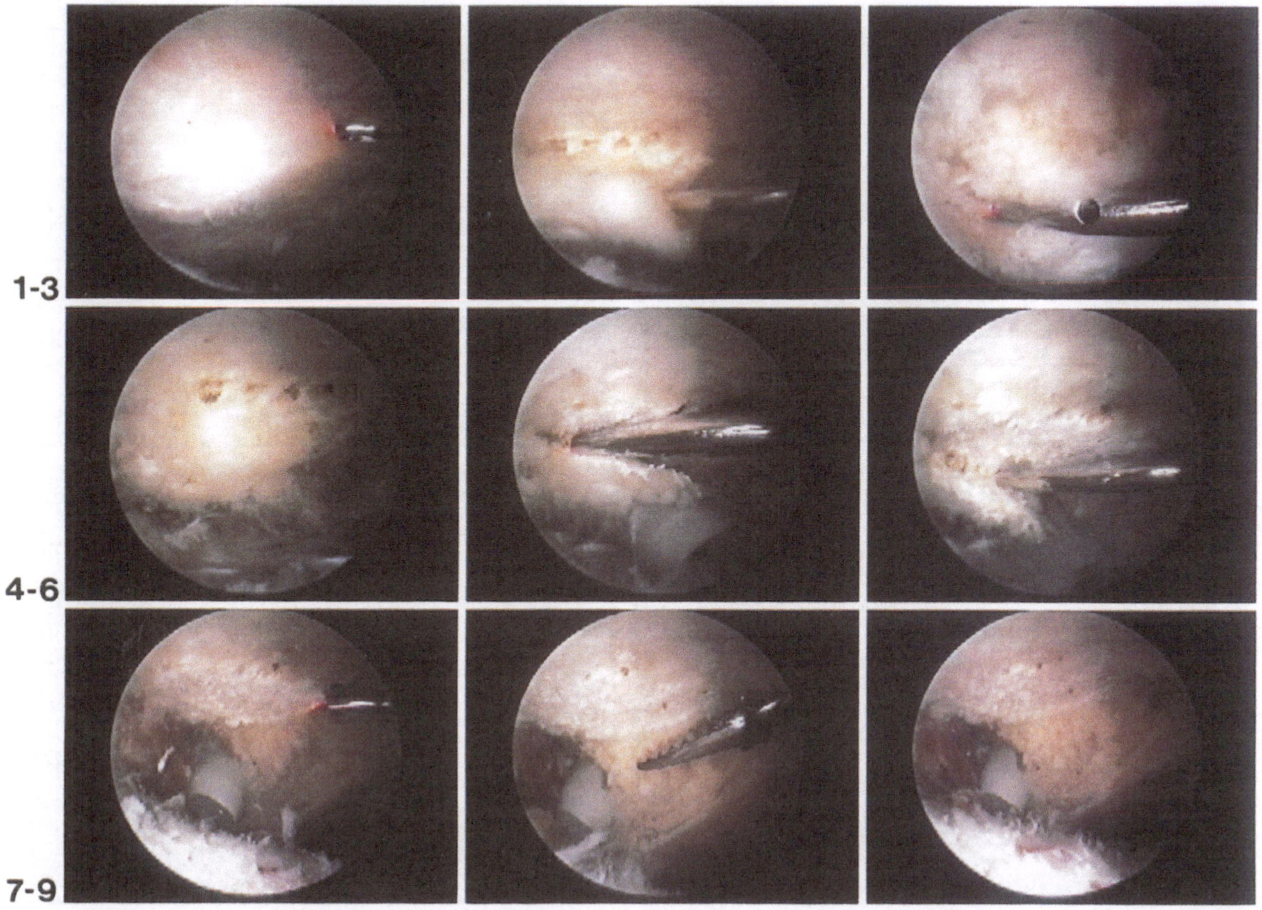

Figure 37-10. Sequential resection of the coracoacromial (CA) ligament and acromioplasty. (Plates 1–3) Incision of the lateral aspect of the CA ligament with dissection of ligament off the undersurface of the acromion. The dissection is taken medially and anteriorly, removing the CA ligament from the acromion and deltoid. (Plates 4–6) Laser incision of the acromion bone, removing a prominent anterior acromial spur. The detached bone fragment is removed with a pituitary rongeur after laser resection. (Plate 7) Laser contouring of the anterior aspect of the acromion bone. (Plate 8) Introduction of an arthroscopic rasp for final acromial smoothing if necessary. (Plate 9) Final appearance of the anterior decompression. Note the clear visualization and lack of bleeding throughout the procedure.

Conclusion

We believe that the 2.1 μm holmium:YAG laser is a valuable tool for arthroscopic shoulder surgery, including labral resection, synovectomy, and coracoacromial arch decompression. The benefits of its use intraoperatively and high patient satisfaction justify its continued application. However, direct comparison studies with mechanical techniques are needed.

Suggested Reading

Berns MW (1991) Laser surgery. Sci Am 264:85–90

Brillhart AT (1991) Arthroscopic laser surgery. Am J Arthrosc 1:5–12

Brillhart AT (1991) Arthroscopic laser surgery: the CO_2 laser and its use. Am J Arthrosc 2:7–12

Brillhart AT (1991) Arthroscopic laser surgery: the Holmium:YAG laser and its use. Am J Arthrosc 3:7–11

Decklebaum LI, Isner JM, Donaldson RF, et al (1985) Reduction of laser-induced pathologic tissue injury using pulsed energy delivery. Am J Cardiol 56:662–667

Fanton GS (1991) Uses of the holmium laser in arthroscopy: multiple joint applications. Presented at the Coherent Symposium on Advances in Laser Arthroscopy: New Techniques in Orthopedic Surgery, Anaheim, CA

Fanton GS, Dillingham MF (1990) Arthroscopic meniscectomy using the holmium:YAG laser: a double-blind study. Presented at the Arthroscopy Association of North America Annual Meeting, Orlando, FL

Fanton GS, Dillingham MF (1992) The use of the holmium laser in arthroscopic surgery. Semin Orthop 7(2):102–116

Goldberg VM (1987) Arthritis. Orthopaedic Knowledge Update II. American Academy of Orthopaedic Surgeons, Chicago, pp 35–47

Goldman JA, Chiapella J, Casey H, et al (1980) Laser therapy of rheumatoid arthritis. Lasers Surg Med 1:93–101

Gross AE, Farine IM (1984) Arthritis. Orthopaedic Knowledge Update I. American Academy of Orthopaedic Surgeons, Chicago, pp 29–40

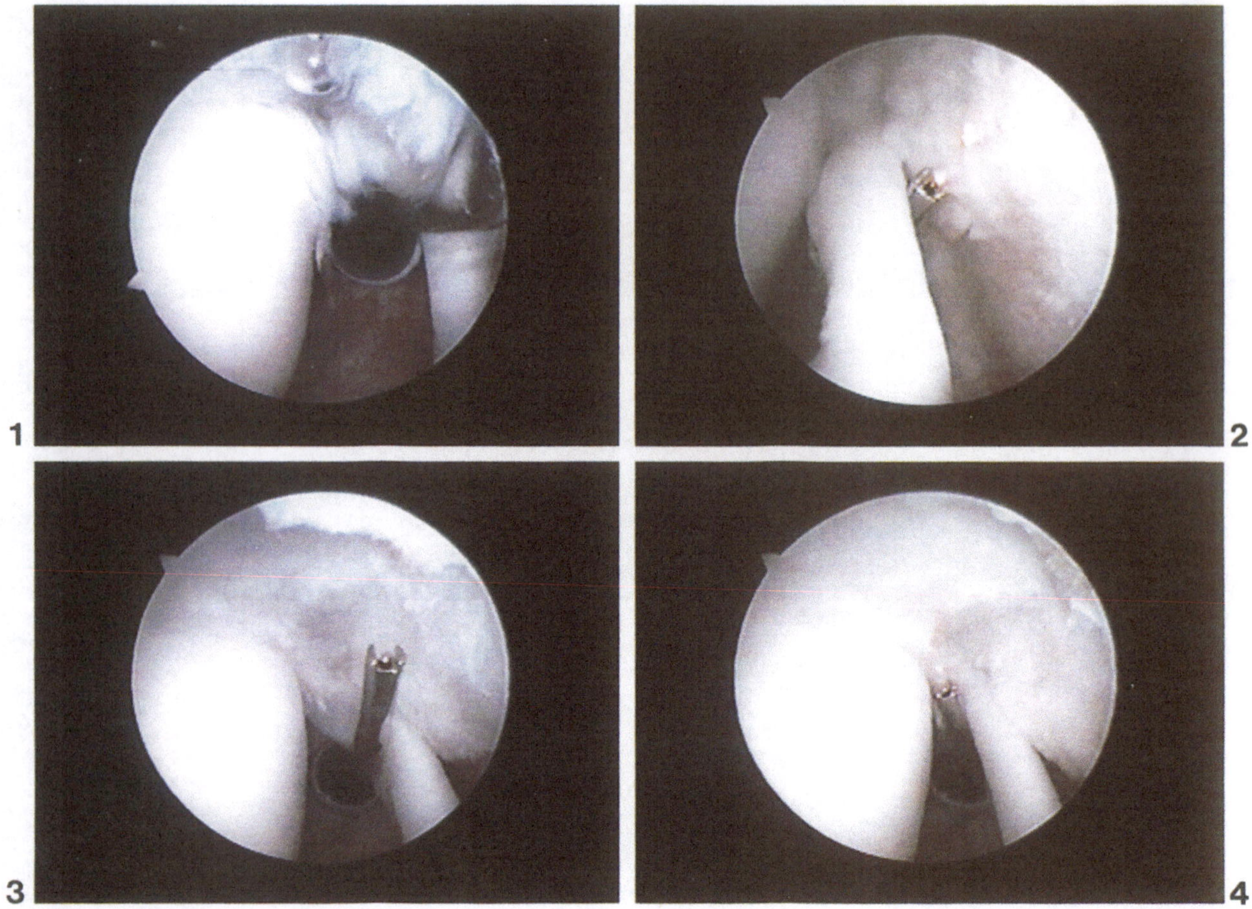

Figure 37-11. Holmium laser débridement and contouring of a partial-thickness rotator cuff tear in the left shoulder. The humeral head is on the left and the biceps tendon on the right. A disposable cannula is introduced below the biceps tendon. (Plate 1) There is extensive degeneration of the undersurface of the rotator cuff at the supraspinatus insertion. (Plate 2) Laser ablation of the degenerative portion of the cuff medial to the biceps tendon. (Plate 3) Laser contouring of fibrillated and degenerative areas of the supraspinatus insertion. (Plate 4) Final appearance after contouring and ablation of the inferior surface of the rotator cuff. Note the smooth transition to the remaining portions of the cuff.

Hobbs ER, Bailin PL, Wheeland RG, et al (1987) Super-pulsed lasers: minimizing thermal damage with short duration, high irradiance pulses. J Dermatol Surg Oncol 13:955–964

Jackson RW (1991) Symposium: lasers in orthopaedic surgery. Contemp Orthop 22:77

Lane GJ, Mooar PA (1991) Holmium:YAG laser arthroscopic débridement [abstract]. Am Soc Laser Med Surg (suppl 3)

Lane GJ, Sherk HH, Mooar PA, et al (1991) CO_2 vs holmium:YAG laser arthroscopic débridement [abstract]. Am Soc Laser Med Surg (suppl 3)

Lord MJ, Maltry JA, Shall LM (1991) Thermal injury resulting from arthroscopic lateral retinacular release by electrocautery: report of three cases and review of the literature. Arthroscopy 7:33–37

Mankin HJ (1982) The response of articular cartilage to mechanical injury: a current concepts review. J Bone Joint Surg [Am] 64:460–465

Meller M, Black H, Sherk H (1991) Wavelength selection in laser arthroscopy. Presented at the American Society for Laser Medicine and Surgery, San Diego

Miller GK, Drennan DB, Maylahn DJ (1987) The effects of technique on histology of arthroscopic partial meniscectomy with electrosurgery. Arthroscopy 3:36

Moller KO, Lind B, Shurman U, et al (1991) Holmium-laser synovectomy of immune synovitis in rabbits [abstract]. Am Soc Laser Med Surg (suppl 3)

Nishioka NS, Domankevitz Y (1989) Reflectance during pulsed holmium laser irradiation of tissue. Lasers Surg Med 9:375–381

Nishioka NS, Domankevitz Y, Flotte TJ, et al (1989) Ablation of rabbit liver, stomach and colon with a pulsed holmium laser. Gastroenterology 96:831–837

Norton LA (1982) Effects of a pulsed electromagnetic field on a mixed chondroblastic tissue culture. Clin Orthop 167:280–290

Rand JA, Gaffey TA (1985) Effect of electrocautery on fresh human articular cartilage. Arthroscopy 1:242–246

Reagan BF, McInerny VK, Treadwell BV, et al (1983) Irrigating solutions for arthroscopy. J Bone Joint Surg [Am] 65:624–631

Schultz RJ, Krishnamurthy S, Thelmo W, et al (1985) Effects of varying intensities of laser energy on articular cartilage: a preliminary study. Lasers Surg Med 5:577–588

Schurman DJ (1990) Arthritis. Orthopaedic Knowledge Update. American Academy of Orthopaedic Surgeons, Chicago, pp 57–66

Sherk HH (1990) Lasers in Orthopedics. Lippincott, Philadelphia
Smith CF, Marshall GJ, Snyder SJ, et al (1984) Comparisons of tissue effects of a surgical scalpel, and electrocautery apparatus and a carbon dioxide laser system when used for making incisions into the menisci of New Zealand rabbits. Laser Surg Med 2:305
Stein E, Sedlacek T, Fabian RL, et al (1990) Acute and chronic effects of bone ablation with a pulsed holmium laser. Lasers Surg Med 10:384–388
Trauner K, Nishioka N, Patel D (1990) Pulsed holmium:yttrium-aluminum-garnet (Ho:YAG) laser ablation of fibrocartilage and articular cartilage. Am J Sports Med 18:316–321
Van Leeuwen TG, van der Veen MJ, Verdasdonk RM, et al (1991) Noncontact tissue ablation by holmium:YSG laser pulses in blood. Lasers Surg Med 11:26–34
Vari SG, Shi WQ, Fishbein MC, et al (1991) Ablation study of the knee structure tissues with a Ho:YAG laser [abstract]. Am Soc Laser Med Surg (suppl 3) p 51
Walsh Jr TJ, Flotte TJ, Anderson RR, et al (1988) Pulsed CO_2 laser tissue ablation: effect of tissue type and pulse duration on thermal damage. Lasers Surg Med 8:108–118

38

2.1 μm Holmium:YAG Arthroscopic Laser Partial Meniscectomy in Athletes: 100 Cases

Pedro Guillén

The 2.1 μm holmium:YAG laser can be used in a conventional operating room. It has become a regular instrument within the surgical armamentarium. At first, the 2.1 μm holmium:YAG laser was used in association with other mechanical instruments, but it now can be used as a single instrument for treating meniscal, synovial, and cartilaginous disease.

Our institution treats a large number of professional athletes as well as recreational athletes. Over a 2.5 year period we have performed arthroscopic surgery with the 2.1 μm holmium:YAG laser. Many of these laser arthroscopy patients participated in the XXV Olympic Games held in Barcelona in 1992 (Figs. 38-1 and 38-2).

Materials and Methods

A review of the first 100 laser arthroscopy cases are presented. The follow-up period ranged from 6 to 18 months. The first arthroscopic laser surgery of the knee was conducted in November 1990. The ages of the patients were from 21 to 30 years of age. With regard to sex, there were more males (79) than females (21). The right side (54 patients) predominated over the left side (46 patients), and there were six cases of bilateral involvement.

With regard to medial or lateral meniscus there were 57 injuries involving the medial meniscus and 43 involving the lateral meniscus. The types of meniscal injuries are as follows:

Bucket-handle tears	15
Posterior longitudinal tears	18
Parrot-beak or transverse tears	14
Degenerative tears	9
Inferior aspect rupture tears	12
Complex rupture tears	11
Discoid lateral meniscus	2
Other unclassified tears	19

There was a predominance of posterior horn lesions of the medial meniscus and transverse lesions of the lateral meniscus. Of the 43 lateral meniscal lesions, 29 presented with associated lesions:

Anterior cruciate ligament tears	2
Posterior cruciate ligament tears	6
Medial meniscal tears	16
Chondral lesions	5

Of the 57 medial meniscal tears, 31 presented with the following associated lesions:

Unspecific synovitis	2
Lateral meniscus	6
Anterior cruciate ligament	8
Chondral lesion	14
Synovial plica	1

The surgeries were carried out with a 22 watt, 2.1 μm holmium:YAG laser. A fiberoptic handpiece was used as a delivery system. Other equipment included special laser safety glasses and standard arthroscopy equipment. The laser probes used were 15 degree probes in 85% of the cases and straight probes in the rest.

Successful local anesthesia was used on 84 patients (Fig. 38-3). Two portals were used in all but four laser cases (Fig. 38-4), in which three portals were used. Four patients had general anesthesia, and 12 had epidural anesthesia.

Results

Regarding surgical time, the laser cases took 5% longer than those with mechanical procedures. This extra time is attributed to the learning curve for the first cases. The

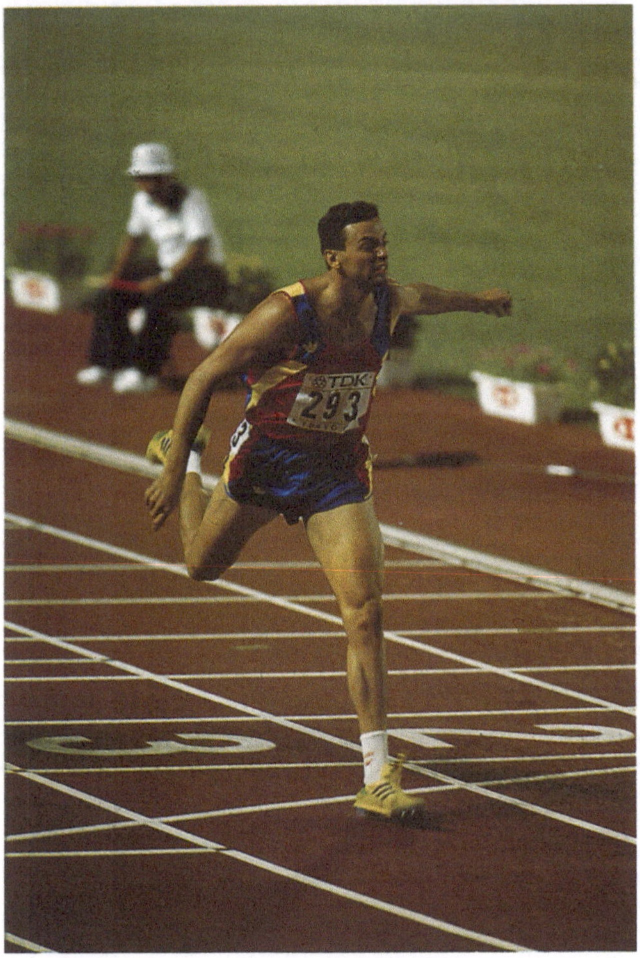

Figure 38-1. Olympic athlete, a silver medalist in the decathlon, underwent surgery on both knees.

duration of hospital stay coincides with that of stays in the "day hospital" (i.e., 6–10 hours) when local anesthesia was used. When the patient requested general or regional anesthesia, the operation was performed early in the morning, and the patient left the hospital in the afternoon in some cases.

Complications were divided into intraoperative and postoperative. Among the intraoperative complications, one was due to failure of local anesthesia and the other to failure of the laser device itself. There were no intraoperative complications that involved the surgeon (e.g. eye damage) or the patient as a result of the laser technique. With regard to postoperative complications, there were six hemarthroses, none of which required arthrocentesis or repeat surgery. Six cases of synovitis resolved uneventfully. There was one case of neuritis of the infrapatellar nerve due to the medial portal placement; it resolved uneventfully. There were two cases of a fistula of the medial portal that remitted without need for suturing. No infections, thrombophlebitis, internal or external burns, or cartilage necrosis were observed.

All professional athletes treated with laser arthroscopy started rehabilitation from the first day after surgery. The patients started with isometric exercises 3 to 6 seconds long and several repetitions every hour, progressing to mobilization exercises when the arthroscope access portals healed. They returned to sports competition within 15 to 30 days of the operation when there was no synovitis. Those with synovitis healed in 8 weeks. On average, this compared favorably with the mechanical technique, according to our experience. Athletes operated on for medial meniscal lesion did much better than those with tears of the lateral meniscus.

Histopathologic study of the one previously laser-treated

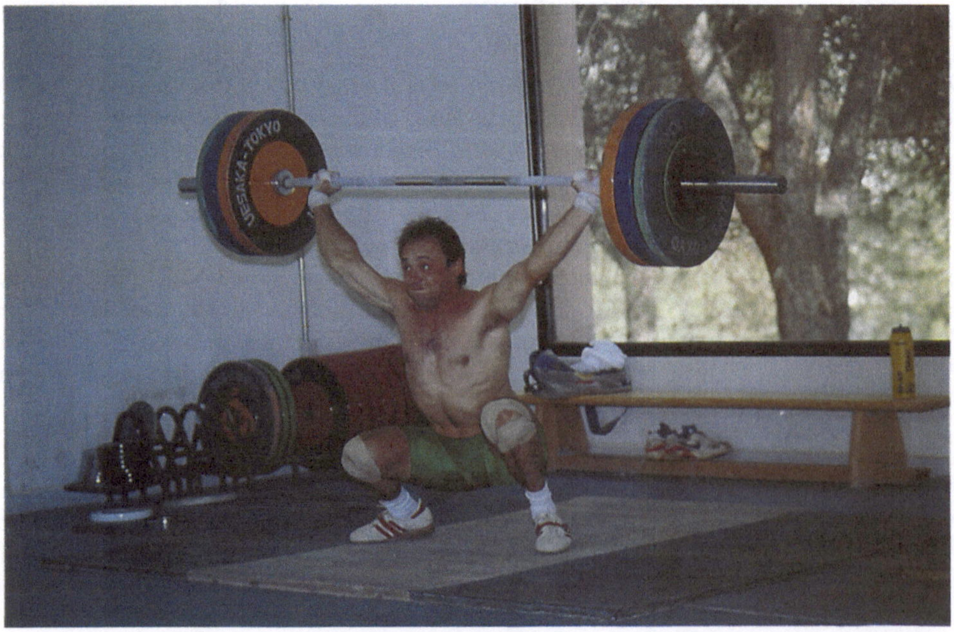

Figure 38-2. Olympic athlete (weight lifting) was operated on the knee with this technique.

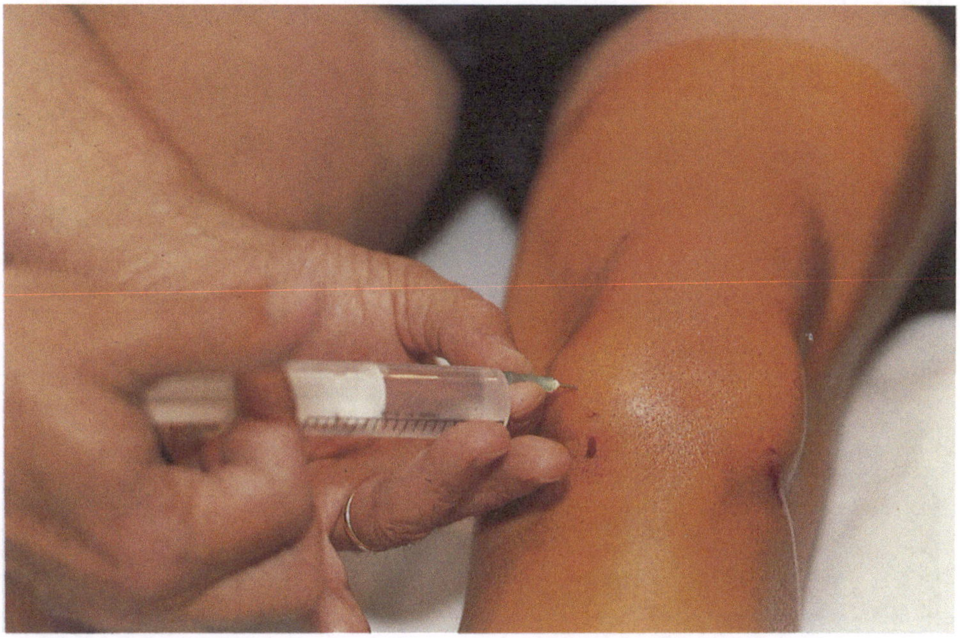

Figure 38-3. Local anethesia being used.

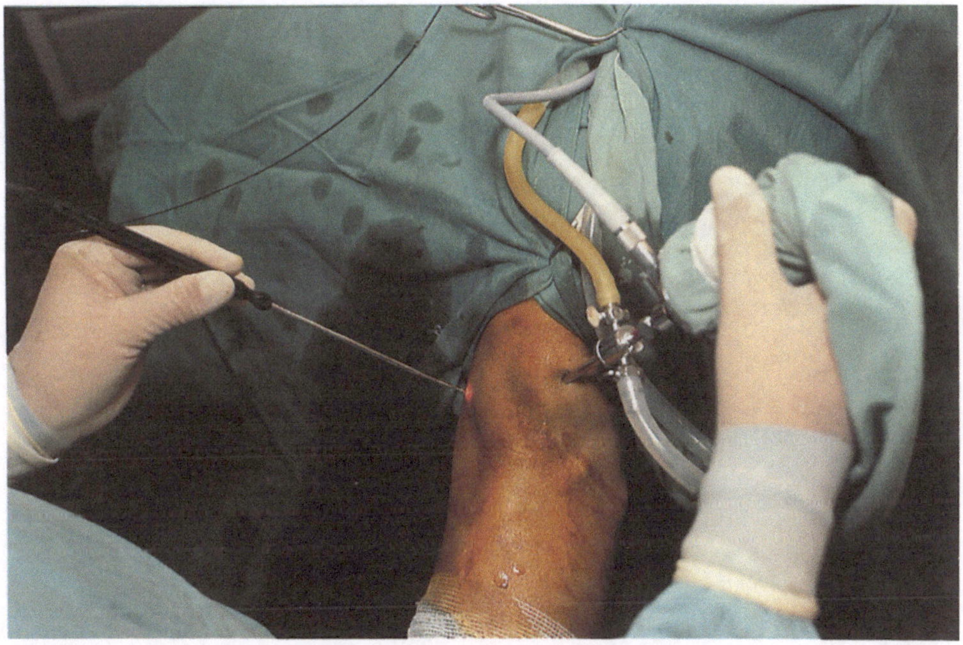

Figure 38-4. Insertion of the laser probe.

meniscal remnant retrieved on the single reoperation did not reveal meniscal degeneration attributed to the technique. That is, this meniscal degeneration could not be differentiated from that seen with the standard mechanical technique (Figs. 38-5 and 38-6) 8 months after the first laser surgery.

Conclusions

The evidence is convincing that the 2.1 μm holmium:YAG laser should become part of the armamentarium of the arthroscopic surgeon. When compared to my results using mechanical tools, recovery times were excellent. It is a superior tool for performing partial meniscectomy in athletes in an outpatient setting with local anesthesia. However, it is important that future equipment become less costly, be smaller, and produce less noise.

References

Brillhart AT (1991) Lasers in arthroscopic surgery. Arthroscopy 7:411–412

Cabot JR (1952) Traumatismes sportifs de l'hemiarticulation externe du genou (fract. exceptees). Presented at the IX Congrés International de Medicine Sportive, Paris, pp 201–207

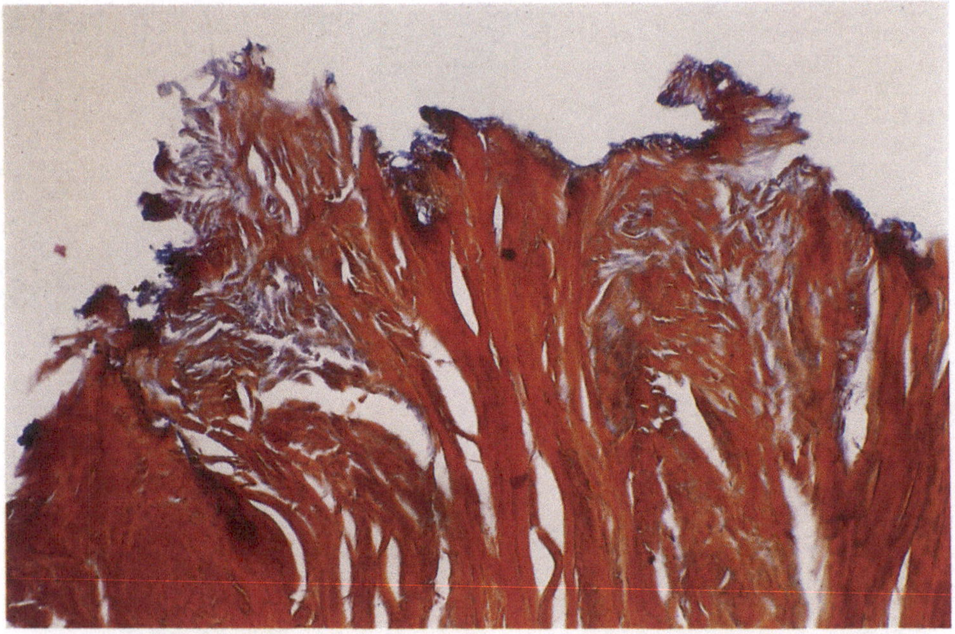

Figure 38-5. Histologic study of the edge of a meniscus cut with a 2.1 μm holmium:YAG laser in which deep thermal damage is not observed.

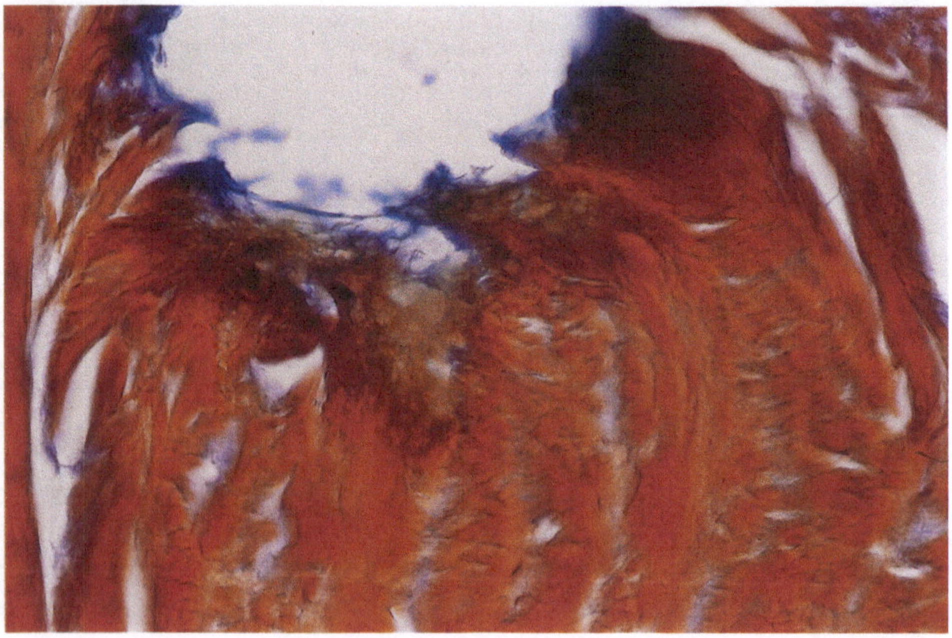

Figure 38-6. Same case as in Figure 38-5, on a larger scale, where thermal damage of a depth of less than 500 μm can be observed.

Guillén-Garcia P (1991) Arthroscopic laser surgery in treating the knee injuries of leading professional athletes. Am J Arthrosc 1(9):15–18

Guillén-Garcia P (1992a) Cirugía artroscópica de rodilla con láser holmium. Rev Ortop Trauma 36(suppl 1):15–18

Guillén-Garcia P (1992b) Surgery with holmium laser in articular orthopaedics. Orthopaedic Product News Jul/Aug/Sept: 35–36

Metcalf RW, Dixon JA (1984) Use of lasers for arthroscopic meniscectomy: a preliminary report on laboratory investigations. Lasers Surg Med 3:305–369

Miller DV, O'Brien SJ, Arnoczky SS, et al (1989) The use of the contact Nd:YAG laser in arthroscopic surgery: effects on articular cartilage and meniscal tissue. Arthroscopy 5:245–253

Monzó E, Ibañez L, Baeza C, et al (1993) Anestesia local y regional para técnicas semi-invasivas en ortopedia. In Monografía del XVIII Symposium Internacional de Traumatología y Ortopedia MAPFRE (in press)

Naves J (1952) Position operatoire pour faciliter l'extirpation de la corne posteriure du menisque externe. Presented at the IX Congrés International de Medicine Sportive, París, pp 173–174

O'Brien SJ, Miller DV (1990) The contact neodymium-yttrium-aluminum-garnet laser: a new approach to arthroscopic laser surgery. Clin Orthop 252:95–100

Ordoñez P, Guillén-Garcia P (1992) Rigidez de rodilla: artrofibrosis. J Fisioter (in press)

Stein E, Sedlacek T, Fabian RL, Nishioka NS (1990) Acute and chronic effects of bone ablation with a pulsed holmium laser. Lasers Surg Med 10:384–388

Toft J (1991) Postoperative morbidity following laser arthroscopic lateral release. Am J Arthrosc 1:23–25

Trauner K, Nishioka N, Patel D (1990) Pulsed holmium: yttrium-aluminum-garnet (Ho:YAG) laser ablation of fibrocartilage and articular cartilage. Am J Sports Med 18:316–320

39

2.1 μm Holmium:YAG Arthroscopic Laser Partial Meniscectomy: 226 Cases

James R. Larson

The development of arthroscopic techniques has dramatically improved our ability to perform minimally invasive procedures. With improved surgical procedures, the injured patient has been able to return to full activity with minimal morbidity and reduced recovery time. As techniques evolved, the limiting factor has been the instruments needed to perform these procedures. In the past, even when the surgeon can easily access the joint and visualize the pathology, the instruments would not allow easy completion of the procedure because of their size, shape, and efficiency. It was natural, therefore, that as lasers evolved with their small delivery systems and no-touch techniques they were found attractive for arthroscopic use.

Materials and Methods

The operating room setup has not been dramatically changed with the addition of the 2.1 μm holmium:YAG laser. The machine is kept in the operating room but is not activated until after the diagnostic portion of the procedure determines that a laser will be necessary. Once it is thought that the laser will be used, the technician is called and it takes only a few minutes to activate the machine. Saline is used for joint distension, but any arthroscopic fluid can be used as it does not affect the efficiency of the laser. A knee holder is used for all procedures, and a tourniquet is placed though it is rarely used. Each portal is injected with 0.25% bupivacaine (Marcaine) with epinephrine to improve hemostasis. The choice of anesthetic is left to the patient, but most patients request general anesthesia. As the handpiece is small and no tourniquet is used, the type of anesthesia does not affect the ability to perform the procedure. For lateral releases, the patient is encouraged to use local anesthesia because it helps evaluate the effectiveness of the release during the procedure. A pump system for joint distention improves clearing the small bubbles created during laser use.

For laser arthroscopic use, the choice of the surgical portals are important. Although the handpieces tolerate some bending during the procedure, it is important not to torque excessively and bend the fibers, which affects the efficiency of the energy delivery system. For medial compartment pathology, it is important to have a working portal near the midline, as it allows the handpiece to be at a right angle to the tissue and more efficiently allows transfer of energy for ablation. In the lateral compartment it is better to have a more medial working portal, again to have the handpiece at a right angle to the tissue. It is therefore important to first perform adequate diagnostic determination before the working portals are created.

Over a 2 year period at Abbott-Northwestern Hospital, 427 arthroscopic laser procedures with the 2.1 μm holmium:YAG laser system have been performed; 226 were isolated meniscectomies. All procedures were performed at the ambulatory surgical center. Most of the procedures were performed under general anesthesia at the request of the patients. Postoperatively it was recommended that the patients bear weight as tolerated and that they remove all dressings at 24 hours. No antibiotics were given during the procedures or the recovery period. The patients were allowed to shower at 24 hours but were not allowed to swim or sit in whirlpools until the puncture sites had sealed. All patients were encouraged to start active range of motion during the first 24 hours. No specific protocol for the use of ice was recommended for the recovery period. By 7 days, they were encouraged to start low impact exercises and could progress to impact activities as tolerated.

Results

Follow-up for the first 226 meniscectomies ranged from 3 to 24 months. Three complications were noted in this series. Twice the handpiece malfunctioned and resulted in fracture of the fiber. The handpieces became warm, and it was quickly apparent that sufficient energy was not being delivered through the handpiece to the meniscal tissue. In both cases, a new handpiece was selected, and the procedure was completed without difficulty. The third complication was a fracture of a free fiberoptic fiber that was inserted through a small cannula when we were developing new handpieces. Approximately 1 cm of the fiber fractured and became a foreign body in the joint. It was easily removed with graspers with no untoward effects.

All patients returned for follow-up at 1, 3, and 6 weeks. In this series, there were no wound infections, thrombophlebitis, or postoperative complications during the recovery period. At the first week of follow-up, all patients presented with a mild effusion that had resolved by the third week of follow-up. By 6 weeks, all patients had returned to their preinjury levels of activity.

For partial medial meniscectomy the average laser time ranged from 18.5 to 20.5 minutes. For the lateral operative meniscus it ranged from 14.0 to 18.5 minutes. As the new higher energy machines became available, the laser operative time decreased. Although the operative time is approximately 25% less than that with mechanical instrument use, the most important improvement with the use of laser has been the easy access to the joint with the small handpiece. The handpiece can easily contour the posterior meniscal pathology without causing iatrogenic trauma to the joint surface during the procedure. In even the tightest, most difficult joint, the pathology can still be easily addressed.

Conclusion

For 226 sequential partial meniscectomies, the procedure was completed with no long-term complications. All sites were accessed for arthroscopy with minimal iatrogenic trauma to the articular surface secondary to the insertion or the use of the handpieces. In this series, the use of the 2.1 μm holmium:YAG laser represents a distinct improvement in the ability to handle even the most complicated meniscal tears.

Suggested Reading

Bickerstaff DR (ed), Wyman A, Laing RW, Smith WD (1991) Partial meniscectomy using the neodymium:YAG laser: an in vitro study. Arthroscopy 7:63–67

Biyikli S, Modest MF (1987) Energy requirements for osteotomy of femora and tibiae with a moving CW CO_2 laser. Lasers Surg Med 7:512–519

Brown JE (1965) The enzyme dissolution of intervertebral disc by the use of chymopapain. Clin Orthop 38:193–197

Choy DS, Saddekni S, Michelson, et al (1991) Percutaneous lumbar disc decompression with Nd:YAG laser. Am J Arthrosc 1(9):9–13

Dandy DJ, Griffiths DD (1989) Lateral release for recurrent dislocation (of the patella. J Bone Joint Surg [Br] 71:121–125

DeLee J (1985) Complications of arthroscopy and arthroscopic surgery: results of a national survey. Arthroscopy 1:214–220

Duffy S, Davis M, Sharp F, Stamp J, Ginsberg R (1992) Preliminary observations of holmium:YAG laser tissue interaction using human uterus. Lasers Surg Med 12:147–152

Fanton G (1992) Lateral retinacular release of the left knee using the VersaPulse surgical laser: a case report. Update in Orthopaedic Laser Surgery (vol 2, no 3)

Fuller JA, Ghadially FN (1972) Ultrastructural observations on surgically produced partial thickness defects in articular cartilage. Clin Orthop 86:193–205

Gottlob C, Kopchok GE, Peng SK, et al (1992) Holmium:YAG laser ablation of human intervertebral disc: preliminary evaluation. Lasers Surg Med 12:86–91

Gropper GR, Robertson JH, McClellan G (1984) Comparative histological and radiographic effects of CO_2 laser versus standard surgical anterior cervical discectomy in the dog. Neurosurgery 14:42–47

Guillen-Garcia P (1991) Arthroscopic laser surgery in treating the knee injuries of leading professional athletes. Am J Arthrosc 1(9):15–18

Jacques SL (1984) Laser–tissue interactions. Cancer Bull 41:211–218

Kettlecamp DB (1981) Management of patellar malalignment. J Bone Joint Surg [Am] 63:1344–1348

Kopchok GE, White RA, Meuller M, Cavaye D (1992) Percutaneous laser discectomy. J Clin Laser Med Surg April: 79–82

Kopchok GE, White RA, Tabbara M, Saadatmanesh V, Peng SK (1990) Holmium:YAG laser ablation of vascular tissue. Lasers Surg Med 10:405–413

Kollmer CE, Sherk HH, Dugan M (1987) Laser use in revision arthroplasty. Surg Forum 38:538

Lesinski SG, Palmer A (1989) Lasers for otosclerosis: CO_2 vs. argon and KTP/532. Laryngoscope 99:1–8

Lord MJ, Maltry JA, Shall LM (1991) Thermal injury resulting from arthroscopic lateral retinacular release by electrocautery: report of three cases and a review of the literature. Arthroscopy 7:33–37

Mankin HJ (1982) The response of articular cartilage to mechanical injury. J Bone Joint Surg [Am] 64:460–465

Miller DV, O'Brien SJ, Arnoczky SS, et al (1989) The use of the contact Nd:YAG laser in arthroscopic surgery: effects on articular cartilage and meniscal tissue. Arthroscopy 5:245–253

Miller GK, Dickason JM, Fox JM, et al (1982) The use of electrosurgery for arthroscopic subcutaneous lateral release. Orthopaedics 5:309–316

Mitchell N, Shepard N (1980) The healing of articular cartilage in intra-articular fractures in rabbits. J Bone Joint Surg [Am] 64:628–634

Nuss RC, Fabian RL, Sarkar R, et al (1988) Infrared laser bone ablation. Lasers Surg Med 8:381–391

Pennino R, Cantor F, O'Connor T, et al (1989) Cartilage sculpting: carbon dioxide laser vs. blade techniques. Lasers Surg Med Suppl 1:7

Rand JA, Gaffey TA (1985) Effect of electrocautery on fresh human cartilage. Arthroscopy 1:242–246

Rothwell AG, Bentley G (1973) Chondrocyte multiplication in osteoarthritic articular cartilage. J Bone Joint Surg [Br] 55:588–594

Schonholtz GJ, Ling B (1985) Arthroscopic chondroplasty of the patella. Arthroscopy 1:92–96

Schonholtz GJ, Zahn MG, Magee CM (1987) Lateral retinacular release of the patella. Arthroscopy 3:269–272

Sherk HH (1991) Orthopedists using lasers in surgery. Am J Arthrosc 9:7–8

Small NC (1988) Complications in arthroscopic surgery performed by experience arthroscopists. Arthroscopy 4:215–221

Small NC (1989) An analysis of complications in lateral retinacular release procedures. Arthroscopy 5:282–286

Smith CF, Johansen WE, Vangsness CT, et al (1989) The carbon dioxide laser: a potential tool for orthopaedic surgery. Clin Orthop 242: 34–50

Stein E, Sedlacek T, Fabian RL, et al (1990) Acute and chronic effects of bone ablation with a pulsed holmium laser. Lasers Surg Med 10:384–386

Stith WJ, Judy MM, Hochschuler, Guyer RD (1991) Choice of lasers for minimally invasive spinal surgery. Orthop Rev 20:137–142

Thomsen S (1989) Medical lasers: how they work and how they affect tissue. Cancer Bull 41:203–210

Toft J (1991) Postoperative morbidity following laser arthroscopic lateral release. Am J Arthrosc 1(9)23–25

Trauner K, Nishioka N, Patel D (1990) Pulsed holmium: yttrium-aluminum-garnet (Ho:YAG) laser ablation of fibrocartilage and cartilage. Am J Sports Med 18:316–320

Whipple TL, Caspari RB, Meyers JF (1983) Laser energy in arthroscopic meniscectomy. Orthopaedics 6:1165–1169

Whipple TL, Caspari RB, Meyers JF (1985) Arthroscopic laser meniscectomy in a gas medium. Arthroscopy 1:2–7

Wolgin M, Finkenberg J, Papaioannou T, et al (1989) Excimer ablation of human intervertebral disc at 308 nanometers. Laser Surg 9:124–131

40

2.1 μm Holmium:YAG Arthroscopic Laser Débridement of Degenerative Knees: 148 Cases

Pekka Mooar

Laser energy has been shown to have biologic effects on articular cartilage (Schultz et al., 1985). It has been demonstrated with several wavelengths that it can be used for arthroscopic applications. It has precision in cutting, making it attractive for the management of articular flap tears. Laser energy appears to preserve more remaining articular cartilage than do mechanical shavers. The combination of cartilage sparing and biostimulation offer theoretic improvements over mechanical instrumentation. The 2.1 μm holmium:YAG laser has the added advantage of versatility and has been my arthroscopic instrument of choice for performing combined partial meniscectomy and chondroplasty in degenerative knees.

Materials and Methods

In 1991 a prospective study was started to evaluate the long-term effects of laser chondroplasty for the treatment of osteoarthritis of the knee. A total of 148 patients were enrolled in the study: 76 were more than 40 years of age and 72 less than 40 years of age. Essentially every knee in this series demonstrated an associated degenerative meniscal tear that was also débrided with the laser.

The use of the 2.1 μm holmium:YAG laser for articular cartilage débridement did not vary much from routine arthroscopic technique. Standard arthroscopic portals were used for visualization of the articular surfaces and laser probe insertion. The procedure was performed under local, regional, or general anesthesia.

Three techniques were used to débride and sculpt the chondral surfaces: (1) a near-contact method directly perpendicular to the surface; (2) a tangential-contact method, with the probe parallel to the surface; and (3) a direct-contact method, with the probe perpendicular to the surface. The near-contact technique was the most useful when the articular cartilage was extensively fibrillated or large flaps existed (Fig. 40-1). An energy setting of 1 joule at a rate of 20 Hz provided rapid, controlled ablation of the loose articular material. The laser fiber is introduced into the knee; and the laser is turned on with the fiber 2 to 4 mm from the articular surface. The laser is advanced slowly toward the chondral surface until a tissue response is observed. Visualization of tissue effects gives the surgeon the best guide to when the energy density has reached the ablation threshold. As seen in Figure 40-2, varying the probe tip's distance from the tissue varies the energy density from 0 to more than 1000 joules/cm^2 within a 0 to 4 mm distance.

The ablation threshold was found by Trauner et al. (1990) to be 50 J/cm^2 for hyaline cartilage. An alternative tangential application prevents the excessive loss of articular tissue, removing only the loose fronds (Fig. 40-3). The loose articular pieces appear to involute and shrink as the laser energy is applied. Care was taken not to remove an excessive amount of cartilage. The ability to precisely control degenerative articular cartilage removal using these techniques is an advantage over the more aggressive mechanical shaving techniques. When large, loose pieces are delaminating from the articular surface, the direct contact technique with the beam perpendicular to the surface is used. The probe is pushed gently throughout the base of the loose piece (Fig. 40-4). The tactile feedback provided by the handpiece in direct contact with the cut surface enhances control. Visualization can be enhanced as the fragment is manipulated with the laser probe tip. After the large fragments have been amputated, the base and edges may be smoothed to a stable margin by tangential application of the laser energy. There were 148 knees operated on in this study using the 2.1 μm holmium:YAG laser for chondroplasty. Virtually every case underwent a simultaneous partial medial or lateral meniscectomy (or both) for

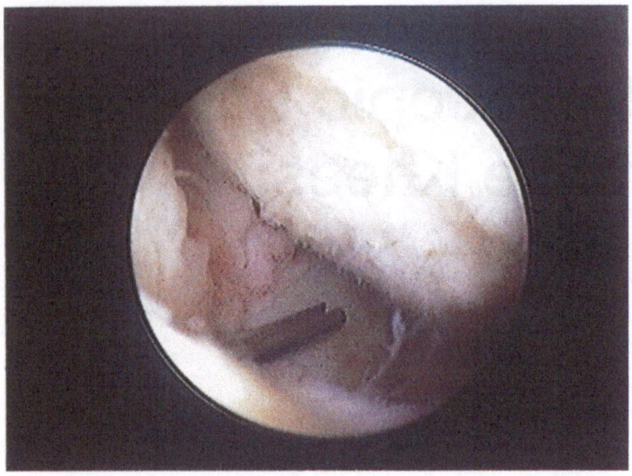

A

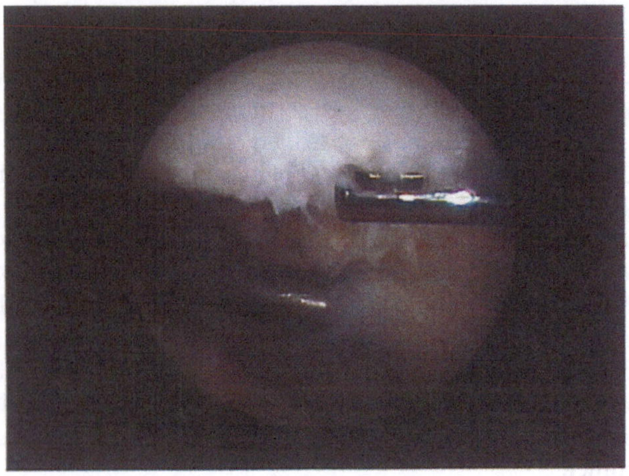

B

Figure 40-1. (a) Partial thickness chondroplasty result. (b) 70-side firing fiber tangential to patella surface.

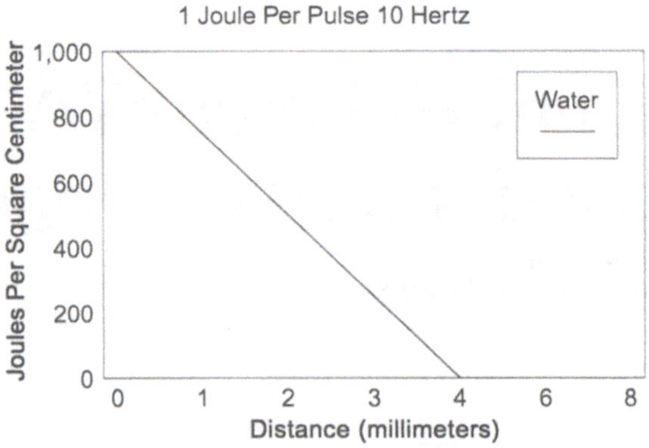

Figure 40-2. Near touch power density curve.

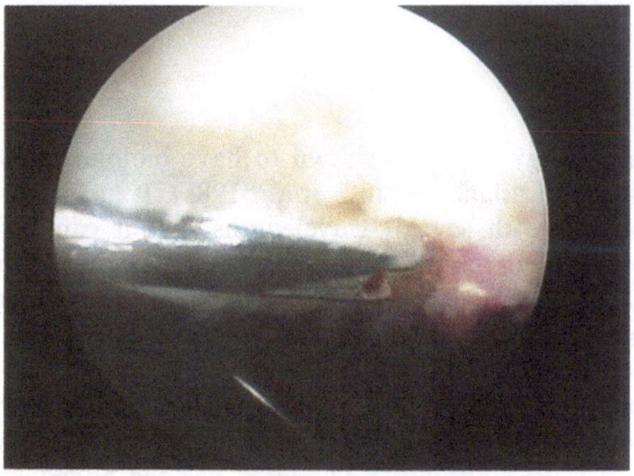

Figure 40-3. Tangential laser application.

degenerative tears using the laser. The technique for partial meniscectomy is discussed elsewhere in this text.

Results

Of the 69 patients under 40 years of age followed for less than 12 months, 2 were subjectively worse, 3 claimed no change symptomatically, and 64 were improved. For those 66 patients over 40 years of age followed less than 1 year, 7 were not improved and 59 were. Only 13 patients were followed more than 12 months, 10 of whom were improved and 3 were not. Ten patients were over 40 years of age, three were not.

Discussion

Degenerative changes in the articular surfaces of the knee are the result of numerous factors (Mankin, 1974a,b). Tidal lavage removes debris, proteolytic enzymes, and prostaglandins. Subjective improvement usually occurs, but complete pain relief is rare. Patient satisfaction shows 75% temporizing benefits at 2 years, but there are no long-term studies (Livesley et al., 1991). Arthroscopic mechanical débridement of the knee has yielded similar results. Rand (1985, 1991) reported 80% improvement at 1 year and 67% improvement at 5 years after mechanical débridement of degenerative menisci and loose articular cartilage. The best results have been obtained in patients with mild degenerative joint disease and mobile meniscal fragments with normal valgus knee alignments. Abrasion chondroplasties have produced variable results, ranging from 80% good results to 33% poor results (Johnson, 1986). In general, the results of abrasion chondroplasties have not been predictable and the results not durable. Rand (1991) reported that 57% of patients who have had abrasion chondroplasties undergo total knee arthroplasties at 3 years, and 6% to 10% of patients are made worse by an abrasion chondroplasty.

As lasers have come into increasing usage in orthopaedic surgery, it is hoped that they will offer a new method of treatment. Vangsness et al. (1992) demonstrated that the 10.6 μm CO_2 laser was an efficient, effective tool for removing articular and meniscal tissue, but there was no dem-

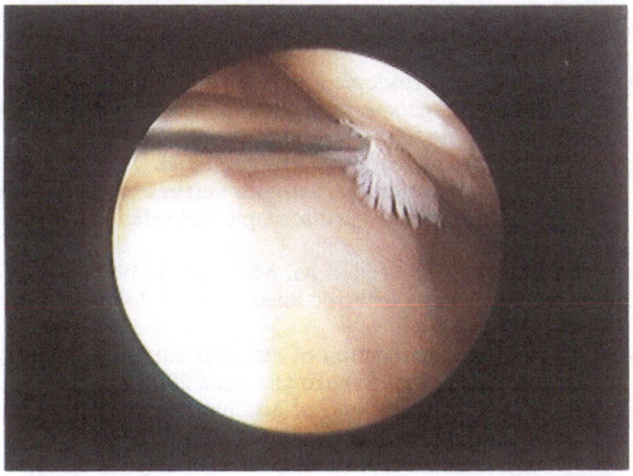

A

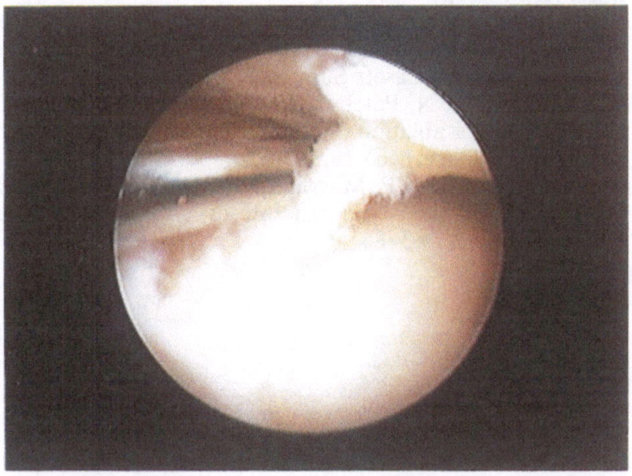

B

Figure 40-4. (a) Direct contact amputation technique for chondral flap lesion. (b) Near contact debulking technique for chondral flap lesion

Table 40-1. Arthroscopic laser débridment months postop

	<3 months	3–6 months	6–12 months	>12 months
<40 Years	47	11	11	3
>40 Years	36	16	14	10

onstrated healing or biostimulation of cartilage repair. Garrick (1992) reported that 10.6 μm CO_2 laser arthroscopy did not have any clinical documentation of enhanced healing, quicker postoperative rehabilitation, or lessened requirement for postoperative analgesia. Lane et al. (1992) compared 10.6 μm CO_2 laser and mechanical débridement techniques in 100 patients. The operative times for the two groups were not statistically different. Although the return to function was the same for both groups, 30% of the CO_2 laser patients compared to 22%

Table 40-2. Arthroscopic laser débridement for patients >40 years of age

<3 months	all showed improvement
3–6 months	15/16 showed improvement
6–9 months	4/10 no change 6/10 improvement
9–12 months	2/4 improvement 2/4 no change
>12 months	2/10 no change 8/10 improvement

Table 40-3. Arthroscopic laser débridement for patients <40 years of age

<3 months	2/47 worse 2/47 no change 43/47 improved
3–6 months	all showed improvement
6–9 months	all showed improvement
9–12 months	2/4 marked improvement 1/4 some 1/4 none
>12 months	2/3 improved 1/3 no change

of the mechanically treated patients had postoperative knee effusions at 4 weeks.

Clinically, the free-beam configuration of the 1.06 μm neodymium:YAG laser has been demonstrated to provide suboptimal cutting of cartilaginous tissue while causing a significant degree of thermal damage to surrounding tissue (Glick, 1984; Inoue et al., 1984). Raunest and Siebert have shown severe degenerative changes in laboratory animals when the 1.06 μm neodymium:YAG laser is used on articular cartilage. The contact tip has been added to the 1.06 μm neodymium:YAG laser to control its depth of penetration, decreasing it to 0.50 μms from 0.85 μm. The contact tip serves as a heat sink and converts the laser to a hot cutting instrument.

Collier et al. (1993) have reported that reparative fibrocartilage adjacent to traumatic equine hyaline cartilage defects that have been irradiated with the 2.1 μm holmium:YAG laser can be seen. This statement did not apply when the subchondral plate was destroyed by irradiation.

Conclusion

Of all the available instruments, I believe that the 2.1 μm holmium:YAG laser is the one that is the easiest to use for combined chondroplasty and partial meniscectomy in degenerative knees. It can be used to sculpt fragmented articular cartilage with more precision than mechanical tools. Laboratory studies have suggested a biostimulatory effect with this wavelength, but there are no clinical studies to confirm this finding. This study shows improvement in symptoms at 1 year in 10 of 13 patients. Of the 135 patients followed for less than 1 year, 123 were improved. However, preliminary data seem to indicate that the 2 year follow-up studies will not be significantly different from historical controls. Obtaining statistically significant data for purposes of accurate comparison to internal and historical controls is an essential goal of this ongoing study. This information is needed before final conclusions are made. A second-look biopsy study is also needed to validate a biostimulatory effect of 2.1 μm holmium:YAG laser energy on degenerative articular cartilage.

Poor prognosticators included obesity, pain as the only preoperative complaint, lack of preoperative mechanical symptoms, and mechanical axis malalignment. It is the same as with mechanical chondroplasty. Therefore patient selection is the key to success with laser chondroplasty. What can be said in favor of laser chondroplasty is that the procedure appears to be facilitated by the 2.1 μm holmium:YAG laser, which allows the surgeon to more easily preserve functional articular cartilage. For all significant grades of chondromalacia, the results appear to be at least as good as when mechanical means are used.

References

Collier MA, Bellamy T, Hangland LM, et al (1993) Initial effects of holmium:YAG laser on equine cartilage adjacent to traumatic lesion: a histopathological assessment. Trans Vet Orthop Res Soc 22:5

Garrick JG (1992) CO_2 laser arthroscopy using ambient gas pressure. Semin Orthop 7(2):90–94

Glick J (1984) Use of the laser beam in arthroscopic surgery. In Casscells SE (ed), Arthroscopy: Diagnostic and Surgical Practice. Lea & Febiger, Philadelphia p 181

Inoue K, et al (1984) Arthroscopic Laser Surgery. IAA, London, pp 29–30.9

Johnson LL (1986) Arthroscopic abrasion arthroplasty historical and pathological perspective: present states. Arthroscopy 2:54–69

Lane G, Sherk HH, Mooar PA, Lee SJ, Black J (1992) Holmium:yttrium-aluminum-garnet laser versus carbon dioxide laser versus mechanical arthroscopic débridement. Semin Orthop 7(2):95–101

Livesley PJ, Doherty M, Needoff M, Moulton A (1991) Arthroscopic lavage of osteoarthritic knees. J Bone Joint Surg [Br] 73:922–926

Mankin HJ (1974a) The reaction of articular cartilage to injury and osteoarthritis: part I. N Engl J Med 291:1285–1292

Mankin HJ (1974b) The reaction of articular cartilage to injury and osteoarthritis: part II. N Engl J Med 291:1335–1340

Rand JA (1985) Arthroscopic management of degenerative meniscus tears in patients with degenerative arthritis. Arthroscopy 1:253

Rand JA (1991) Role of arthroscopy in osteoarthritis of the knee. Arthroscopy 7:358–363

Schultz RJ, Krishnamurthy S, Thelmo W, et al (1985) Effects of varying intensities of laser energy on articular cartilage: a preliminary study. Lasers Surg Med 5:577–588

Trauner K, Nishioka N, Patel D (1990) Pulsed holmium:YAG (Ho:YAG) laser ablation of fibrocartilage and articular cartilage. Am J Sports Med 18:316–320

Vangsness Jr CT, Smith CF, Marshall GJ, Sweeny JR, Johansen E (1992) CO_2 laser vaporization of articular cartilage. Semin Orthop 7(2)83–85

41

2.1 μm Holmium:YAG Arthroscopic Laser Chondroplasty: 262 Cases

William P. Thorpe

The purpose of chondroplasty is to reduce pain and improve the function of a joint that has been damaged by trauma or an arthritic process (Magnuson 1941; Insall, 1967; Ewing, 1980; Sprague, 1981; Johnson, 1986). Laser chondroplasty, particularly 2.1 μm holmium:YAG laser chondroplasty, has distinct attractions in my opinion. In general, 2.1 μm holmium:YAG laser chondroplasty patients are satisfied. Second, the depth of penetration of the 2.1 μm holmium:YAG laser is easier to control than that with a mechanical device (Decklebaum et al., 1985; Hobbs et al., 1987; Burns and Nelson 1988; Walsh et al., 1988; Sherk 1990; Trauner, 1990; Burns, 1991). Third, the 2.1 μm holmium:YAG laser allows better immediate intraoperative appearance of the treated chondral surface than when mechanical tools are used.

The efficacy of chondroplasty is mostly due to removal of abnormal tissue, but there is a role for changes in surface structure (Magnuson, 1941; Insall, 1967). It is not essential to remove all diseased tissue to the edge of relatively normal cartilage. There has been a tendency with mechanical tools to remove too much tissue including normal cartilage to make smoother edges. However, the least amount of tissue removed the better, so long as the bulk of the unstable tissue is removed. The 2.1 μm holmium:YAG laser makes this easier.

Materials and Methods

A total of 262 arthroscopic laser chondroplasties were performed between July 1991 and December 1992. There were 10 cases of ankle arthroscopy, 5 cases of elbow arthroscopy, and 21 cases of shoulder arthroscopy in which chondral lesions were noted. A total of 226 knee laser chondroplasties were performed: 43 of the knee cases (19%) were patients with nondegenerative disorders and 183 (81%) were patients with degenerative disorders. Most of the patients with degenerative disorders demonstrated some damage to the meniscus. The age distribution of this group is 18 to 74 years; most of the nondegenerative cases were in patients under age 25 years, and most of those with degenerative damage were over age 45. Males outnumbered females in a ratio of 2:1.

Follow-up ranged from 1 to 18 months. All patients were seen within 72 hours after surgery, some at 6 weeks, at 3 months, and at approximately 1 year or more postoperatively.

A pulse rate of 20 pulses per second and an energy per pulse of 1 joule were most commonly used. This is because high pulse rates and low energy per pulse yielded better results subjectively, especially with superficial "shaggy" lesions. The better results indicated that a lesser depth of thermal damage was advantageous.

The orientation of the delivery system was important. The probe was placed tangential or parallel to the surface when possible. When the portal placement did not permit, the probe was withdrawn to the point (usually 3–5 mm) that little tissue effect was noted. The purpose of both these techniques was to deliver the minimal amount of energy to the unstable cartilage to vaporize it, at the same time minimizing unwanted effects on stable articular cartilage. With less discoloration the results seemed better.

Laser chondroplasty for grade IV lesions (bone exposed) (Outerbridge, 1961) has not been very effective. Therefore, these lesions were dealt with by using abrasive chondroplasty, osteotomy, or replacement arthroplasty if conservative measures failed.

Patients with chondromalacia lesions of the patella underwent realignment procedures only as indicated by patellofemoral malalignment. If a patient had no lateral subluxation of the patella, patellofemoral realignment was not done even in the presence of a chondromalacia lesion, because results of chondroplasty of the patella without lateral release in those patients with patello-femoral congruence are better, in my opinion, than those with lateral release.

All patients who had chondral lesions of the knee and ankle were instructed about partial weight-bearing with crutches for a period of 6 weeks postoperatively. All patients were begun on immediate postoperative active range of motion. They were not allowed on exercise machinery until 6 weeks. No sports were allowed for 3 months in athletes, and no squatting or climbing was allowed for 6 weeks with any patient.

Results

In athletic patients, postoperative pain was not significantly reduced, but overall functional results seemed to be improved. Rehabilitation time was sometimes better compared to mechanical methods. There was often less swelling. In the degenerative group, the results were favorable. Most patients who had undergone laser chondroplasty had significant improvement postoperatively. Most patients had mild postoperative swelling. Pain reduction was obvious to virtually every patient. Most patients required very little pain medication after surgery. The range of motion was usually full 72 hours after surgery. No long-term loss of motion was encountered. Preoperative night pain subsided in the majority. Most patients who had a limp preoperatively improved significantly. Many either reduced the dose or stopped using antiinflammatory medication. The results in patients who had been offered knee reconstruction but opted to have laser chondroplasty were exceptionally good. Two patients who underwent mechanical chondroplasty prior to July 1991 subsequently underwent a laser chondroplasty for the opposite knee after July 1991. Both indicated the preferance of laser chondroplasty. Two patients underwent bilateral chondroplasty, one with mechanical means and the other with laser. Both patients indicated a preference to laser chondroplasty postoperatively. One of the two patients subsequently underwent a second arthroscopic chondroplasty with the laser in the knee that had undergone original mechanical chondroplasty. The results were satisfactory. Several patients indicated a threefold increase in their walking distance as required by their cardiologist for exercise programs. Many indicated a weight loss of 5 to 10 pounds and a general improvement in overall well-being.

Remarkably, there were no infections, no evidence of persistent effusion, no thrombophlebitis, and no evidence of severe pain. No cases of arthrotomy or repeat laser arthroscopy were required. There has been no expressed patient dissatisfaction with the procedure. There were two cases of laser probe failure. One 2 mm burn was produced when the laser was inappropriately applied to the undersurface of the skin during a lateral release. It healed without sequelae.

Conclusions

As with many surgical procedures, results are clinically observed often before a complete understanding of the scientific basis is present. This situation is definitely the case with laser-assisted chondroplasty but also remains true of mechanical chondroplasty. Further scientific investigation is needed.

The 2.1 μm holmium:YAG laser chondroplasty is effective in reducing pain associated with grade I, grade II, and some cases of grade III chondromalacia. It offers no advantage over mechanical techniques for grade IV chondromalacia, especially in malaligned knees. The short-term results are good. The future of arthroscopic laser chondroplasty with the 2.1 μm holmium:YAG laser is encouraging. If long-term results are found at least equal to mechanical means, the short-term benefits appear to justify continued use for chondroplasty.

References

Burns MW (1991) Laser surgery. Sci Am 264:85–90

Burns MW, Nelson J (1988) Laser application in biomedicine. I. Biophysics, cell biology, and biostimulation. J Laser Appl 1:34–39

Decklebaum LI, Isner JM, Donaldson RF, et al (1985) Reduction of laser induced pathologic tissue injury using pulse energy. Am J Cardiol 56:662–667

Ewing JW (1990) Arthroscopic treatment of degenerative meniscus lesions and early degenerative arthritis of the knee. In Articular Cartilage and Knee Joint Function: Basic Science and Arthroscopy. Raven Press, New York 137–145

Hobbs ER, Balin PL, Wheeland RG, et al (1987) Super pulsed lasers: minimizing thermal damage with short duration, higher irradiance pulses. J Dermatol Surg Oncol 13:955–964

Insall J (1967) Intraarticular surgery for degenerative osteoarthritis of the knee. J Bone Joint Surg [Br] 49:211

Johnson LL (1986) Arthroscopic abrasion arthroplasty: historical and pathologic perspective: present status. Arthroscopy 2:54–69

Magnuson PB (1941) Joint débridement and surgical treatment of degenerative arthritis. Surg Gynecol Obstet 73:1–9

Outerbridge RE (1961) The etiology of chondromalacia patella. J Bone Joint Surg [Br] 43:752–757

Sherk HH (1990) Lasers in Orthopaedics. Lippincott, Philadelphia

Sprague NF (1981) Arthroscopic treatment for degenerative knee joint disease. Clin Orthop 160:118–123

Trauner K (1990) Pulsed holmium:yttrium-aluminum-garnet (Ho:YAG): laser ablation of fibrocartilage in articular cartilage. Am J Sports M 18:316–320

Walsh JT, Flotte TJ, Anderson RR, et al (1988) Pulsed CO_2 laser tissue ablation: effect of tissue type and pulse duration on thermal damage. Lasers Surg Med 8:108–118

42

2.1 μm Holmium:YAG Arthroscopic Laser Surgery: Prospective Report of 100 Cases

Thomas M. Walker

This report describes a prospective study of 100 consecutive arthroscopies using the 2.1 μm holmium:YAG laser compared to a retrospective analysis of 100 conventional arthroscopies with the same procedural mix. Included in each group were 43 acute meniscectomies, 27 meniscectomies for chronic pain, 13 lateral releases, 4 plica resections, and 4 adhesion resections. Also included were 9 subacromial shoulder decompressions.

Materials and Methods

Beginning with our most recent conventional procedures, the same number of cases for each category were retrospectively reviewed and compared with the laser procedures with regard to: level of postoperative pain, degree of effusion, range of motion, and complications. Initial postoperative and long-term results were evaluated.

All knee surgeries were performed under either epidural blocks ($n = 86$) or general anesthesia ($n = 5$). Shoulder arthroscopies were performed under either general anesthesia ($n = 7$) or scalene blocks ($n = 2$). Thigh tourniquets were inflated in all conventional knee procedures. No tourniquet was inflated for any of the laser knee procedures. Arthroscopy was performed using standard three-portal techniques, with additional portals as needed. An attempt was made to use the laser exclusively where possible to evaluate the flexibility of this instrument and compare the duration of surgery. However, whenever it was clearly more efficient or time-saving, conventional instrumentation was utilized as an adjunct to the laser.

In all cases an arthroscopy pump with pressure levels of approximately 60 mm Hg was used. Ringer's lactate irrigation was used with 1 g of cefazolin or 1 cc of 1:100,000 epinephrine in alternating 2000 cc bags of irrigant. Postoperatively, the wounds were dressed with 4 × 4 inch gauze squares, a single gauze roll, and an overlying 6 inch Ace wrap bandage. Straight-leg-raising exercises and range of motion to allowable limits were initiated immediately in the recovery room. The patients were encouraged to ambulate to comfort with the use of crutches as necessary. Activities were minimized for the first 48 hours postoperatively.

Patients were seen for initial follow-up between the third and fifth postoperative days. They were then seen 1 week later and again at 4 weeks postoperatively. Subsequent visits were dictated either at 6 weeks or continued weekly as necessary until symptoms had been satisfactorily resolved.

In cases where multiple procedures were performed, only the primary diagnosis was used to compare the data. Pain levels were measured by the type of medication required postoperatively and the duration of their use.

"No pain" meant that the patient reported taking no pain medication postoperatively. "Mild pain" meant that over-the-counter analgesics were used. "Moderate pain" indicated the use of Darvocet, and "severe pain" indicated that the patient required codeine derivatives or analogs.

Effusion levels were recorded as "none" if no ballotment could be appreciated; "mild" if ballotment was present but the range of motion exceeded 110 degrees and caused no pain: "moderate" if the effusion was easily ballotable and flexion was limited to less than 90 degrees with discomfort. Effusions were judged "severe" if the patient showed tense, painful distention requiring aspiration.

Motion levels were initially measured 3 to 5 days postoperatively when the compression bandages were removed. Subsequent measurements were made at approximately 10 days, 3 weeks, and 6 weeks, or on a weekly basis as necessary if the motion had not returned fully prior to that time. Elapsed times from surgery until the

Table 42.1. Age and sex of patients undergoing arthroscopic laser surgery.

		Sex of patients (no.)					
		Conventional		Laser		Average age (years)	
Procedure	Series	Male	Female	Male	Female	Conventional	Laser
Meniscectomy, acute	43	33	10	28	15	34	36
Meniscectomy, chronic	27	12	15	18	9	49	52
Lateral release	13	3	10	4	9	18	24
Plicae	4	1	3	3	1	29	24
Adhesions	4	2	2	2	2	33	35
Subacromial decompression	9	4	5	6	3	41	43

patient reached a level of no or negligible pain, full range of motion, and no or trace effusion were recorded and compared. Complications were noted for each group and a determination made as to whether they were related directly or indirectly to any instrument failure.

All laser procedures were performed with a 2.1 μm holmium:YAG laser. The first 64 cases were performed with 15 watts maximum power. For the remaining 36 procedures, a 20 watt maximum power instrument was used.

The age and sex distributions for each of the patient categories were found to be similar in each instance (Table 42-1).

Results

Initially, it was thought that use of the laser compared to conventional arthroscopy until a learning curve of approximately 50 cases had been accomplished. Subsequent surgery times were considerably shorter and improved over standard techniques for many procedures using the laser with conventional instrumentation.

Acute Meniscal Tears

Patients with meniscal lesions who reported a history of symptoms for less than 6 months or a definitive injury or insult were classified as having acute meniscal tears. There were 43 cases in this category. Repairable lesions were excluded. There were 10 bucket-handle tears, 6 radial tears, 7 parrot-beak tears, 8 horizontal tears, and 12 complex tears.

Pain after acute meniscectomy was reported to be marked in 30 cases of conventional arthroscopies and in 3 laser-treated patients. Pain levels were reported moderate following 7 conventional and 1 laser procedure. Mild pain was reported in 6 conventionally treated patients and 31 laser-treated patients. None of the conventionally treated group was pain-free, whereas nine patients treated with the laser reported no pain requiring medication. The average time from surgery to no or negligible pain was 5 days for the laser-treated group and 12 days for the conventionally treated group.

Marked effusions were recorded in one laser-treated and two conventionally treated patients. Moderate effusions were seen following 2 laser and 11 conventional arthroscopies; 34 laser-treated and 29 conventionally treated patients had mild effusions; and 6 laser patients and 1 conventional patient had no measurable effusions. Laser-treated patients required an average of 9 days until resolution of the effusion compared with 19 days for the control group.

Initial postoperative range of motion for the laser-treated group was 126 degrees compared to 110 degrees for conventional treatment. The laser group averaged 12 days to achieve full range of motion and the conventional group 23 days.

Chronic Meniscal Tears

There were 27 lesions classified as chronic meniscal tears: The patients had described symptoms of more than 12 months' duration and could not recall any single known insult.

Only two laser-treated patients reported marked pain postoperatively in the chronic meniscectomy group, compared to 23 conventionally treated patients. Moderate pain was present in only one of the laser group and in four of the conventional group. Seventeen patients treated with the laser reported mild pain and seven of the laser group said they had no pain. None of the conventionally treated patients reported no or mild pain.

Marked effusions were noted in two patients following conventional procedures and in one after laser treatment. Moderate effusions were seen in 12 of the conventional group and in three of the laser-treated patients. Mild effusions were present in 13 with conventional treatment and 20 with laser procedures. Three laser patients showed no effusions, whereas no conventional patient was effusion-free. It took an average of 11 days for resolution of the effusion in the laser group and 26 days in the conventional group.

The initial range of motion following laser treatment with chronic meniscectomy was 117 degrees compared to 87 degrees for patients treated with conventional arthroscopy. The average time to regain full motion postoperatively following arthroscopy for chronic meniscus tear was 21 days for the laser group and 28 days for the conventional group.

Lateral Release

Of the 13 lateral release procedures performed with the laser, 2 patients reported no pain, 10 said they had mild pain, and 1 had moderate pain. None of the patients reported marked pain. In the conventional lateral release group, 1 patient had mild pain, 2 had moderate pain, and 10 had marked pain. Laser release patients reported negligible or no pain on average of 7 days postoperatively compared to 26 days for the conventionally treated group.

In the lateral release laser group, 1 patient showed no effusion, mild effusions were seen in 10 patients, and moderate effusions in 2. No patient in which the release was performed with the laser developed a marked effusion. Conventionally performed lateral release resulted in 10 moderate and 3 marked effusions. No patient had a level of mild or no effusion postoperatively. It took an average of 11 days to resolve the effusion in the laser lateral release group compared to 30 days for the conventional release group.

Initial postoperative range of motion following lateral release with the laser was 128 degrees compared to 81 degrees after conventional release. It took an average of 11 days to regain full motion after the laser procedure and 30 days following conventional release.

Plicae

Only four cases of isolated plica resection were encountered in this series. After laser ablation of plicae, three patients reported no pain and one reported mild pain. After conventional plica resection, two patients reported marked pain: one moderate and one mild pain. It took an average of 6 days for the laser group to be pain-free compared to 22 days for the conventionally treated group.

There were three patients with mild effusion and one with no effusion following the laser plica ablation. Conventional excision resulted in two mild, one moderate, and two marked effusions. An average of 6 days was required to resolve the effusions following laser ablation of the plicae compared with 21 days for the conventional technique.

The average postoperative motion following laser plica excision was 102 degrees compared with 90 degrees using conventional instruments. It took an average of 9 days to regain full motion following the laser techniques and 18 days with conventional resection.

Adhesions

Four cases of isolated adhesion removal were treated in this series. Using the laser for adhesion ablation, three patients reported mild postoperative pain, and one claimed no pain. After conventional excision, two patients reported marked pain, and two patients reported moderate pain. Laser-treated patients averaged 10 days to pain-free status, whereas the conventionally treated group took an average of 17 days until pain was deemed negligible.

One patient after laser ablation of adhesions showed no effusion, two patients had mild effusions, and one patient had a moderate effusion. After conventional excision, three patients had moderate effusions and one had marked effusion. The effusions noted after adhesion resection lasted an average of 12 days after the laser technique compared to 26 days after conventional excision.

The initial postoperative motion was 110 degrees in the laser-treated group and 90 degrees in the conventionally treated group. It took an average of 15 days for the laser group to reach a full range of motion compared to 26 for the conventionally treated patients.

Subacromial Decompression

In this series, nine patients were treated with subacromial decompression. The laser was used to effect hemostasis and assist in ablation of the bursa and to release and partially resect the coracoacromial ligament. The soft tissues of the undersurface of the acromion were also ablated, exposing the bone for burring, which was carried out in standard fashion.

Pain levels following the laser-assisted decompression technique were reported as mild in four cases, moderate in four cases, and marked in one case. Two patients reported mild levels of pain following conventional decompression, six had moderate pain, and one marked. The average time to pain-free status was 16 days using the laser and 18 days using the conventional technique.

The motion measured after arthroscopy of the shoulder involved abduction only. Initial postoperative abduction following subacromial decompression averaged 85 degrees for both the laser and the conventional treatment groups. Time required to regain full abduction was 24 days using the laser and 25 days using the conventional technique.

Complications

There were two instances of fiber tip breakage using the laser that resulted in release of free fiber fragments into the joint. In each case, a motorized shaver was used to remove these fragments. There was no complication observed as a result of either of these incidents, and in each case the healing process was uneventful. One case was an acute meniscus tear and the other a chronic meniscus tear. No other complications were directly or indirectly attributable to use of the laser.

There were two cases of deep vein thrombosis in the conventional group. Each was treated with heparin, and no sequelae have been noted.

Two cases of fibrosis, each after lateral release, occurred after conventional procedures. Each was treated with repeat arthroscopy and débridement after physical therapy and other conservative measures had failed.

Six cases of back pain were noted. All occurred in patients who had undergone epidural blocks and were thought to be unrelated to the arthroscopic technique.

One patient in the laser group required repeat arthroscopy. She had had a chronic discoid meniscus tear and had sustained a repeat injury 16 weeks after her first surgery. At the second arthroscopy, a new peripheral tear was identified and repaired. The patient had a good recovery after the second procedure. Although it is thought that the second tear was not a result of the laser treatment with the first surgery, hers was the only reoperation required and so is included for that purpose.

No case of deep vein thrombosis, fibrosis, or back pain was experienced in any category of the laser group.

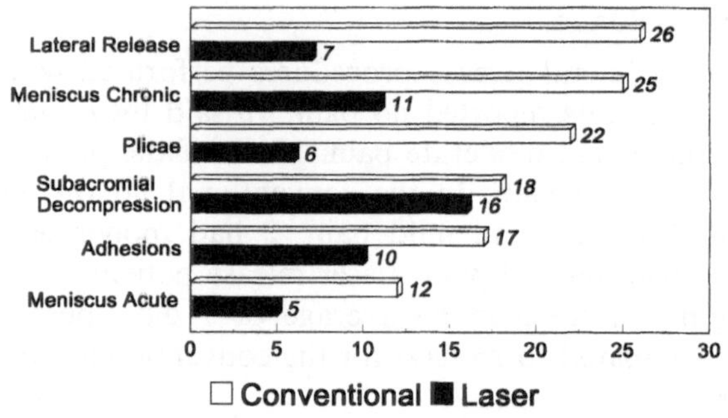

Figure 42-1. Postoperative days to negligible pain, conventional (open bars) versus laser (filled bars) surgery.

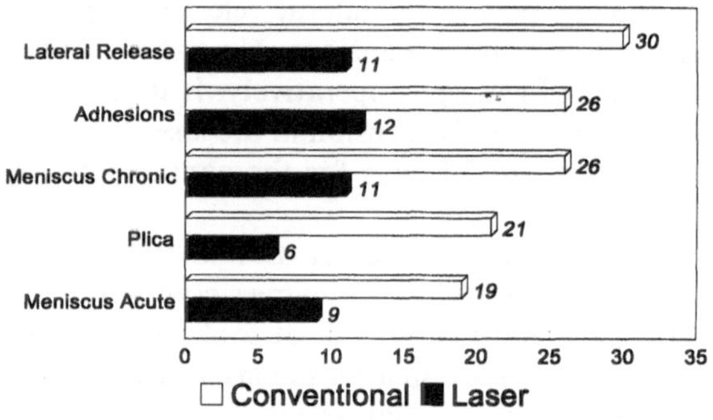

Figure 42-2. Days to trace effusion, conventional (open bars) versus laser (filled bars) surgery.

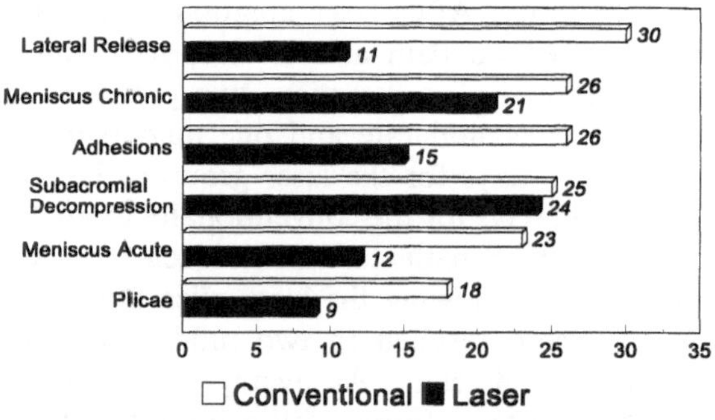

Figure 42-3. Days to free range of motion, conventional (open bars) versus laser (filled bars) surgery.

Summary and Discussion

This report presents the findings of 100 consecutive cases utilizing the 2.1 μm holmium:YAG laser for arthroscopy. The study deals mainly with the initial postoperative findings, although the series now has an 18 month average follow-up since surgery. In none of the cases has further surgery been required. No late complications attributable to the laser have been observed.

Reviewing the data, it is apparent that for each of the parameters studied—postoperative pain (Fig. 42-1), effusions (Fig. 42-2), and range of motion (Fig. 42-3)—the patients treated with the laser showed at least equal or better overall results than those treated conventionally.

The most notable differences between laser and conventional technique were seen in patients who underwent lateral release. In this group, each of the parameters evaluated suggested significant benefit using the laser for lateral release instead of conventional techniques. It is of particular note that no patient showed a marked effusion, and only two patients had a moderate effusion. Also, no patient had marked pain, and only one patient had moderate pain. The fact that none of these patients has required further surgery for this condition (average 18 months follow-up) suggests that the technique is as effective as conventional, mechanical lateral release. It was also noted that these patients generally had a much lower level of disability throughout their recuperation. They required crutches for only a few days in most cases, and initiation of therapy was not only earlier but progressed much faster than those using the conventional release technique.

No comparisons were made in this study between the laser and electrocautery for lateral release, but these comparisons are currently in progress.

After meniscectomy, there appeared to be benefits with respect to postoperative pain as well as to the level of effusion, but they were not as dramatic as those noted for the lateral release group of patients. It was our general impression that the type of tear encountered affected the observed degree of effusion and pain. Acute bucket-handle meniscal tears seemed to recover quickly, but complex meniscal tears showed a slower response rate.

Clinical observations suggested that the use of the laser in posterior horn tears, especially those complex types that are difficult to access, were much more easily treated with the laser. Iatrogenic scuffing of the articular surface was markedly reduced because of the small size of the laser instrumentation. It is also possible that the small size of the laser handpiece negates the need for excessive stress on the joint, which may be a source of postoperative pain and inflammation. Indeed, the question arises as to why resection of fragments of a nonvascular structure, such as an easily accessible bucket-handle tear, would be different in the conventionally treated versus the laser-treated group. Again it is possible that elimination of the need for a tourniquet and the reduction in the amount of stress applied to the knee to allow visualization and access may play a role.

Cases involving excisions of plicae or adhesions demonstrated a general trend similar to that of other categories in this series. However, insufficient numbers make any conclusions speculative. Further follow-up on a larger series of these categories is required. Similarly, it is thought that the number of subacromial decompressions was too small to draw any specific conclusions. However, it did not appear that the use of the laser caused any statistically significant improvement with regard to levels of pain or postoperative motion. It should be noted that the use of the laser did seem to allow better visualization of the structures within the subacromial space than when using the conventional technique.

The only complication attributable to the laser per se was fiber breakage in the two cases noted above. It did not seem to cause any clinical sequelae during the healing process. This problem is of concern, however, as it is thought that it could potentially be a source of joint irritation and inflammation and possibly require repeat arthroscopy or arthrotomy if not noted at the time of occurrence. It was thought that the tip breakage resulted, at least in one of the instances, when the laser abutted the bony surface and created a backfire effect, perhaps creating enough energy to burst the fiber tip. The second instance of breakage appeared to be related to pure fiber failure, as no difficulty was encountered when placing the handpiece into the joint, and failure occurred in an unencumbered portion of the joint cavity.

The question as to whether eliminating the need for a tourniquet would improve or eliminate the incidence of deep vein thrombosis was highlighted in two cases of conventional arthroscopy during this study. In each of these cases in which a tourniquet had been used, the patient complained of no thigh symptoms during the initial postoperative period, and no prophylaxis was used.

It is thought that the two instances of fibrosis in the conventionally treated group that required repeat arthroscopy were at least in part due to the hemiarthrosis with accompanying pain and limitation of motion, which led to a delay in mobilization and a prolonged recovery time in each case. The laser eliminates much of the bleeding encountered with conventional techniques and may therefore offer an alternative procedure that reduces or eliminates the incidence of fibrosis, thereby expediting recovery and avoiding the possible need for further surgical treatment.

The instances of back pain, which occurred in six patients after conventional treatment and four patients following laser treatment, seemed unrelated to the type of procedure performed. Rather, they seemed to be due to the epidural block technique.

Conclusions

Based on the results of this study, it appears that the 2.1 μm holmium:YAG laser is an effective device that in and of itself can be used without fear of significant instrument-induced complications. It is further concluded that the use of this instrument can be as effective or more effective than conventional instrumentation in the treatment of several lesions encountered in knee arthroscopy. The benefits noted after laser-assisted lateral release were so impressive that we believe laser release is the procedure of choice for a lateral release at this time.

It is also our belief that the use of the laser for certain types of meniscal lesions can be beneficial in terms of technical efficiency and for patient comfort and rehabilitation. This conclusion applies most to posterior horn tears, which are difficult to access behind the condyle or reflected into the posterior aspects of the intercondylar notch. Such lesions can be approached and ablated with minimal stress or iatrogenic damage to the knee.

The results of our limited number of procedures performed on plicae and adhesions are encouraging, but we do not believe the numbers are adequate to draw any specific conclusions at this time. Although it is clear that the laser was helpful for allowing good visualization during subacromial decompressions in the limited number of cases we compared, the initial long-term results did not seem to differ significantly from those obtained with the conventional technique.

It is our conclusion from this study that the 2.1 μm holmium:YAG laser appears to offer an effective alternative or adjunct to conventional instrumentation for the treatment of a variety of joint lesions.

Suggested Reading

Dillingham MF, Price JM, Fanton GS (1993) Holmium laser surgery. Orthopaedics 16:563–566

Trauner K, Nishioka N, Patel D (1990) Pulsed Ho:YAG laser ablation of fibrocartilage and articular cartilage. Am J Sports Med 3:316–320

43

Use of the 2.1 μm Holmium:YAG Laser in Arthroscopic Temporomandibular Joint Surgery

James H. Quinn

The minimally invasive procedure of temporomandibular joint (TMJ) arthroscopic surgery was first performed by McCain in the United States in 1985 (McCain, 1985) This technique has met with documented success. The largest retrospective study was a 6-year, multicenter evaluation of 4,681 joints reported in 1992 with an average of 91% success rate in range of motion, reduction of pain, ability to masticate a normal diet, and disability reduction (McCain et al., 1992). Identification in the TMJ of chondromalacia (Quinn, 1989) identical with that which occurs in the knee and significant concentrations of pain mediators prosthoglandin E_2 and leukotriene B_4 (Quinn and Bazan, 1990), found in other inflamed synovial joints, emphasizes the biologic and pathologic analogies of the TMJ with the other joints of the body. TMJ arthroscopic surgical procedures employed are those that have been successfully performed by orthopaedic surgeons for the past 15 to 20 years. These procedures consist of the surgical anterior release of anterior displaced articular discs with posterior cauterization of the retrodiscal tissues to maintain the disc in the reduced position, motorized shaving of the fibrillated fibrocartilage of chondromalacia grade III, synovectomy, removal of osteophytes, and débridement of arthrofibrotic joints with motorized shavers.

Although the results of these surgical procedures performed with mechanical instrumentation were successful there was still a need for a nonmechanical energy source which could be delivered by a small delivery probe resulting in less iatrogenic traumatic damage within the joint. Approximately 3 years ago, the 2.1 μm holmium:YAG laser was first utilized in the TMJ by Koslin (Koslin and Martin, 1993) with considerable success. Indications for arthroscopic TMJ laser surgery are: (1) disabling TMJ pain, unrelieved by appropriate nonsurgical therapy; (2) anterior disc dislocations without reduction in the open position; (3) hypomobility (less than 35 mm interincisal range of motion); (4) hypermobility; (5) fibroankylosis/arthrofibrosis; and (6) degenerative TMJ disease.

Surgical Techniques

The technique of TMJ arthroscopic surgery utilized (McCain et al., 1991), employs a double portal with a cannula in the posterior recess and one anterior recess of the superior joint space. A 2.1 μm holmium:YAG laser has been utilized in all of the surgical procedures by me. A small joint surgical probe was designed for the 2.1 μm holmium:YAG laser unit for use in the TMJ as well as other small joints and was employed in the surgical procedures performed.

Anterior TMJ Disc Dislocations

The technique uses the small joint probe to work through the operating cannula in the anterior recess. The laser settings used are 10 pulses per second and 1.5 Joules (15 watts). The incision is begun at the most anterior medial aspect of the dislocated disc continuing anteriorly along the disc margin as far laterally as possible (Fig. 43-1). The incision is deepened until the longitudinal fibers of the superior head of the lateral pterygoid muscle is observed, indicating that the disc has been released (Fig. 43-2). With an obturator in the operating anterior recess cannula the disc is pushed posteriorly and superiorly as far as possible, moving the disc over the condyle. Moving the anterior cannula and obturator into the posterior recess, posterior and inferior pressure is placed on the retrodiscal tissues, further reducing the disc into functional position. With reduced laser energy, 9.0 pulses per second and 0.5 Joules (4.5 watts), laser energy is directed into the retro-

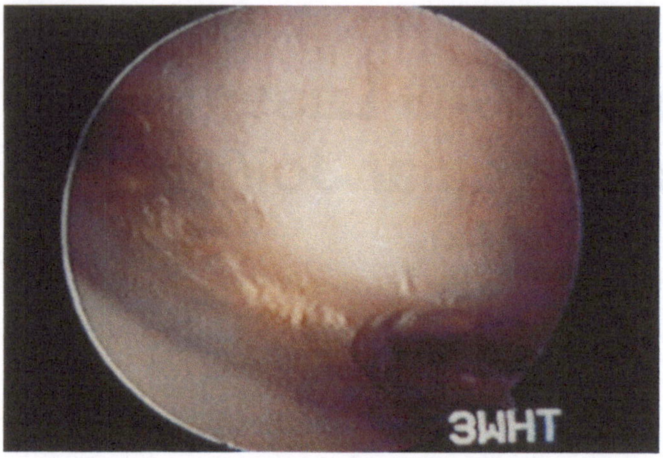

Figure 43-1. Use of the 2.1 μm holmium:YAG laser joint probe to release the anteriorly dislocated TMJ disc. Incision begins medially continuing along the anterior disc margin as far laterally as possible (right TMJ).

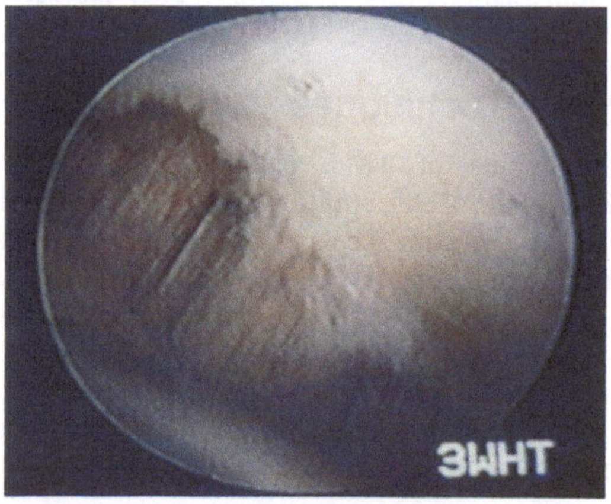

Figure 43-2. This reveals the longitudinal fibers of the superior head of the lateral pterygoid muscle, indicating that the disc has been released from its attachment (right TMJ).

discal tissue which produces fusion of the deeper connective tissue to help immobilize the disc (Fig. 43-3).

TMJ Disc Perforations

The 2.1 μm holmium:YAG laser is used to vaporize fibrillated cartilage around the periphery of the disc perforation using 10 pulses per second and 1 Joule (10 watts) followed by sculpting to round the margins of the disc, thus reducing the friction created by movement of the disc against the articular surfaces. Any attached adhesions are also vaporized to assure adequate discal mobility.

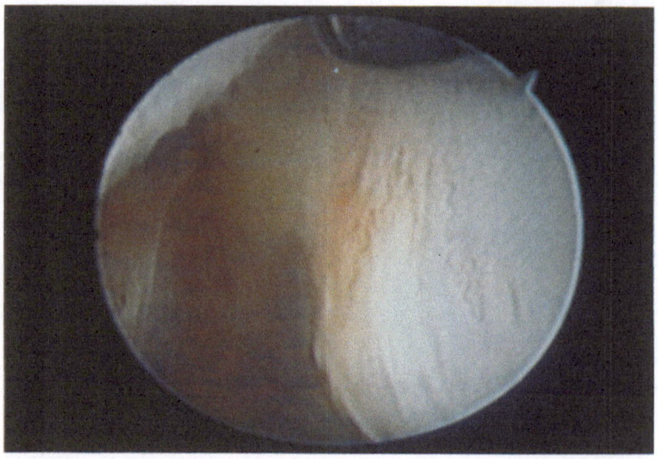

Figure 43-3. The 2.1 μm holmium:YAG laser probe has created a trough in the retrodiscal tissue with reduced energy levels to produce fusion of the deeper connective tissues tightening this area to aid in immobilizing the reduced disc (right TMJ).

Grade III Chondromalacia with Fibrillation of the Articular Fibrocartilage

The 2.1 μm holmium:YAG laser is used to vaporize the fibrillating cartilage instead of using a motorized shaver using 10 pulses per second and 1 Joule (10 watts). The advantage of the 2.1 μm holmium:YAG laser in this procedure is that the operating probe handpiece is very small and the limited joint space is easily accessed, leading to less scuffing than occurs with the use of a motorized shaver. The laser does not pull on the fibrillated cartilage as does the motorized shaver, which can result in undesirable removal of normal tissue.

Fibroankylosis/Arthrofibrosis

This is an excellent use for the 2.1 μm holmium:YAG laser over the motorized shaver in that it vaporizes and completely removes the fibrous tissue instead of leaving shreds of fibrous tissue attached to the articular surfaces (Fig. 43-4). Complete joint débridement can be accomplished more rapidly with less instrumentation. Vaporization of arthrofibrosis utilizes 10 pulses per second and 1.5 Joules (15 watts).

Ablation of Osteophytes

The 2.1 μm holmium:YAG laser can be used to completely ablate bony osteophytes which are frequently found on the condyle or articular eminence or both in association with advanced degenerative TMJ disease with disc perforation (Fig. 43-5). The recommended setting would be 10 pulses per second and 1.5 Joules (15 watts). This removes the osteophytes but leaves a somewhat

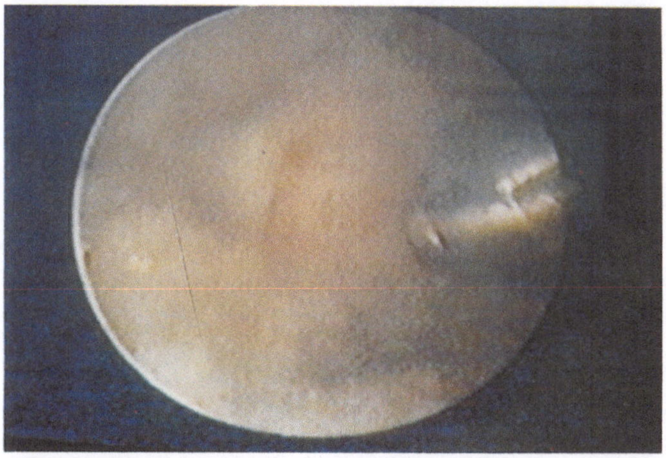

Figure 43-4. Vaporization of arthrofibrosis in the posterior aspect of the TMJ with the 2.1 μm holmium:YAG laser probe in place (right TMJ).

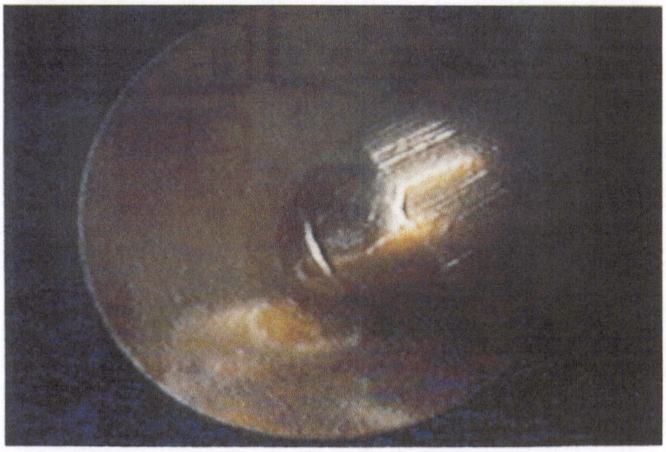

Figure 43-5. Ablation of a condylar osteophyte with the 2.1 μm holmium:YAG laser probe (right TMJ).

roughened base. It is necessary to use an abrader bur to smooth the remaining bony base.

Summary

The advantages of the 2.1 μm holmium:YAG laser over mechanical surgical instruments are: (1) fewer instruments are required; (2) less scuffing of tissue; (3) work can be done in smaller areas; and (4) surgery can be performed rapidly with precision and minimal tissue damage. Reports in the oral and maxillofacial literature support the success of the use of the 2.1 μm holmium:YAG laser in TMJ surgery (Koslin and Martin, 1993; Hendler et al., 1992). My 2.1 μm holmium:YAG laser TMJ arthroscopic surgical preliminary results on 69 joints beginning 2.5 years ago are most gratifying. Findings have been consistent with those described by Fanton and Dillingham (1992) of a substantial reduction in inflammation and pain with earlier rehabilitation than with conventional arthroscopy. Although the use of the 2.1 μm holmium:YAG laser in TMJ surgery is relatively new, the preliminary results have been most gratifying.

References

Fanton GS, Dillingham MF (1992) The use of the holmium laser in arthroscopic surgery. Semin Orthop 7:102–116

Hendler B, Gateno J, et al. (1992) Holmium:YAG laser arthroscopy of the temporomandibular joint. J Oral Maxillofac Surg

Koslin MG, Martin JC (1993) The use of the holmium laser for temporomandibular joint arthroscopic surgery. J Oral Maxillofac Surg 51:122–123

McCain JP (1985) Arthroscopy of the human temporomandibular joint. Proceedings, Annual Meeting, American Association of Oral and Maxillofacial Surgeons, Oct. 4–7, Washington, D.C.

McCain JP, de la Rua H, LeBlanc WG (1991) Puncture technique and portals of entry for diagnostic and operative arthroscopy of the temporomandibular joint. Arthroscopy 7:221

McCain JP, Sanders B, Koslin MG, et al (1992) Temporomandibular joint arthroscopy: A 6-year multicenter retrospective study of 4,831 joints. J Oral Maxillofac Surg 50:926–930

Quinn JH (1989) Pathogenesis of temporomandibular joint chondromalacia and arthralgia. Oral Maxillofac Clin North Am 1:

Quinn JH, Bazan NG (1990) Identification of prosthoglandin E_2 and leukotriene B_4 in the synovial fluid of painful, dysfunctional temporomandibular joints. J Oral Maxillofac Surg 48:968–971

44

Future of Arthroscopic Laser Surgery

Allen T. Brillhart

The most significant events in the future of arthroscopic laser surgery will involve publication of results of blinded prospective clinical studies. Information gathering and education are more important than improvements in technology at this point. There is so much new information to be learned, applied, and analyzed that the artroscopist must grasp the current state of technology before looking too far into the future.

The wait-and-see concept no longer applies to today's technology. Many systems are now workable and beneficial. The immediate future will involve use of state of the art systems by more surgeons. Fine-tuning of present applications will definitely occur, and it will be as much for cost reduction as for ease of use. Systems will emerge that will entice arthroscopists, but they are not likely to cause the present systems to be immediately abandoned.

Nevertheless, advancements in technology will lead to the production of more powerful and versatile systems, and more durable fiberoptic delivery systems will accompany these changes. Tissue-specific applications will be better understood and utilized. Long-term effects and patient outcomes will ultimately define the permanent role for arthroscopic laser surgery.

Appendix A: Related Nobel Prizes in Physics

1918 **Max Planck** for discovering energy quanta (1900).
1921 **Albert Einstein** for explaining the photoelectric effect and for his services to theoretical physics (1905).
1922 **Niels Bohr** for his model of the atom and its radiation (1913).
1964 **Charles H. Townes, Nikolai G. Basov**, and **Alexandr M. Prokhorov** for developing masers (1951–1952) and lasers.
1981 **Nicolaas Bloembergen** and **Arthur L. Schawlow** for developing laser spectroscopy and **Kai M. Siegbahn** for developing high-resolution electron spectroscopy (1958).

Appendix B: Greek Alphabet

Alpha	A	α	Nu	N	ν
Beta	B	β	Xi	Ξ	ξ
Gamma	Γ	γ	Omicron	O	o
Delta	Δ	δ	Pi	Π	π
Epsilon	E	ε	Rho	P	ρ
Zeta	Z	ζ	Sigma	Σ	σ
Eta	H	η	Tau	T	τ
Theta	Θ	θ	Upsilon	Y	υ
Iota	I	ι	Phi	Φ	ϕ
Kappa	K	κ	Chi	X	χ
Lambda	Λ	λ	Psi	Ψ	ψ
Mu	M	μ	Omega	Ω	ω

Appendix C: Laser Safety Reference Sources

Laser Institute of America [publishes ANSI standards]
12424 Research Parkway, Suite 130
Orlando, FL 32826
(407)380-1553

American National Standards Institute (ANSI)
1430 Broadway
New York, NY 10018
(212)354-3300

Association of Operating Room Nurses (AORN)
10170 E. Mississippi Avenue
Denver, CO 80231
(303)755-6300

American Society for Laser Medicine and Surgery (ASLMS)
2404 Stewart Square
Wausau, WI 54401
(715)845-9283

Center for Devices and Radiological Health (CDRH)
Food and Drug Administration
5600 Fishers Lane
Rockville, MD 20857
(301)443-3403

Occupational Safety and Health Administration (OSHA)
Bureau of National Affairs
1231 25th Street NW
Washington, DC 20037
(202)452-4200

Appendix D: Arthroscopic Laser Wavelengths Discussed in This Book

Laser	Spectrum	Wavelength (μm)
Carbon dioxide (CO_2)	Far-infrared	10.6
Holmium:YAG (Ho:YAG)	Mid-infrared	2.1
Erbium: YAG (Er:YAG) (Developmental)	Mid-infrared	2.94
Neodymium:YAG (Nd:YAG); contact mode recommended	Near-infrared	1.06
Neodymium:YAG (Nd:YAG); investigational	Near-infrared	1.32
Neodymium: YAG (Nd:YAG)	Near-infrared	1.44
Helium-neon (HeNe); aiming beam	Red	0.632
KTP: investigational—potassium titanyl phosphate (a frequency-doubled 1.06 μm neodymium:YAG)	Green	0.532
Excimer: investigational in the United States but not in Europe; XeCl	Ultraviolet	0.308

Appendix E: Contributing Arthroscopic Laser System Manufacturers

Coherent
3270 West Bayshore Road
P.O. Box 10122
Palo Alto, CA 94303-0810
(800)227-1914

Eclipse Surgical Technologies, Inc.
P.O. Box 50875
Palo Alto, CA 94303
(800)238-2205

Laser Photonics, Inc.
12351 Research Parkway
Orlando, FL 32826
(800)624-3628

Luxar Corporation
19204 N. Creek Parkway, Suite 100
Bothell, WA 98011
(800)548-1482

Premier Laser Systems
3 Morgan
Irvine, CA 92718
(800)544-8044

Sharplan Lasers, Inc.
1 Pearl Court
Allendale, NJ 07401
(800)394-2000

Sunrise Technologies, Inc.
47257 Fremont Boulevard
Fremont, CA 94538
(510)623-9001

Surgical Laser Technologies
200 Cresson Boulevard
P.O. Box 880
Oaks, PA 19456-0880
(800)366-4758

Surgilase, Inc. (Laser Photonics Distributor)
I-95 Corporate Park
33 Plan Way
Warwick, RI 02886
(800)537-5273

Trimedyne, Inc.
2801 Barranca Road
Irvine, CA 92714
(800)733-5273

Carl Zeiss, Inc.
1 Zeiss Drive
Thornwood, NY 10594
(800)642-7675

Appendix F: Representative Laser Safety Products Manufacturers

American Allsafe, 99 Wales Avenue, Tonawanda, NY 14150; (716)695-8300

American Optical Company, Safety Products Group, 14 Mechanics Street, Southbridge, MA 01550; (508)765-9711

Arbor Technologies, Inc., 3728 Plaza Drive, Ann Arbor, MI 48108; (313)665-3516

Aura Lens Products, Inc., P.O. Box 763, St. Cloud, MN 56302

Baxter Healthcare Corp., Technology and Ventures Division, 2132 Michelson Drive, Irvine, CA 92715; (714)474-6400

Bolle, rue Tacon, B.P. 139, F-01104 Oyannex, France

Class, Inc., 840 Avenue F (#104), Plano, TX 75074; (214)423-7099

Ealing Electro-Optics, Inc., New Englander Industrial Park, Holliston, MA 01746; (508)429-8370

Edmund Scientific, Edmund Building, Barrington, NJ 08007; (609)547-3488

Energy Technology, Inc., P. O. Box 1038, San Luis Obispo, CA 93406; (805)544-7770

Engineering Technology, Inc., P.O. Box 8859, Waco, TX 76714-8859; (817)772-0082

Fish-Schurman Corp., P.O. Box 319, New Rochelle, NY 10802; (914)636-1300

General Scientific Equipment Co., 525 Spring Garden, Philadelphia, PA 19123; (215)922-5710

Glendale Protective Technologies, 130 Crossways Park Drive, Woodbury, NY 11797; (516)921-5800

Lab Safety Supply, P.O. Box 13689, Janesville, WI 53547-1368; (800)356-0783

Lase, Inc., 7209 East Kemper Road, Cincinnati, OH 45249; (800)543-4288

Laser Institute of America, 12424 Research Parkway (#130), Orlando, FL 32826; (407)380-1553

Laser-R Shield Inc., P.O. Box 91957, Albuquerque, NM 87199; (800)288-1164

Laser Safety Associates, 1435 Acadia Street, Durham, NC 27701; (919)684-2032

Laser Sense, P.O. Box 163, Yorktown Heights, NY 10598; (914)245-6708

LaserVision GmbH [in USA: UVEX Winter Optical], Berliner Strasse, D-8550 Forchheim, Germany

Hubert LeBodo, Laboratoire d'Energetique Laser et de Thermophysique, Guidel-Plages, 56520 Guidel, France

Litechnica International, Inc., 4801 Massachusettes Avenue NW (#400), Washington, DC 20016; (202)895-1563

Merocel Corp., 950 Flanders Road, Mystic, CT 06355; (203)572-9586

MIRA, Inc., 87 Rumford Avenue, Waltham, MA 02154; (800)847-6472

Omicron Eye Safety Corp., 73 Main Street, Brattleboro, VT 05301; (802)257-7363

Phase-R Co., Box G-2, New Durham, NH 03855; (603)859-3800

Fred Reed Optical, P.O. Box 27010, Albuquerque, NM 87125-7010; (505)265-3531

Rockwell Associates, Inc., P.O. Box 43010, Cnicinnati, OH 45243; (513)271-1568

Rodenstock USA, Inc., 246 Main Street, East Greenwich, RI 02818; (800)225-8141

Seton Name Plate Corp., PO Drawer DC-1331, New Haven, CT 06505; (513)271-1568

Simpson-Bayse, 430 Ayre Street, Wilmington, DE 19804; (302)995-7191

David H. Sliney, Consulting Physicist, 406 Streamside Drive, Fallston, MD 21047; (301)877-1646

Spectra-Optics, 12317 Gladstone Avenue, Sylmar, CA 91342; (213)361-0949

Stackhouse Associates, Inc., 150 Sierra Street, El Segundo, CA 90245; (213)322-6676

Sun Medical, 1179 Corporate Drive West (#100), Arlington, TX 76006; (817)633-1373

Sunstone, Inc., 2235 Route 130, Dayton. NJ 08810; (201)329-0140

Surgimedics/SLP, 2828 North Crescent Ridge Drive, The Woodlands, TX 77381; (713)363-4949

TTI Medical, 7026 Koll Center Parkway (#207), Pleasanton, CA 94566; (800)322-7373

U.S. Laser Corp., PO Box 609, 825 Windham Court North, Wyckoff, NJ 07481; (201)848-9200

U.V. Products, Inc., PO Box 1501, San Gabriel, CA 91778; (213)285-3123

UVEX Winter Optical, Inc., 10 Thurber Boulevard, Smithfield, RI 02917; (401)232-1200

Ximed Medical Systems, 2855 Kifer Road (#200), Santa Clara, CA 95050; (408)727-9483

Yamamoto Kogaku Co., Safety and Healthcare Division, 1-2 Chodo-3, Higashiosaka City, Osaka 577, Japan

Appendix G: Recommended Laser Texts

Absten GT, Joffe SN (1989) Lasers In Medicine, An Introductory Guide (2nd ed). Chapman & Hall, London

Ball KA (1990) Lasers, The Perioperative Challenge. Mosby, St. Louis

Sherk HH (1990) Lasers in Orthopaedics. Lippincott, Philadelphia

Siebert WE, Wirth CJ (1991) Laser in der Orthopädie. Thieme, Stuttgart

Sliney DH, Trokell SL (1993) Medical Lasers and Their Safe Use. Springer-Verlag, New York

Appendix H: Prefixes for Powers of Ten

Power	Prefix	Abbreviation
10^{-18}	atto	a
10^{-15}	femto	f
10^{-12}	pico	p
10^{-9}	nano	n
10^{-6}	micro	μ
10^{-3}	milli	m
10^{-2}	centi	c
10^{-1}	deci	d
10^{3}	kilo	k
10^{6}	mega	M
10^{9}	giga	G
10^{12}	tera	T
10^{15}	peta	P
10^{18}	exa	E

Appendix I

Periodic Table of the Elements

Symbol Atomic mass†	Ca 20 40.08 $4s^2$	Atomic number Electron configuration

Group I	Group II	Transition elements										Group III	Group IV	Group V	Group VI	Group VII	Group 0
H 1 1.0080 $1s^1$																H 1 1.0080 $2s^4$	He 2 4.0026 $1s^2$
Li 3 6.94 $2s^1$	Be 4 9.012 $2s^2$											B 5 10.81 $2p^1$	C 6 12.011 $2p^2$	N 7 14.007 $2p^3$	O 8 15.999 $2p^4$	F 9 18.998 $2p^5$	Ne 10 20.18 $2p^6$
Na 11 22.99 $3s^1$	Mg 12 24.31 $3s^2$											Al 13 26.98 $3p^1$	Si 14 28.09 $3p^2$	P 15 30.97 $3p^3$	S 16 32.06 $3p^4$	Cl 17 35.453 $3p^5$	Ar 18 39.948 $3p^6$
K 19 39.102 $4s^1$	Ca 20 40.08 $4s^2$	Sc 21 44.96 $3d^14s^2$	Ti 22 47.90 $3d^24s^2$	V 23 50.94 $3d^34s^2$	Cr 24 51.996 $3d^54s^1$	Mn 25 54.94 $3d^54s^2$	Fe 26 55.85 $3d^64s^2$	Co 27 58.93 $3d^74s^2$	Ni 28 58.71 $3d^84s^2$	Cu 29 63.54 $3d^{10}4s^1$	Zn 30 65.37 $3d^{10}4s^2$	Ga 31 69.72 $4p^1$	Ge 32 72.59 $4p^2$	As 33 74.92 $4p^3$	Se 34 78.96 $4p^4$	Br 35 79.91 $4p^5$	Kr 36 83.80 $4p^6$
Rb 37 85.47 $5s^1$	Sr 38 87.62 $5s^2$	Y 39 88.906 $4d^15s^2$	Zr 40 91.22 $4d^25s^2$	Nb 41 92.91 $4d^45s^1$	Mo 42 95.94 $4d^55s^1$	Tc 43 (99) $4d^55s^2$	Ru 44 101.1 $4d^75s^1$	Rh 45 102.91 $4d^85s^1$	Pd 46 106.4 $4d^{10}5s^6$	Ag 47 107.87 $4d^{10}5s^1$	Cd 48 112.40 $4d^{10}5s^2$	In 49 114.82 $5p^1$	Sn 50 118.69 $5p^2$	Sb 51 121.75 $5p^3$	Te 52 127.60 $5p^4$	I 53 126.90 $5p^5$	Xe 54 131.30 $5p^6$
Cs 55 132.91 $6s^1$	Ba 56 137.34 $6s^2$	57 - 71‡	Hf 72 178.49 $5d^26s^2$	Ta 73 180.95 $5d^36s^2$	W 74 183.85 $5d^46s^2$	Re 75 186.2 $5d^56s^2$	Os 76 190.2 $5d^66s^2$	Ir 77 192.2 $5d^76s^2$	Pt 78 195.09 $5d^96s^1$	Au 79 196.97 $5d^{10}6s^1$	Hg 80 200.59 $5d^{10}6s^2$	Tl 81 204.37 $6p^1$	Pb 82 207.2 $6p^2$	Bi 83 208.98 $6p^3$	Po 84 (210) $6p^4$	At 85 (218) $6p^5$	Rn 86 (222) $6p^6$
Fr 87 (223) $7s^1$	Ra 88 (226) $7s^2$	89 - 103§	Rf 104 (261) $6d^27s^2$	Ha 105 (262) $6d^37s^2$	Unh 106 (263)	Uns 107 (261)											

‡Lanthanide series	La 57 138.91 $5d^16s^2$	Ce 58 140.12 $5d^14f^16s^2$	Pr 59 140.91 $4f^36s^2$	Nd 60 144.24 $4f^46s^2$	Pm 61 (147) $4f^56s^2$	Sm 62 150.4 $4f^66s^2$	Eu 63 152.0 $4f^76s^2$	Gd 64 157.25 $5d^14f^76s^2$	Tb 65 158.92 $5d^14f^86s^2$	Dy 66 162.50 $4f^{10}6s^2$	Ho 67 164.93 $4f^{11}6s^2$	Er 68 167.26 $4f^{12}6s^2$	Tm 69 168.93 $4f^{13}6s^2$	Yb 70 173.04 $4f^{14}6s^2$	Lu 71 174.97 $5d^14f^{14}6s^2$
§Actinide series	Ac 89 (227) $6d^17s^2$	Th 90 (232) $6d^27s^2$	Pa 91 (231) $5f^26d^17s^2$	U 92 (238) $5f^36d^17s^2$	Np 93 (239) $5f^36d^07s^2$	Pu 94 (239) $5f^66d^07s^2$	Am 95 (243) $5f^76d^07s^2$	Cm 96 (245) $5f^76d^17s^2$	Bk 97 (247) $5f^86d^17s^2$	Cf 98 (249) $5f^{10}6d^07s^2$	Es 99 (254) $5s^{11}6d^07s^2$	Fm 100 (253) $5f^{12}6d^07s^2$	Md 101 (255) $5f^{13}6d^07s^2$	No 102 (255) $6d^07s^2$	Lr 103 (257) $6d^17s^2$

Glossary

Ablation Volume removal of tissue by vaporization.

Absorption Action of the tissue in taking up the laser energy, causing a reaction within the tissue.

Absorption coefficient Factors describing light's ability to be absorbed. Optical properties of different tissues after the absorption.

Absorption length Depth the laser energy travels beyond the defect created.

Absorption, thermal Uptake of light energy by tissue, converting it into heat.

Accessible radiation Radiation to which it is possible for the human eye or skin to be exposed during normal usage.

Aiming beam A 0.632 μm helium-neon laser (or other light source) used as a guide light. Used coaxially with infrared or other invisible light.

Amplitude Height of the wave from the top of one peak to the bottom of the next; measures the power of the wave.

Apparent visual angle Angular subtense of the source as calculated from source size and distance from the eye. It is not the beam divergence of the source.

Articulated arm Laser delivery device consisting of hollow metal tubes with joints that allow the "arm" to move. Mirrors are located at each joint to reflect the laser beam.

Attenuation Decreasing the intensity (power) of light as it passes through a medium.

Average power Total amount of laser energy delivered divided by the duration of the laser exposure.

Aversion response Movement of the eyelid or the head to avoid an exposure to a noxious stimulant or bright light. It can occur within 0.25 second, including the blink reflex time.

Biostimulation Use of low power light (milliwatts), usually laser, to stimulate metabolic activity on a subcellar level. Experimentally examined for meniscal repair and cartilage regeneration.

Blink reflex See *Aversion response*.

Carbon dioxide (CO_2) laser Emits far infrared light at 10.6 μm. Lasers are made as a sealed tube or flowing gas units. Handheld resonator or articulated arm delivery systems are used for arthroscopy.

Chromophore Optically active (colored) material in tissue that acts as the target for laser light.

Coherence Orderliness of wave patterns by being in phase in time and space (temporally and spatially).

Collimated beam Effectively, a "parallel" beam of light with low divergence or convergence.

Collimation Ability of the laser beam to not spread (low divergence) with distance.

Contact probe Synthetic material used to tip

laser fibers to allow touch of tissue with the probe, intensifying its effect and allowing cutting and coagulation of tissue at relatively low powers and with a high degree of control.

Continuous wave (CW) Constant, steady-state delivery of laser power.

Controlled area Area that requires control and supervision for protection from radiation hazards.

Delivery system Method used to deliver the light energy from the laser system to the target area.

Diffraction Deviation of part of a beam, determined by the wave nature of radiation and occurring when the radiation passes the edge of an opaque obstacle.

Diffuse reflection Change in the spatial distribution of the laser beam in many directions (scattering) after it hits a surface.

Divergence Increase in the diameter of the beam as the beam gets further away from the exit aperture of the laser.

Dosimetry Measuring the amount (joules) and intensity (watts/cm^2) of light delivered to tissue.

Electromagnetic spectrum Span of frequencies (wavelengths) considered to be light—from radio and television waves to gamma and cosmic rays.

Embedded laser Laser with an assigned class number higher than the inherent capability of the laser system in which it is incorporated, where the system's lower classification is the result of engineering features that limit the accessible emission.

Energy Capacity for doing work. Energy content is commonly used to characterize the output from pulsed lasers and is generally expressed in joules (J).

Erbium:YAG Infrared laser of 2.94 μm wavelength.

Excimer Excited dimer. A gas mixture used as the basis of lasers emitting ultraviolet light.

Excitation Energizing a material into a state of population inversion.

Excited state State of an atom in which it has an electron orbiting in a higher shell, causing a high energy state.

Extended source Source of radiation that can be resolved by the eye into a geometric image, in contrast to a point source of radiation, which cannot be resolved into a geometric image.

Failsafe interlock Interlock where the failure of a single mechanical or electrical component of the interlock causes the system to go into, or remain in, a safe mode.

FDA United States Food and Drug Administration.

Feedback mechanism System of mirrors in the laser head that promotes population inversion by amplifying the light energy.

Fiberoptics System of flexible quartz or glass fibers with internal reflective surfaces that pass light through thousands of glancing reflections. Many hundreds or thousands of individual fibers are needed to transmit an image, but only single fibers are used to transmit laser light during treatment.

Fluence Amount of energy delivered to the tissue, determined by watts multiplied by time divided by the spot size (in square centimeters).

Focal length Distance between the lens and the focal point (point at which the beam is most intense).

Focal point Exact point where the laser beam has converged and is most intense.

Frequency Number of wave peaks that pass a given point per second; inversely related to wavelength.

Gas laser Laser system that uses gas as the active medium.

Gated pulse Discontinuous burst of laser light; made by timing (gating) a continuous wave output, usually in fractions of a second.

Ground state State of an atom at a low energy level.

Half-power point Value on either the leading or trailing edge of a laser pulse at which the power is one-half its maximum value.

HeNe laser Helium-neon laser that emits

a 0.632 μm wavelength. Laser producing low power (milliwatts) red light; used as a guide light for infrared lasers or experimentally for biostimulation.

Hertz (Hz) Frequency measurement of a wave in cycles per second.

Holmium:YAG laser Laser that emits a 2.1 μm wavelength. Holmium is the primary rare earth element that is used in the laser medium. It is a solid-state laser with a YAG crystal doped with holmium but also chromium and thulium.

Impact size Size of crater or width of incision left by a laser hit. It is related to the spot size of the beam, except the impact size varies depending on how the energy is applied.

Infrared radiation Electromagnetic radiation with a wavelength in the range of 0.7 μm to 1 mm.

Installation Procedure for supplying and connecting electrical power to a health care laser system.

Integrated radiance Integral of the radiance over the exposure duration in joules per square centimeter per steradian ($J \cdot cm^{-2} \cdot sr^{-1}$). Also known as pulsed radiance.

Intrabeam viewing Viewing condition whereby the eye is exposed to all or part of a laser beam.

Ionizing radiation Radiation commonly associated with an x-ray that is of a high enough energy to cause DNA damage with no direct, immediate thermal effect. Contrasts with nonionizing radiation of surgical lasers.

Irradiance See *Power density*

Joule Unit of energy. One joule equals one watt multiplied by one second. Laser powers are sometimes described in joules per second. A power of one joule per second equals one watt. Therefore a joule is the rate of energy delivery.

KTP Potassium titanyl phosphate. Crystal used to change the wavelength of a neodymium: YAG laser from 1.06 μm (infrared) to 0.532 μm (green). Not used in arthroscopy as of now.

Lambertian surface Ideal surface whose emitted or reflected radiance is independent of the viewing angle.

Laser Light amplification by the stimulated emission of radiation. Device that produces intense beams of pure colors of light.

Laser energy Expressed in joules (watt-seconds).

Laser medium (Active medium) material used to emit the laser light and for which the laser is named.

Laser safety officer Individual who has the authority and responsibility to monitor and enforce the control of laser hazards during laser procedures. This person can be a physician, nurse, or technician.

Laser system Assembly of electrical, mechanical, and optical components, including a laser.

Limiting angular subtense (α_{min}) Apparent visual angle that divides intrabeam viewing from extended-source viewing.

Maximum permissible exposure Radiation level to which a person may be exposed without causing hazardous effects to the skin or eye.

Metastable state State of an atom, just below a higher excited state, that an electron occupies momentarily before destabilizing and emitting light.

Micron One-millionth (10^{-6}) of a meter; symbol μ.

Mode Term used to describe how the power of a laser beam is distributed within the geometry of the beam. Also used to describe the operating mode of a laser, such as continuous or pulsed.

Mode locking Process similar to Q-switching except the pulses produced are even shorter (about 10^{-12} second) and emerge in short trains of pulses instead of singularly. It is usually achieved with a dye cell.

Monochromatic Composed of photons of one color *or* wavelength.

Monochromaticity Waves are monochromatic when they are all of the same wavelength (color).

Nanometer (nm) Measure of length. One nanometer equals 10^{-9} meter (one billionth of a meter) and is the usual measure of light wavelength. Visible light ranges from about 400 nm in the purple to about 750 nm in the deep red; 1000 nm = 1 μm.

Nanosecond One billionth 10^{-9} of a second. Longer than a picosecond or femtosecond but shorter than a microsecond. Associated with Q-switched ophthalmic neodymium:YAG lasers.

Neodymium Rare earth element that is the active element in a neodymium:YAG laser.

Neodymium:YAG Nd:YAG; neodymium:yttrium-aluminum-garnet. A mineral crystal used as a laser medium to produce three commonly used wavelengths: 1.06, 1.3, and 1.44 μm.

Nominal hazard zone (NHZ) Space near the laser impact area where direct, scattered, or reflected radiation exceeds the applicable MPE. Special eye and skin precautions must be enforced.

Nominal ocular hazard distance (NOHD) Distance along the axis of the unobstructed beam from the laser to the human eye beyond which the irradiance or radiant exposure during normal operation is not expected to exceed the appropriate MPE.

Operation Performance of the laser or laser system over the full range of its intended functions (normal operation). It does not include maintenance or service as defined in this section.

Optical density (OD, D_λ) Logarithm to the base 10 of the reciprocal of the transmittance: $D_\lambda = -\log_{10} t_\lambda$, where t_λ is transmittance.

Phase Waves are in phase with each other when all the troughs and peaks coincide and are "locked" together. The result is a reinforced wave of increased amplitude (brightness).

Photocoagulation Tissue coagulation caused by light (laser).

Photodisruption Creating an acoustic shock wave through Q-switching or mode-locking to gently "snap" apart membranes. It is a "cold cutting" technique with laser.

Photon Basic particle of light. Light energy given off by an excited atom.

Point source Source of radiation whose dimensions are small enough, compared with the distance between source and receptor, to be neglected in calculations.

Population inversion When the number of excited atoms in a laser medium exceeds the number of atoms not excited.

Power Rate of energy delivery (expressed in watts) at which energy is transferred, received, or emitted (joules per second).

Power density (irradiance) Amount of energy concentrated in a spot of particular size. It is expressed in watts per square centimeter and is the brightness of the spot.

PRF Abbreviation for pulse-repetition frequency. See Repetitively pulsed laser.

Protective housing Enclosure that surrounds a laser or laser system that prevents access to laser radiation above the applicable maximum permissible exposure level. The aperture through which the useful beam is emitted is not part of the protective housing. The protective housing may enclose associated optics and a work station, and it limits access to other associated radiant energy emissions and to electrical hazards associated with components and terminals.

Pulse Discontinuous burst of laser, in contrast to a continuous beam. A true pulse achieves higher peak powers than that attainable in a continuous wave output—usually pulsed in microseconds or shorter (see *Gated pulse*).

Pulse duration Duration of a laser pulse; usually measured as the time interval between the half-power points on the leading and trailing edges of the pulse.

Pulsed laser Laser that delivers its energy in the form of a single pulse or a train of pulses; in this standard, the duration of a pulse less than 0.25 second.

Pulse width Amount of time (in microseconds) of the pulse duration.

Q-switching Switching the "quality" of a resonator, producing high peak powers (millions of watts) but for short bursts (nanoseconds)—usually achieved with a pockel's cell. It creates a "sparking" and shock wave effect (see Photodisruption, Mode locking).

Radian (rad) Unit of angular measure equal to the angle subtended at the center of a circle by an arc whose length is equal to the radius of the circle. 1 radian $\approx$ 57.3 degrees; 2π radians = 360 degrees.

Radiance Radiant flux or power output per unit solid angle per unit area, in watts per square centimeter per steradian ($W \cdot cm^{-2} \cdot sr^{-1}$)

Radiant energy Energy emitted, transferred, or received in the form of radiation (in joules).

Radiant exposure Surface density of the radiant energy received (in joules per square centimeter: $J \cdot cm^{-2}$).

Radiant flux Power emitted, transferred, or received in the form of radiation (in watts). Also called radiant power.

Radiant intensity (of a source in a given direction) Quotient of the radiant flux leaving a source and propagated in an element of solid angle containing the given direction, by the element of solid angle (in watts per steradian: $W \cdot sr^{-1}$).

Radiant power See *Radiant flux*.

Reflectance Ratio of the total reflected energy to the total energy that hits the reflective substance.

Repetitively pulsed laser Laser with multiple pulses of radiant energy occurring in sequence with a pulse-repetition frequency of 1 Hz or more.

Resonator Space between the laser mirrors where lasing action occurs.

Scattering Process by which the beam of light is distributed in many different paths after striking a surface.

Service Performance of those procedures or adjustments described in the manufacturer's service instructions that may affect any aspect of the performance of the laser or laser system. It does not include maintenance or operation as defined in this section.

SMA Subminiature adaptor.

Solid angle Three-dimensional angular spread at the vertex of a cone measured by the area intercepted by the cone on a unit sphere whose center is the vertex of the cone. It is expressed in steradians (sr).

Specular reflection Mirror-like reflection.

Spontaneous emission Release of a photon of absorbed energy from an atom without stimulation of another photon.

Spot size Mathematic measurement of a focused laser spot. In a TEM_{00} beam it is the area that contains 86% of the incident power. This is the optical spot size and does not necessarily indicate the size of the laser crater that will be made. The latter is the impact size.

Steradian (sr) Unit of measure for a solid angle. There are 4π steradians about any point in space.

Stimulated emission Release of photon energy from an atom already in the excited state after being struck by a photon of equal energy.

Superpulse Operating mode on the 10.6 μm CO_2 laser describing a fast pulsing output (250–1000 times per second), with peak powers per pulse higher than the maximum attainable in the continuous wave mode. Average powers of superpulse (speed of tissue removal) are always lower than the maximum in continuous wave.

TEM Transverse electromagnetic mode; determines the precision of the laser beam from the power distribution over the spot area.

Thermal relaxation time Rate at which a structure can conduct heat. When pulse times of a laser are shorter than the time required for heat to spread out of a target, the heat damage is confined to that target.

Thulium Rare earth element that can be used in solid-state YAG lasers.

TIR Total internal reflection.

Transmission Passage of energy through a medium.

Transmittance Ratio of total transmitted radiant power to total incident radiant power.

Ultraviolet radiation Electromagnetic radiation with wavelengths that are shorter than those of the visible wavelengths.

Vaporization Converting a solid or a liquid into a vapor; usually occurs in tissue at 100°C.

Velocity Rate of speed at which a wave travels; approximately 186, 300 miles per second.

Visible radiation Electromagnetic radiation detectable by the human eye ranging from 0.4 to 0.7 μm in wavelength.

Watt Unit of power; one watt equals one joule per second.

Wavelength Distance between two successive peaks on a wave, usually measured in millimeters, micrometers, nanometers, or Ångstrom units; determines the color of the light.

X-ray Short wavelength of light, producing ionization effects commonly associated with radiation hazards. Not a problem with surgical laser units.

YAG Yttrium-aluminum-garnet crystal used to suspend rare earth elements such as holmium or neodymium in the laser cavity.

Index